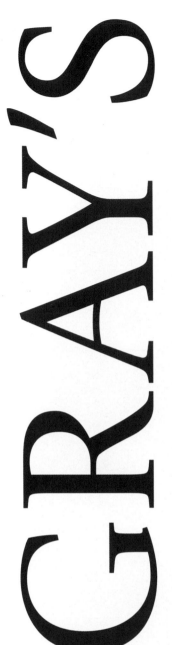

CLINICAL PHOTOGRAPHIC DISSECTOR OF THE HUMAN BODY

T0127828

Second Edition

Marios Loukas, MD, PhD
Dean of Basic Sciences
Dean of Research
Professor, Department of Anatomical Sciences
St. George's University School of Medicine
Grenada, West Indies

R. Shane Tubbs, PhD, MSc, PA-C
Professor, Chief Scientific Officer and Vice President
Seattle Science Foundation
Seattle, Washington;
Professor, Department of Anatomical Sciences
St. George's University School of Medicine
Grenada, West Indies;
Honorary Faculty, California Neuroscience Institute
Professor and Affiliate Faculty, Institute for Systems Biology
Seattle, Washington;
Professor, Centre of Anatomy and Human Identification
University of Dundee
Scotland, United Kingdom;
Adjunct Professor, Department of Neurosurgery
Vanderbilt University
Nashville, Tennessee

Brion Benninger, MD, MSc
Professor of Medical Innovation, Technology & Research
Professor of Clinical Anatomy
Executive Director, Medical Anatomy Center
Western University of Health Sciences
Lebanon, Oregon;
Faculty, Samaritan Orthopaedic and Surgery Residencies
Faculty, Samaritan Sports Medicine Fellows
Samaritan Health Services
Corvallis, Oregon
President, Alps Innovative Medical
Healthcare and Education Futurist

ELSEVIER

ELSEVIER

1600 John F. Kennedy Blvd.
Ste. 1600
Philadelphia, PA 19103-2899

GRAY'S CLINICAL PHOTOGRAPHIC DISSECTOR
OF THE HUMAN BODY, SECOND EDITION

ISBN: 978-0-323-54417-7

Copyright © 2019 by Elsevier Inc.

All rights reserved. No part of this publication may be reproduced or transmitted in any form or by any means, electronic or mechanical, including photocopying, recording, or any information storage and retrieval system, without permission in writing from the publisher. Details on how to seek permission, further information about the Publisher's permissions policies and our arrangements with organizations such as the Copyright Clearance Center and the Copyright Licensing Agency, can be found at our website: www.elsevier.com/permissions.

This book and the individual contributions contained in it are protected under copyright by the Publisher (other than as may be noted herein).

Notices

Knowledge and best practice in this field are constantly changing. As new research and experience broaden our understanding, changes in research methods, professional practices, or medical treatment may become necessary.

Practitioners and researchers must always rely on their own experience and knowledge in evaluating and using any information, methods, compounds, or experiments described herein. In using such information or methods they should be mindful of their own safety and the safety of others, including parties for whom they have a professional responsibility.

With respect to any drug or pharmaceutical products identified, readers are advised to check the most current information provided (i) on procedures featured or (ii) by the manufacturer of each product to be administered, to verify the recommended dose or formula, the method and duration of administration, and contraindications. It is the responsibility of practitioners, relying on their own experience and knowledge of their patients, to make diagnoses, to determine dosages and the best treatment for each individual patient, and to take all appropriate safety precautions.

To the fullest extent of the law, neither the Publisher nor the authors, contributors, or editors, assume any liability for any injury and/or damage to persons or property as a matter of products liability, negligence or otherwise, or from any use or operation of any methods, products, instructions, or ideas contained in the material herein.

The Publisher

Previous edition copyrighted 2013 by Saunders, an imprint of Elsevier Inc.

Library of Congress Control Number: 2018951822

Senior Content Strategist: Jeremy Bowes
Director, Content Development: Rebecca Gruliow
Publishing Services Manager: Catherine Jackson
Senior Project Manager: John Casey
Senior Designer: Amy Buxton

  Working together to grow libraries in developing countries

www.elsevier.com • www.bookaid.org

Printed in China

9 8 7 6 5

I would like to dedicate this book to my brilliant and wonderful wife, Joanna, who has been the bright star of my life. Her continuous support, dedication, love, and affection give me the energy and courage to fulfill all of our dreams.

ML

I would like to thank my wife, Susan, and son, Isaiah, for their support and patience during the writing of this dissector. All that I do, I do for them. I also want to dedicate this book in memory of my brother-in-law, Nelson Jones, whose intellect, engagement of others, and curiosity about life have been examples for me.

RST

It's an honor to dedicate this work to Bill Bryan, Jim McDaniel, and Gail Hendricks, who always fought for what is right. I would also like to extend my gratitude to those who provided me with clinical pearls and critical thinking in my training during medical school and as lifelong learners—Gerald Tressidor, Peter Bell, Chris Colton, Harold Ellis, and Lynn Loriaux. Special thanks to Erik Szeto and his family for always thinking of community service and providing for all. Lastly, I am indebted to my wife, Alison, who supports my passions, my son, Jack, who remains forever inquisitive, my father, Roger, for his engineering mind and love of life, and my mother for her fight for equality and education.

BB

Credits

The following plates are from Drake RL et al: *Gray's Atlas of Anatomy*, 2nd edition, Philadelphia, Elsevier, 2015.

Plates 2.1, 2.2, 3.1, 3.2, 4.1, 4.2, 5.2, 7.1, 7.2, 8.1 to 8.3, 9.1, 9.2, 10.1 to 10.3, 11.1, 12.2 to 12.4, 13.2, 13.3, 14.1, 14.2, 15.1, 15.2, 16.1 to 16.3, 17.1, 17.2, 18.2 to 18.5, 19.1, 19.2, 20.1, 20.2, 21.1, 21.2, 22.1, 22.2, 23.1, 23.2, 24.1, 24.2, 25.1, 26.2, 27.1 to 27.3, 28.1, 28.2, 29.1 to 29.4

The following plates are from Drake RL et al: *Gray's Anatomy for Students*, 3rd edition, Philadelphia, Elsevier, 2015.

Plates 5.1, 6.1 to 6.4, 12.1, 13.1, 18.1, 22.3, 23.3, 24.3, 24.4, 26.1

Dissection of the human body, even in the twenty-first century, continues to be the best way of learning the intricacies of the human body. The tactility involved with dissection and the variations in structures between specimens allows the student to gain a much deeper appreciation of human morphology. However, as the time allotted for anatomical education continues to be whittled down in most curricula, courses must continually evolve. Therefore, courses that continue to dissect the human cadaver must utilize all available time wisely. Traditionally, in most anatomy courses that use cadavers, students begin their dissections with the aid of a dissector and follow step-by-step instructions of how to dissect the human body. Such guides, in general, are written much like cookbooks and usually do not provide students with a pictorial step-by-step guide of what to expect during their exploration of the human body. When figures are used by such resources, they are almost always schematic drawings that often look nothing like the actual anatomical structures that are seen by the students. It is this deficit in the extant literature that compelled us to compile dissection photographs with accompanying text to better assist the student of anatomy. It is our hope that being able to see what students are expected to find during their dissection, from superficial to deep, will allow them to be more efficient not only in their learning experience but also with their time.

Marios Loukas
R. Shane Tubbs
Brion Benninger

Acknowledgments

This dissection book is the work not only of the authors but also of numerous scientific and clinical friends and colleagues who have been so generous with their knowledge and have given significant feedback and help. This book would not have been possible were it not for the contributions of the colleagues and friends listed below.

The following instructors of the Department of Anatomical Sciences, St. George's University, School of Medicine, Grenada, West Indies for their incredible artistic talents and significant contribution throughout the book to numerous illustrations:
Jessica Holland, MS
Brandon Holt, MS
David Nahabedian, MS
Angelica Ortiz, MS
Charles Price, MS
Xochitl Vinaja, MS
Katie Yost, MS

A very special group of medical students, members of the Student Clinical Research Society in the Department of Anatomical Sciences at St. George's University, helped enormously with the completion of this project through their comments and criticism:
Theofanis Kollias
Elizabeth Hogan
Frank Scali

We would also like to thank the following colleagues for their technical expertise in dissections and their enormous help with this project:
Alysia Tucker, MD
Kathleen Bubb, MD
Ewarld Marshall, MD
William Merbs
Michael Snosek (PhD candidate)
Benjamin Turner (PhD candidate)
Maira DuPlessis (PhD candidate)

The following St. George's University alumni and current research fellows of the Department of Anatomical Sciences have been great friends and colleagues. Their continuous support, comments, criticism, and enthusiasm have contributed enormously to the completion of this project:
Denzil Etienne, MD
Alana John, MD
Mitchell Muhlman, MD
Stephen Osiro, MD
Andrew Walters, MD

The following individuals from the Department of Anatomical Sciences at St. George's University have also been very helpful with their comments and criticisms:
Olufemi Bogunjoko, MBBS
Danny Burns, MD, PhD
Cathleen Bubb, MD
James Coey, MBBS
Maira DuPlessis, MSc
Deon Forrester, MD
Rachel George, MD
Mathangi Gilkes, MBBS MSc
Robert Hage, MD, PhD
Robert Jordan, PhD
Temitope Kehinde, MBChB
Theofannis Kollias, MD
Ahmed Mahgoub, MBBS
Ewarld Marshall, MD
Kazzara Raeburn, MD
Ramesh, Rao
Vish Rao, PhD
Deepak Sharma, MD
Feimatta Sowa, MD
Kristna Thompson, MD
Alana Wade, MD

We are also grateful to the following members of St. George's University for their photographic and technical expertise and lab assistance:
Joanna Loukas (photography and design)
Rayn Jacobs (design)
Carlson Dominique (laboratory technician)
Rodon Marast (laboratory technician)
Christopher Belgrave (laboratory technician)
Rodon Marrast (laboratory technician)
Seikou Phillip (laboratory technician)
Shiva Mathurin (laboratory technician)
Romeo Cox (laboratory technician)
Nelson Davis (laboratory technician)
Travis Joseph (laboratory technician)
Marlon Jodeph (laboratory technician)
Chad Phillip (laboratory technician)
Simone Lewis (laboratory technician)
Arnelle Gibbs (laboratory technician)
Cheryce Fraser (laboratory technician)

Also, Mrs Nadica Thomas-Dominique, Ms. Tracy Shabazz, and Ms. Yvonne James for their invaluable assistance.

The following great friends have been very instrumental over the years with their enthusiasm, continuous support, and most important, mentoring in the completion of this and many other projects:

Allen Pensick, PhD
Peter Abrahams, MD
†Gene Colborn, PhD
Vid Persaud, MD, PhD

The authors would also like to thank *Shivayogi Bhusnurmath, MD,* and *Bhati Bhusnurmath, MD,* for their important comments on the pathological specimens.

The authors would also like to give a very special thank you to *Drs. George Salter, Jerzy Walocha, Jerzy Gielecki,* and *Anna Zurada* for their generous efforts in reviewing this book.

A special thanks to our friends and partners in Elsevier for this project — *Jeremy Bowes, Rebecca Gruliow, John Casey,* and *Madelene Hyde.*

We would like to acknowledge all our former and current students who have kept us thinking fresh and edgy with all their comments to improve the learning and teaching of anatomy.

Finally, we would like to thank those who donated their bodies to anatomical science; without them this project would not have been possible.

---

†Deceased.

Reviewers

In addition to the reviewers listed below, we would also like to acknowledge the valuable contributions of the reviewers of the first edition.

ARGENTINA

Susana Biasutto, PhD
Professor, Anatomical Institute
National University of Cordoba
Cordoba, Argentina

AUSTRALIA

Fiona Stewart, MBBS, BSc
Associate Professor, School of Rural Medicine
University of New England
Armidale, NSW, Australia

AUSTRIA

Andreas H. Weiglein, MD
Vice Chair, Institute of Anatomy
Medical University of Graz
Graz, Austria

CANADA

Vid Persaud, MD, PhD, DSc, FRCPath (Lond.)
Professor Emeritus and Former Head
Department of Human Anatomy and Cell Science
University of Manitoba
Winnipeg, Manitoba, Canada

CHINA

Changman Zhou, MD, PhD
Professor, Department of Anatomy and Embryology
Peking University Health Science Center
Beijing, China

CZECH REPUBLIC

J. Stingl, PhD
3rd Faculty of Medicine
Institute of Anatomy
Charles University
Prague, Czech Republic

FRANCE

Fabrice DuParc, MD, PhD
Professor of Anatomy
Department of Medicine and Pharmacy
University of Rouen
Rouen, France

GERMANY

Reinhard Putz, MD
Professor, Institute of Anatomy
Ludwig-Maximilians-University of Munich
Munich, Germany

INDIA

Subhash D. Joshi, MBBS, MS
Dean, SAIMS Medical College
Indore, India

IRAN

Mohammadali M. Shoja, MD
Medical Philosophy and History Research Center
Tabriz University of Medical Sciences
Tabriz, Iran

ITALY

Raffaele De Caro, MD
Full Professor, Director of Institute of Human Anatomy
University of Padova
Padova, Italy

JAPAN

Tatsuo Sato, MD, PhD
President
Tokyo Ariake University of Medicine and Health Sciences
Tokyo, Japan

NEW ZEALAND

Helen Nicholson, BSc (Hons), MBChB, MD (Bristol)
Professor and Dean
Otago School of Medical Sciences
University of Otago
Otago, New Zealand

Mark Stringer, BSc (Hons), MBBS, MS (Lond), MRCP (UK)
Professor, Department of Anatomy
Otago School of Medical Sciences
University of Otago
Otago, New Zealand

POLAND

Jerzy Gielecki, MD, PhD
Dean for English Division
University of Warmia and Mazury
Olsztyn, Poland

Anna Zurada, MD, PhD
Medical Faculty
Department of Anatomy
University of Warmia and Mazury
Olsztyn, Poland

SAUDI ARABIA

Abdullah M. Aldahmash
Chairman of Anatomy and Director of Stem Cell Unit
College of Medicine
King Saud University
Riyadh, Saudi Arabia

SOUTH AFRICA

Dr. Albert van Schoor, PhD
Senior Lecturer, Department of Anatomy
University of Pretoria
Johannesburg, South Africa

TURKEY

Nihal Apaydin, MD
Associate Professor, Department of
  Anatomy
Ankara University
Ankara, Turkey

UNITED KINGDOM

**Bernard Moxham, BDS, PhD,
FHEA, FSB**
Professor of Anatomy and Head of
  Teaching in Biosciences
President of the International
  Federation of Associations of
  Anatomists (IFAA)
Cardiff School of Biosciences
Cardiff, United Kingdom

**Jonathan Spratt, MA(Cantab),
FRCS (Eng), FRCS (Glasg), FRCR**
Consultant Clinical Radiologist
University of North Durham
Durham, United Kingdom

UNITED STATES

**Anthony V. D'Antoni, MS, DC,
PhD**
Assistant Professor of Anatomy in
  Radiology
Department of Radiology
Weill Cornell Medicine
New York, New York, United States

†Camille DiLullo, PhD
Professor, Department of Anatomy
Philadelphia College of Osteopathic
  Medicine
Philadelphia, Pennsylvania, United
  States

Anthony Olinger, PhD
Assistant Professor
Department of Anatomy
Kansas City University of Medicine
  and Biosciences
Kansas City, Missouri, United States

David J. Porta, PhD
Professor, Department of Biology
Bellarmine University
Louisville, Kentucky, United States

Kyle E. Rarey, PhD
Professor, Departments of Anatomy
  & Cell Biology and
  Otolaryngology
University of Florida College of
  Medicine
Gainesville, Florida, United States

George Salter Jr, PhD
Professor Emeritus of Anatomy
University of Alabama at
  Birmingham
Birmingham, Alabama, United
  States

Carol E.H. Scott-Conner, MD, PhD
Professor, Division of Surgical
  Oncology and Endocrine Surgery
Department of Surgery
University of Iowa Carver College of
  Medicine
Iowa City, Iowa, United States

Joel Vilensky, PhD
Professor Emeritus of Anatomy and
  Cell Biology
Indiana University School of
  Medicine
Fort Wayne, Indiana, United States

†Deceased

Contents

NOTE: This dissection guide is cross-referenced to the following atlases: Netter, *Atlas of Human Anatomy,* ed 7 (Netter); *McMinn's Clinical Atlas of Human Anatomy,* ed 7 (McMinn); and *Gray's Atlas of Anatomy,* ed 2 (Gray's). Page references from each atlas are provided at the beginning of Chapters 2 through 29 to give you the opportunity to study the relevant anatomy in depth to aid in your dissection.

Get the most out of your Gray's Dissector!

Included in your purchase are **BONUS dissection videos** + (for print purchasers) the **complete enhanced eBook**

See inside front cover for access details

SECTION I

INTRODUCTION

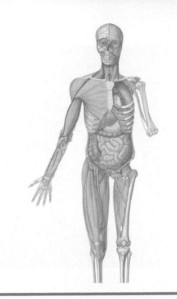

CHAPTER 1   DISSECTION LABORATORY MATERIALS, TOOLS, AND TECHNIQUES

Using appropriate dissection laboratory materials and tools is essential in making the dissection of a cadaver as rewarding as possible. Many experienced dissectors have their favorite tools. Obtaining the following materials and dissection tools allows dissectors to care for their cadaver donor while acquiring experience and knowledge of a successful dissection. Although not comprehensive, this list provides appropriate tools to dissect a cadaver donor in the anatomy teaching laboratory.

MATERIALS
Cadaver Materials

- Blocks
  Plastic or wooden blocks of different shapes and sizes (6–18 inches) can be used to position the cadaver (Fig. 1.1).
- Stands
  Removable stands that either bridge or attach to dissection tables are useful for holding dissection guides, texts, and atlases for dissection.
- Plastic sheets
  Plastic sheets can be used to cover the cadaver, which usually comes with a shroud and a cotton sheet. This helps maintain moisture within the cadaver, to prevent drying, and to allow dissection of appropriately hydrated tissues.
- Cotton sheets
  Surgical green or blue sheets covering a plastic sheet help preserve the cadaver and create a professional working environment.
- Spray bottle with wetting solution
  An individual plastic spray bottle (1 quart) at each cadaver station allows dissectors to maintain good-quality tissue (see Fig. 1.1). An alternative is a 2- to

3-gallon pressure spray unit shared among the dissection laboratory stations.
- Holding container
  The plastic 5- to 10-gallon container with a spigot stores cadaver hydration solution.
- Cadaver hydrating solution
  Several types of mixtures are available to hydrate and maintain cadaver tissue. The authors use a solution with 3000 mL of propylene glycol, 500 mL of ethyl alcohol, and 300 mL of fabric softener, in a 10-gallon holding unit, with the remainder filled with water.
- Cadaver bag
  The bag helps to maintain hydration of the cadaver (Fig. 1.2).

Dissector Materials

- Scrubs
  Comfortable clothing also can be worn with scrubs or under a lab coat.
- Disposable shoe covers
  Shoe covers protect shoes worn in the laboratory during dissection and can be disposed of on exiting the lab, ensuring cleanliness inside and outside the laboratory (Fig. 1.3). Closed-toed shoes should be worn in the dissecting laboratory.
- Goggles
  Protective safety goggles or glasses should be worn at all times during dissection (see Fig. 1.3).
- Face shields
  Shields can be worn when using bone saws or when excessive fluids are present (see Fig. 1.3).
- Gloves
  Gloves vary in the type of synthetic material used; powdered gloves and powder-free gloves are available. (Fig. 1.4). Offer both types to protect dissectors with

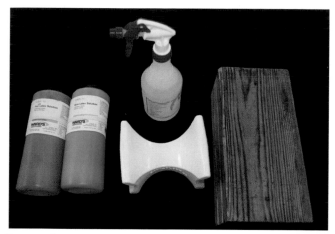

Fig. 1.1 Red and blue latex wrap (to keep cadaver moist); spray bottle; plastic and wooden blocks.

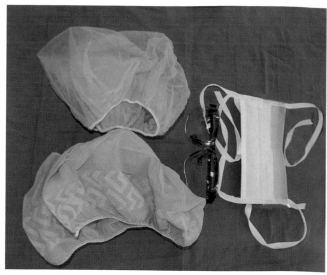

Fig. 1.3 Disposable hair and shoe covers; mask with eye shield; goggles.

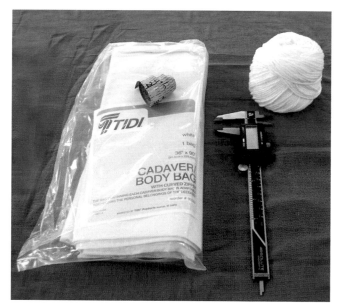

Fig. 1.2 Cadaver bag and cloth measuring tape; ball of string; digital calipers.

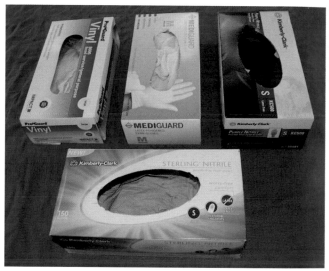

Fig. 1.4 Laboratory gloves differentiated by powder and powder free, latex and latex free.

different skin sensitivities. *Double gloving* helps to prevent contact with cadaver embalming fluids, which may irritate sensitive skin.

- First-aid kit

In a dissection laboratory, nicks and pricks are inevitable, so an up-to-date first-aid kit is essential. It should contain adhesive strips (e.g., Band-Aids), cleansing solutions (e.g., hydrogen peroxide), gauze rolls/pads, and eyewash solution. The phone number of the lab director and/or physician should be posted on a wall inside the lab so that users can contact them to answer any emergency issues that may arise if students are allowed to dissect during nonformal hours.

Dissection Tools

- Cloth/measuring tape

A cloth or paper measuring tape can be invaluable when measuring distances from landmarks of surface anatomy (see Fig. 1.2).

- Skin marker

Marking pens can be helpful tools for tracing out the incision before dissection. Markers can also be used to highlight surface anatomy (Fig. 1.5).

- Disposable scalpels

Disposable scalpels have an advantage because the blade is already secured to the handle. Have a disposable sharps bin in the laboratory (see Fig. 1.5).

- Scalpel handles and blades

Metal scalpel blades are relatively standardized. Many different blade shapes and sizes are available; however, dissectors should experiment to determine which best suits them and the targets to be dissected. The authors prefer larger blades for their students. Scalpels are used primarily to make skin incisions but also can be used to reflect the dermis and areas with dense connective tissue.

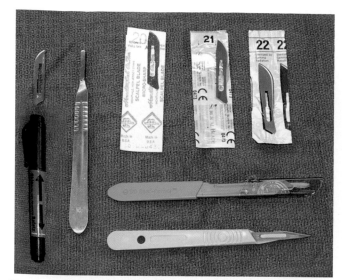

Fig. 1.5 Various scalpel blades and handles (metal and disposable scalpels). An example of a skin marker that can be used for outlining skin incisions is shown.

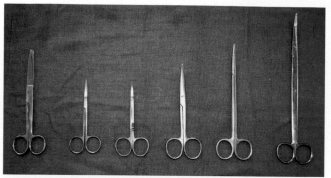

Fig. 1.6 Various scissors differentiated by length and blade type (straight or curved, pointed or blunted): 6-inch Deaver, straight fine scissors, curved fine scissors, 5-inch Mayo, 7-inch Metzenbaum, 9-inch Metzenbaum.

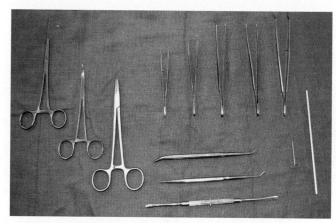

Fig. 1.7 *Left,* Hemostat or artery clamps (straight and curved). *Upper,* Needle holder; various forceps differentiated by length, toothed and nontoothed. *Lower,* Probes and dissectors. *Right,* T-pin and orange stick.

- Sharps bin or container

  For safety compliance, all dissection laboratories should have a sharps bin to dispose of scalpel blades, disposable scalpels, pins, and needles.

- Scissors

  Both 5-inch and 7-inch straight and curved scissors may be used. It is important that the scissors used for each dissection are appropriate in size (Fig. 1.6). Generally, head and neck dissection can be conducted with 5-inch scissors. The remainder of the body can be dissected with 7-inch scissors. The classic scissor dissection technique is a *reverse dissection*. Straight and curved scissors tend to be user specific.

- Hemostat clamps

  Corrugated and smooth, 5-inch and 7-inch hemostat clamps are available (Fig. 1.7). The corrugated type can be used to clamp onto the edge of skin incisions to aid in flap removal. Smooth clamps can be used to hold onto delicate structures during dissection. Hemostat clamps can be used when retracting tissue over relatively long dissection periods.

- Needle holders

  The needle holder allows the user to secure and remove scalpel blades (see Fig. 1.7).

- Forceps

  Toothed and nontoothed forceps are either 5 inches or greater than 5 inches long. Toothed forceps enable the dissector to grip tissue without it sliding out of the hands. Nontoothed forceps allow the dissector to control delicate tissues during meticulous dissection without damaging the tissue (see Fig. 1.7).

- Spatula probe/pointer

  Instruments that have a probe or tip on one end and spatula on the other can be used to highlight dissected structures. The spatula can aid blunt dissection (see Fig. 1.7).

- T-pins

  T-pins (1½–2 inches) are useful in securing structures away from the desired dissection region. T-pins also can be used when setting up laboratory examinations (see Fig. 1.7).

- Chisel (osteotome)

  Narrow-blade and broad-blade chisels are important for performing osteotomies and can help dissect, for example, between the occipital condyles and various vertebrae (Fig. 1.8). Chisels can be used to break up a bone surface to view the soft tissue deep to it (e.g., anterior cranial fossa).

- Rubber mallet

  A mallet is used when striking the chisel to crack surface areas, such as when performing osteotomies (see Fig. 1.8).

- Electric Stryker saw

  Used when cutting bone, the Stryker saw has a safety mechanism that prevents the blade from cutting the user's skin and soft tissue.

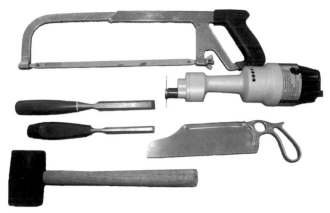

Fig. 1.8 Handsaws (long and short) for bone; electric Stryker bone saw; chisel (broad and narrow blades); rubber mallet.

- Handsaw

  A simple bone saw can be used to customize various dissections and amputations for plastination (see Fig. 1.8). A handsaw is important for hemipelvectomy dissections.

DISSECTION TECHNIQUES

Using the proper technique during dissection is important when developing good dissection skills. Initially, holding the instruments correctly and practicing the techniques may not feel natural. The authors believe that cadaver dissection techniques should reflect the techniques used during surgical procedures. Learning to hold forceps and scissors is fundamental during dissection. These techniques also can be used in the operating room and certain office settings during interventional procedures.

- Scalpel

  The technique for placing a blade onto a scalpel handle requires a hemostat to hold the blade and then place it onto the handle while holding the forceps (Figs. 1.9 and 1.10). When cutting with the blade, use the tip and the first centimeter of the blade. Direct the scalpel using smooth, sweeping motions (Fig. 1.11). Avoid "sawing" and "woodpecker" techniques. Dull blades that require "pushing" the scalpel are dangerous; therefore maintain a sharp blade at all times.

- Forceps

  Hold the forceps as you would hold a pencil, with a pincer grip. The classic mistake is holding the forceps in the palm of the hand as if grasping. Hold the forceps vertically and perpendicularly to the target tissue to allow a 360-degree window of use (Fig. 1.12).

- Scissors

  The appropriate technique when dissecting with scissors is called *reverse dissection* (Fig. 1.13). This requires the user to keep the scissor blades closed when entering into the tissue to be dissected, then opening

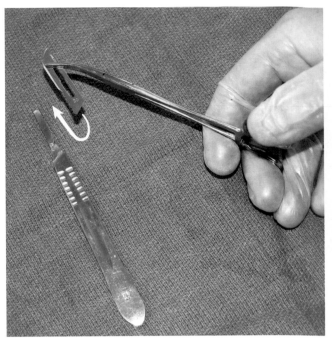

Fig. 1.9 Placing or replacing scalpel blades onto a scalpel handle. Use hemostat or needle holder to grip the scalpel blade. Line up the base angle of the blade with the tip-of-handle angle.

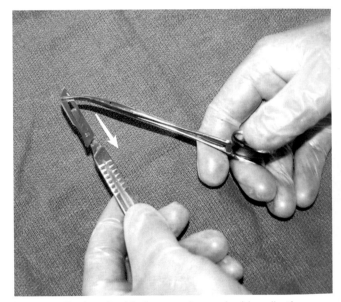

Fig. 1.10 Placing the blade onto the scalpel handle tip. Generally, a clicking sound confirms the blade is secured correctly.

the blades to create a splaying of the tissue. This results in natural separation of tissue structures and planes. Cut only tissue that is fully exposed so that the desired tissue can be preserved.

- Buttonhole maneuver

  A buttonhole maneuver is helpful when dissecting a flap of dermis. Create a 2-cm parallel incision along the original skin incision, 2 to 3 cm from the edge.

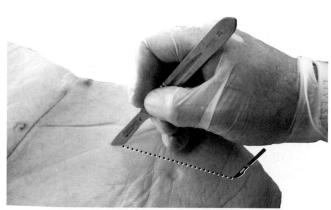

Fig. 1.11 Using the scalpel tip to create skin incisions. Note the grip of the scalpel provides side-to-side and back-to-front blade stability.

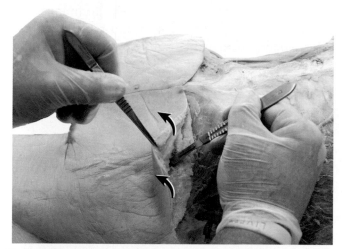

Fig. 1.12 Holding toothed forceps with a 360-degree view and using the scalpel tip between tissue layers while maintaining tension of superficial tissue layer.

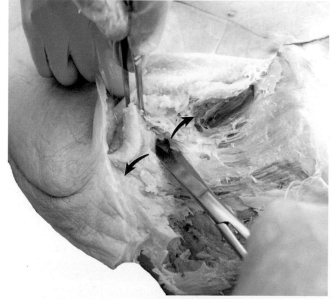

Fig. 1.13 Blunt dissection introduces the scissor tips into the tissue, and then reverse dissection opens the tissue planes.

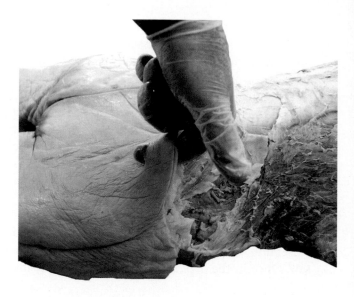

Fig. 1.14 The buttonhole maneuver is helpful when dissecting large skin flaps and provides appropriate tension to expedite dissection. Place your fingertip(s) into the parallel incision and retract with appropriate tension.

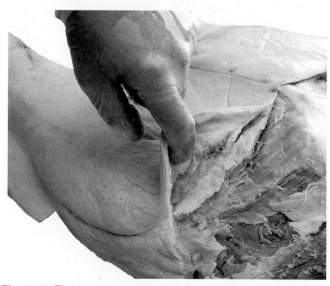

Fig. 1.15 The buttonhole maneuver for retraction of the skin allows adequate visualization of the underlying tissue for further dissection.

Repeat this, generally near the corners of the skin flap. Place your index finger into the parallel incision, and retract the skin flap with appropriate tension that would allow either blunt dissection or a sharp edge to cut the apex of the flap (Figs. 1.14 and 1.15).
- Surface fracturing technique
  The surface fracturing technique requires placing the broad blade of a chisel parallel to the bone and with as much of the blade along the bone. Strike the chisel head with a mallet using a technique that does *not* follow through once the head is struck. The objective is to direct the energy through the blade onto the

bony surface, causing multiple fractured segments while protecting the soft tissue beneath the bone (e.g., fracturing anterior cranial fossa plate before superior orbit dissection) (Fig. 1.16).

- Direct fracturing technique
  The direct fracturing technique can be performed using a narrow-bladed chisel or by tilting a broad-bladed chisel so that a direct point touches the bone to be fractured. Strike the chisel head with the mallet as if driving a nail. This technique will fracture through a specific part of outer layer of bone (Fig. 1.17).

- Prying technique
  The prying technique requires placing the blade of a chisel into the gap created by a handsaw or electric saw. Once in the gap, rotate the chisel blade using a circular motion of the wrist while gripping the chisel to pry the two bony edges apart. Prying is especially useful when performing a craniotomy (see Chapter 23).

- Stryker saw
  The technique for using the electric bone saw is performed by placing the blade directly perpendicular to the bone. Place enough pressure onto the bony surface until the blade has gone through the thickness of the bone. Once through the bone, remove the blade, and assess whether the prying technique is required.

- Stryker saw scoring
  The scoring technique requires using a Stryker electric saw blade to score the surface of the bone region to be removed. Often an "X" pattern of scoring can weaken the bony cortex. Once the scoring is completed, use the surface fracturing technique. This allows fracture of the cortex and removal of bony fragments without damaging soft tissue beneath the cortex (e.g., removing outer cortex of mandibular ramus; see Chapter 22).

SPECIALIZED MATERIALS TO HIGHLIGHT STRUCTURES

- Latex solutions
  Use latex solutions as an injection to highlight vessels, especially small vessels that may not be easily dissectible.

- Needle and syringe
  Multiple syringe sizes and needle sizes are used to inject latex or dye into spaces (Fig. 1.18). Injection of the globe (eyeball) with water also may be useful to obtain lifelike qualities.

- Suture material
  Multiple sizes of suture material to reattach dissected structures can be useful when demonstrating

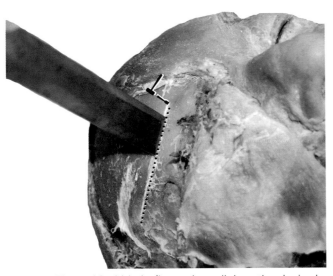

Fig. 1.16 Place chisel blade flat and parallel on the desired bone surface. The surface fracturing technique generally results in multiple fragments protecting the deep tissue.

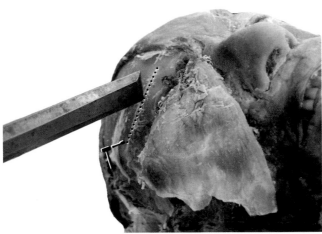

Fig. 1.17 Place chisel blade at an angle on the desired bone surface. The direct fracturing technique creates a specific fracture at the point of the chisel blade.

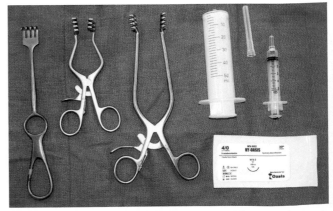

Fig. 1.18 *Left to right,* Handheld retractor (Volkmann); dynamic self-retaining retractors (Weitlaner); syringes (50 mL and 5 mL); suture material.

superficial and deep structures after dissection (see Fig. 1.18).

- Retractors

  Types include (1) single-handled manual retractor for dynamic traction and (2) self-retractor used to retract two sides simultaneously, allowing the dissector to practice surgical procedures without needing others to retract structures manually (see Fig. 1.18).

- Food coloring

  Mix with a solution to inject into the body, to fill up potential spaces and to highlight others.

- Electronic digital calipers

  Use to measure specific length, size, and shape of anatomic structures (see Fig. 1.2).

- Plastination

  The plastination technique preserves dissected regions or structures to be used as *prosected material,* with a life span of 6 months to 20 years,

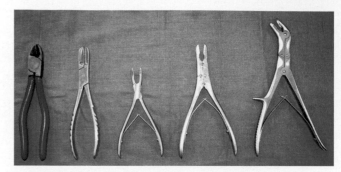

Fig. 1.19 *Left to right,* Metal wire cutters (2), bone cutter (Liston), 5-inch bone-cutter forceps, 7-inch bone-cutter rongeur (Stille).

depending on technique, body part, and frequency of use.

- Rongeur and rib cutters

  These can be used to cut through small- to medium-sized bones and to customize cut ends of all bone sizes (Fig. 1.19).

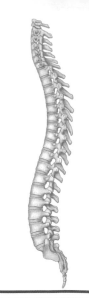

CHAPTER 2 MUSCLES OF THE BACK AND SCAPULA

ATLAS REFERENCES*
Netter: 180–183, 257, 413–418
McMinn: 101–103, 131–136, 144
Gray's Atlas: 20–32, 36–42, 399, 400

BEFORE YOU BEGIN
Make sure that you have palpated the following anatomic landmarks on yourself and classmates:
- Superior nuchal line
- External occipital protuberance (inion)
- Mastoid process
- Spinous process of the 7th cervical vertebra (C7, vertebra prominens)
- Spinous process of the thoracic and lumbar vertebrae, the sacrum, and the coccyx
- Medial and lateral parts of the clavicles
- Iliac crests
- Trapezius muscle
- Latissimus dorsi muscle
- Deltoid muscle
- Triceps brachii muscle
- Acromion

SKIN AND SUPERFICIAL FASCIA
○ Begin by palpating bony landmarks. With a marker, draw the following lines on the skin of the cadaver (Fig. 2.1):
   1. From the external occipital protuberance, down the midline of the back to the sacrum.
   2. Laterally, from the external occipital protuberance to the mastoid process on each side of the cadaver.

3. Laterally, from the spinous process of the vertebra prominens to the acromion of each shoulder.
   4. Superiorly from the sacrum, curving obliquely over the iliac crests to the midaxillary line on each side of the body; that is, to a point about halfway around the upper edge of each iliac crest.
○ Incise the skin along the lines just described, beginning at the point where the incisions for the midline and from the shoulders meet (Fig. 2.2).
○ Retract the skin carefully (with toothed forceps), leaving the fat (superficial fascia) intact (see Fig. 2.2).

DISSECTION **TIP**
Place absorptive cloths at the inferolateral spaces of the iliac crest. Excessive amounts of embalming fluid often accumulate at this location.

DISSECTION **TIP**
Make necessary "buttonholes" in the skin to facilitate the dissection (Fig. 2.3), as indicated in Chapter 1.

○ On one side of the body, the dissectors should first reflect only the skin, leaving the superficial fascia (tela subcutanea) in place.
○ Start the separation of the superficial fascia from the underlying deep fascia in the midline, by identifying a small part of the trapezius muscle.
○ Carefully scrape off the superficial fascia from the surface of the muscle with your scalpel (Fig. 2.4).

DISSECTION **TIP**
As the superficial fascia is reflected, watch for the passage of neurovascular bundles from the deep fascia into the deep surface of the superficial fascia. Save short segments of several of these for later demonstration and review.

*NOTE: This dissection guide is cross-referenced to the following atlases: Netter, *Atlas of Human Anatomy*, ed 7 (Netter); *McMinn's Clinical Atlas of Human Anatomy*, ed 7 (McMinn); and *Gray's Atlas of Anatomy*, ed 2 (Gray's). Page references from each atlas are provided at the beginning of Chapters 2 through 29 to give you the opportunity to study the relevant anatomy in depth to aid in your dissection.

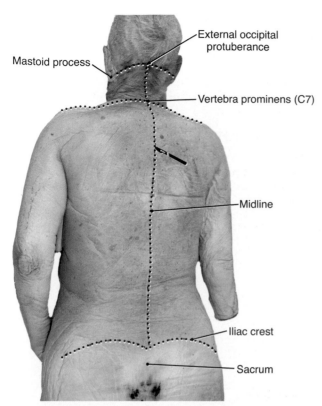

Fig. 2.1 Skin markings for incision lines: neck and back.

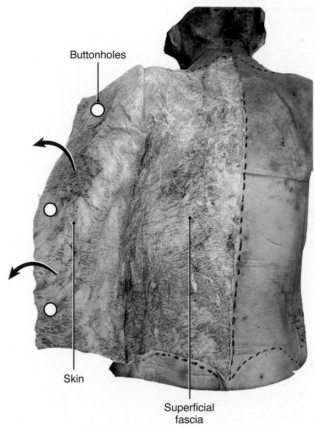

Fig. 2.3 Make "buttonholes" in the skin to facilitate its reflection from the superficial fascia.

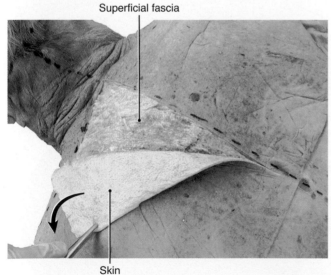

Fig. 2.2 Reflection of skin from superficial fascia.

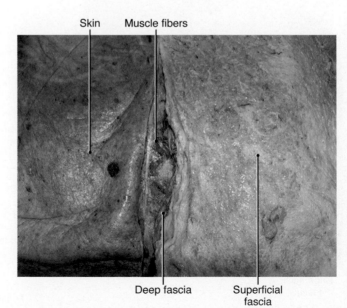

Fig. 2.4 Deep skin incisions showing deep fascia and muscle fibers.

DISSECTION TIP

Take precautions to avoid cutting too deeply with the scalpel. In some cadavers, the superficial fascia is very thin, and more deeply situated structures can be cut and destroyed (Figs. 2.5 and 2.6).

○ Completely remove superficial fascia over the latissimus dorsi muscle.
○ On the other side of the body, the skin and superficial fascia can be reflected together.

DISSECTION TIP

Care must be taken in this latter approach to avoid damage to the underlying muscles, especially the trapezius and latissimus dorsi muscles and their aponeuroses. Identify these before the skin and fascia are reflected more than a few centimeters.

SUPERFICIAL MUSCLES OF THE BACK: PART 1

○ Remove enough deep fascia to clarify the borders of the two most superficial muscles of the back, the trapezius and latissimus dorsi (Fig. 2.7).

ANATOMY NOTE

Note the diamond-shaped aponeurotic area of the trapezius at the upper middle thoracic region (see Fig. 2.7). The skin, superficial fascia, and deep fascia are relatively thin here. This is in contrast to the lateral lumbar region, where the amount of subcutaneous fat is increased (see Fig. 2.6).

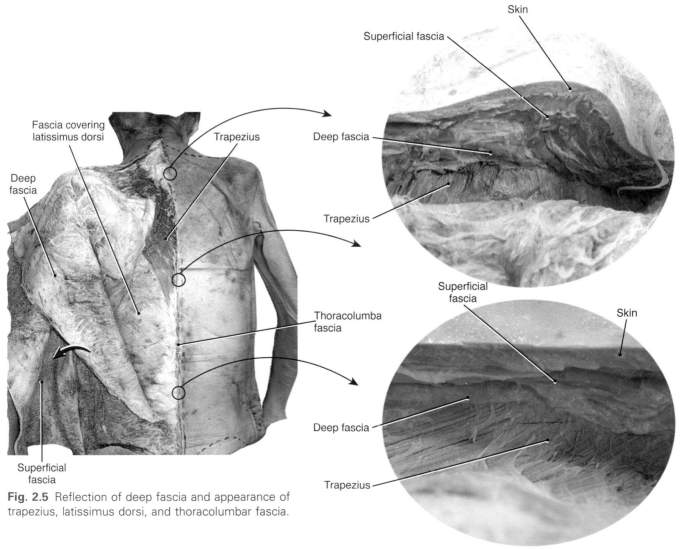

Fig. 2.5 Reflection of deep fascia and appearance of trapezius, latissimus dorsi, and thoracolumbar fascia.

Fig. 2.6 Note possible differences in thickness of the skin and fascia. Avoid cutting too deeply with the scalpel to prevent damage to superficial structures when exposing them.

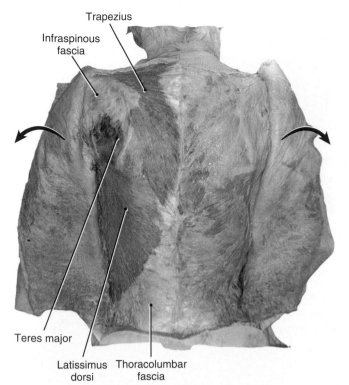

Fig. 2.7 Complete removal of superficial fascia over trapezius, latissimus dorsi, and posterior layer of thoracolumbar fascia on left side of cadaver. Deep fascia and some adipose tissue have been left intact on right side.

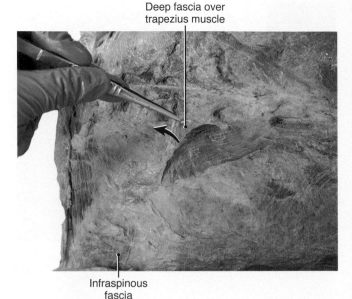

Fig. 2.8 Careful separation of deep fascia covering trapezius muscle.

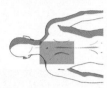

○ Identify the teres major muscle and the infraspinous fascia (see Fig. 2.7).

ANATOMY **NOTE**

This fascia covering the infraspinatus muscle is attached to the margins of the infraspinous fossa and is continuous with the deltoid fascia along the posterior border of the muscle.

○ Carefully separate the deep fascia covering the trapezius muscle (Fig. 2.8).
○ While cleaning away the fascia that overlies the most cranial portion of the trapezius (Figs. 2.9 and 2.10), look for the greater occipital nerve.
○ This nerve usually can be found approximately 1 inch (2.5 cm) from the midline and 1 inch inferior to the superior nuchal line, as the nerve pierces the trapezius (Figs. 2.11 and 2.12).
○ Also at this location, locate the occipital artery, and preserve it as the trapezius is reflected (see Fig. 2.12).

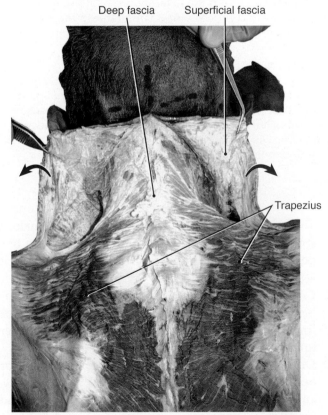

Fig. 2.9 Exposure of superior part of trapezius with portions of deep fascia still covering its uppermost portion.

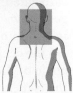

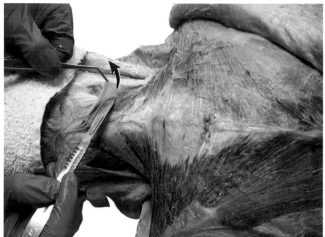

Fig. 2.10 Exposure of deep fascia covering the upper portion of trapezius.

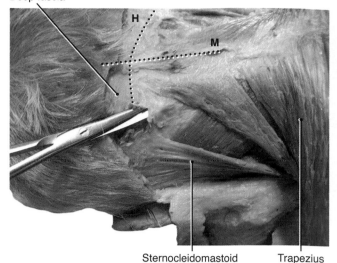

Deep fascia

Sternocleidomastoid Trapezius

Fig. 2.11 After identifying the greater occipital nerve, separate and remove the deep fascia; *M*, midline; *H*, horizontal line.

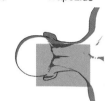

DISSECTION TIP

GREATER OCCIPITAL NERVE
To identify the greater occipital nerve, draw a horizontal imaginary line from the external occipital protuberance to the mastoid process. At 3 cm lateral to the external occipital protuberance on the imaginary line, remove the deep fascia to identify this nerve.

3RD OCCIPITAL NERVE
Usually the deep fascia over the trapezius muscle below the superior nuchal line is very thick and difficult to cut until the 7th cervical vertebra (C7) level. Pay special attention to the dissection process. Intermingled with the deep fascia over this area is the **3rd occipital nerve;** try to expose and save it (Fig. 2.13).

Greater occipital nerve

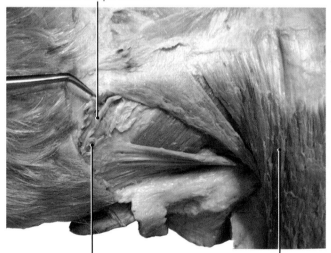

Occipital artery Trapezius

Fig. 2.12 Deep fascia is cut, and the greater occipital nerve and occipital artery are visible.

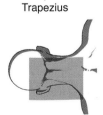

○ To detach the trapezius from its origin, first make a small vertical cut through the lower part of the trapezius at the 12th thoracic vertebra (T12) level as it attaches to the midline.

○ Continue the incision to the external occipital protuberance. Define and loosen the trapezius with your fingers or with scissors before you proceed further upward along the midline (Fig. 2.14).

○ Detach the trapezius from its origin on the superior nuchal line and the external occipital protuberance, and sever the fibers that arise from the spines and associated ligaments of the cervical and thoracic vertebrae. Reflect the trapezius laterally toward its insertion onto the scapula (Fig. 2.15).

○ On the deep surface of the trapezius, near the superior angle of the scapula, look for the nerve that supplies the trapezius, the accessory nerve.

○ Note the artery that supplies the trapezius muscle, the ascending branch of the transverse cervical artery.

○ Identify the levator scapulae, rhomboid minor and major muscles, and neurovascular bundle (Fig. 2.16).

○ Clean the fascia from these muscles so that their fibers can be seen clearly.

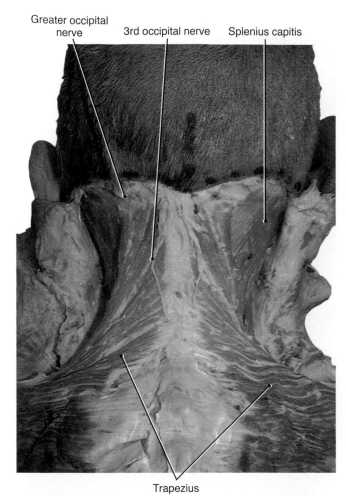

Greater occipital nerve 3rd occipital nerve Splenius capitis

Trapezius

Fig. 2.13 Complete exposure and detachment of the superior part of the trapezius from the deep fascia. Observe the 3rd occipital nerve.

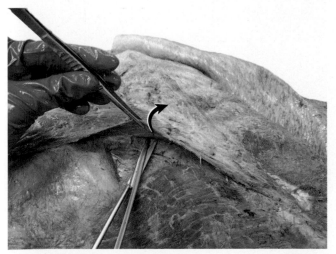

Fig. 2.14 Dissection of lateral trapezius muscle facilitated by a separation technique using dissecting scissors.

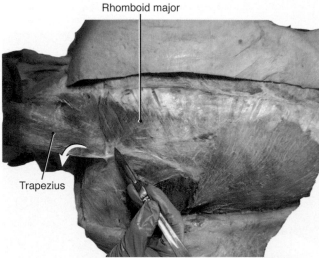

Rhomboid major

Trapezius

Fig. 2.15 Separation of the connective tissue on the deep surface of trapezius.

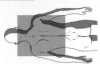

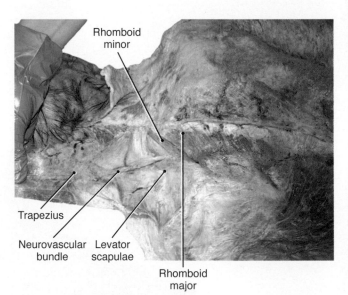

Rhomboid minor

Trapezius

Neurovascular bundle   Levator scapulae

Rhomboid major

Fig. 2.16 Complete reflection of the trapezius and appearance of the underlying levator scapulae and rhomboid muscles, and neuromuscular bundle.

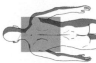

○ Gently retract the levator scapulae muscle medially. At the midpoint of the levator, you will see the accessory nerve exit and run on the internal surface of the trapezius muscle (Figs. 2.17 and 2.18).

○ Carefully separate the neurovascular bundle to identify the accessory nerve, ascending branch of the transverse cervical artery, and tributaries of transverse cervical vein (Figs. 2.19 and 2.20).

○ Carefully expose the deep fascia over the rhomboid major and minor muscles. In some specimens the line

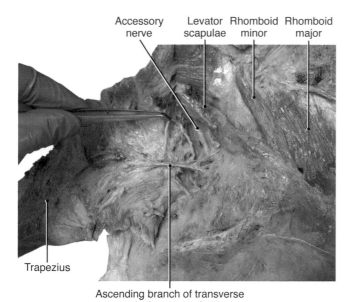

Accessory nerve | Levator scapulae | Rhomboid minor | Rhomboid major

Trapezius

Ascending branch of transverse cervical artery and vein

Fig. 2.17 Identification of accessory nerve, emerging deep from medial side at midpoint of levator scapulae muscle.

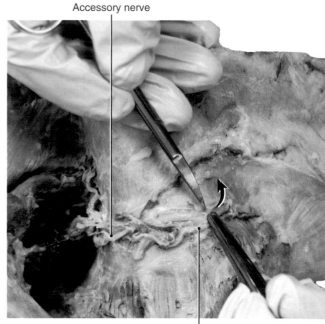

Accessory nerve

Ascending branch of transverse cervical artery and vein

Fig. 2.18 Careful separation of neurovascular bundle to identify accessory nerve, ascending branch of transverse cervical artery, and tributaries of transverse cervical vein.

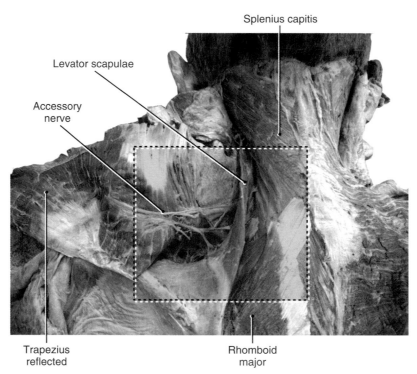

Splenius capitis

Levator scapulae

Accessory nerve

Trapezius reflected

Rhomboid major

Fig. 2.19 After careful dissection of connective tissue, trapezius muscle is reflected and accessory nerve identified.

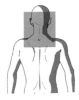

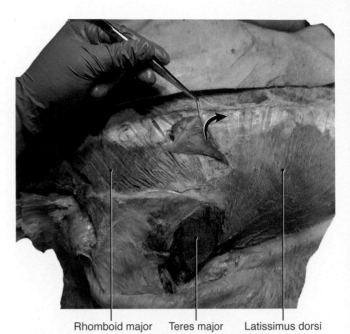

Fig. 2.20 Trapezius muscle is reflected and the accessory nerve identified.

Labels on Fig. 2.20:
- Trapezius reflected
- Accessory nerve
- Transverse cervical artery
- Transverse cervical vein
- Levator scapulae

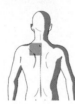

Fig. 2.21 Carefully expose deep fascia over the rhomboid major and minor muscles.

Labels on Fig. 2.21:
- Rhomboid major
- Teres major
- Latissimus dorsi

ANATOMY **NOTE**

In about 50% of the specimens, the dorsal scapular artery is absent, and the deep branch of the transverse cervical artery replaces it. The dorsal scapular artery typically arises from the 3rd part of the subclavian artery and runs posteriorly through the brachial plexus.

MUSCLES OF THE SCAPULA

ANATOMY **NOTE**

The infraspinous fascia is attached to the scapula around the boundaries of the attachments of the infraspinatus, teres minor and major, long head of triceps brachii, and deltoid muscles.

- Clean the teres major muscle (Fig. 2.25).
- Identify the teres minor and deltoid muscles and the long head of triceps brachii (Fig. 2.26).

ANATOMY **NOTE**

The fibers of the teres minor muscle run more or less parallel to the fibers of the teres major and are medial to the long head of the triceps brachii and deltoid muscles (see Fig. 2.25).

- Beginning superiorly, reflect the infraspinous fascia to expose the long head of triceps and deltoid muscles (Figs. 2.27 and 2.28).

of cleavage between the rhomboid muscles may be unclear (Figs. 2.21 and 2.22).

- Reflect the rhomboid muscles laterally toward their insertion onto the medial border of the scapula (Fig. 2.23) (Plate 2.1).
- Deep to the rhomboids, identify the serratus posterior superior muscle, which inserts onto the ribs rather than onto the scapula. (This fact will assist you in its identification.)
- On the deep surface of the rhomboids, try to identify the dorsal scapular nerve and dorsal scapular artery (Fig. 2.24).

ANATOMY **NOTE**

The dorsal scapular nerve innervates the rhomboid and levator scapulae muscles (in addition to branches from C3 and C4). The dorsal scapular nerve arises from C5, one of the two nerves that arise directly from the ventral rami of the brachial plexus.

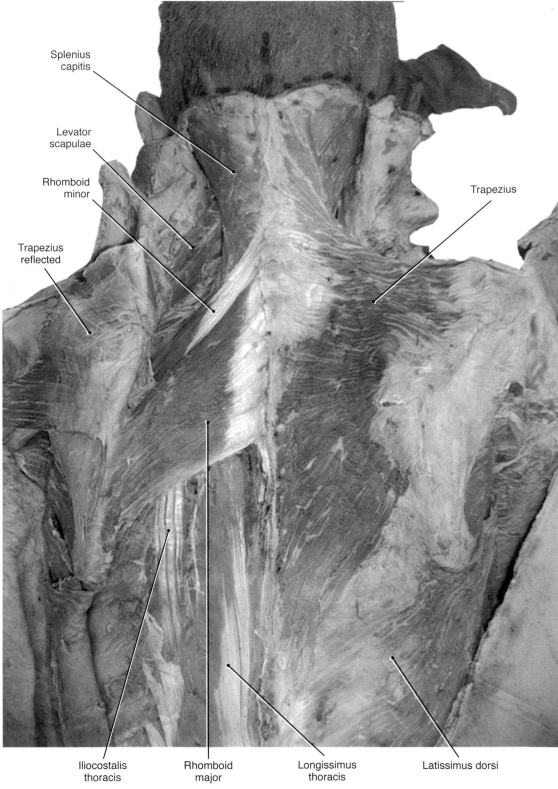

Splenius
capitis

Levator
scapulae

Rhomboid
minor

Trapezius
reflected

Trapezius

Iliocostalis
thoracis

Rhomboid
major

Longissimus
thoracis

Latissimus dorsi

Fig. 2.22 Trapezius and latissimus dorsi muscles are reflected. Underlying intermediate extrinsic muscles of the back are exposed.

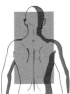

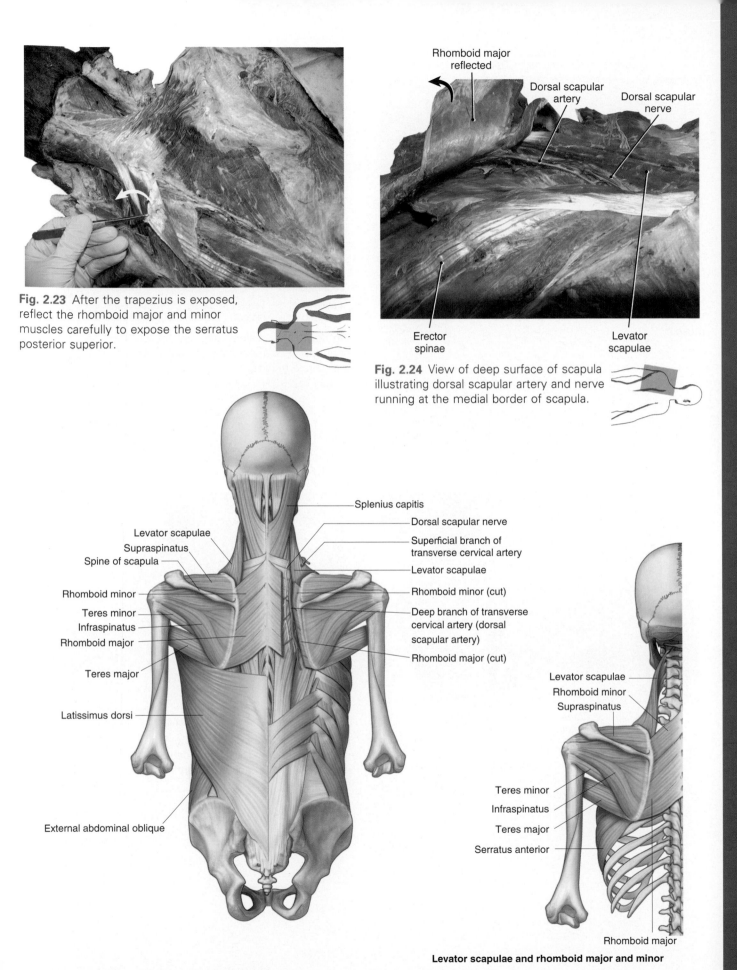

Fig. 2.23 After the trapezius is exposed, reflect the rhomboid major and minor muscles carefully to expose the serratus posterior superior.

Rhomboid major reflected

Dorsal scapular artery

Dorsal scapular nerve

Erector spinae

Levator scapulae

Fig. 2.24 View of deep surface of scapula illustrating dorsal scapular artery and nerve running at the medial border of scapula.

Splenius capitis

Dorsal scapular nerve

Superficial branch of transverse cervical artery

Levator scapulae

Rhomboid minor (cut)

Deep branch of transverse cervical artery (dorsal scapular artery)

Rhomboid major (cut)

Levator scapulae

Supraspinatus

Spine of scapula

Rhomboid minor

Teres minor

Infraspinatus

Rhomboid major

Teres major

Latissimus dorsi

External abdominal oblique

Levator scapulae

Rhomboid minor

Supraspinatus

Teres minor

Infraspinatus

Teres major

Serratus anterior

Rhomboid major

Levator scapulae and rhomboid major and minor

Plate 2.1 Superficial musculature of the back.

Latissimus dorsi Teres major Trapezius Infraspinous fascia

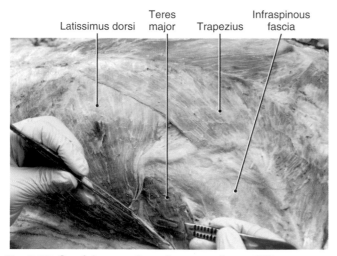

Fig. 2.25 Careful separation of teres major from upper border of latissimus dorsi muscle.

Trapezius

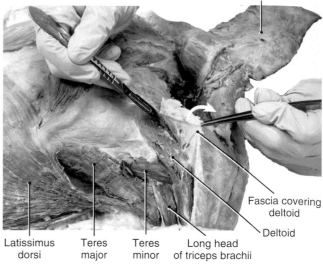

Fascia covering deltoid

Deltoid

Latissimus dorsi Teres major Teres minor Long head of triceps brachii

Fig. 2.27 With scalpel, carefully detach deep fascia covering the posterior fibers of the deltoid muscle.

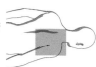

Latissimus dorsi Rhomboid major Trapezius

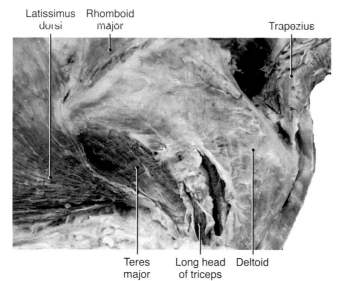

Teres major Long head of triceps Deltoid

Fig. 2.26 View of deltoscapular region. Long head of triceps brachii and deltoid muscles are exposed after careful separation from infraspinous fascia.

Rhomboid major Teres minor Deltoid Trapezius

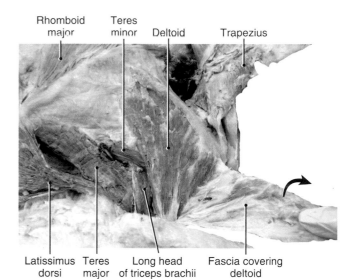

Latissimus dorsi Teres major Long head of triceps brachii Fascia covering deltoid

Fig. 2.28 Deep fascia covering deltoid muscle is reflected, exposing deltoid muscle with its attachments onto spine of scapula.

- Insert your index finger under the deltoid muscle (Fig. 2.29).
- Using toothed forceps, scalpel, and scissors, reflect the posterior border of the deltoid laterally, separating it at its attachment on the spine of the scapular and acromion (Fig. 2.30).
- Continue reflecting the muscle laterally and posteriorly until the surgical neck of the humerus is visible, but leave the deltoid muscle attached to the deltoid tuberosity, the insertion of the muscle.
- Identify the quadrangular space bordered posteriorly by the teres major and minor muscles, long head of triceps brachii, and surgical neck of the humerus (see Fig. 2.30).
- Identify the axillary nerve as it appears posterior to the surgical neck of the humerus (see Fig. 2.30). The nerve is accompanied by the posterior circumflex humeral artery, a branch of the third portion of the axillary artery. The axillary nerve and posterior circumflex humeral artery appear in the field by emerging through the quadrangular space.
- Thoroughly clean the axillary nerve and the posterior circumflex humeral vessels at their entrance into the deltoid muscle behind the surgical neck of the humerus. Protect these as you clean connective tissue away from the muscles that help form the boundaries of the quadrangular space.

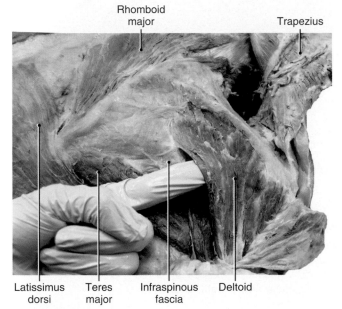

Rhomboid major Trapezius

Latissimus dorsi Teres major Infraspinous fascia Deltoid

Fig. 2.29 Insert your index finger under deltoid muscle, and with a scalpel, detach its attachments to scapula.

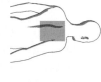

DISSECTION TIP

The axillary nerve typically branches off to several smaller branches and is usually superior to the posterior circumflex humeral artery.

- Identify the triangular space between the teres minor, teres major, and the long head of the triceps (see Fig. 2.30).
- Identify the scapular circumflex artery within the triangular space.

ANATOMY NOTE

This artery originates from the subscapular artery, one of the three branches of the third part of the axillary artery. The scapular circumflex artery branches to the overlying skin of the triangular space before turning around the lateral border of the scapula and passing deep to the infraspinatus muscle.

DISSECTION TIP

The scapular circumflex artery typically is located at the midpoint of the lateral border of the scapula (see Fig. 2.33).

ANATOMY NOTE

The infraspinous and supraspinous fasciae are attached to the scapula around the boundaries of the attachments of the infraspinatus and supraspinatus muscles, respectively.

- Identify the medial border of the infraspinatus muscle.
- With a scalpel, carefully detach deep fascia (infraspinous fascia) covering infraspinatus muscle (Fig. 2.31).

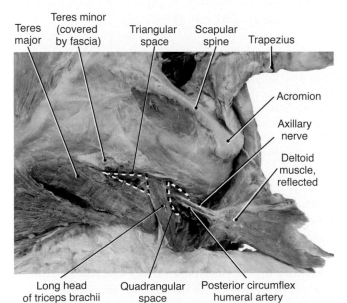

Teres major Teres minor (covered by fascia) Triangular space Scapular spine Trapezius

Acromion

Axillary nerve

Deltoid muscle, reflected

Long head of triceps brachii Quadrangular space Posterior circumflex humeral artery

Fig. 2.30 View of internal surface of reflected deltoid muscle with posterior circumflex humeral artery and axillary nerve exposed. Note quadrangular and triangular spaces.

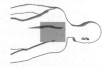

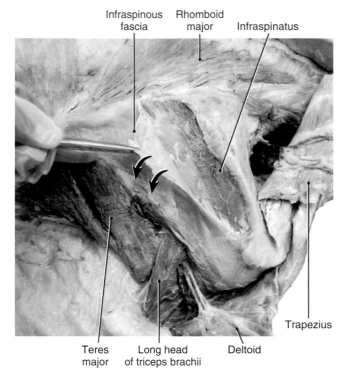

Infraspinous fascia — Rhomboid major — Infraspinatus

Teres major — Long head of triceps brachii — Deltoid — Trapezius

Fig. 2.31 With a scalpel, carefully detach deep fascia (infraspinous fascia) covering infraspinatus muscle.

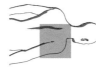

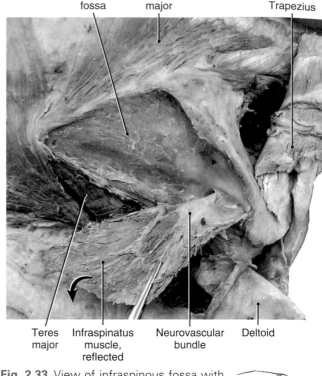

Infraspinous fossa — Rhomboid major — Trapezius

Teres major — Infraspinatus muscle, reflected — Neurovascular bundle — Deltoid

Fig. 2.33 View of infraspinous fossa with infraspinatus muscle reflected. Note the neurovascular bundle covered with connective tissue, which contains the suprascapular artery, vein, and nerve.

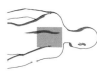

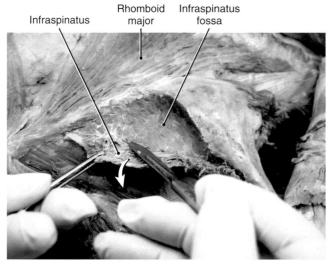

Infraspinatus — Rhomboid major — Infraspinatus fossa

Fig. 2.32 With scalpel, carefully detach infraspinatus muscle from infraspinous fossa.

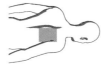

○ Carefully detach infraspinatus muscle from infraspinous fossa (Fig. 2.32).
○ Reflect the infraspinatus muscle laterally from the infraspinous fossa toward its humeral insertion (Fig. 2.33). Note the neurovascular bundle covered with

connective tissue, which contains the suprascapular artery, vein, and nerve.
○ Carefully separate the connective tissue over the neurovascular bundle to expose the suprascapular artery, nerve, and vein (Fig. 2.34).

ANATOMY **NOTE**

The suprascapular artery has a rich anastomosis with the scapular circumflex artery. This arrangement allows strong collateral arterial supply to develop between the subclavian artery and the third part of the axillary artery in the event of occlusion of the more proximal portions of the axillary artery.

○ Identify and clean the supraspinatus muscle (Fig. 2.35).
○ Beginning medially, reflect the muscle laterally from the supraspinous fossa far enough to expose the suprascapular nerve and artery.
○ Identify the suprascapular artery and trace it from its origin to its crossing of the superior transverse scapular ligament to enter the supraspinous fossa, deep to the supraspinatus muscle (Fig. 2.36). Note the passage of the suprascapular nerve and vessels around the greater scapular notch, where they enter the infraspinatus muscle (Plate 2.2).

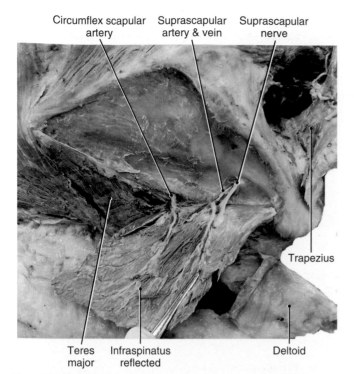

Circumflex scapular artery | Suprascapular artery & vein | Suprascapular nerve

Trapezius

Teres major | Infraspinatus reflected | Deltoid

Fig. 2.34 Connective tissue is dissected out, exposing the suprascapular artery, vein, and nerve, as well as the scapular circumflex artery.

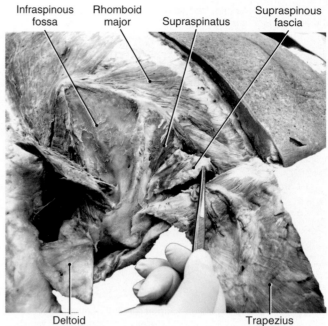

Infraspinous fossa | Rhomboid major | Supraspinatus | Supraspinous fascia

Deltoid | Trapezius

Fig. 2.35 Supraspinous fascia is reflected and the supraspinatus muscle exposed.

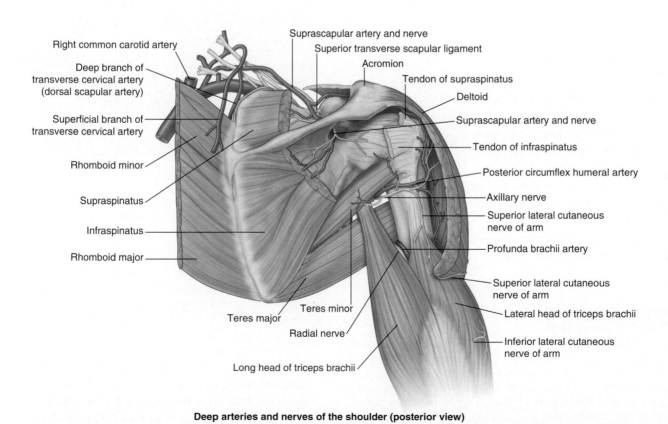

Right common carotid artery
Deep branch of transverse cervical artery (dorsal scapular artery)
Superficial branch of transverse cervical artery
Rhomboid minor
Supraspinatus
Infraspinatus
Rhomboid major

Suprascapular artery and nerve
Superior transverse scapular ligament
Acromion
Tendon of supraspinatus
Deltoid
Suprascapular artery and nerve
Tendon of infraspinatus
Posterior circumflex humeral artery
Axillary nerve
Superior lateral cutaneous nerve of arm
Profunda brachii artery
Superior lateral cutaneous nerve of arm
Lateral head of triceps brachii
Inferior lateral cutaneous nerve of arm

Teres major
Teres minor
Radial nerve
Long head of triceps brachii

Deep arteries and nerves of the shoulder (posterior view)

Plate 2.2 Collateral arterial supply between the subclavian artery and the third part of the axillary artery through anastomoses of the scapular circumflex artery and the suprascapular artery.

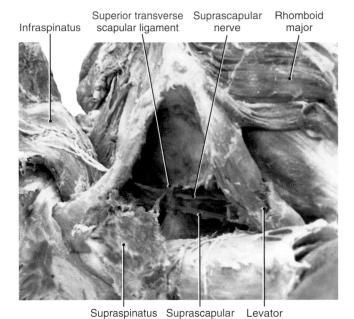

Infraspinatus — Superior transverse scapular ligament — Suprascapular nerve — Rhomboid major

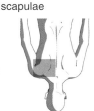

Supraspinatus — Suprascapular artery — Levator scapulae

Fig. 2.36 View of internal surface of the supraspinous fossa. Notice suprascapular artery passing over superior transverse scapular ligament and suprascapular nerve underneath it.

SUPERFICIAL MUSCLES OF THE BACK: PART 2

- ○ Completely remove the deep fascia to expose the latissimus dorsi muscle.
- ○ Make an incision through the aponeurosis of the latissimus dorsi muscle about ½ inch (1.25 cm) from the midline of the back, and cut its attachments to the crest of the ilium.
- ○ Reflect the latissimus dorsi muscle superiorly and laterally (Fig. 2.37).
- ○ Reflection of the trapezius and latissimus dorsi muscles exposes underlying intermediate extrinsic muscles of the back.
- ○ Identify the serratus anterior and the serratus posterior inferior muscles (Fig. 2.38).

DISSECTION **TIP**

If you do not exercise care, you will reflect the serratus posterior inferior muscle with the latissimus dorsi. The key to their separation lies in the recognition that although the serratus posterior inferior arises in common with part of the latissimus dorsi, the serratus inserts onto the lower ribs. These fibers can be observed as they diverge from those of the latissimus to pass to their insertion (Fig. 2.39).

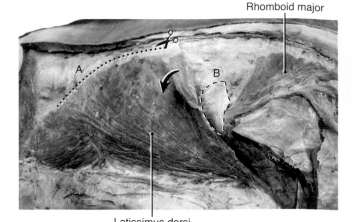

Rhomboid major

Latissimus dorsi

Fig. 2.37 *Dotted line A* shows location of incision through aponeurosis of latissimus dorsi muscle. *Dotted line B* shows area of connective/adipose tissue covering serratus anterior muscle.

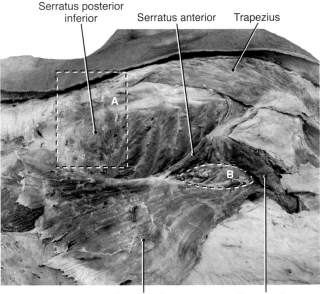

Serratus posterior inferior — Serratus anterior — Trapezius

Latissimus dorsi, reflected — Teres major

Fig. 2.38 Latissimus dorsi muscle is reflected, and *dotted outline A* shows serratus posterior inferior muscle. Connective/adipose tissue of Fig. 2.33 is removed and serratus anterior muscle exposed. *Dotted line B* shows second area of connective/adipose tissue between serratus anterior and latissimus dorsi muscles.

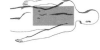

- ○ Pay special attention when removing the connective adipose tissue between the latissimus dorsi, serratus anterior, and teres major muscles so as not to injure the thoracodorsal artery and vein (Figs. 2.40 and 2.41).
- ○ Cut the origin of the serratus posterior inferior muscle and reflect it toward its insertion.

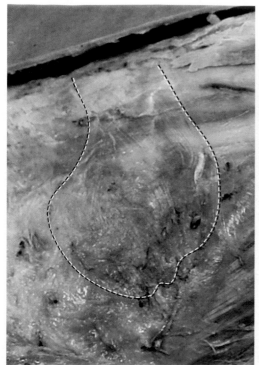

Fig. 2.39 *Dotted lines* show borders of serratus posterior inferior muscle.

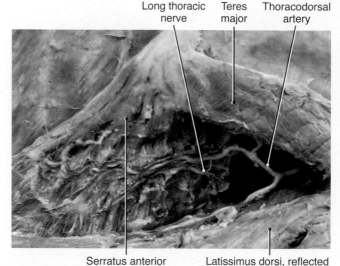

Long thoracic nerve Teres major Thoracodorsal artery

Serratus anterior Latissimus dorsi, reflected

Fig. 2.41 Close-up view of space between teres major, serratus anterior, and latissimus dorsi muscles (area *B* in Fig. 2.38). Note the thoracodorsal artery and long thoracic nerve supplying the serratus anterior muscle.

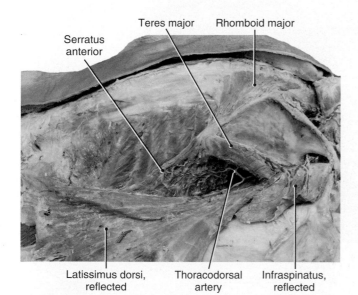

Serratus anterior Teres major Rhomboid major

Latissimus dorsi, reflected Thoracodorsal artery Infraspinatus, reflected

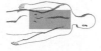

Fig. 2.40 View of the internal surface of the scapula and dorsal scapular artery traveling at the medial border of the scapula.

○ Make a longitudinal incision through the lumbar part of the thoracolumbar fascia near the midline. Then, by cutting its attachments to the underlying musculature, reflect this thick fascia/aponeurosis combination laterally far enough to expose the erector spinae muscle layer (Figs. 2.42 and 2.43).

DISSECTION **TIP**

The reflection of the thoracolumbar fascia is performed in the lumbar region only. For the thoracic region, it is unnecessary because the fascia is much thinner there. In this specimen, the fascia in the thoracic region was thick enough to be reflected (see Fig. 2.42).

○ Identify and separate the three longitudinally oriented columns of the erector spinae muscle: the spinalis, longissimus, and iliocostalis (Fig. 2.44).

ANATOMY **NOTE**

The spinalis is the more medial muscle; the longissimus is the longest muscle, extending to the neck; and the iliocostalis is the most lateral of the three muscles, attaching the iliac crest to the ribs.

DEEP MUSCLES OF THE BACK

○ To expose the deeper musculature, remove a block of the erector spinae muscle several inches long from the lower thoracic and upper lumbar region, and identify the transversospinalis musculature (Figs. 2.45 and 2.46). The transversospinalis muscles include the semispinalis, multifidus, and rotators.

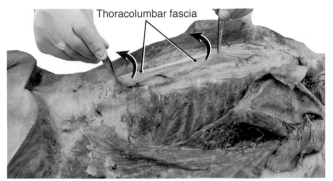

Thoracolumbar fascia

Fig. 2.42 Reflection of thoracolumbar fascia.

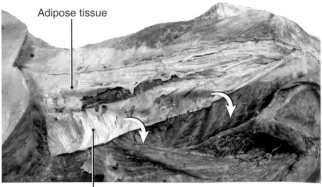

Adipose tissue

Thoracolumbar fascia, reflected

Fig. 2.43 Thoracolumbar fascia is reflected, and erector spinae muscle is exposed. Note adipose tissue overlying erector spinae. *Dotted line* represents longitudinal incision of thoracolumbar fascia from the midline.

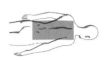

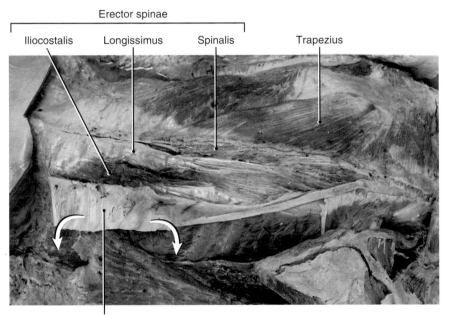

Erector spinae

Iliocostalis   Longissimus   Spinalis   Trapezius

Thoracolumbar fascia, reflected

Fig. 2.44 The thoracolumbar fascia is reflected, and the erector spinae muscle is exposed.

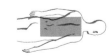

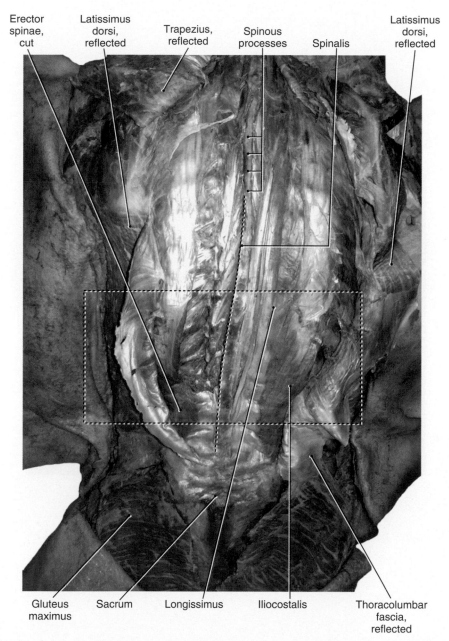

Erector
spinae,
cut

Latissimus
dorsi,
reflected

Trapezius,
reflected

Spinous
processes

Spinalis

Latissimus
dorsi,
reflected

Gluteus
maximus

Sacrum

Longissimus

Iliocostalis

Thoracolumbar
fascia,
reflected

Fig. 2.45 The thoracolumbar fascia is reflected laterally, and the erector spinae muscle (spinalis, longissimus, iliocostalis) are exposed on the right. On the left, the erector spinae muscles are cut to expose the deeper muscles of back.

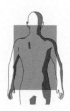

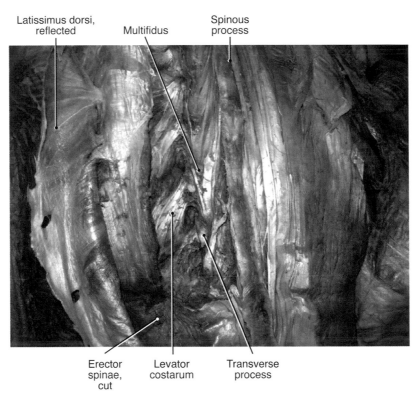

Latissimus dorsi, reflected

Multifidus

Spinous process

Erector spinae, cut

Levator costarum

Transverse process

Fig. 2.46 Multifidus and levator costarum muscles are exposed.

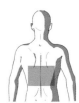

LABORATORY IDENTIFICATION CHECKLIST

OSTEOLOGY
☐ Skull and vertebrae
☐ Superior nuchal line
☐ External occipital protuberance
☐ Mastoid process
☐ Vertebra prominens (C7)
☐ Spinous processes of thoracic and lumbar vertebrae, and sacrum and coccyx

CLAVICLE
☐ Medial and lateral ends, body, and curvatures

SCAPULA
☐ Acromion
☐ Spine of scapula
☐ Medial or vertebral border
☐ Superior border
☐ Suprascapular notch
☐ Inferior angle
☐ Superior angle
☐ Lateral or axillary border
☐ Coracoid process

OTHER
☐ Iliac crests

MUSCLES
☐ Trapezius
☐ Latissimus dorsi
☐ Serratus posterior inferior
☐ Serratus posterior superior
☐ Levator scapulae
☐ Rhomboid minor
☐ Rhomboid major
☐ Deltoid
☐ Triceps brachii, long head
☐ Supraspinatus
☐ Infraspinatus

☐ Teres major
☐ Teres minor
☐ Transversospinalis
  ☐ Semispinalis
  ☐ Multifidus
  ☐ Rotatores
☐ Semispinalis
☐ Splenius capitis
☐ Erector spinae
  ☐ Spinalis
  ☐ Longissimus
  ☐ Iliocostalis

NERVES
☐ Greater occipital
☐ Accessory
☐ Dorsal scapular
☐ Suprascapular
☐ Axillary

FASCIAE
☐ Thoracolumbar
☐ Supraspinous/infraspinous

LIGAMENT
☐ Superior transverse scapular

ARTERIES
☐ Occipital
☐ Suprascapular
☐ Scapular circumflex
☐ Transverse cervical
☐ Dorsal scapular
☐ Posterior circumflex humeral

VEIN
☐ Transverse cervical

ATLAS REFERENCES

Netter: 170, 174–178, 184
McMinn: 94–99, 104, 105
Gray's Atlas: 20–32, 36–42, 399, 400

SUBOCCIPITAL TRIANGLE

- Make a midline skin incision from the spinous process of the 7th cervical vertebra (C7) to the external occipital protuberance (Fig. 3.1).
- At the level of the external occipital protuberance, make a horizontal skin incision connecting the right and left mastoid processes.
- Reflect the skin and the subcutaneous fat as one layer.
- Beneath the subcutaneous tissue, a connective tissue layer covers the upper portion of the trapezius muscle (Fig. 3.2); dissect away this layer and expose the trapezius (Fig. 3.3).
- While cleaning out the fascia that overlies the most cephalic portion of the trapezius muscle (see Fig. 2.10), look for the greater occipital nerve (Fig. 3.4).
- Also at this location, locate the occipital artery and preserve it as the trapezius is reflected.

ANATOMY **NOTE**

The greater occipital nerve usually can be found about 1 inch (2.5 cm) from the midline of the neck and 1 inch inferior to the superior nuchal line, as this nerve pierces the trapezius muscle (see Figs. 2.11 to 2.12).

DISSECTION **TIP**

Usually, the deep fascia over the trapezius muscle, below the superior nuchal line, is thick and difficult to cut until the C7 level. About 1 cm lateral to the midline, the 3rd occipital nerve (medial branch of dorsal ramus of C3 spinal nerve) is seen along the nuchal ligament (ligamentum nuchae) intermingled with the deep fascia over this area (see Figs. 3.3 and 3.4). Generally, the 3rd occipital nerve is very small and often is cut during routine dissections.

- Identify the greater occipital nerve and the 3rd occipital nerve, and preserve them after reflecting the trapezius away from its cranial and cervical attachments. Carefully reflect the trapezius muscle from its cranial and cervical attachments (Figs. 3.5 to 3.7).

DISSECTION **TIP**

The trapezius is thin at its cephalic and cervical attachments (see Fig. 3.6). Be careful during its reflection. While reflecting the trapezius up from its distal end, keep the scalpel blade facing downward toward the vertebrae, not upward, in order to prevent damage to the muscle.

- The small amount of connective tissue between the trapezius and splenius capitis muscles can be removed.
- At the lateral border of the splenius capitis, identify the lesser occipital nerve (see Fig. 3.7).
- Identify the splenius capitis and splenius cervicis muscles; divide them at their origins from the spines of the cervical and upper thoracic vertebrae and reflect them laterally, exposing the semispinalis capitis muscle (Figs. 3.8 through 3.10).
- Cut the attachment of the semispinalis capitis muscle from the skull and the ligamentum nuchae to reveal the suboccipital triangle. Preserve the greater occipital and lesser occipital nerves as the semispinalis muscle is reflected.

DISSECTION **TIP**

Make one small cut on the semispinalis capitis muscle medial to the greater and lesser occipital nerves (Fig. 3.11). In this way, the semispinalis capitis muscle easily can be reflected laterally without disturbing the course of the nerves (Fig. 3.12).

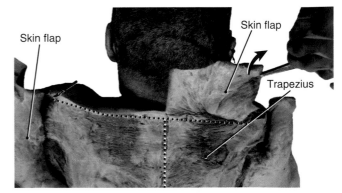

Fig. 3.1 Once the overlying skin is reflected, the deeper lying trapezius muscle is seen.

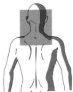

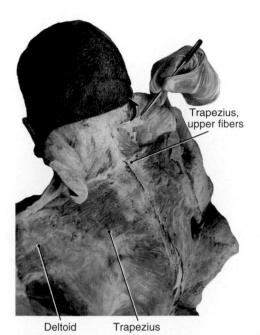

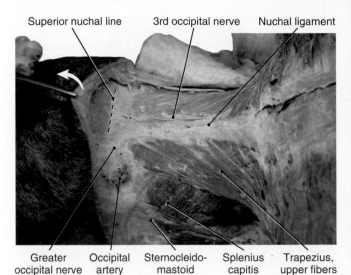

Fig. 3.2 Reflected skin and fascia revealing upper, middle, and lower fibers of the trapezius muscle.

Trapezius, upper fibers

Deltoid   Trapezius

Superior nuchal line   3rd occipital nerve   Nuchal ligament

Greater occipital nerve   Occipital artery   Sternocleido-mastoid   Splenius capitis   Trapezius, upper fibers

Fig. 3.4 Structures superficial to suboccipital triangle: nuchal ligament, trapezius (upper fibers), splenius capitis, sternocleidomastoid, 3rd occipital nerve, and occipital artery.

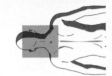

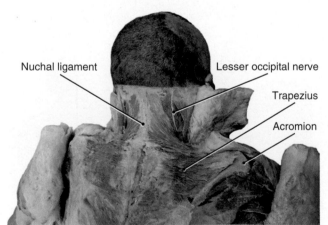

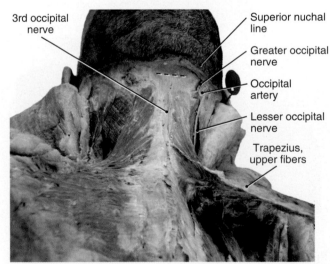

Nuchal ligament   Lesser occipital nerve

Trapezius

Acromion

Fig. 3.3 Superficial upper back and suboccipital regions: upper, middle, and lower fibers of trapezius muscle and nuchal ligament (ligamentum nuchae).

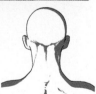

3rd occipital nerve

Superior nuchal line

Greater occipital nerve

Occipital artery

Lesser occipital nerve

Trapezius, upper fibers

Fig. 3.5 Initial reflection of the trapezius muscle.

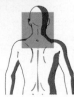

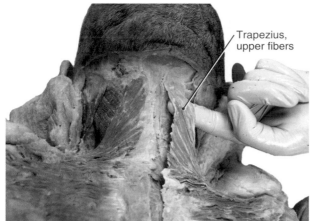

Fig. 3.6 Elevation of upper fibers of the trapezius muscle reflected away from the nuchal ligament.

Trapezius, upper fibers

Greater occipital nerve

Occipital artery

Lesser occipital nerve

Splenius capitis

Splenius cervicis

Fig. 3.8 Insert the scissors deep to the splenius capitis muscle at the midline and continue the incision inferiorly along the nuchal ligament.

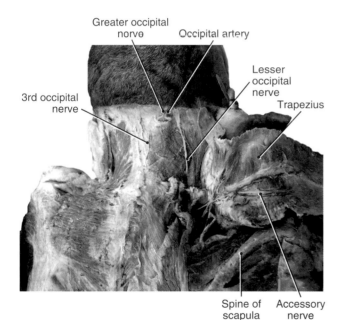

Greater occipital nerve

Occipital artery

3rd occipital nerve

Lesser occipital nerve

Trapezius

Spine of scapula

Accessory nerve

Fig. 3.7 Posterolateral view of superficial suboccipital region with reflected trapezius muscle and its associated neurovascular bundle pasted on its undersurface.

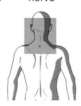

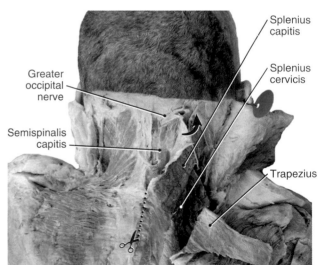

Splenius capitis

Splenius cervicis

Greater occipital nerve

Semispinalis capitis

Trapezius

Fig. 3.9 Reflect splenius capitis laterally, and continue incision toward 1st thoracic vertebra (T1) level.

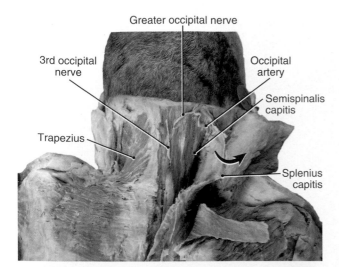

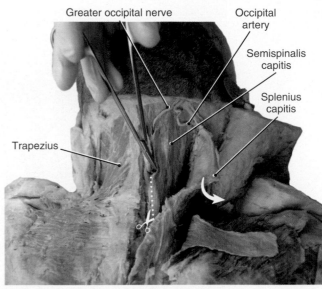

Fig. 3.10 Complete reflection of the splenius capitis muscle laterally.

Fig. 3.11 Make an incision into the semispinalis capitis muscle near the midline down to approximately the T1 level. Preserve the greater and 3rd occipital nerves.

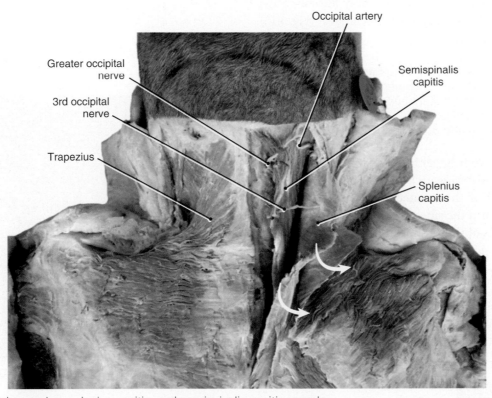

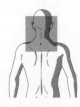

Fig. 3.12 Reflected trapezius, splenius capitis, and semispinalis capitis muscles.

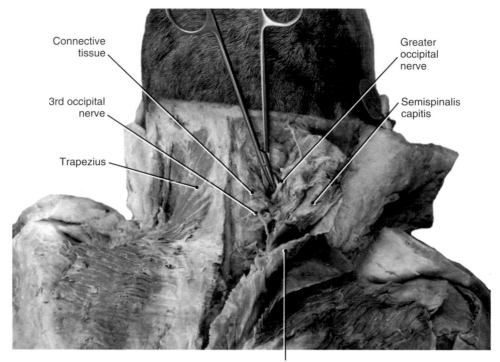

Fig. 3.13 Remove fat and connective tissues from around the greater and 3rd occipital nerves. Use the separation technique with your scissors.

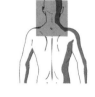

○ Trace the occipital nerves down through the underlying fat and connective tissue, clearing away the connective tissue using the "separating scissors technique" (Fig. 3.13).

DISSECTION **TIP**

Even after the semispinalis capitis muscle is reflected, generally the boundaries or contents of the suboccipital triangle are not immediately apparent and are hidden by overlying connective tissue. Remove these tissues carefully (Figs. 3.14 and 3.15).

○ Place the tip of your finger into the suboccipital triangle to locate the posterior arch of the atlas.
○ After removal of the connective tissue, identify the muscles that form the sides of the suboccipital triangle: inferior capitis oblique, superior capitis oblique, and rectus capitis posterior major (Fig. 3.16) (Plate 3.1).

ANATOMY **NOTE**

The rectus capitis posterior major is found superficial to the rectus capitis posterior minor. Although the rectus capitis posterior minor is considered a "suboccipital" muscle, it does not contribute to the margins of the suboccipital triangle.

DISSECTION **TIP**

Use fine scissors and take your time to expose and clearly demonstrate the vertebral artery. Besides the connective tissue over the vertebral artery, a rich venous plexus is also present. Clean away the connective tissue and venous plexus. You will see only the posterior wall of the vertebral artery.

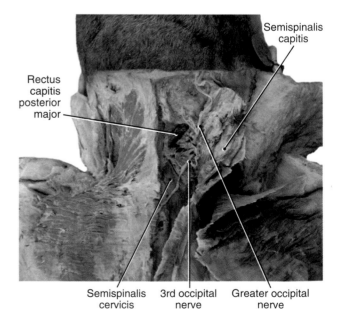

Fig. 3.14 Dissection of suboccipital triangle demonstrating the rectus capitis posterior major muscle and greater and 3rd occipital nerves. Remove all fat and connective tissue.

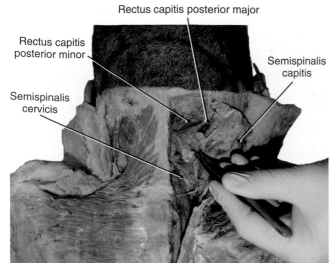

Fig. 3.15 Dissection of suboccipital triangle revealing surrounding muscles, including the rectus capitis posterior major and minor and semispinalis capitis muscles.

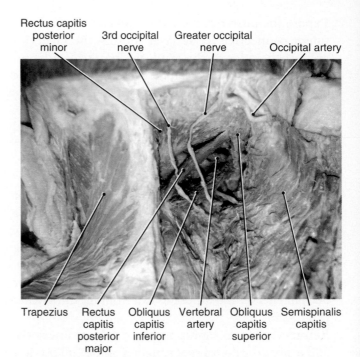

Fig. 3.16 Dissection of the suboccipital triangle highlighting borders and contents.

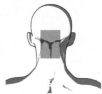

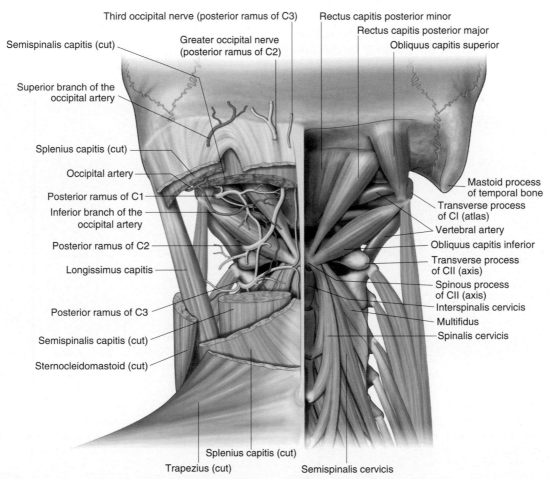

Plate 3.1 The suboccipital triangle and associated structures.

Expose the posterior arch of the atlas, and identify a tough connective tissue layer joining the posterior arch of the atlas to the skull, the posterior atlanto-occipital membrane. Clean the loose connective tissue away from the arch and expose the vertebral artery, which lies in the sulcus of the posterior arch of the atlas. Between the sulcus of the posterior arch and the vertebral artery, identify the suboccipital nerve, which innervates the suboccipital muscles and overlying semispinalis capitis muscle (Fig. 3.17).

○ Using a scalpel, cut the rectus capitis posterior major and inferior capitis oblique muscles from the spinous process of the axis, and reflect them laterally (Fig. 3.18).

○ Note the exit of the greater occipital nerve emerging from even deeper tough connective tissue (Fig. 3.19).

○ Remove this connective tissue surrounding the greater occipital nerve, and expose its exit from the dura mater (Fig. 3.20).

○ Retract the rectus capitis posterior minor superiorly, and expose the dorsal root ganglion of the 2nd cervical (C2) spinal nerve (Fig. 3.21).

LAMINECTOMY

○ In preparation for the laminectomy, reflect or cut away the muscles of the back from the spines and transverse processes of the vertebrae as completely as possible using a scalpel, scissors, and chisel (Fig. 3.22).

○ Clean away as much as possible all of the intrinsic muscles of the back from the laminae of the lower

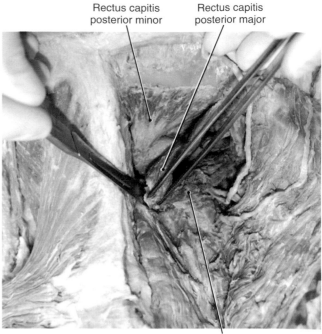

Rectus capitis posterior minor   Rectus capitis posterior major

Obliquus capitis inferior

Fig. 3.18 Dissection of suboccipital triangle, reflecting rectus capitis posterior major and obliquus capitis inferior muscles laterally.

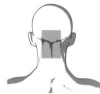

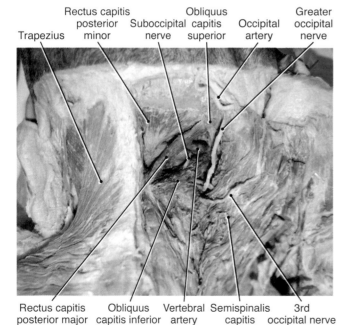

Trapezius   Rectus capitis posterior minor   Suboccipital nerve   Obliquus capitis superior   Occipital artery   Greater occipital nerve

Rectus capitis posterior major   Obliquus capitis inferior   Vertebral artery   Semispinalis capitis   3rd occipital nerve

Fig. 3.17 Suboccipital triangle borders (rectus capitis posterior major, superior and inferior capitis oblique muscles) and contents (vertebral artery, suboccipital nerve).

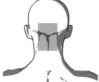

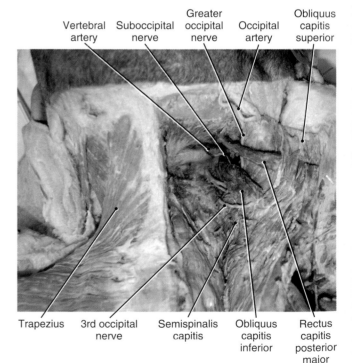

Vertebral artery   Suboccipital nerve   Greater occipital nerve   Occipital artery   Obliquus capitis superior

Trapezius   3rd occipital nerve   Semispinalis capitis   Obliquus capitis inferior   Rectus capitis posterior major

Fig. 3.19 Dissection of suboccipital triangle illustrating the obliquus capitis inferior and rectus capitis posterior major muscles, and revealing suboccipital nerve and vertebral artery.

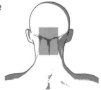

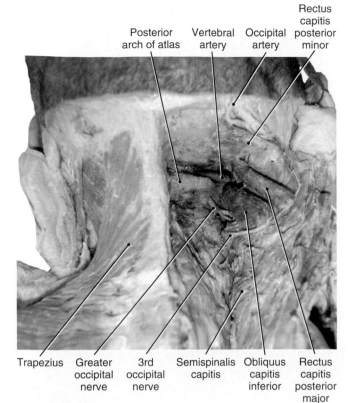

Fig. 3.20 Dissection of suboccipital triangle, with reflected rectus capitis posterior minor exposing posterior arch of atlas.

Labels (top): Posterior arch of atlas | Vertebral artery | Occipital artery | Rectus capitis posterior minor

Labels (bottom): Trapezius | Greater occipital nerve | 3rd occipital nerve | Semispinalis capitis | Obliquus capitis inferior | Rectus capitis posterior major

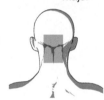

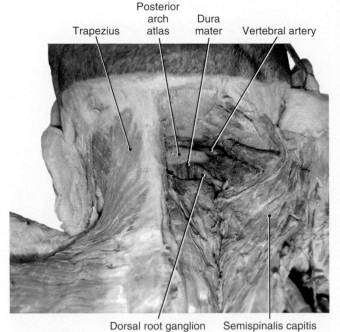

Fig. 3.21 Dissection of suboccipital triangle exposing dura mater of spinal cord, dorsal root ganglion, vertebral artery, and posterior arch of atlas.

Labels (top): Trapezius | Posterior arch atlas | Dura mater | Vertebral artery

Labels (bottom): Dorsal root ganglion C2 spinal nerve | Semispinalis capitis

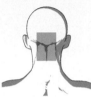

cervical, thoracic, and upper lumbar regions (Fig. 3.23).

○ With a bone saw or chisel and mallet, cut through the laminae longitudinally from the lower cervical to the lower lumbar regions (Figs. 3.24 through Fig. 3.26).

○ Angle the saw or chisel laterally.

DISSECTION TIP

If using a chisel and mallet, perform the surface fracturing technique. Short tapping blows of the mallet are used until the lamina is felt to fracture. Do not allow the chisel to be driven too deeply, or injury to the spinal cord or its rootlets will occur.

○ Direct the blade of the saw or chisel anteromedially to avoid cutting the spinal nerves (see Fig. 3.25) (Plate 3.2).

○ Complete the dissection bilaterally (see Fig. 3.26).

○ Using toothed forceps, gently lift spinous process–lamina unit away from spinal canal, revealing dura mater, dorsal root ganglia, and spinal cord (Fig. 3.27).

○ Remove the spinous process–lamina unit from the lumbar region, exposing dura mater (Fig. 3.28).

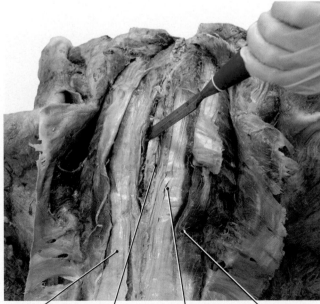

Labels: Erector spinae | Spinalis | Longissimus | Iliocostalis

Fig. 3.22 Superficial and intermediate muscles of back region reflected, revealing superficial layer of deep or native back muscles (erector spinae: spinalis, longissimus, iliocostalis).

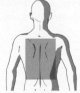

Lamina

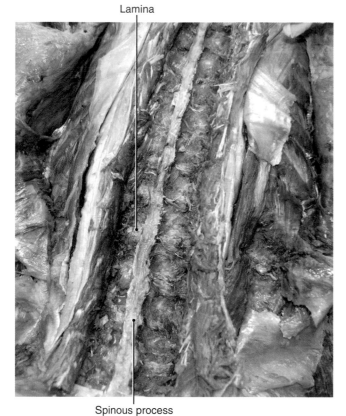

Spinous process

Fig. 3.23 After removal of all muscles from the paraspinous region, the spinous processes and laminae are seen.

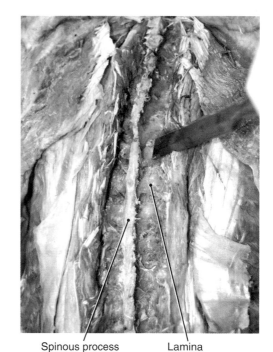

Spinous process   Lamina

Fig. 3.24 The chisel is placed flat onto each lamina and angled away from the midline.

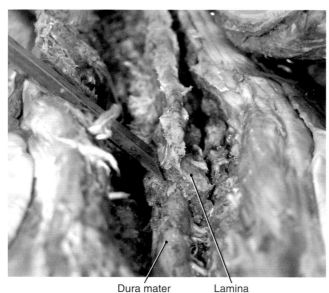

Dura mater   Lamina

Fig. 3.25 Direct blade of saw or chisel anteromedially to avoid cutting spinal nerves.

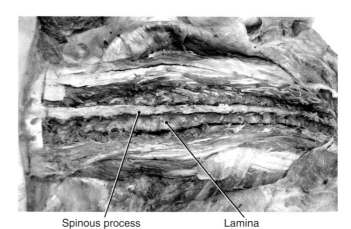

Spinous process   Lamina

Fig. 3.26 Bilateral dissection through laminae of vertebrae using chisel and mallet technique to reveal dura mater and spinal cord (Stryker-type electric saw also can be used).

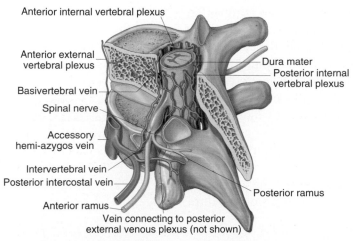

Anterior internal vertebral plexus

Anterior external vertebral plexus

Basivertebral vein

Spinal nerve

Accessory hemi-azygos vein

Intervertebral vein

Posterior intercostal vein

Anterior ramus

Dura mater

Posterior internal vertebral plexus

Posterior ramus

Vein connecting to posterior external venous plexus (not shown)

Plate 3.2 A lateral view of the hemisected vertebra exposing the spinal cord.

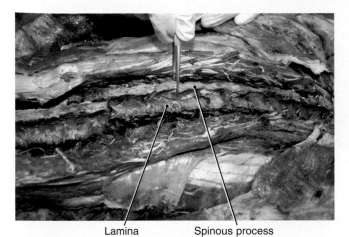

Lamina   Spinous process

Fig. 3.27 Using toothed forceps, gently lift spinous process–lamina unit away from spinal canal, revealing dura mater, dorsal root ganglia, and spinal cord.

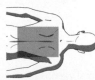

DISSECTION **TIP**

To facilitate the process, several laminae can be removed together as a block (see Figs. 3.26 to 3.28). After excision of the vertebral laminae and spinous processes, the vertebral canal may not be exposed widely enough for clear visualization of its contents. If this is the case, remove additional bone as necessary with bone rongeurs or with a mallet and chisel. Exercise particular care in the regions of the intervertebral foramina to avoid cutting or tearing away the spinal nerve rootlets. Sharply pointed edges of bone may be present in the dissection field after the laminectomy is completed. Identify any sharp spicules and remove them to avoid injuries to your hands.

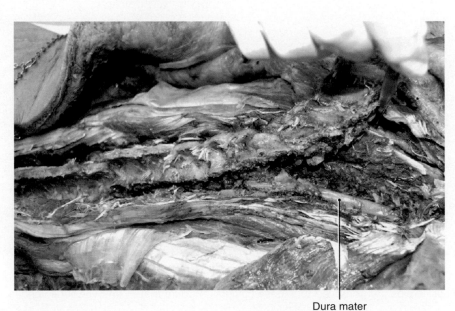

Dura mater

Fig. 3.28 Removal of spinous process–lamina unit from lumbar region, exposing dura mater.

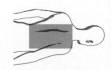

- Remove the spinous processes and the laminae en bloc from the spinal canal (Fig. 3.29).
- Note the contents of the spinal canal: the epidural fat and the vertebral venous plexus of Batson (Fig. 3.30).
- Remove the fat and the venous plexus from the epidural space to expose the dura mater. Lift a part of the dura in the midline, and make a small, slit-like incision with scissors or a scalpel (Fig. 3.31).
- Continue the midline incision throughout the entire length of the dura mater (Fig. 3.32).
- If possible, avoid incising the underlying arachnoid layer by lifting and maintaining tension on the dura mater. Reflect the dura laterally to expose the contents of the dural sac. If the incision in the dura is made successfully, the arachnoid will appear as a thin, almost transparent layer (see Fig. 3.32).

DISSECTION TIP

Sometimes, arachnoid calcifications (plaques) may be present (Fig. 3.33). These are usually incidental findings and have been attributed to trauma, myelography, subarachnoid hemorrhage (see Fig. 3.32), and spinal anesthesia.

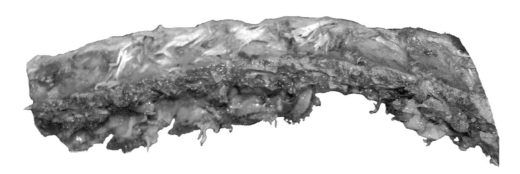

Fig. 3.29 Section of spinous process–lamina unit removed from vertebral column.

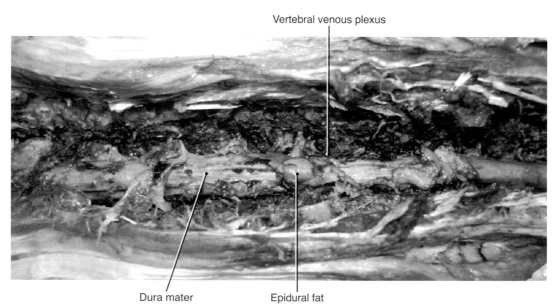

Fig. 3.30 Spinous process–lamina unit removed to expose epidural fat, dura mater, and vertebral venous plexus.

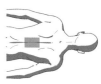

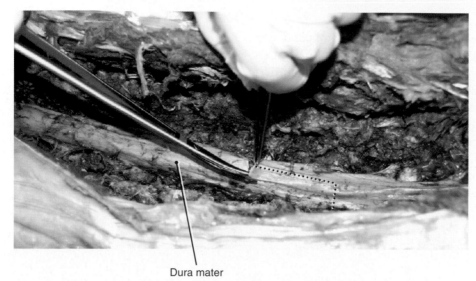
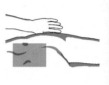

Dura mater

Fig. 3.31 Spinous process–lamina unit removed from lumbar region, revealing dura mater covering spinal cord and cauda equina. Elevate dura mater while making the transverse cut.

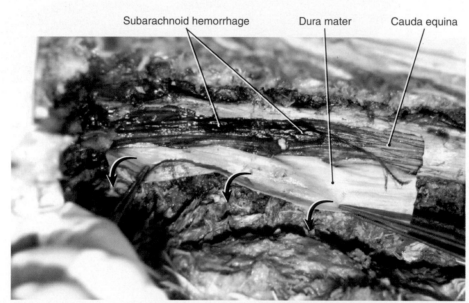

Subarachnoid hemorrhage   Dura mater   Cauda equina

Fig. 3.32 Transverse and vertical incisions reflecting dura mater, revealing cauda equina and subarachnoid hemorrhage.

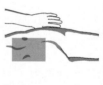

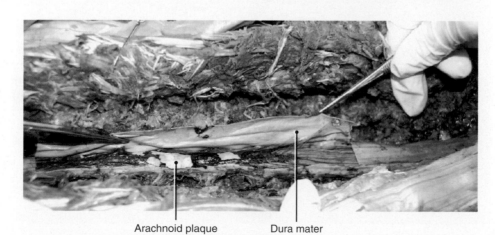

Arachnoid plaque   Dura mater

Fig. 3.33 Transverse and vertical incisions reflecting dura mater, revealing arachnoid plaque among cauda equina.

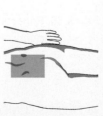

○ Identify the spinal cord and its covering of pia mater. Observe the beginning of the filum terminale at its origin from the conus medullaris, the terminal part of the spinal cord. Note the cluster of nerve roots on either side of the conus medullaris, the *cauda equina* (Fig. 3.34; see also Figs. 3.31, 3.32, and 3.38).

○ Transect and remove the spinal cord with its dural covering (Fig. 3.35).

○ Look for the tooth-like denticulate ligaments on each side of the spinal cord, lifting the cord carefully with forceps for inspection. These projections occur at the level of each vertebra, from the occipital bone to the last thoracic spinal nerve. The denticulate ligaments pierce the arachnoid mater to attach to the dura mater (Figs. 3.36 and 3.37).

○ Identify the posterior longitudinal ligament on the vertebral bodies after the removal of the spinal cord and dura mater (Fig. 3.38).

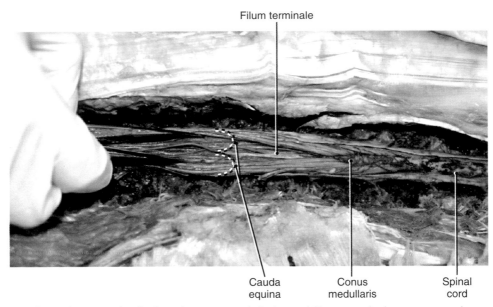

Filum terminale

Cauda equina

Conus medullaris

Spinal cord

Fig. 3.34 Dura mater reflected to reveal spinal cord, conus medullaris, and filum terminale among cauda equina.

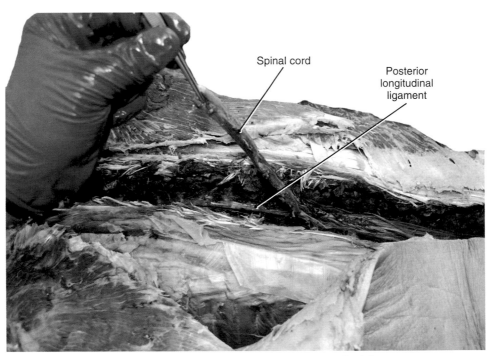

Spinal cord

Posterior longitudinal ligament

Fig. 3.35 Reflecting spinal cord from cephalad to caudal reveals posterior longitudinal ligament.

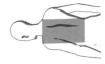

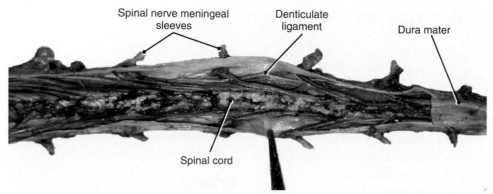

Fig. 3.36 Transverse and vertical incisions reflecting dura mater, revealing spinal cord, denticulate ligament, and spinal nerve dural sleeves.

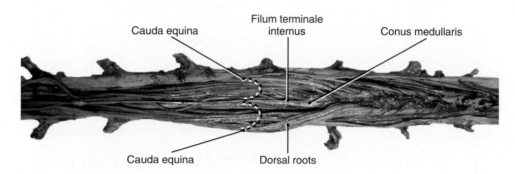

Fig. 3.37 Transverse and vertical incisions reflecting dura mater, revealing conus medullaris, dorsal roots, and filum terminale.

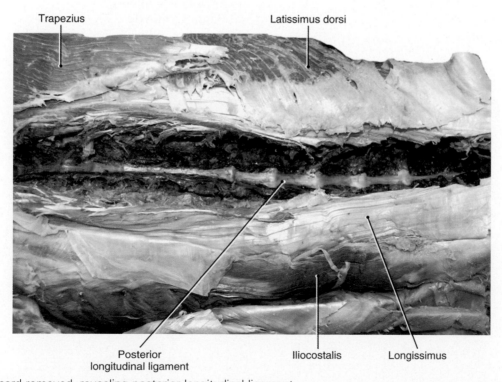

Fig. 3.38 Spinal cord removed, revealing posterior longitudinal ligament.

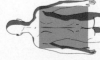

LABORATORY IDENTIFICATION CHECKLIST

NERVES
☐ Greater occipital nerve (dorsal ramus C2)
☐ Lesser occipital nerve (ventral rami of C2 and C3)
☐ 3rd occipital nerve (dorsal ramus C3)
☐ Suboccipital nerve (dorsal ramus C1)
☐ Dorsal root ganglion
☐ Spinal nerve

ARTERIES
☐ Occipital artery
☐ Vertebral artery

VEIN
☐ Vertebral venous plexus (Batson)

MUSCLES
☐ Trapezius
☐ Splenius capitis
☐ Semispinalis capitis
☐ Sternocleidomastoid
☐ Rectus capitis posterior major
☐ Rectus capitis posterior minor
☐ Obliquus capitis superior
☐ Obliquus capitis inferior
☐ Semispinalis capitis
☐ Erector spinae
☐ Spinalis
☐ Longissimus
☐ Iliocostalis
☐ Multifidus

BONES
☐ Atlas
   ☐ Posterior arch
☐ Spinous processes
☐ Lamina
☐ Transverse processes
☐ Body
☐ Vertebral foramen

LIGAMENTS
☐ Nuchal ligament (ligamentum nuchae)
☐ Ligamentum flavum
☐ Posterior longitudinal ligament

SPINAL CORD AND LAYERS
☐ Dura mater
☐ Arachnoid mater
☐ Pia mater
☐ Denticulate ligaments
☐ Filum terminale
☐ Conus medullaris
☐ Cauda equina
☐ Spinal nerve meningeal sleeve

LUMBAR PUNCTURE

Gray's Anatomy for Students: 44, 45, 48
Netter: 166–169*

Clinical Application

A lumbar puncture uses a spinal needle to access the subarachnoid space between the 2nd and 4th lumbar vertebrae (L2 and L4) to withdraw cerebrospinal fluid for analysis (Fig. II.1).

Anatomic Landmarks

- Below the L2 vertebra. Feel spinous processes and space between processes (Fig. II.2).
- Supracristal plane crosses L4/L5 junction. Puncture is safe just superior or inferior to this point, which avoids the spinal cord.
- Superficial to deep:
  Skin
  Subcutaneous tissue
  Supraspinous ligament
  Interspinous ligament
  Ligamentum flavum (provides increased resistance to needle)
  Dura mater
  Subarachnoid space–cerebrospinal fluid

EXTRADURAL ANESTHESIA (CAUDAL OR SACRAL BLOCK)

Gray's Anatomy for Students: 44, 45, 48
Netter: 166, 169

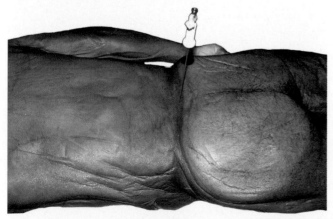

Fig. II.1

*The Clinical Applications in each section are cross-referenced to the following sources: Drake: *Gray's Anatomy for Students*, ed 2, and Netter: *Atlas of Human Anatomy*, ed 7. Page references from each source are provided for procedures in the Clinical Applications.

Clinical Application

Introduce anesthetic solutions into the epidural space, which will anesthetize the spinal nerves exiting the dura mater.

Anatomic Landmarks (Figs. II.4 and II.5)

- Natal cleft
- Sacral cornu
- Superficial to deep:
  Skin
  Subcutaneous tissue
  Posterior sacrococcygeal ligament (increased resistance)
  Sacral canal
- Sacralization is the anomalous fusion of the 5th lumbar vertebra (L5) to the 1st sacral vertebra (S1) (Fig. II.3).

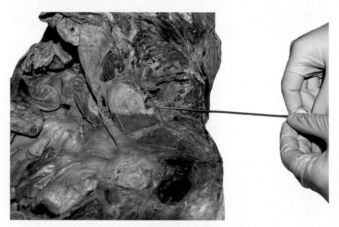

Fig. II.2

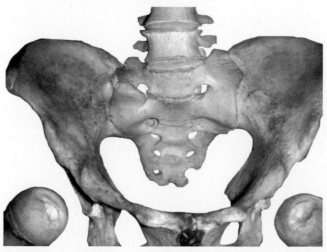

Fig. II.3

TRIANGLE OF AUSCULTATION

Gray's Anatomy for Students: 37
Netter: 183

Clinical Application

The triangle of auscultation defines an area that allows better auscultation with a stethoscope (because of less overlying muscle mass), to maximize listening to the lungs, 6th intercostal space, and the gastroesophageal junction on the left and assessing potential pathology.

Anatomic Landmarks

- Medial border of scapula
- Lateral border of trapezius
- Superior border of latissimus dorsi

Note: Area of triangle increases when arms are crossed and trunk is flexed.

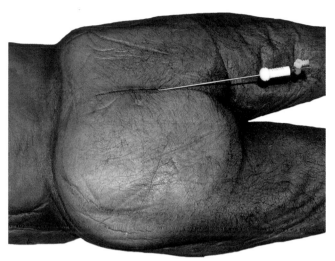

Fig. II.4

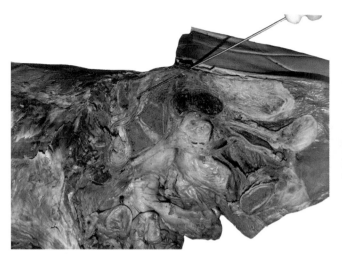

Fig. II.5

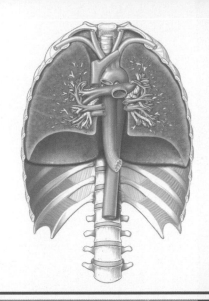

CHAPTER 4   PECTORAL REGION AND FEMALE BREAST

ATLAS REFERENCES
Netter: 187–191, 194, 195, 258–260, 416, 418
McMinn: 126–129, 178–181
Gray's Atlas: 62–72, 394–396, 402

SKIN AND SUPERFICIAL FASCIA
○ Make an incision from the jugular notch over the clavicle to the shoulder (Fig. 4.1a).
○ Make a midline incision from the jugular notch to the xiphoid process (Fig. 4.1b).

○ Extend the incision across the border of the costal margin toward the midaxillary line (Fig. 4.1c).
○ Continue the incision from the shoulder distally to the upper one third of the arm. An encircling incision around the midportion of the arm permits removal of the skin from the upper arm (Fig. 4.1d).
○ Start the dissection at the junction of the jugular notch and the clavicle. Reflect the skin of anterior thoracic wall, medial to lateral using combined blunt and sharp dissection (Fig. 4.2).

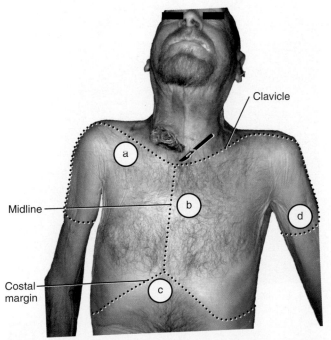

Fig. 4.1 Skin tracing of anterior thoracic wall for superficial dissection incisions. *a,* clavicle; *b,* midline; *c,* xiphoid process; *d,* upper arm.

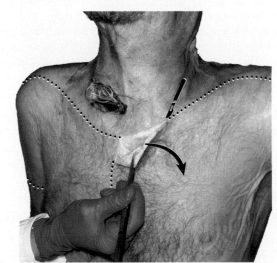

Fig. 4.2 Skin reflection of anterior thoracic wall, exposing deltopectoral region.

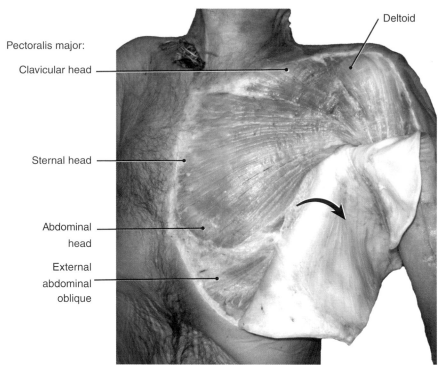

Pectoralis major:

Clavicular head

Sternal head

Abdominal head

External abdominal oblique

Deltoid

Fig. 4.3 Skin reflection of anterior thoracic wall, exposing the deltopectoral triangle, serratus anterior, and external abdominal oblique muscles.

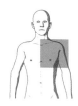

DISSECTION **TIP**

As the superficial fascia and skin are retracted, you will encounter anterior cutaneous branches of ventral primary rami and vessels emerging near the sternum. The vessels are the perforating branches of the internal thoracic artery and the perforating tributaries to the internal thoracic vein. Cut through these cutaneous nerves and vessels.

○ Reflect the skin and remove the superficial fascia from the thorax, shoulders, axillae, and proximal portions of the arms medially to the axilla (Figs. 4.3 and 4.4). Continue to use combined blunt and sharp dissection.

FEMALES

○ In addition to the aforementioned incisions described in the reflection of the skin, make an oblique incision through the skin of the breast from the midpoint of the clavicle toward the anterior axillary line, encircling the areola (Fig. 4.5).

○ Lift the skin at the edge of the incision with your forceps and reflect medially to the axilla.

○ Start reflecting the adipose tissue from the pectoralis major with a scalpel (Figs. 4.6 and 4.7).

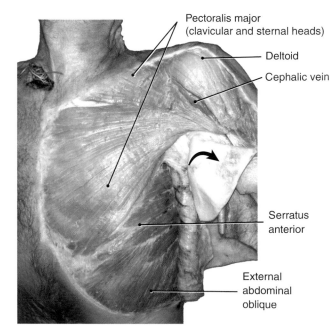

Pectoralis major (clavicular and sternal heads)

Deltoid

Cephalic vein

Serratus anterior

External abdominal oblique

Fig. 4.4 Skin reflection of anterior thoracic wall, medial to lateral.

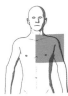

ANATOMY **NOTE**

Note the retinacula cutis, which begins at the dermis and extends deeply into the breast, forming fibrous septae and irregular bands of dense connective tissue.

○ Cut through the middle of the areola, making a sagittal incision through the nipple-areolar complex, revealing glandular tissue, ducts, connective tissue, and fat of the breast (Fig. 4.8). Partially remove the breast (Fig. 4.9). Try to identify one or more lactiferous ducts (Fig. 4.10).

ANATOMY **NOTE**

The lactiferous ducts may possess an expanded part (the lactiferous sinus or ampulla) deep to the nipple. The ducts become very narrow as they pass through the nipple, each terminating separately upon its surface. In most aged cadavers, little will remain of the duct system or glandular tissue, being replaced with fibrous tissue infiltrated with fat.

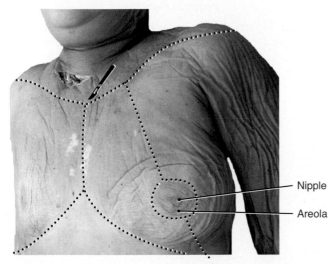

— Nipple

— Areola

Fig. 4.5 Skin of female breast with nipple-areolar complex.

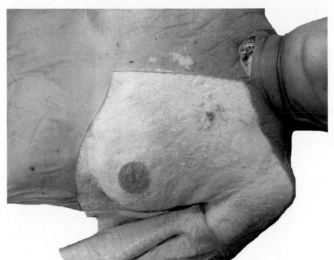

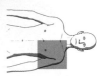

Fig. 4.6 Skin reflection from anterior thoracic wall (same technique as Fig. 4.2), revealing superficial fascia and nipple-areolar complex.

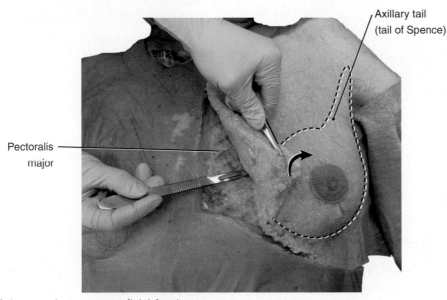

Axillary tail (tail of Spence)

Pectoralis major —

Fig. 4.7 Reflecting left breast, deep to superficial fascia.

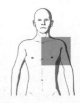

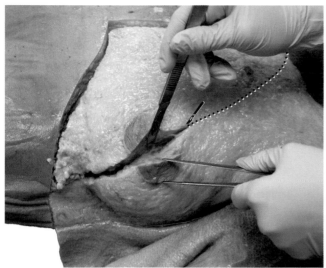

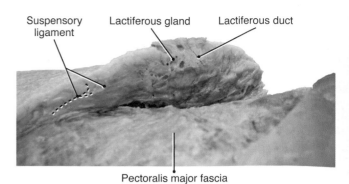

Fig. 4.10 Sagittal incision through the nipple-areolar complex, revealing gland, duct, and suspensory ligament of breast (see dashed square in Fig. 4.9).

Fig. 4.8 Sagittal incision through the nipple-areolar complex, revealing glandular tissue, ducts, connective tissue, and fat of breast.

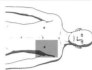

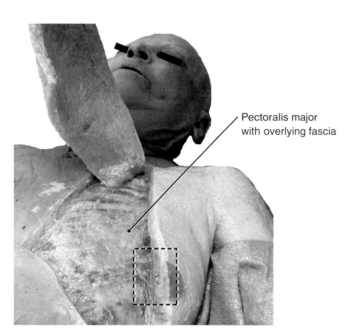

Fig. 4.9 Partial removal of left breast, revealing pectoralis major and fascia lying deep to breast.

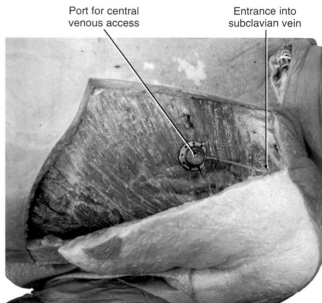

Fig. 4.11 Left pectoralis major with overlying central venous port.

DISSECTION **TIP**

Sometimes it is possible to identify an injection reservoir under the subcutaneous tissue (Fig. 4.11). These allow direct access to a large vein without having to "stick" the vein each time and are used for long-term injections such as for chemotherapy.

SUPERFICIAL DISSECTION

○ Identify the pectoralis major muscle, which is invested in a thin tough fascia, the pectoral fascia (part of the deep fascia system) (Fig. 4.12).

○ After cleaning the fascia from the pectoralis major, notice the separation of the pectoralis major from the deltoid muscle by the deltopectoral triangle (see Fig. 4.12).

ANATOMY **NOTE**

The clavicle, the clavicular head of the pectoralis major muscle, and the deltoid muscle form this triangle. Within the deltopectoral triangle, the cephalic vein is found.

○ Dividing the fascia that lies superficial to it will expose the cephalic vein. The cephalic vein is an important landmark for identifying the first part of the axillary artery (see Fig. 4.12).

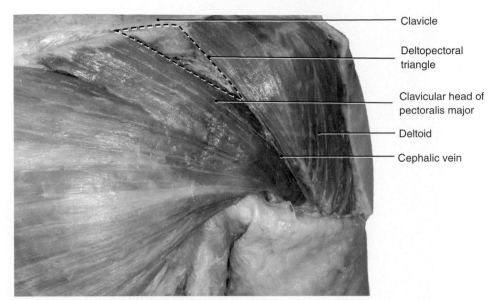

Fig. 4.12 Skin reflected from left anterolateral thoracic wall, revealing deltopectoral muscles, deltopectoral triangle, and cephalic vein.

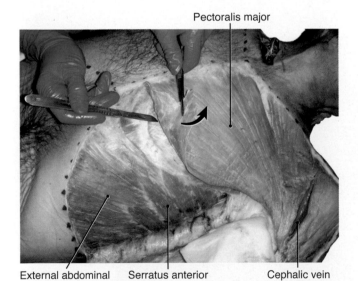

Fig. 4.13 Left pectoralis major muscle reflected from anterior chest wall.

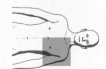

○ Detach the clavicular, sternal, and abdominal parts of the pectoralis major with a scalpel and reflect the muscle laterally to its insertion onto the humerus (Fig. 4.13).

○ Transect the clavicular portion of the pectoralis major muscle to the midclavicular line to avoid cutting important vessels and nerves, including the medial and lateral pectoral nerves (Fig. 4.14).

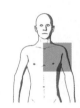

DISSECTION **TIP**

When the pectoralis major is reflected, pay special attention so as not to transect the medial pectoral nerve as it passes through (or lies lateral or inferior to) the pectoralis minor muscle to enter the pectoralis major.

DEEP DISSECTION

○ After the pectoralis major has been reflected, identify the upper border of pectoralis minor and dissect the clavipectoral fascia to expose the subclavian and axillary vein (Fig. 4.15).

ANATOMY **NOTE**

The clavipectoral fascia attaches proximally to the clavicle and invests the subclavius muscle. It then passes as a sheet toward the pectoralis minor, invests it, and then blends distally with axillary fascia forming the so-called suspensory ligament of the axilla.

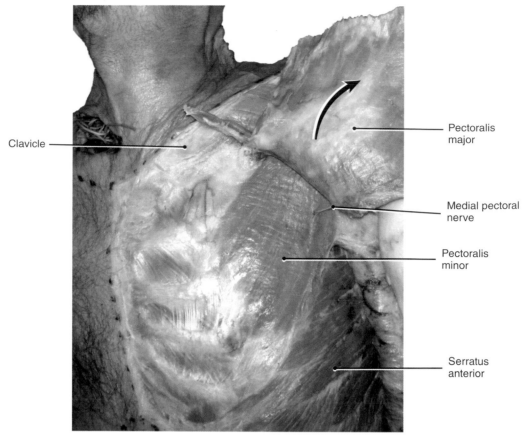

Clavicle

Pectoralis major

Medial pectoral nerve

Pectoralis minor

Serratus anterior

Fig. 4.14 Reflection of pectoralis major muscle highlighting pectoralis minor attachment to ribs 3 through 5.

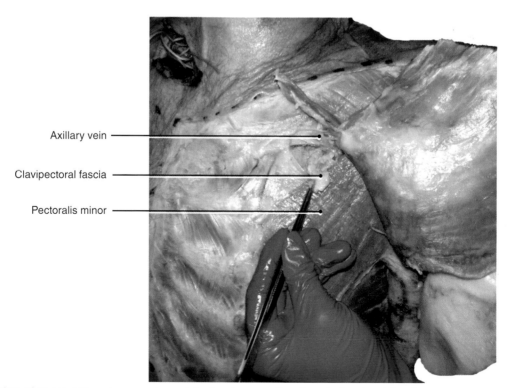

Axillary vein

Clavipectoral fascia

Pectoralis minor

Fig. 4.15 Reflection of pectoralis major muscle and its fascia, revealing the clavipectoral fascia.

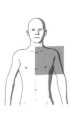

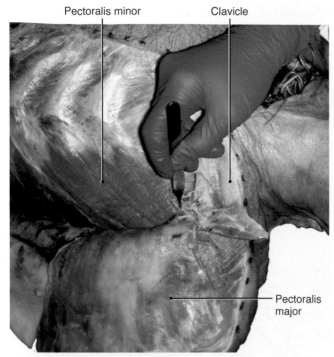

Pectoralis minor   Clavicle

Pectoralis major

Fig. 4.16 Removal of clavipectoral fascia and identification of axillary vein.

- Next observe the subclavian vein, the lateral pectoral nerves, and the pectoral branches of the thoracoacromial artery as they emerge to reach the pectoralis major muscle (Figs. 4.16 and 4.17).
- Trace the pectoral arteries to their origin from the thoracoacromial artery, and preserve these as the dissection proceeds.
- Insert the scissors under the inferior border of the pectoralis minor and cut the connective tissue underneath (Fig. 4.18). Reflect the pectoralis minor anteriorly.
- With a scalpel, reflect the pectoralis minor from ribs 3 through 5 (Fig. 4.19).

DISSECTION **TIP**

Often, in older cadavers, large lymph nodes located deep to the pectoralis minor (retropectoral nodes) may be evident.

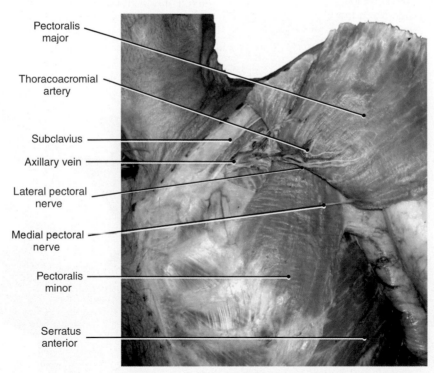

Pectoralis major

Thoracoacromial artery

Subclavius

Axillary vein

Lateral pectoral nerve

Medial pectoral nerve

Pectoralis minor

Serratus anterior

Fig. 4.17 Reflection of pectoralis major and its fascia, revealing medial and lateral pectoral nerves.

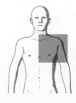

○ As the superficial fascia is reflected from the anterolateral aspect of the thoracic wall, look for the thoracoepigastric vein. The thoracoepigastric vein is a tributary to the axillary vein by direct or indirect connections. During the reflection of the fascia near the midaxillary line, lateral cutaneous branches of ventral primary rami may be exposed where they enter the superficial fascia (Fig. 4.20). Try to preserve as many of these as possible.

○ Identify the long thoracic nerve, which innervates the serratus anterior muscle (see Fig. 4.20). Trace the nerve a few centimeters inferior to the junction of the T2 ventral primary ramus (intercostobrachial nerve) and the thoracoepigastric vein at the midaxillary line over the serratus anterior muscle.

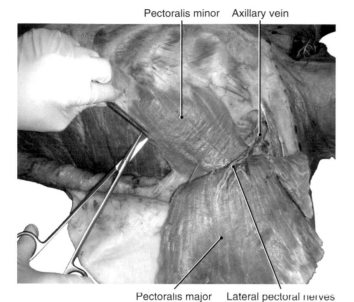

Pectoralis minor   Axillary vein

Pectoralis major   Lateral pectoral nerves

Fig. 4.18 Reflection of pectoralis major and its fascia, revealing pectoralis minor muscle. Scissors are positioned along the lateral inferior border of pectoralis minor.

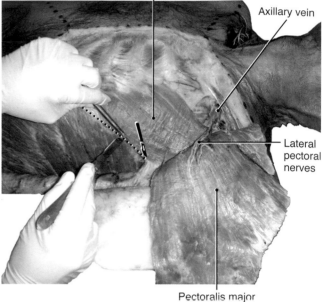

Pectoralis minor

Axillary vein

Lateral pectoral nerves

Pectoralis major

Fig. 4.19 Reflection of pectoralis major and its fascia, revealing pectoralis minor muscle. Place scalpel tip under lateral inferior border of pectoralis minor.

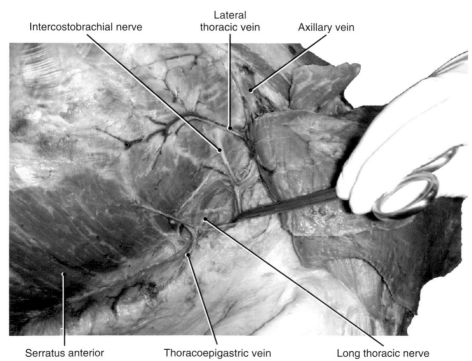

Intercostobrachial nerve   Lateral thoracic vein   Axillary vein

Serratus anterior   Thoracoepigastric vein   Long thoracic nerve

Fig. 4.20 Reflection of pectoralis major and minor muscles and deep fascia, revealing veins and, intercostobrachial and long thoracic nerves.

○ Remove part of the axillary sheath and the axillary fascia deep to the pectoralis major. This tube-like fascia covers the axillary artery, axillary vein, and the brachial plexus and is derived from the prevertebral fascia. With your scissors separate the fascia and remove most of it (Figs. 4.21 and 4.22). Once the fascia is removed, replace the pectoralis minor over the axillary artery.

○ Clean the intercostobrachial nerve (T2), which emerges from the 2nd intercostal space. This nerve supplies the skin of the axilla and the proximal medial aspect of the arm. In some specimens, the 3rd intercostal nerve may communicate with the intercostobrachial nerve. Clean this nerve toward the skin of the axilla (Fig. 4.23).

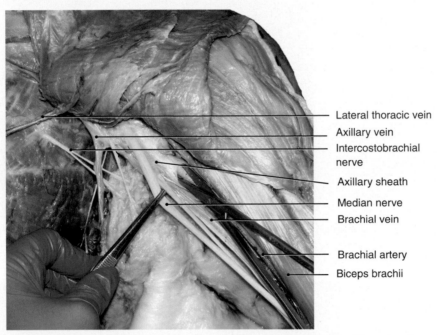

Lateral thoracic vein
Axillary vein
Intercostobrachial nerve
Axillary sheath
Median nerve
Brachial vein

Brachial artery
Biceps brachii

Fig. 4.21 Reflection of pectoralis major and minor muscles and deep fascia, revealing axillary sheath, axillary and brachial veins, and the median nerve.

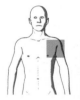

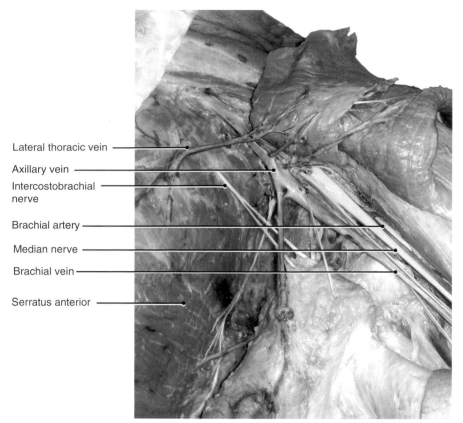

Lateral thoracic vein —

Axillary vein —

Intercostobrachial nerve —

Brachial artery —

Median nerve —

Brachial vein —

Serratus anterior —

Fig. 4.22 Reflection of pectoralis major and minor muscles and deep fascia, revealing neurovascular structures of the axillary region.

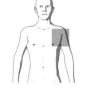

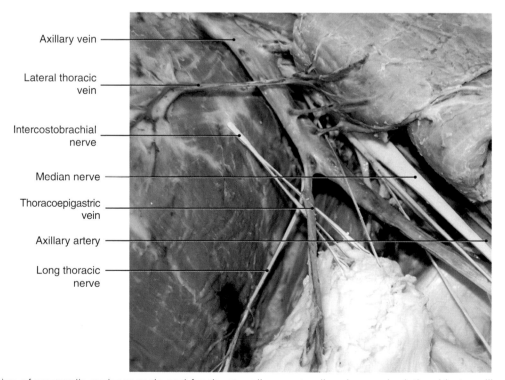

Axillary vein —

Lateral thoracic vein —

Intercostobrachial nerve —

Median nerve —

Thoracoepigastric vein —

Axillary artery —

Long thoracic nerve —

Fig. 4.23 Reflection of pectoralis major muscle and fascia, revealing pectoralis minor and relationship to axillary and long thoracic arteries.

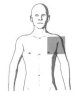

○ The pectoralis minor muscle divides the axillary artery into three parts (Fig. 4.24).

○ At the lateral border of the pectoralis minor on the surface of the serratus anterior, expose the lateral thoracic artery (see Fig. 4.24).

○ Its origin is typically from the 2nd portion of the axillary artery; however, this may vary. Look carefully for a small artery penetrating the musculature of the 1st or 2nd intercostal spaces. This is the superior thoracic artery that arises from the 1st part of the axillary artery (Fig. 4.25, Plates 4.1 and 4.2).

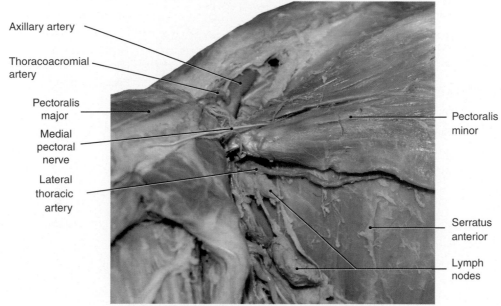

Fig. 4.24 Reflection of pectoralis major muscle exposing lateral thoracic artery, seen traveling along the lateral border of the pectoralis minor muscle.

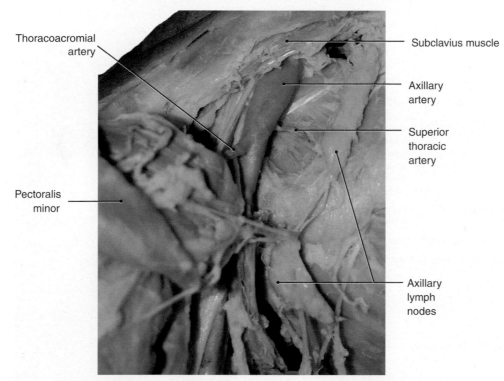

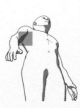

Fig. 4.25 Dissection of axillary region, revealing reflected pectoralis minor muscle, axillary and superior thoracic arteries, and axillary lymph nodes.

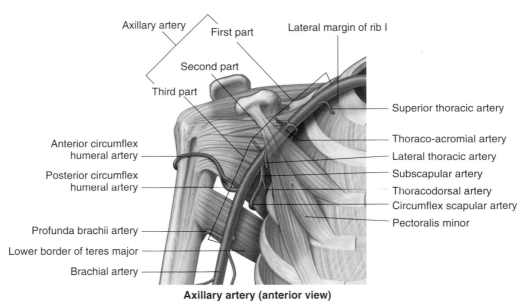

Axillary artery (anterior view)

Plate 4.1 Divisions of axillary artery.

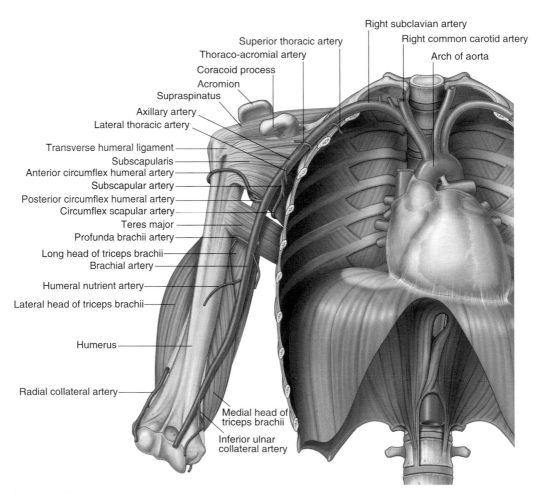

Plate 4.2 Branches of axillary artery.

○ Place a probe or your scissors between the external intercostal membrane and the internal intercostal muscle (Fig. 4.26).

ANATOMY **NOTE**

The external intercostal membrane travels between the lateral border of the sternum and the midclavicular line.

○ Cut this membrane and expose the internal intercostal muscle (Figs. 4.26 and 4.27).

ANATOMY **NOTE**

This muscle layer runs in a direction opposite to the external intercostals, like "hands in your back pockets." The external intercostal muscles are oriented in a direction medially and downward, like "hands in your front pockets" (Fig. 4.28). Near the sternum, the external intercostal muscles are continued medially as the external intercostal membrane.

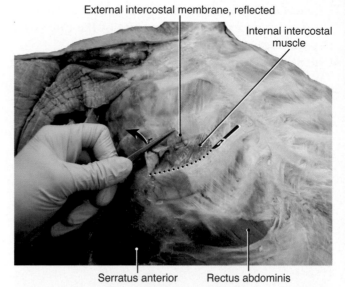

External intercostal membrane, reflected

Internal intercostal muscle

Serratus anterior   Rectus abdominis

Fig. 4.27 The external intercostal membrane is cut and reflected laterally to reveal internal intercostal muscle.

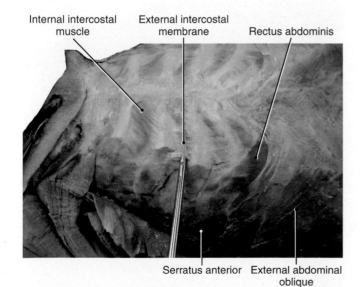

Internal intercostal muscle   External intercostal membrane   Rectus abdominis

Serratus anterior   External abdominal oblique

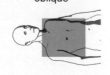

Fig. 4.26 Anterior thoracic wall musculature, revealing external intercostal membrane (over the scissors), internal intercostal, external abdominal oblique, rectus abdominis, and serratus anterior muscles.

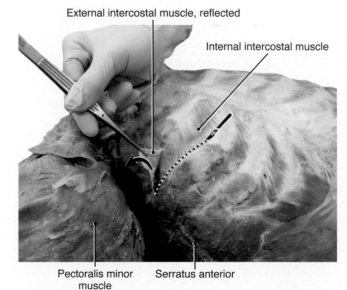

External intercostal muscle, reflected

Internal intercostal muscle

Pectoralis minor muscle   Serratus anterior

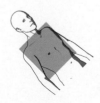

Fig. 4.28 Anterolateral chest wall with reflected pectoralis muscle and fascia, revealing external intercostal, internal intercostal, and serratus anterior muscles.

- Reflect the internal intercostal muscle adjacent to the sternum and expose the contents of the intercostal space (Figs. 4.29 and 4.30).
- Identify the endothoracic fascia and carefully reflect it (Fig. 4.31).
- Identify the internal thoracic artery and vein (Figs. 4.32 and 4.33).

External intercostal   Endothoracic
muscle   fascia

Internal intercostal muscles

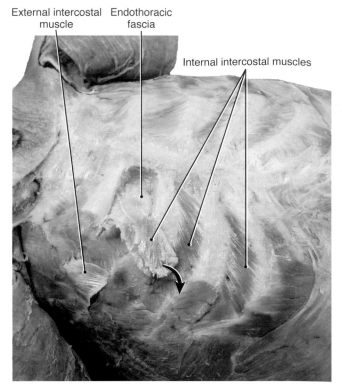

Fig. 4.30 Anterolateral chest wall with reflected internal intercostal, revealing endothoracic fascia and external and internal intercostal muscles.

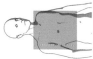

Internal intercostal
muscle

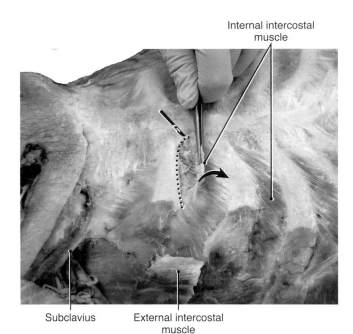
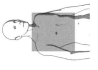

Subclavius   External intercostal
                  muscle

Fig. 4.29 Anterolateral chest wall revealing subclavius, external intercostal, and internal intercostal muscles. The internal intercostal muscle is cut superiorly and reflected inferiorly to expose the endothoracic fascia.

External intercostal muscle   Endothoracic fascia

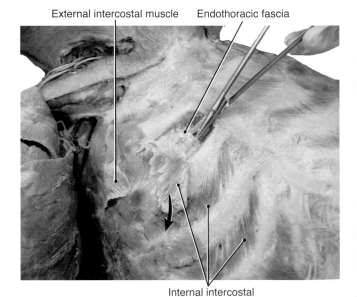

Internal intercostal
muscle

Fig. 4.31 Anterolateral chest wall with reflected internal intercostal, revealing endothoracic fascia with external and internal intercostal muscles.

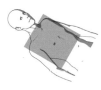

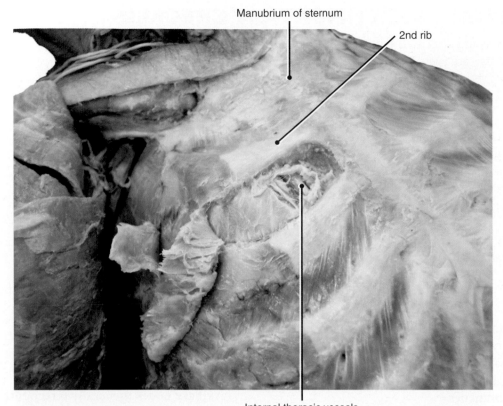

Manubrium of sternum

2nd rib

Internal thoracic vessels

Fig. 4.32 Anterior chest wall with reflected internal intercostal muscle and endothoracic fascia, revealing internal thoracic artery and vein.

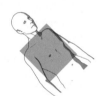

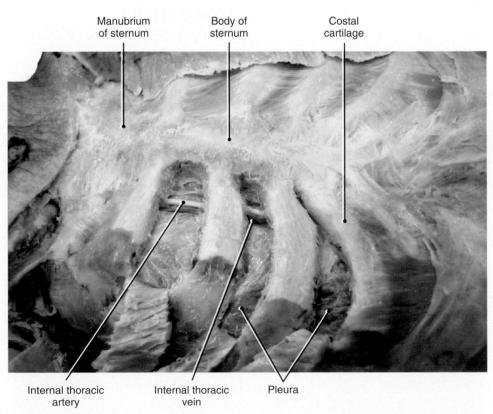

Manubrium of sternum

Body of sternum

Costal cartilage

Internal thoracic artery

Internal thoracic vein

Pleura

Fig. 4.33 Anterior chest wall with reflected internal intercostal muscle and endothoracic fascia, revealing internal thoracic artery and vein.

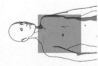

LABORATORY IDENTIFICATION CHECKLIST

Some of the nerves and arteries listed here will have been dissected during the laboratory for the superficial back (and upper limb) but also are seen when dissecting the breast.

NERVES
- ☐ Anterior cutaneous branches of intercostal
- ☐ Intercostobrachial (T2)
- ☐ Lateral cutaneous branches of intercostal (T3-T7)
- ☐ Lateral pectoral
- ☐ Medial pectoral
- ☐ Axillary
- ☐ Long thoracic
- ☐ Thoracodorsal
- ☐ Subscapular

ARTERIES
- ☐ Thoracoacromial
  - ☐ Pectoral branches
  - ☐ Deltoid branches
  - ☐ Clavicular branches
  - ☐ Acromial branches
- ☐ Internal thoracic
- ☐ Lateral thoracic
- ☐ Anterior intercostal
- ☐ Posterior intercostal

VEINS
- ☐ Axillary
- ☐ Internal thoracic
- ☐ Intercostal

MUSCLES
- ☐ Pectoralis major
  - ☐ Clavicular part
  - ☐ Sternal part
  - ☐ Abdominal part (not always present)
- ☐ Pectoralis minor
- ☐ Subclavius
- ☐ Serratus anterior
- ☐ External/internal intercostals

BONES
- ☐ Sternum
  - ☐ Manubrium
  - ☐ Body
  - ☐ Xiphoid process
  - ☐ Manubriosternal joint (angle of Louis, T4-T5)
- ☐ Clavicle
- ☐ 1st rib
- ☐ Ribs 2–12

LYMPHATICS
- ☐ Axillary nodes (generally 6 recognized nodal groups with total of 35–40 nodes)
- ☐ Internal thoracic node drainage (~5 per side)
- ☐ Thoracic duct

LIGAMENTS
- ☐ Suspensory ligaments (of Cooper)

BREAST
- ☐ Areolar-nipple complex
- ☐ Superficial fascia (from anterior chest wall)
- ☐ Lobes (15–20)
- ☐ Tail of breast (Spence)
- ☐ Deep fascia

ATLAS REFERENCES

Netter: 212–217
McMinn: 182–184, 192–211
Gray's Atlas: 72–92, 108–119

OPENING THE THORACIC CAVITY

○ With a scalpel, transect the intercostal muscles, serratus anterior muscle, and a portion of the external abdominal oblique muscle (Figs. 5.1 and 5.2).

○ Make sure that you start your dissection above the emergence of the intercostobrachial nerve (T2) and then descend toward the midaxillary line.

○ With a saw or bone cutter, carefully cut the intercostal musculature from the first intercostal space lateral to the manubrium, then extend these incisions downward, just anterior to the emergence of the anterior cutaneous branches of the intercostal nerves, cutting the ribs and intercostal musculature down to the level of the 10th rib (Fig. 5.3).

○ Divide the manubrium transversely above the sternal angle using a bone saw, cutters, or scalpel (Fig. 5.4).

○ After making the saw cuts, use a scalpel and bone cutters or mallet and chisel to free the anterior thoracic wall (Fig. 5.5).

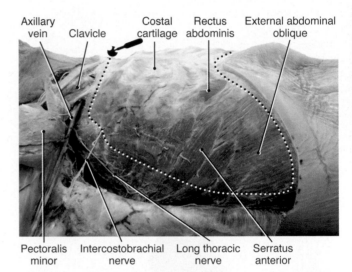
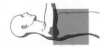

Fig. 5.2 Anterolateral view of chest with tracing for incision to reveal deep chest structures.

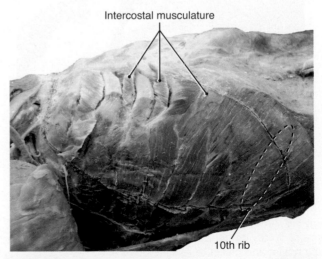

Fig. 5.3 Anterolateral view of thorax with incision to allow for thoracotomy.

Fig. 5.1 Anterior chest wall with skin, fascia, and pectoralis major and minor reflected, revealing tracing of rib cage for deep dissection of thorax.

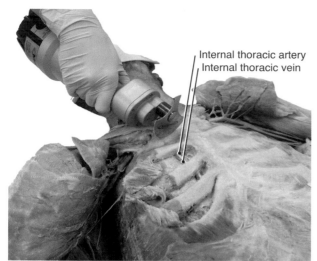

Internal thoracic artery
Internal thoracic vein

Fig. 5.4 Skin, fascia, and pectoral muscles reflected from anterior chest wall to reveal intercostal dissection of intercostal muscles, as well as internal thoracic artery and vein. Bone saw, cutters, or scalpel is used to make the bone incisions.

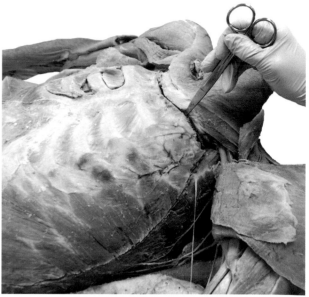

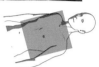

Fig. 5.6 Anterolateral view of chest with incision to reveal deep chest structures. Once bone and connective tissue have been transected, use blunt scissors to lift chest plate.

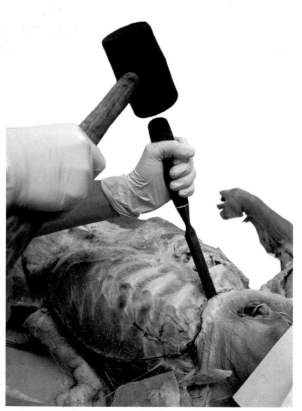

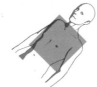

Fig. 5.5 Anterolateral view of chest with incision to reveal deep chest structures. Use mallet and chisel to release bone and connective tissue to allow removal of anterior chest wall plate.

○ Once bone and connective tissue have been transected, use blunt scissors to lift the anterior thoracic wall. Try to avoid damage to the underlying lungs (Fig. 5.6).

> ### DISSECTION **TIP**
>
> Often, in the first and second intercostal spaces, you will be able to place your fingertips underneath the internal surface of the anterior thoracic wall and lift it up (Fig. 5.7).
>
> If some parts are still connected to the wall, use a scalpel and bone cutters to free the anterior thoracic wall (Fig. 5.8).
>
> Be careful when you place your fingertips under the exposed ribs; sharp bone spicules are often present and may cause injury. Use a bone cutter or rongeur to remove these.

○ Place your fingertips underneath the openings of the thoracic wall and pull up (Fig. 5.9).

○ If the internal thoracic vessels are still intact, cut them and then pull the chest wall inferiorly, exposing the thoracic contents.

○ As you reflect the wall inferiorly, incise the parietal pleura from the internal surface of the anterior thoracic wall with a scalpel, leaving it intact over the lungs (Fig. 5.10).

○ Cut the sternopericardial ligaments that connect the pericardial sac to the posterior surface of the sternum.

○ Continue the reflection of the anterior thoracic wall downward until the thoracic viscerae can be clearly seen (Fig. 5.11).

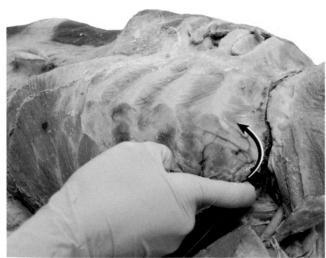

Fig. 5.7 Anterolateral chest wall can be removed manually.

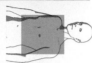

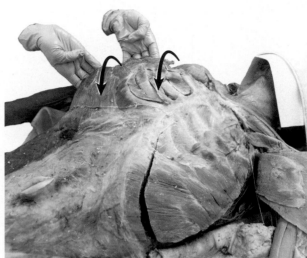

Fig. 5.9 Anterolateral chest wall reflected manually. Release connective tissue deep to anterior chest wall bilaterally.

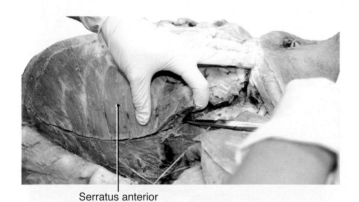

Serratus anterior

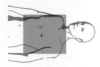

Fig. 5.8 Anterolateral view of thorax with incision to reveal deeper structures. Use blunt dissection with scissors to remove the chest wall.

Pericardial cavity and mediastinal pleura

Transected rib

Diaphragm

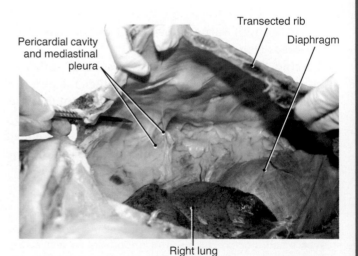

Right lung

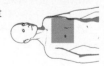

Fig. 5.10 Partial reflection of anterior chest wall plate, revealing deep structures.

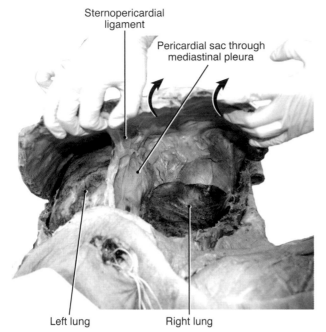

Fig. 5.11 Bilateral reflection of anterior chest wall plate, revealing deep internal structures.

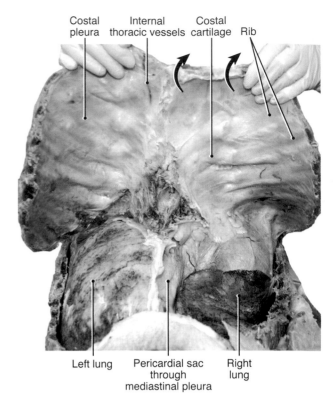

Costal pleura — Internal thoracic vessels — Costal cartilage — Rib

Left lung — Pericardial sac through mediastinal pleura — Right lung

Fig. 5.12 Bilateral reflection of anterior chest wall, revealing deep internal structures.

○ Keep the wall turned downward as the dissection proceeds (Fig. 5.12).

○ Forcing the wall down usually results in sufficient stretching or tearing of tissues so that the anterior wall remains reflected inferiorly. If this is not the case, you can remove the anterior thoracic wall (Fig. 5.13). Using blunt dissection with your hand or blunt-ended scissors from superior to inferior helps guide the anterior connective tissue as desired.

DISSECTION **TIP**

The pleura is attached to the thoracic wall by a continuous layer of connective tissue, the endothoracic fascia. In some cadavers with previous pathology of the thorax, such as infections, the pleura may be thickened and adherent to the thoracic walls, making efforts to preserve it difficult.

○ Observe the internal surface of the anterior thoracic wall, and identify the internal thoracic arteries and veins and their branches (Fig. 5.14).

○ Reflect the parietal pleura to expose the intercostal muscles.

○ Reflecting the parietal pleura in the 1st and 2nd intercostal spaces exposes the internal thoracic artery. Identify it.

○ To expose the internal thoracic artery and vein further, reflect the transversus thoracis muscles.

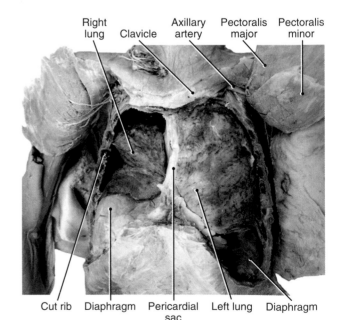

Right lung — Clavicle — Axillary artery — Pectoralis major — Pectoralis minor

Cut rib — Diaphragm — Pericardial sac — Left lung — Diaphragm

Fig. 5.13 Anterior thoracic wall removed, revealing internal thoracic structures. Note that the right lung is collapsed. This is probably due to a pneumothorax that occurred during life.

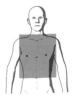

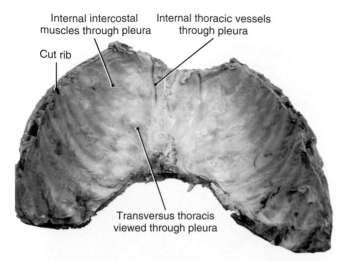

Internal intercostal muscles through pleura
Internal thoracic vessels through pleura
Cut rib
Transversus thoracis viewed through pleura

Fig. 5.14 Undersurface of removed chest plate, revealing structures intimate with the chest plate.

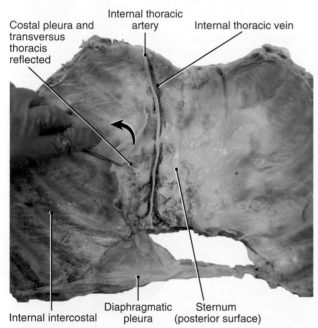

Costal pleura and transversus thoracis reflected
Internal thoracic artery
Internal thoracic vein
Internal intercostal
Diaphragmatic pleura
Sternum (posterior surface)

Fig. 5.15 Undersurface of removed chest wall, highlighting internal thoracic artery.

○ **Identify the branches of the internal thoracic artery, such as the perforating and anterior intercostal branches (Fig. 5.15).**

ANATOMY **NOTE**

Typically, the terminal branches of the internal thoracic artery—the superior epigastric and musculophrenic branches—are located close to the xiphoid process.

○ **Identify the costodiaphragmatic and costomediastinal recesses.**
○ **After inspecting the subdivisions of the parietal pleura, push the lung away from the heart with your fingertips.**
○ **Identify the mediastinal pleura separating the lung from the pericardial sac.**

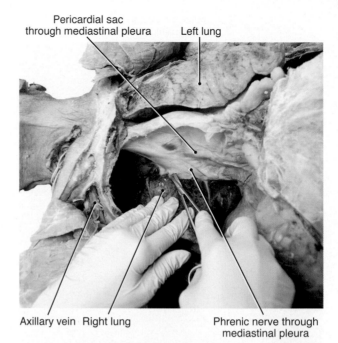

Pericardial sac through mediastinal pleura
Left lung
Axillary vein   Right lung
Phrenic nerve through mediastinal pleura

Fig. 5.16 Anterior thoracic structures with right lung reflected to expose mediastinum to dissect for lung removal.

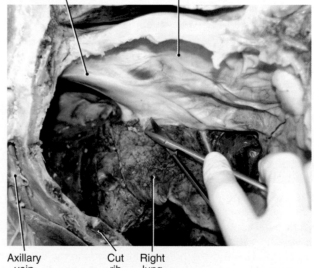

Phrenic nerve through mediastinal pleura   Pericardial sac through mediastinal pleura
Axillary vein
Cut rib
Right lung

Fig. 5.17 Anterior chest structures with right lung reflected to expose mediastinum.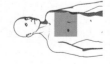

○ **Insert the scissors and separate the mediastinal pleura from the pericardium (Figs. 5.16 and 5.17).**
○ **Identify the phrenic nerve traveling anterior to the hilum of the lung and preserve it (Fig. 5.18).**
○ **Use the separation technique to expose the pulmonary arteries and veins (Fig. 5.19).**

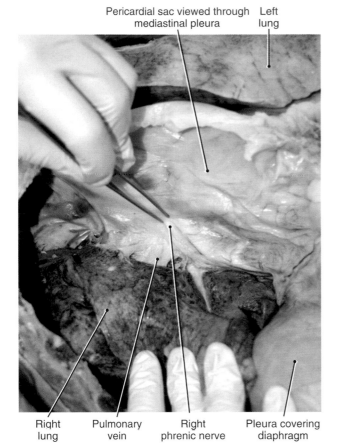

Pericardial sac viewed through mediastinal pleura   Left lung

Right lung   Pulmonary vein   Right phrenic nerve   Pleura covering diaphragm

Fig. 5.18 Anterior chest structures with right lung reflected to reveal mediastinum, highlighting phrenic nerve through the mediastinal pleura.

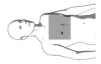

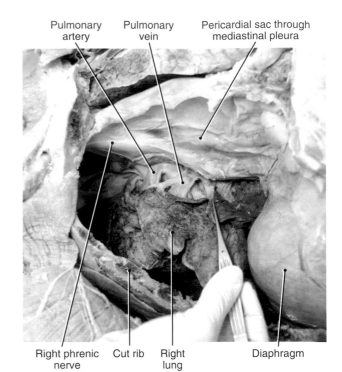

Pulmonary artery   Pulmonary vein   Pericardial sac through mediastinal pleura

Right phrenic nerve   Cut rib   Right lung   Diaphragm

Fig. 5.19 In the right pleural cavity, the pulmonary artery and vein are seen.

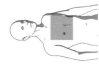

○ Use the same technique for the contralateral lung (Figs. 5.20 and 5.21).

DISSECTION **TIP**

The costodiaphragmatic recess is usually the location where excess embalming fluids accumulate during dissection. Drain the fluid using a syringe, and place paper towels into the recess (Figs. 5.22 and 5.23). Also, once the lungs are removed, holes can be made in the posterior intercostal spaces so that fluid exits onto the dissection table. This method may necessitate placing a wedge or block under the thorax to lift the body slightly off of the dissecting table.

○ After exposing the pulmonary veins, pulmonary arteries, and primary bronchi at the hila of the left and right lungs, transect them with scissors or a scalpel (Figs. 5.24, 5.25, 5.26, and Plate 5.1).
○ Remove the lungs from the thoracic cavity, and observe the posterior mediastinum covered with parietal pleura (Figs. 5.27 to 5.30).

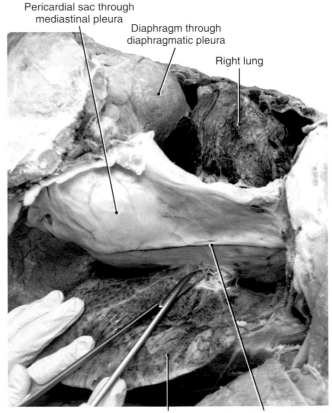

Pericardial sac through mediastinal pleura   Diaphragm through diaphragmatic pleura   Right lung

Left lung   Left phrenic nerve through mediastinal pleura

Fig. 5.20 Anterior thoracic structures with left lung reflected for hilar dissection.

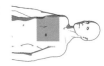

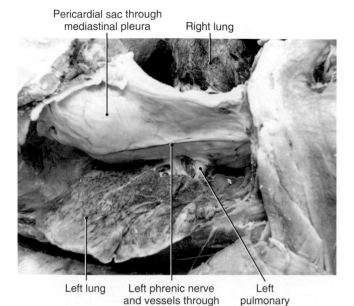

Pericardial sac through mediastinal pleura   Right lung

Left lung   Left phrenic nerve and vessels through mediastinal pleura   Left pulmonary artery

Fig. 5.21 Anterior thoracic structures with left lung reflected for hilar dissection, revealing pulmonary vessels.

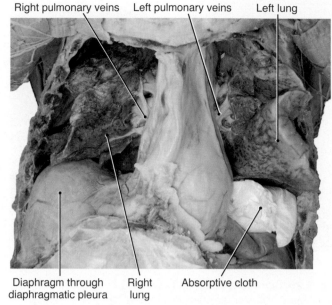

Right pulmonary veins   Left pulmonary veins   Left lung

Diaphragm through diaphragmatic pleura   Right lung   Absorptive cloth

Fig. 5.23 Anterior thoracic wall removed, revealing deep structures. Right and left pulmonary veins are exposed.

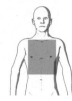

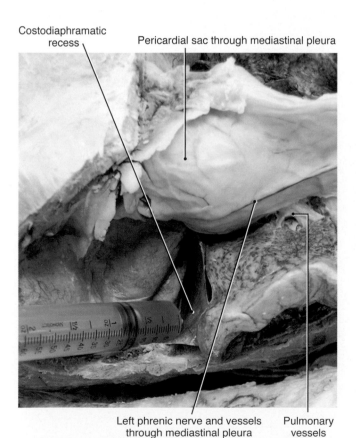

Costodiaphramatic recess   Pericardial sac through mediastinal pleura

Left phrenic nerve and vessels through mediastinal pleura   Pulmonary vessels

Fig. 5.22 Anterolateral view of deep chest dissection. Syringe is placed into the costodiaphragmatic recess, and excess fluid is aspirated.

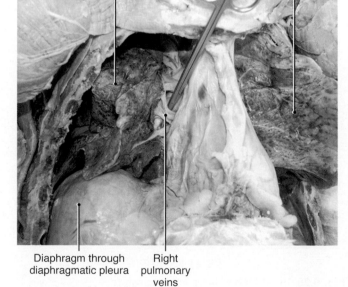

Right lung   Left lung

Diaphragm through diaphragmatic pleura   Right pulmonary veins

Fig. 5.24 Right pulmonary vein exposed and lifted upward for transection.

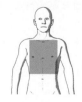

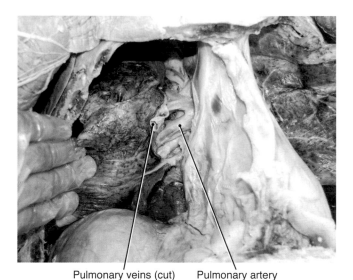

Pulmonary veins (cut)   Pulmonary artery

Fig. 5.25 Right lung retraction revealing pulmonary artery after pulmonary veins have been cut.

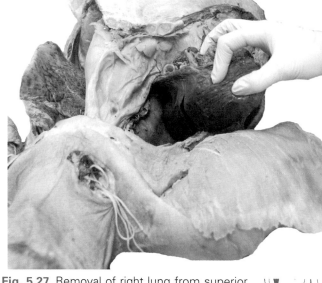

Fig. 5.27 Removal of right lung from superior to inferior with medial retraction.

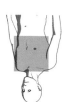

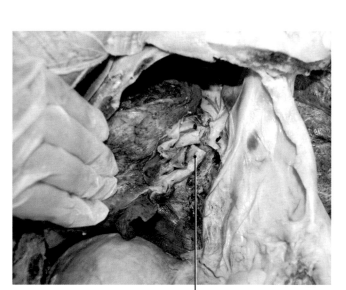

Right primary bronchus (cut)

Fig. 5.26 Right lung pulmonary vasculature and airway (primary bronchus) transected.

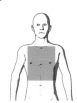

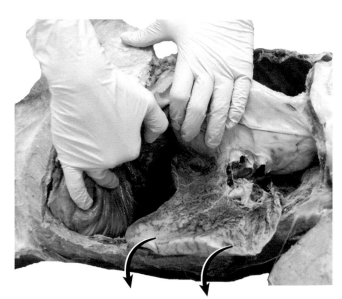

Fig. 5.28 Removal of left lung with pulmonary vasculature and bronchi transected, using medial retraction.

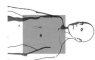

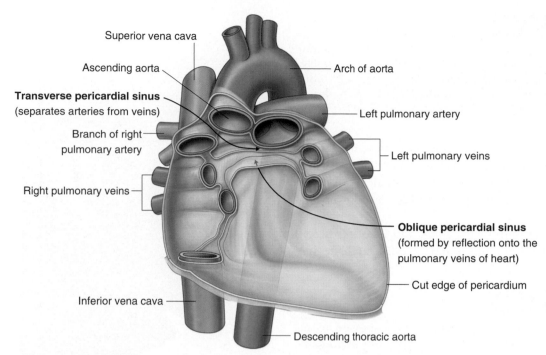

Superior vena cava

Ascending aorta

Arch of aorta

Transverse pericardial sinus
(separates arteries from veins)

Left pulmonary artery

Branch of right
pulmonary artery

Left pulmonary veins

Right pulmonary veins

Oblique pericardial sinus
(formed by reflection onto the
pulmonary veins of heart)

Cut edge of pericardium

Inferior vena cava

Descending thoracic aorta

Plate 5.1 Pericardial sac with heart removed.

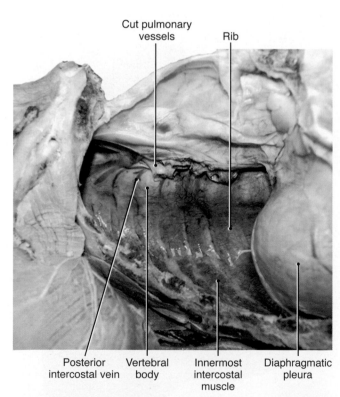

Cut pulmonary
vessels

Rib

Posterior
intercostal vein

Vertebral
body

Innermost
intercostal
muscle

Diaphragmatic
pleura

Fig. 5.29 Right hemithorax with lung
removed, revealing vertebral column and
posterior chest wall.

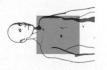

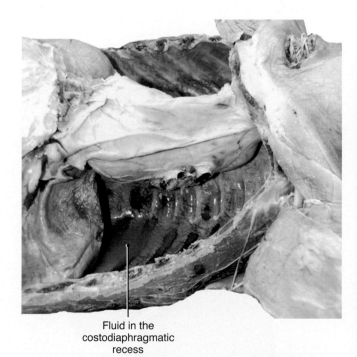

Fluid in the
costodiaphragmatic
recess

Fig. 5.30 Bilateral lung removal with intact
pericardial sac and contents.

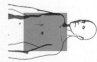

DISSECTION TIP

Often the lungs have adhesions far inferior and posterior to the hilum of the lung. To remove the lung completely, push the diaphragm inferiorly and explore with your fingertips the area posterior and inferior to the hilum so that such adhesions can be dissected free (see Fig. 5.30).

○ Place the lungs onto a tray, and examine the internal surface of each lung separately. For the right lung, identify the oblique and horizontal fissures and their corresponding upper, middle, and lower lobes (Fig. 5.31).

○ Inspect the hilum of the lung, and identify the pulmonary arteries, pulmonary veins, and primary bronchi (Fig. 5.32).

DISSECTION TIP

Note that the horizontal fissure often appears to be incomplete in right lungs. To identify the pulmonary arteries and pulmonary veins at the hilum of the lung, note that the pulmonary veins are located along the anterior aspect of the hilum, where the pulmonary arteries usually are located superior and anterior to the bronchi (see Fig. 5.32).

○ Similar to the right lung, identify the oblique fissure in the left lung and the corresponding upper and lower lobes (Fig. 5.33).

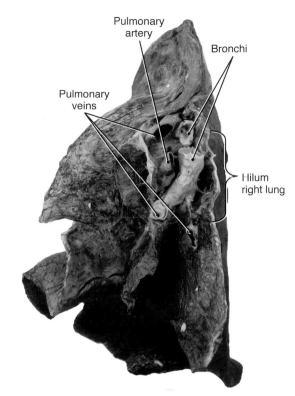

Fig. 5.32 Right lung (medial view) highlighting structures of the hilum.

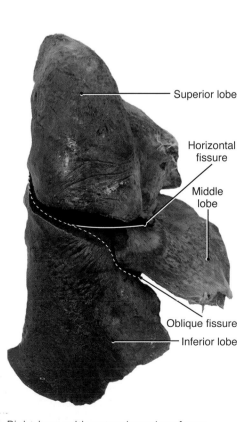

Fig. 5.31 Right lung with anterolateral surfaces.

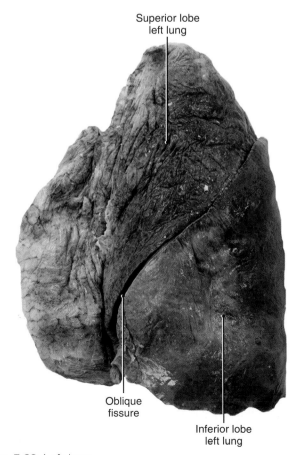

Fig. 5.33 Left lung.

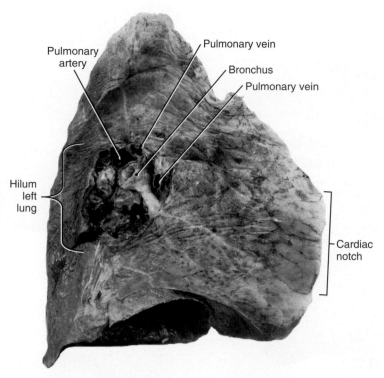

Fig. 5.34 Removal of left lung with medial view highlighting hilum structures.

○ Inspect the hilum of the lung, and identify the pulmonary arteries, pulmonary veins, and primary bronchi (Fig. 5.34).

○ Identify the cardiac notch on the superior lobe of the left lung and lingula.

○ Inferior to the hilum, trace the two layers of visceral pleura fusing together to form the pulmonary ligament (Fig. 5.35).

OPTIONAL LUNG DISSECTION
ANATOMY **NOTE**

The lung contents can be dissected to expose a single segmental bronchus, segmental artery, and segmental vein. The portion of lung supplied by the segmental bronchus, artery, and vein is defined as a *bronchopulmonary segment.*

○ With your forceps, lift the bronchus, and using blunt dissection, separate it from the lung parenchyma.

○ Remove most of the internal lung parenchyma with your forceps and scissors, leaving its borders and lateral walls intact (Fig. 5.36).

○ In the right lung, you will be able to dissect the superior, middle, and inferior lobar bronchi.

ANATOMY **NOTE**

Each lobar bronchus branches off into several segmental bronchi, and each of these supplies one bronchopulmonary segment. The right lung contains 10 to 12 bronchopulmonary segments, and the left lung contains 10.

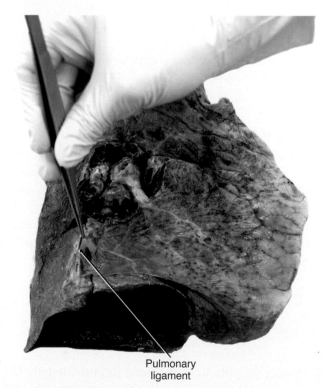

Fig. 5.35 Removal of left lung with medial view highlighting pulmonary ligament.

ANATOMY **NOTE**

When you reach a bronchopulmonary segment, note the relationships among the artery, vein, and bronchus. The segmental arteries are located posterior to the segmental bronchi, and the segmental veins are between two adjacent bronchopulmonary segments.

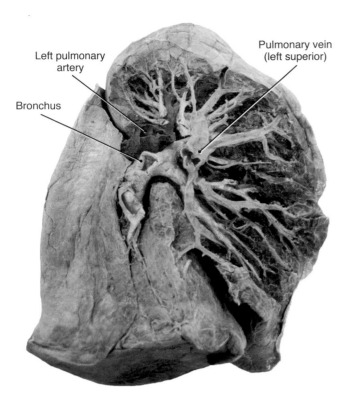

Left pulmonary artery

Bronchus

Pulmonary vein (left superior)

Fig. 5.36 Removal of left lung with medial view illustrating bronchopulmonary segments.

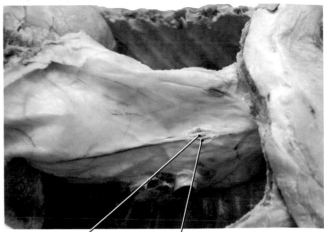

Left phrenic nerve   Pericardiacophrenic vein

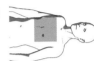

Fig. 5.37 Bilateral lung removal with intact pericardial sac and contents.

ANATOMY **NOTE**

As it passes superior to the right pulmonary artery, the right superior lobar bronchus is termed the *eparterial bronchus.*

REMOVAL OF THE HEART

○ Before removing the heart from the pericardial cavity, the phrenic nerves must be identified and preserved. Observe the pericardiacophrenic vein at the lateral border of the pericardial sac bilaterally.

○ Dissect the pericardium next to the pericardiaco-phrenic vein, and identify the phrenic nerve (Figs. 5.37 and 5.38).

ANATOMY **NOTE**

The phrenic nerve is accompanied by the pericardiaco-phrenic artery, a branch of the internal thoracic artery.

○ Dissect the phrenic nerve along its entire length, from the top of the thoracic cavity to its penetration of the diaphragm (Figs. 5.39 and 5.40).

○ With toothed forceps, lift the right inferolateral edge of the pericardium near the diaphragm, and make a small incision (Fig. 5.41).

○ Note the attachment of the pericardium to the central tendon of the diaphragm.

○ Make a transverse incision in the pericardium parallel to the diaphragmatic surface (Fig. 5.42).

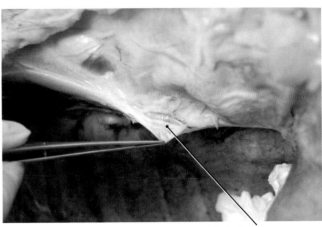

Left phrenic nerve

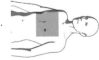

Fig. 5.38 Left hemithorax with intact pericardial sac, revealing left phrenic nerve.

DISSECTION **TIP**

When the pericardial sac is first opened, a small amount of serous fluid is often seen.

○ Make a second, connecting vertical incision through the pericardium along the side of the right atrium (Fig. 5.43) and along the side of the left ventricle (Fig. 5.44).

○ Note that the parietal pericardium and the visceral pericardium (epicardium) are continuous with the great vessels as they pierce the fibrous pericardium.

EXTERNAL INSPECTION

○ For orientation of the heart within the pericardial cavity, observe the position of the right atrium, right

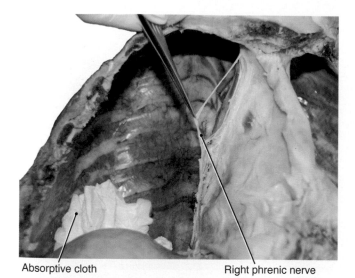

Absorptive cloth   Right phrenic nerve

Fig. 5.39 Bilateral lung removal with intact pericardial sac and contents, exposing the right phrenic nerve.

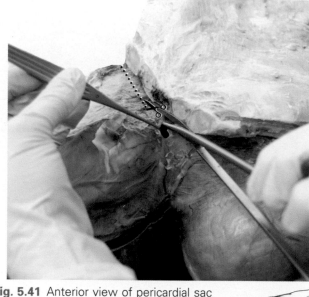

Fig. 5.41 Anterior view of pericardial sac with tracing for transverse incision *(dotted line)* of pericardial sac.

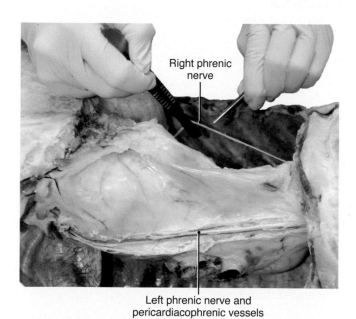

Right phrenic nerve

Left phrenic nerve and pericardiacophrenic vessels

Fig. 5.40 Intact pericardial sac and contents with dissected phrenic nerve and pericardiacophrenic vessels.

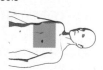

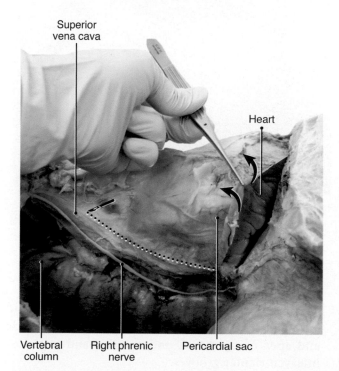

Superior vena cava

Heart

Vertebral column   Right phrenic nerve   Pericardial sac

Fig. 5.42 Anterolateral view of pericardial sac with base reflected (black arrows) and tracing for lateral vertical incision *(dotted line)*.

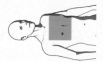

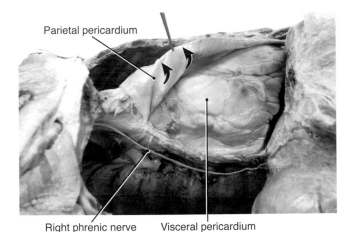

Parietal pericardium

Right phrenic nerve   Visceral pericardium

Fig. 5.43 Reflected pericardial sac revealing visceral pericardium of heart.

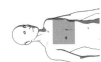

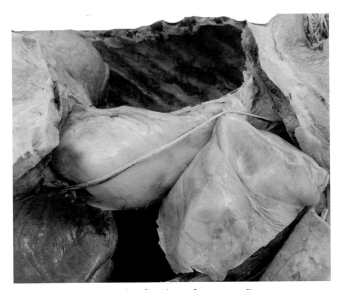

Fig. 5.44 Anterolateral reflection of pericardial sac while maintaining an intact left phrenic nerve.

auricle, right ventricle and its outflow tract, and pulmonary trunk. Note the left atrium, left ventricle and apex of the heart, and anterior and posterior interventricular grooves.

ANATOMY **NOTE**

The right ventricle forms the sternocostal surface and part of the diaphragmatic surface of the heart. The left or pulmonary surface is composed mainly of the left ventricle. The right ventricle forms the sternocostal surface and part of the diaphragmatic surface of the heart. Note that the right ventricle is the most anterior part of the heart and is almost in contact with the sternum.

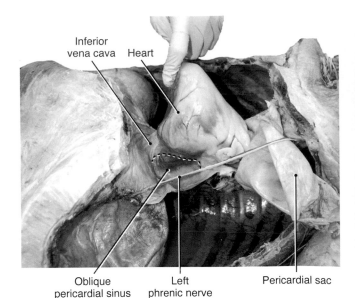

Inferior
vena cava   Heart

Oblique   Left   Pericardial sac
pericardial sinus   phrenic nerve

Fig. 5.45 Reflected pericardial sac with apex of heart reflected anteriorly to reveal the oblique sinus *(dotted line)*.

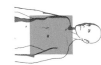

SINUSES

ANATOMY **NOTE**

Note the position of the inferior vena cava, which is located inferior and to the right between the heart and the diaphragm.

ANATOMY **NOTE**

The reflections of the pericardium lead to the formation of two so-called sinuses within the pericardial cavity, the transverse and oblique pericardial sinuses.

○ To identify the oblique pericardial sinus, lift the apex of the heart laterally and to the right with your fingertips, and expose the blindly ending space in the pericardial cavity behind the heart and below the venous hilum (Fig. 5.45).

ANATOMY **NOTE**

The venous hilum contains the four pulmonary veins and the superior and inferior vena cava. The sleeve-like investment of visceral pericardium around these vessels and the roof of the left atrium reflects to show the parietal pericardial sac, forming the inverted, U-shaped oblique sinus.

○ If you place your fingers in front of the atria and directly behind the aorta and pulmonary artery, you will occupy the space known as the *transverse pericardial sinus* (Fig. 5.46).

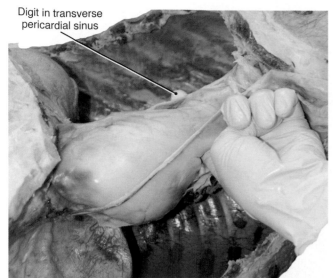

Fig. 5.46 Reflected pericardial sac with placement of digit through transverse sinus.

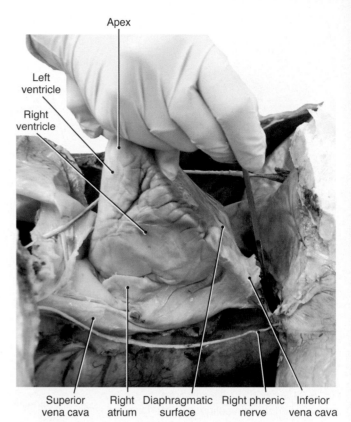

Fig. 5.48 Apex of heart reflected anteriorly to allow transection of inferior vena cava.

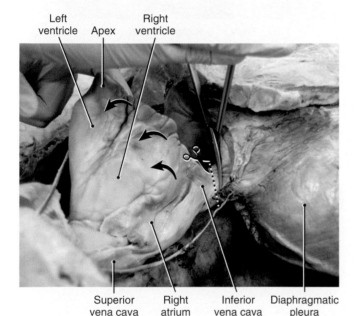

Fig. 5.47 Apex of heart reflected anteriorly to allow transection of inferior vena cava.

TECHNIQUE

○ To remove the heart, first lift its apex upward and expose the inferior vena cava, then transect it (Figs. 5.47 and 5.48).

○ With scissors, separate the adhesions between the heart (posteriorly) and pericardium, and lift the heart upward to expose the left atrium (Figs. 5.49 and 5.50).

○ Cut the superior vena cava. Next, cut the ascending aorta and the pulmonary trunk (Figs. 5.51 to 5.53). Remove the heart from the pericardial cavity.

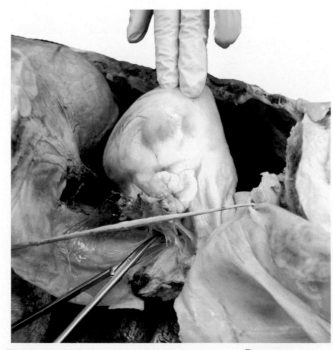

Fig. 5.49 With the apex of the heart elevated, scissors are used to separate the pericardium from the posterior surface of heart.

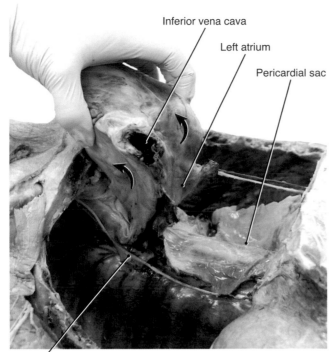

Inferior vena cava

Left atrium

Pericardial sac

Right phrenic nerve

Fig. 5.50 Apex of heart reflected anterosuperiorly, revealing cut inferior vena cava, left atrium, and posterior pericardial structures.

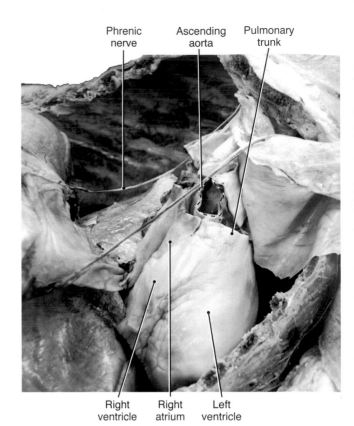

Phrenic nerve   Ascending aorta   Pulmonary trunk

Right ventricle   Right atrium   Left ventricle

Fig. 5.52 External view of heart with transected great vessels.

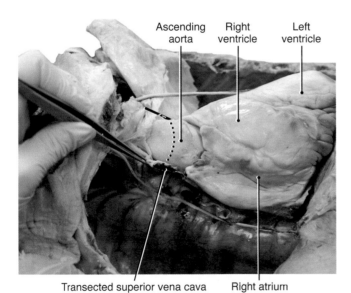

Ascending aorta   Right ventricle   Left ventricle

Transected superior vena cava   Right atrium

Fig. 5.51 With the pericardial sac displaced laterally and the superior vena cava cut, the ascending aorta is identified. The *dotted line* notes the region of the aorta to be transected.

DISSECTION **TIP**

In some hearts, the pulmonary veins are adherent to the pericardium. Place some tension on the heart and lift it upward. If necessary, place the scissors between the pulmonary veins and the pericardium and separate the two.

○ Observe the left side of the thoracic cavity, specifically the lateral side of the aortic arch and the pulmonary trunk (Figs. 5.54 and 5.55).
○ Identify and trace the left vagus nerve over the arch of the aorta (Fig. 5.56). Note the relationship between the vagus and phrenic nerves.

ANATOMY **NOTE**

Identify the ligamentum arteriosum, the connection between the left pulmonary artery and the arch of the aorta. Identify the trachea and its bifurcation into the left and right bronchi. The vagus nerves give rise to the recurrent laryngeal nerves. On the left side, as the nerve crosses the aorta, it gives rise to the recurrent laryngeal nerve (Figs. 5.57 and 5.58).

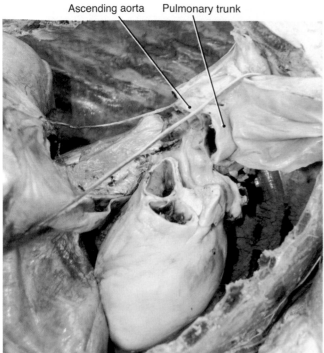

Ascending aorta   Pulmonary trunk

Fig. 5.53 External view of heart with transected great vessels.

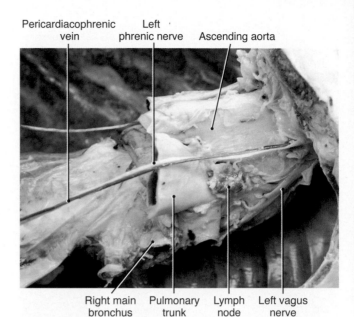

Pericardiacophrenic   Left
vein   phrenic nerve   Ascending aorta

Right main   Pulmonary   Lymph   Left vagus
bronchus   trunk   node   nerve

Fig. 5.55 A closer view of Fig. 5.60 shows the left vagus nerve and a regional lymph node.

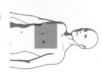

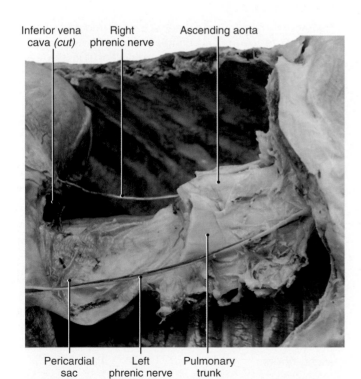

Inferior vena   Right   Ascending aorta
cava *(cut)*   phrenic nerve

Pericardial   Left   Pulmonary
sac   phrenic nerve   trunk

Fig. 5.54 Bilateral lung removal, with the anterior part of the pericardial sac and heart removed.

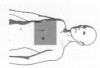

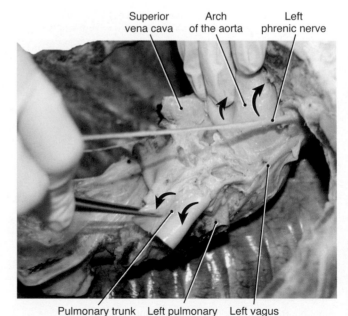

Superior   Arch   Left
vena cava   of the aorta   phrenic nerve

Pulmonary trunk   Left pulmonary   Left vagus
pulled inferiorly   artery   nerve

Fig. 5.56 With the pulmonary trunk displaced inferiorly, note the relationship of the phrenic and vagus nerves to the hilum of the lung. The phrenic nerve travels anterior and the vagus nerve posterior to the hilum of the lung.

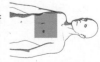

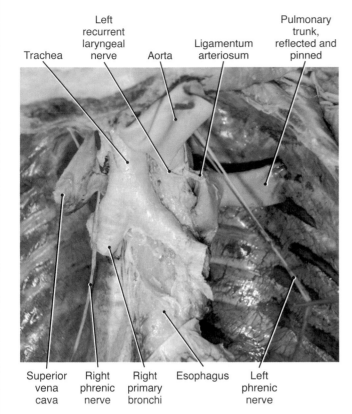

Left
recurrent
laryngeal
Trachea   nerve   Aorta   Ligamentum   Pulmonary
arteriosum   trunk,
reflected and
pinned

Superior   Right   Right   Esophagus   Left
vena   phrenic   primary   phrenic
cava   nerve   bronchi   nerve

Fig. 5.57 Anterior view of mediastinal structures, including the aorta, trachea, and esophagus.

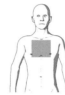

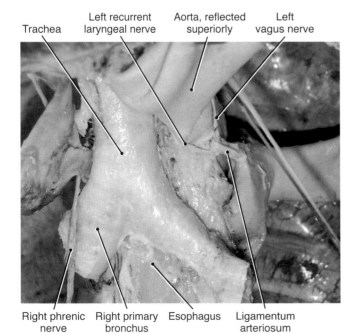

Left recurrent   Aorta, reflected   Left
laryngeal nerve   superiorly   vagus nerve
Trachea

Right phrenic   Right primary   Esophagus   Ligamentum
nerve   bronchus   arteriosum

Fig. 5.58 Deep mediastinal structures include right and left bronchus and vagus, phrenic, and recurrent laryngeal nerves.

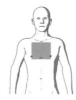

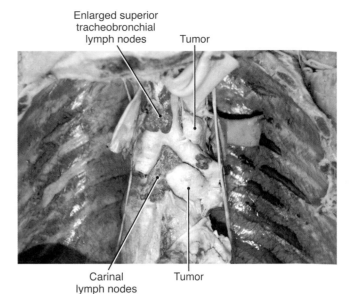

Enlarged superior
tracheobronchial
lymph nodes   Tumor

Carinal   Tumor
lymph nodes

Fig. 5.59 Anterior view of mediastinal structures, revealing lymph nodes, right and left bronchus, reflected ascending aorta, and tumor intimate with left bronchus.

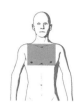

○ Clean the left vagus nerve, and where the left vagus crosses the aortic arch, locate the left recurrent laryngeal nerve.

ANATOMY **NOTE**

The left recurrent laryngeal nerve passes under the ligamentum arteriosum and courses upward between the trachea/esophagus and the ascending aorta in the tracheoesophageal groove. The right recurrent laryngeal nerve arises from the right vagus nerve at the level of the right subclavian artery and turns back superiorly behind this vessel, to pass upward and medially toward the larynx to enter the tracheoesophageal groove.

○ Along the right side of the trachea (or esophagus) identify and clean the right vagus nerve. This nerve can be found by probing between the azygos vein and the lateral aspect of the trachea, at which point the right vagus nerve begins to pass posterior to the root of the right lung.
○ Expose the tracheal bifurcation, and identify the carinal (inferior tracheobronchial) lymph nodes. A nerve plexus anterior to the carina can be seen by cutting into the trachea at its bifurcation. The nerves represent the deep cardiac plexus formed by sympathetic and vagal fibers.

DISSECTION **TIP**

Dissect the tracheobronchial lymph nodes; these nodes often are enlarged from malignant disease (Fig. 5.59).

- Remove the pericardium over the esophagus. With forceps, lift the esophagus and remove the pleura from over the esophagus and the vertebral column (Figs. 5.60 and 5.61).
- After removal of the pleura, dissect the fatty layer present over the vertebral bodies. Dissect between the esophagus and the vertebral bodies to identify the thoracic duct (Fig. 5.62), which often looks similar to adipose tissue.
- Clean and preserve the thoracic duct (Fig. 5.63).
- With forceps, lift the pleura, and with the aid of scissors, separate the pleura from the underlying tissues over the ribs (Figs. 5.64 and 5.65).

DISSECTION **TIP**

To reflect the pleura, use the tip of the scissors or a probe, and scrape the tissue between the pleura and the ribs. Do not cut any tissue with the forceps; use it as a probe (see Figs. 5.64 and 5.65).

- Remove the majority of pleura from the thoracic cavity (Fig. 5.66). Trace the intercostal vein, artery, and nerve traveling in one of the posterior intercostal spaces.

DISSECTION **TIP**

Use the handle of your scissors to remove fat over the intercostal space (Fig. 5.67).

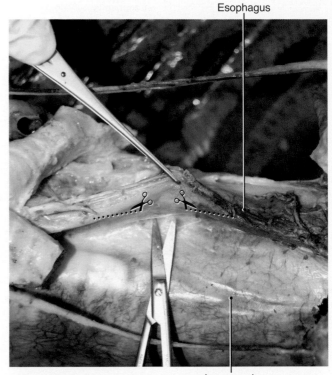

Fig. 5.61 Anterolateral view of deep posterior mediastinal structures with tension on mediastinal pleura.

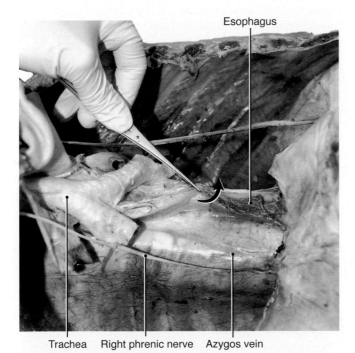

Fig. 5.60 Anterolateral view of the posterior mediastinum. Note that the esophagus is being retracted laterally.

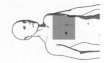

Fig. 5.62 Anterolateral view of deep posterior mediastinal structures, highlighting the thoracic duct, esophagus, and azygos vein.

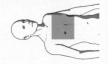

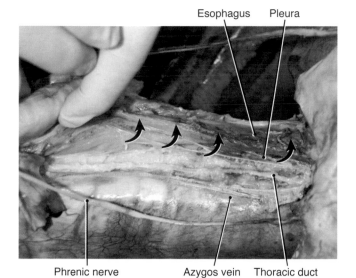

Esophagus   Pleura

Phrenic nerve   Azygos vein   Thoracic duct

Fig. 5.63 Anterolateral view of deep posterior mediastinal structures, demonstrating the thoracic duct, esophagus, and azygos vein.

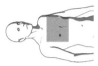

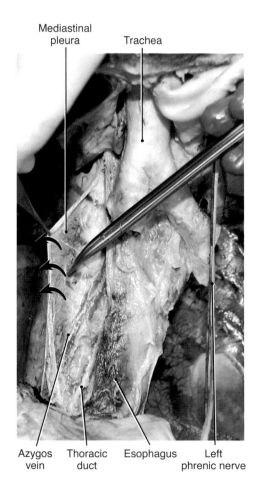

Mediastinal pleura   Trachea

Azygos vein   Thoracic duct   Esophagus   Left phrenic nerve

Fig. 5.64 Anterior view of deep mediastinal structures, revealing azygos vein, thoracic duct, and esophagus.

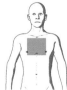

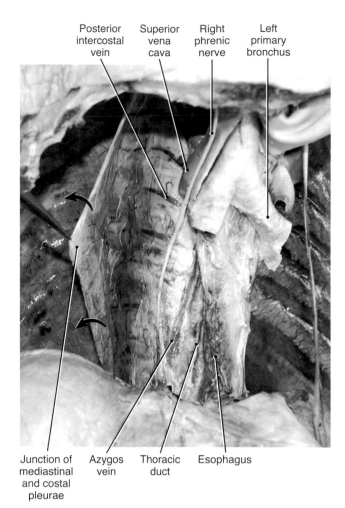

Posterior intercostal vein   Superior vena cava   Right phrenic nerve   Left primary bronchus

Junction of mediastinal and costal pleurae   Azygos vein   Thoracic duct   Esophagus

Fig. 5.65 Anterior view of posterior chest wall structures, revealing posterior intercostal vein, azygos vein, superior vena cava, and interface between mediastinal and costal pleurae.

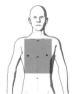

○ Trace and identify the sympathetic trunk that runs along the junction between the vertebral bodies and ribs and appears as a white line. Near the midportion of the thoracic vertebral column, identify a bundle of nerve fibers originating from the sympathetic chain and running obliquely toward the midline (Fig. 5.68). This is the *greater splanchnic nerve*, formed primarily from fibers of the sympathetic trunk.

○ Clean the sympathetic trunk and identify the greater (T5-T9), lesser (T10-T11), and least (T12) splanchnic nerves (Fig. 5.69, Plate 5.2).

DISSECTION TIP

The origin of the greater, lesser, and least splanchnic nerves is subject to variation. Also, the lesser and least splanchnic nerves are often difficult to see in the thorax before removal of the liver on the right, and because of an immobile descending thoracic aorta on the left.

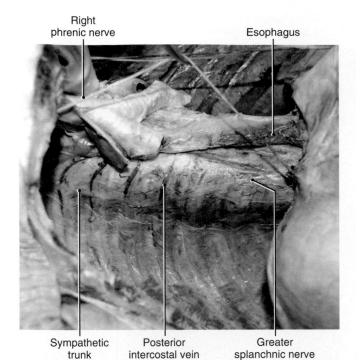

Right
phrenic nerve

Esophagus

Sympathetic
trunk

Posterior
intercostal vein

Greater
splanchnic nerve

Fig. 5.66 Right lateral view of posterior chest wall, revealing sympathetic trunk, greater splanchnic nerves, and posterior intercostal vein.

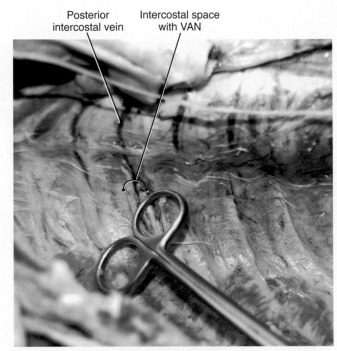

Posterior
intercostal vein

Intercostal space
with VAN

Fig. 5.67 Right lateral view of posterior chest wall, revealing neurovascular structures of the intercostal space at T4. *VAN*, Vein, artery, nerve.

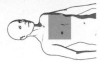

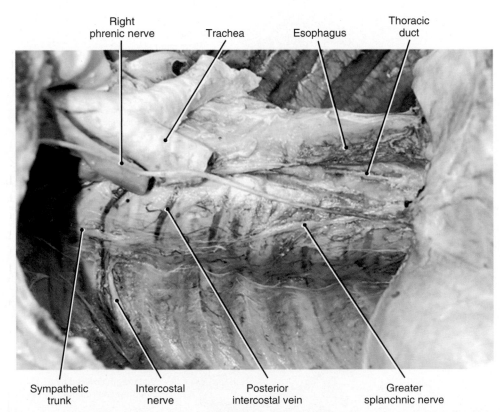

Right
phrenic nerve

Trachea

Esophagus

Thoracic
duct

Sympathetic
trunk

Intercostal
nerve

Posterior
intercostal vein

Greater
splanchnic nerve

Fig. 5.68 Right lateral view of posterior chest wall, demonstrating the sympathetic trunk, greater splanchnic nerve, and intercostal nerve.

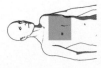

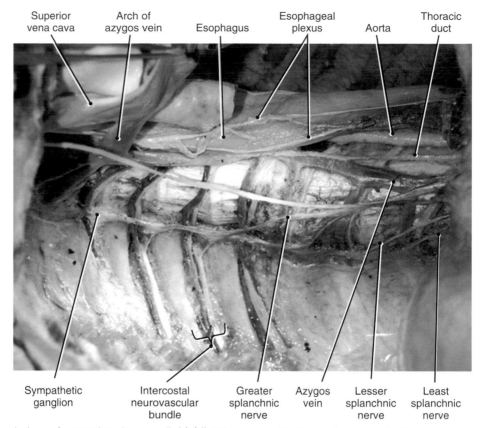

Superior vena cava • Arch of azygos vein • Esophagus • Esophageal plexus • Aorta • Thoracic duct

Sympathetic ganglion • Intercostal neurovascular bundle • Greater splanchnic nerve • Azygos vein • Lesser splanchnic nerve • Least splanchnic nerve

Fig. 5.69 Right lateral view of posterior chest wall, highlighting sympathetic trunk, sympathetic ganglion, and greater and lesser splanchnic nerves.

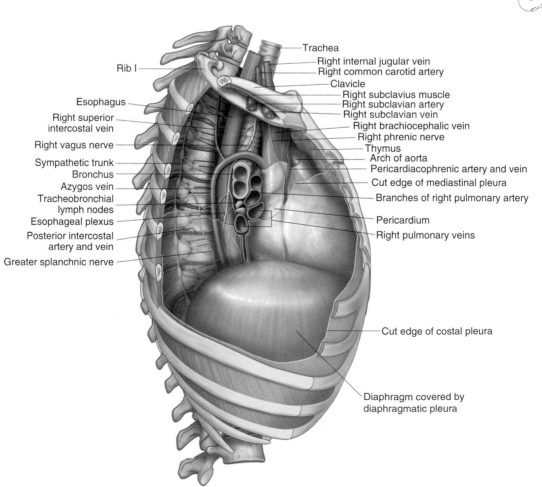

Trachea
Right internal jugular vein
Right common carotid artery
Clavicle
Right subclavius muscle
Right subclavian artery
Right subclavian vein
Right brachiocephalic vein
Right phrenic nerve
Thymus
Arch of aorta
Pericardiacophrenic artery and vein
Cut edge of mediastinal pleura
Branches of right pulmonary artery
Pericardium
Right pulmonary veins

Rib I
Esophagus
Right superior intercostal vein
Right vagus nerve
Sympathetic trunk
Bronchus
Azygos vein
Tracheobronchial lymph nodes
Esophageal plexus
Posterior intercostal artery and vein
Greater splanchnic nerve

Cut edge of costal pleura

Diaphragm covered by diaphragmatic pleura

Plate 5.2 Right side of hemithorax and mediastinum.

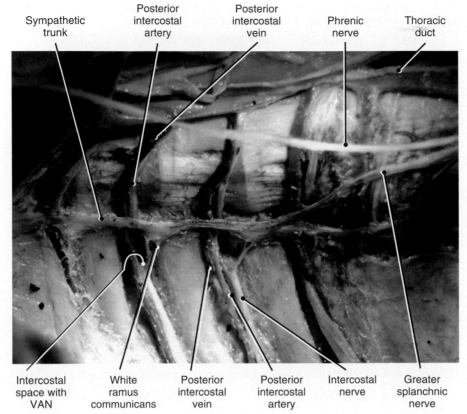

Sympathetic trunk | Posterior intercostal artery | Posterior intercostal vein | Phrenic nerve | Thoracic duct

Intercostal space with VAN | White ramus communicans | Posterior intercostal vein | Posterior intercostal artery | Intercostal nerve | Greater splanchnic nerve

Fig. 5.70 Right lateral view of posterior chest wall with sympathetic trunk, white ramus communicans, and intercostal nerve. *VAN,* Vein, artery, nerve.

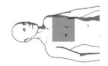

○ After cleaning out the sympathetic trunk and thoracic splanchnic nerves, dissect and clean the communicating rami connecting the sympathetic trunk with the intercostal nerves. Identify the white and gray rami communicantes (Fig. 5.70).

○ Trace the left and right vagus nerves as they descend behind the right and left primary bronchi to form the esophageal plexus on the anterior surface of the esophagus (Fig. 5.71).

○ Trace the superior vena cava and the veins draining into it. To the right of the superior vena cava, find the azygos vein draining into it (see Fig. 5.71). Identify the right posterior intercostal veins anterior and superior to the vertebral bodies.

○ On the left side of the thorax, identify the hemiazygos vein with the lowest three or four left posterior intercostal venous tributaries. Lift the esophagus at the midline, and note the accessory hemiazygos vein crossing the midline to join the azygos vein (Fig. 5.72).

DISSECTION TIP

The arch of the aorta and the descending thoracic aorta can be displaced or atherosclerotic, making the dissection of the left posterior thorax difficult. Often the greater, lesser, and least splanchnic nerves, as well as the hemiazygos and accessory hemiazygos veins, are hidden behind the aorta.

○ Lift the midportion the thoracic aorta, and note the origin of the posterior intercostal arteries. Identify the esophageal and bronchial arteries arising from the anterior aspect of the aorta (Figs. 5.73 and 5.74).

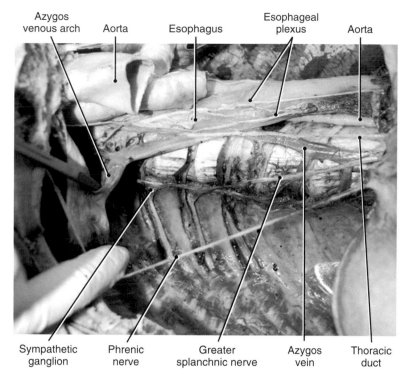

Fig. 5.71 Right lateral view of posterior chest wall, revealing azygos vein, sympathetic trunk, ganglion, and splanchnic nerve.

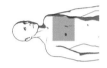

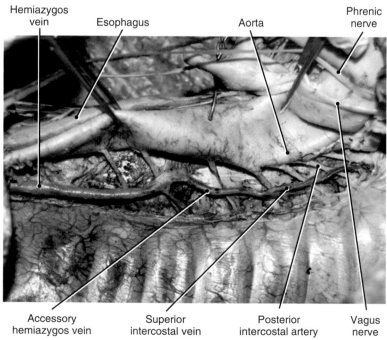

Fig. 5.72 Left lateral view of posterior thoracic wall, revealing accessory azygos and accessory hemiazygos veins.

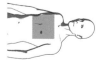

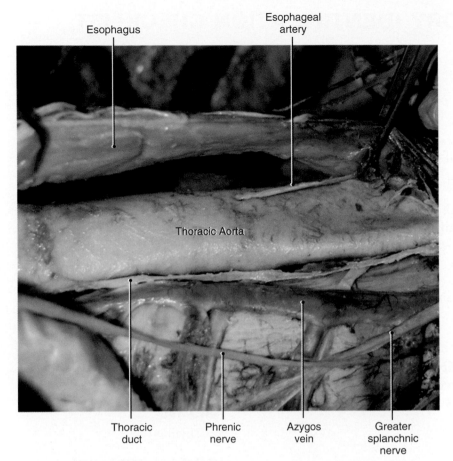

Esophagus   Esophageal artery

Thoracic Aorta

Thoracic duct   Phrenic nerve   Azygos vein   Greater splanchnic nerve

Fig. 5.73 Right lateral view of posterior chest wall, demonstrating the esophagus, esophageal artery, aorta, thoracic duct, and azygos vein.

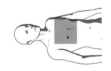

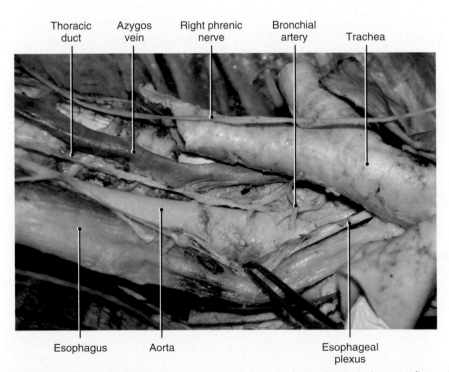

Thoracic duct   Azygos vein   Right phrenic nerve   Bronchial artery   Trachea

Esophagus   Aorta   Esophageal plexus

Fig. 5.74 Left lateral view of posterior mediastinum with the esophagus and esophageal plexus reflected, demonstrating the aorta, thoracic duct, and azygos vein.

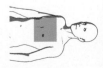

LABORATORY IDENTIFICATION CHECKLIST

NERVES
- ☐ Anterior intercostal
- ☐ Intercostobrachial (T2)
- ☐ Lateral intercostal T3-T7
- ☐ Intercostal
- ☐ Sympathetic trunk
- ☐ Sympathetic ganglia
- ☐ Greater splanchnic
- ☐ Lesser splanchnic
- ☐ Least splanchnic
- ☐ Gray and white rami communicantes
- ☐ Stellate ganglion
- ☐ Phrenic
- ☐ Vagus
- ☐ Right recurrent laryngeal
- ☐ Left recurrent laryngeal
- ☐ Esophageal plexus
- ☐ Cardiac plexus

ARTERIES
- ☐ Aorta
- ☐ Subclavian
- ☐ Internal thoracic
- ☐ Superior epigastric
- ☐ Musculophrenic
- ☐ Pericardiacophrenic
- ☐ Pulmonary
- ☐ Bronchial
- ☐ Esophageal
- ☐ Anterior intercostal
- ☐ Posterior intercostal

VEINS
- ☐ Superior vena cava
- ☐ Inferior vena cava
- ☐ Subclavian
- ☐ Internal thoracic
- ☐ Superior epigastric
- ☐ Brachiocephalic
- ☐ Anterior intercostal
- ☐ Posterior intercostal
- ☐ Azygos
- ☐ Accessory hemiazygos
- ☐ Hemiazygos

MUSCLES
- ☐ External intercostal
- ☐ Internal intercostal
- ☐ Innermost intercostal
- ☐ Transversus thoracis
- ☐ Subcostals
- ☐ Diaphragm

LYMPHATICS
- ☐ Thoracic duct

LIGAMENT
- ☐ Ligamentum arteriosum

GLAND
- ☐ Thymus

ORGAN TISSUES
- ☐ Lung
  - ☐ Hilum
  - ☐ Lingula
  - ☐ Oblique fissure
- ☐ Parietal pleura
- ☐ Visceral pleura
- ☐ Pulmonary ligament
- ☐ Lobes of right and left lungs
- ☐ Primary bronchi
- ☐ Secondary bronchi
- ☐ Tertiary bronchi
- ☐ Apex of heart
- ☐ Base of heart
- ☐ Esophagus

BONES
- ☐ Sternum
- ☐ Ribs
- ☐ Bodies of thoracic vertebrae with intervertebral discs

ATLAS REFERENCES

Netter: 216–230
McMinn: 185–191
Gray's Atlas: 92–107

BEFORE YOU BEGIN
Inspection

Inspect the heart externally and identify the following:

- Right atrium
- Right auricle
- Superior vena cava (SVC)
- Inferior vena cava (IVC)
- Subpulmonary infundibulum or conus
- Pulmonary artery
- Ascending aorta
- Left atrium
- Pulmonary veins
- Left auricle (Figs. 6.1 to 6.4)

Identify the *sulcus terminalis,* a shallow groove on the surface of the right atrium, which extends between the right side of the orifice of the SVC and that of the IVC.

> ### DISSECTION TIP
>
> The dissection typically begins with the exposure and identification of the coronary arteries. Note the apex of the left ventricle and the *acute* (right) (see Fig. 6.1) and *obtuse* (left) (see Fig. 6.4) margins of the heart.

CORONARY ARTERIES

- To remove the epicardium (visceral pericardium) and the fat covering the right coronary artery, identify the right auricle and retract it laterally.
- Palpate the space between the right auricle and the atrioventricular (AV, coronary) groove or sulcus, and expose the proximal part of the right coronary artery (Fig. 6.5).

> ### DISSECTION TIP
>
> Most of the coronary arteries in adults can be felt with palpation because of their increased hardening from atherosclerotic changes of aging.

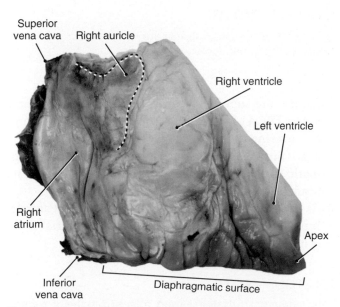

Fig. 6.1 Anterior view of external surfaces of the heart; *dotted outline,* right auricle.

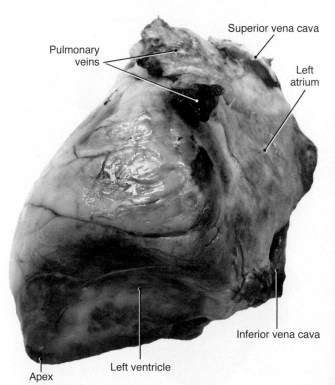

Fig. 6.2 Topographic view of left atrium and ventricle.

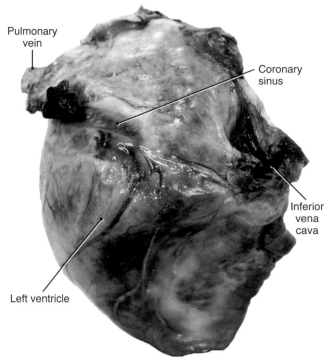

Pulmonary vein

Coronary sinus

Inferior vena cava

Left ventricle

Fig. 6.3 Topographic view of the posterior heart.

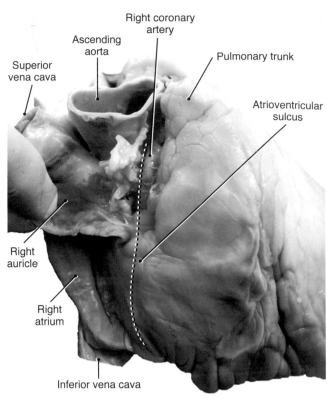

Right coronary artery

Ascending aorta

Superior vena cava

Pulmonary trunk

Atrioventricular sulcus

Right auricle

Right atrium

Inferior vena cava

Fig. 6.5 Topographic view of base of heart structures; *dotted line,* tracing of right coronary artery.

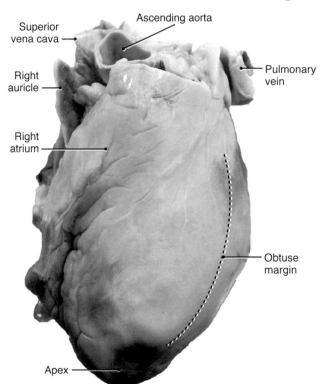

Ascending aorta

Superior vena cava

Right auricle

Right atrium

Pulmonary vein

Obtuse margin

Apex

Fig. 6.4 Base, margin, and apex of topographic heart; *dotted line,* obtuse margin.

ANATOMY **NOTE**

The terms *atrium* and *auricle* are not synonymous. The auricles are appendages of the atria.

○ Expose the superficial portion of the *right coronary artery* (RCA) by cleaning away the epicardium and fat covering the vessel (Fig. 6.6).
○ Trace the RCA toward the right side of the diaphragmatic surface of the heart, taking care to protect its branches.
○ As the artery passes near the edge of the right auricle, it usually gives off the artery of the sinu-atrial node (Fig. 6.7).

ANATOMY **NOTE**

The sinu-atrial (SA) nodal artery arises from the proximal portion of the RCA in 65% of cases, traveling upward to the right atrium at the junction of the SVC and the right auricle, where it enters the sinu-atrial node. In the remaining cases, the SA nodal artery arises from the proximal portion of the left coronary artery.

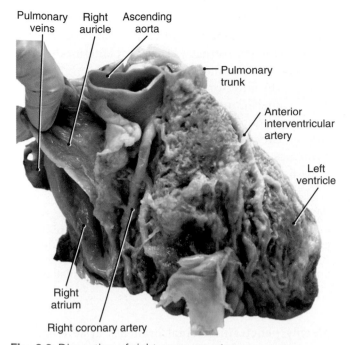

Fig. 6.6 Dissection of right coronary artery from its origin.

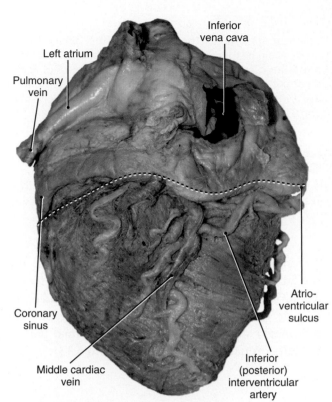

Fig. 6.8 Posterior view of heart with the inferior (posterior) interventricular artery and middle cardiac vein exposed.

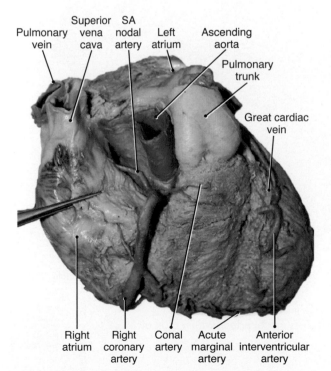

Fig. 6.7 Dissection of right coronary artery from its origin. *SA,* Sinu-atrial.

○ The second branch of the RCA is the artery of the conus, or *conal artery.* The conal artery arises from the proximal part of the RCA and passes to the left, around the right ventricle, at the level of the subpulmonary infundibulum (see Fig. 6.7). Close to the diaphragmatic surface of the heart, the RCA typically gives rise to the right marginal artery, which supplies the inferior border of the right ventricle.

○ The RCA continues posteriorly in the AV (atrioventricular) groove and in most cases descends and terminates in the inferior (posterior) interventricular groove as the inferior (posterior) interventricular (descending) artery (Fig. 6.8).

ANATOMY NOTE

This artery supplies the inferior third of the interventricular septum and a portion of the inferior wall of the left ventricle.

○ Before it becomes the inferior (posterior) interventricular artery, the RCA will give off the artery of the atrioventricular (AV) node.

ANATOMY **NOTE**

In 80% of specimens, the AV nodal artery arises from the RCA near the inferior (posterior) interventricular groove as it crosses the "crux" of the heart (Fig. 6.9). The crux of the heart is the center point of the anatomic base where the atria and ventricles are most closely approximated posteriorly.

DISSECTION **TIP**

To identify the artery to the AV node, carefully lift the left atrium at the inferior (posterior) AV groove, and clean away the fat (see Fig. 6.9B).

○ To remove the epicardium (visceral pericardium) and the fat covering the left coronary artery, identify the left auricle and retract it laterally (Figs. 6.10 and 6.11).
○ Palpate the space between the left auricle, the AV (coronary) sulcus, and expose the proximal part of the left coronary artery (Figs. 6.12 and 6.13).

○ The left coronary artery is typically very small (a few centimeters in length) and divides into the anterior interventricular coronary artery (left anterior descending) and left circumflex artery.
○ Palpate the anterior interventricular groove, and feel for the anterior interventricular artery. Use the separation technique to expose the anterior interventricular artery. This vessel gives off relatively large diagonal branches to the anterior surface of the left ventricle (Fig. 6.14).

ANATOMY **NOTE**

An often-encountered variation is the presence of myocardial bridges covering the left anterior interventricular artery, which penetrates the myocardium for a few centimeters and emerges distally as an epicardial artery (see Fig. 6.14).

○ Deeply penetrating septal branches arise from the deep surface of the anterior interventricular artery

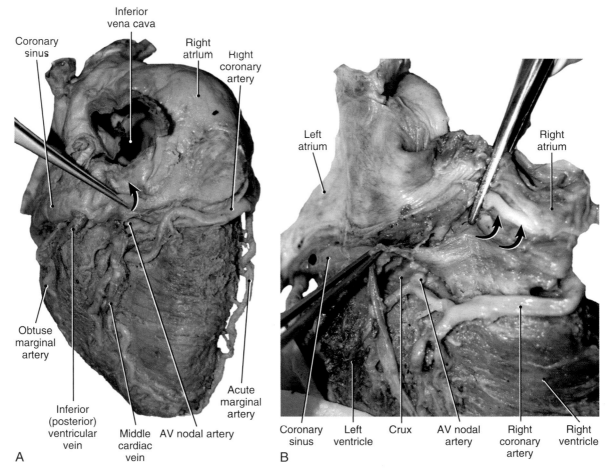

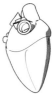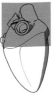

Fig. 6.9 A, Posterior view of heart with inferior (posterior) interventricular artery and artery to the atrioventricular (AV) node exposed. B, Left atrium pulled back to reveal AV nodal artery within crux of heart.

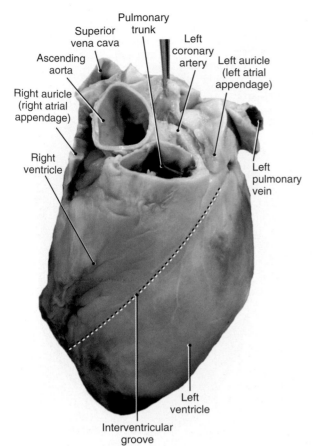

Fig. 6.10 Vertical tilt of heart revealing its base and apex.

Labels: Superior vena cava, Pulmonary trunk, Ascending aorta, Left coronary artery, Left auricle (left atrial appendage), Right auricle (right atrial appendage), Right ventricle, Left pulmonary vein, Left ventricle, Interventricular groove

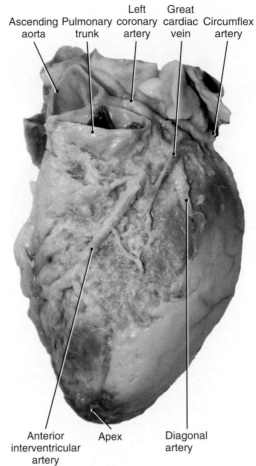

Fig. 6.12 Epicardial fat is removed from the surface of the left ventricle and the anterior interventricular artery is exposed.

Labels: Ascending aorta, Pulmonary trunk, Left coronary artery, Great cardiac vein, Circumflex artery, Anterior interventricular artery, Apex, Diagonal artery

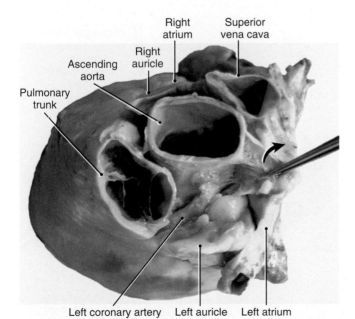

Fig. 6.11 Superior view of the great vessels. To the left of the great vessels, fat is reflected and the origin of the left coronary artery is exposed.

Labels: Right atrium, Superior vena cava, Right auricle, Ascending aorta, Pulmonary trunk, Left coronary artery, Left auricle, Left atrium

and enter the muscular interventricular septum (Figs. 6.15 and 6.16) at the level of the subpulmonary infundibulum to supply the proximal parts of the left and right bundle branches.

o The circumflex coronary artery runs in the left AV groove toward the left border and around to the base of the heart. This vessel typically gives off the left marginal artery crossing the left border of the heart, supplying the left ventricular free wall (Fig. 6.17).

ANATOMY **NOTE**

Numerous variations exist in the pattern of distribution of the right and left coronary arteries. Among the most common of the variations is the source of the inferior (posterior) interventricular coronary artery. In the majority of cases, the RCA provides the source for this artery. In about 15% of cases, however, the left circumflex artery gives off this branch.

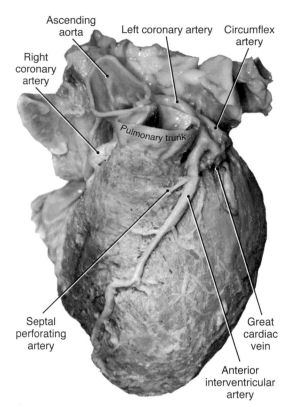

Fig. 6.13 Epicardial fat removed from left ventricle with the anterior interventricular artery exposed.

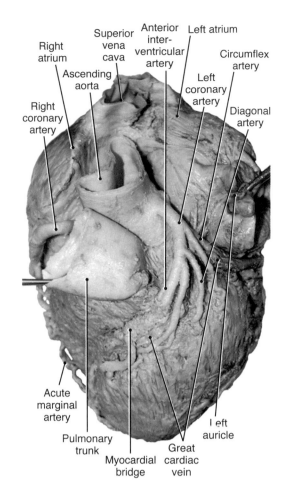

Fig. 6.14 Removing epicardial fat from the left ventricle and exposing the anterior interventricular artery to reveal diagonal branches and a myocardial bridge.

DISSECTION **TIP**

At many times during this dissection, it is possible to identify hearts that have undergone coronary artery bypass graft (CABG) procedures (Figs. 6.18 and 6.19).

○ Try to expose the graft vessel and identify to which vessel it is connected.

○ On the posterior surface of the heart at the AV sulcus between the IVC and the left atrium, identify the *coronary sinus*, a small confluence of veins approximately 2 cm long.

ANATOMY **NOTE**

The coronary sinus receives the great cardiac vein, the middle cardiac vein, and occasionally, the small cardiac vein and the oblique vein of the left atrium.

○ Identify the **great cardiac vein**, which lies in the anterior interventricular groove, accompanying the left anterior interventricular artery.

○ The **middle cardiac vein** lies in the inferior (posterior) interventricular groove and accompanies the inferior (posterior) interventricular artery.

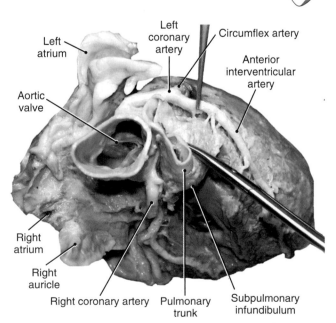

Fig. 6.15 Anterior interventricular artery is retracted, and septal perforating branches are exposed.

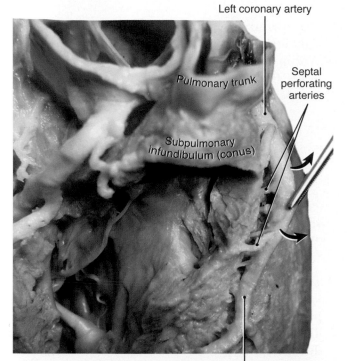

Left coronary artery

Pulmonary trunk

Septal perforating arteries

Subpulmonary infundibulum (conus)

Anterior interventricular artery

Fig. 6.16 Left coronary artery with septal and anterior interventricular branches.

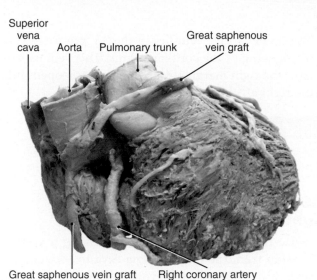

Superior vena cava

Aorta

Pulmonary trunk

Great saphenous vein graft

Great saphenous vein graft

Right coronary artery

Fig. 6.18 Anterior view of the heart demonstrating a great saphenous vein graft.

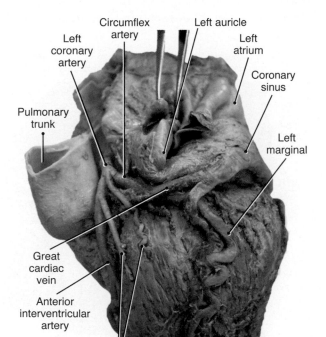

Circumflex artery

Left auricle

Left atrium

Coronary sinus

Left marginal

Left coronary artery

Pulmonary trunk

Great cardiac vein

Anterior interventricular artery

Diagonal arteries

Fig. 6.17 Lateral view with vertical tilt revealing left coronary artery, circumflex and marginal branches.

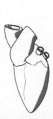

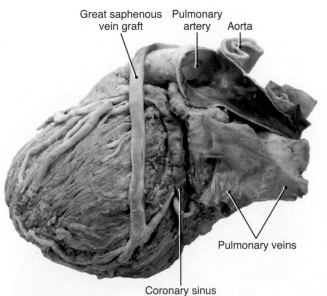

Great saphenous vein graft

Pulmonary artery

Aorta

Pulmonary veins

Coronary sinus

Fig. 6.19 Posterior view revealing the great saphenous vein graft.

○ The small cardiac vein lies in the AV groove next to the opening of the coronary sinus. This vein usually joins the right marginal vein or separately opens into the right atrium.

DISSECTION TIP

The cardiac veins have very thin walls and are often damaged during dissection.

DISSECTION OF HEART
Right Atrium

○ Incise the right atrium laterally, making a vertical incision from the inferior vena cava to the superior vena cava (Fig. 6.20), and avoid cutting the IVC valve.

○ With forceps, reflect the flap made by the lateral incision in the right atrium, and observe the muscular ridge within the chamber, the *crista terminalis* (Fig. 6.21 and Plate 6.1).

○ Note the **pectinate muscles** arising from the crista terminalis and fanning out through the wall of the right auricle.

○ Observe the smooth roof of the right atrium between the orifices of the two venae cavae, the *sinus venarum*.

○ Within the right atrium, note the valve of the IVC (eustachian valve), medial to the opening of the IVC. Note the valve (thebesian valve) and ostium of the coronary sinus (coronary os).

○ Note also the venae cordis minimae (thebesian veins), which are small openings in the internal surface of the right atrium.

○ The interatrial septum forms the medial wall of the right atrium.

○ Within the septum is a depressed region, the *fossa ovalis* (fossa ovale), bordered by a thicker rim of muscle, the superior limbus fossa ovalis (Fig. 6.22).

ANATOMY NOTE

The fossa ovalis marks the line of fusion between the original embryonic septum secundum with the septum primum, closing the ostium secundum. In 20% of cases, the area of fusion in the interatrial septum is incomplete, and an oblique fissure of communication between the two atria is retained. This is known as a "probe-patent foramen ovale" (Fig. 6.23).

○ Turn the right atrium upward, and note the *tricuspid valve* and its three leaflets: septal, anterior, and posterior.

○ The separation of the three leaflets may not be well delineated.

○ Identify the membranous septum between the septal and anterior leaflets of the tricuspid valve.

○ Place one finger deeply within the aorta (below the level of its valve) while palpating the base of the interatrial septum with the thumb of the same hand. The small area where the thumb and the finger are separated by the thinnest amount of tissue marks the site of the membranous septum (Figs. 6.24 and 6.25).

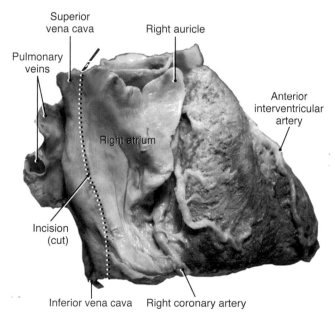

Fig. 6.20 Anterior view of the right atrium with incision landmark between the inferior and superior venae cavae.

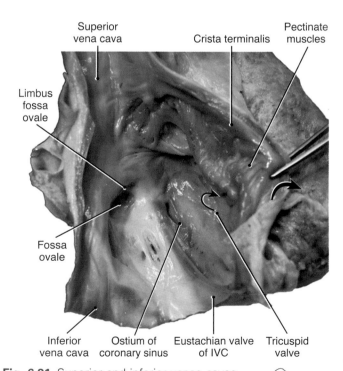

Fig. 6.21 Superior and inferior venae cavae opened with a vertical incision, revealing internal structures of the right atrium *IVC*, Inferior vena cava.

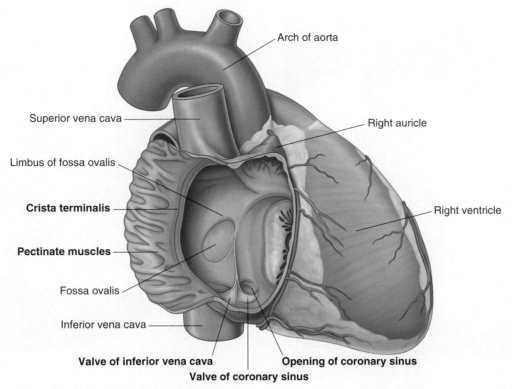

Plate 6.1 A view of the structures of the right atrium.

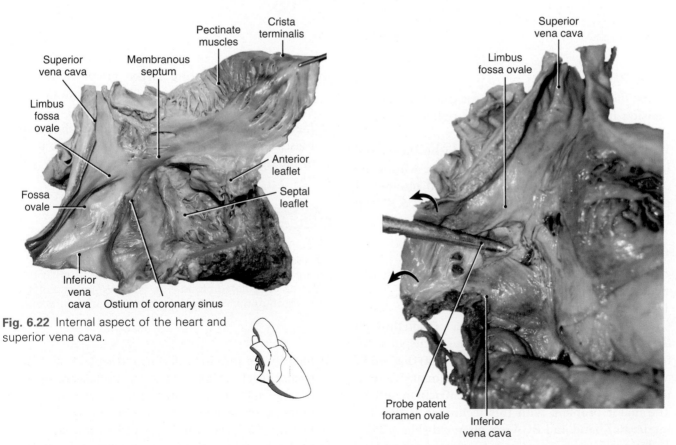

Fig. 6.22 Internal aspect of the heart and superior vena cava.

Fig. 6.23 Right atrium reflected to reveal patent foramen ovale.

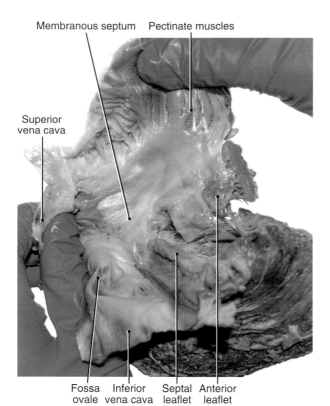

Membranous septum   Pectinate muscles

Superior
vena cava

Fossa   Inferior   Septal   Anterior
ovale   vena cava   leaflet   leaflet

Fig. 6.24 Anterior atrial wall is lifted upward, and with a light behind it (transillumination), the membranous septum is seen.

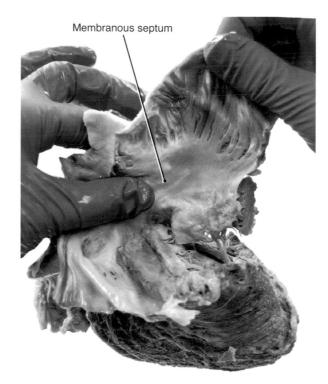

Membranous septum

Fig. 6.25 Right atrium reflected with dissector's left thumb palpating the membranous septum.

Left Atrium

○ Incise the left atrium laterally, making a horizontal incision from the right to the left pulmonary veins (Fig. 6.26).

○ With forceps, reflect the flap made by the lateral incision in the left atrium, and observe within the chamber a smooth surface and limited number of pectinate muscles in the left auricle (Fig. 6.27 and Plate 6.2).

Right Ventricle

The following two techniques are used to expose the contents of the right ventricle:

Technique 1:

○ Open the right ventricle by making an incision through the right atrium to expose fully the tricuspid valve toward the right ventricle (ventricular inlet) (Fig. 6.28).

○ Make a second incision from the pulmonary valve to the apex of the right ventricle (ventricular outlet). The major problem with this technique is that the moderator band and RCA are often cut (Fig. 6.29).

Technique 2:

○ Make a small, circular incision a few centimeters below the subpulmonary infundibulum. This area typically is occupied by the right ventricular free wall (Fig. 6.30).

○ Carefully, start cutting larger pieces of the right ventricular free wall, keeping in mind not to cut the moderator band (Fig. 6.31 and Plate 6.3).

○ Identify the moderator band, cut around the papillary muscle toward the tricuspid valve, and expose as much of the right ventricle as possible (Fig. 6.32).

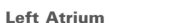

DISSECTION **TIP**

The majority of hearts have a significant amount of coagulated blood around the cordae tendineae and the papillary muscles (Fig. 6.33). With forceps, carefully clean out the coagulated blood (Fig. 6.34). Water also may be run through the heart to aid in this cleaning process.

○ Identify the anterior, inferior, and septal leaflets of the tricuspid valve. Observe that the leaflets are anchored to papillary muscles within the ventricle by slender, tough, chordae tendineae (see Fig. 6.34).

○ Identify the large **anterior papillary** muscle.

○ Posterior and inferior to this muscle is the **posterior papillary muscle**.

○ The **septal papillary muscle** may consist of several small, septal papillary muscles arising from the interventricular septum, with short chordae tendineae

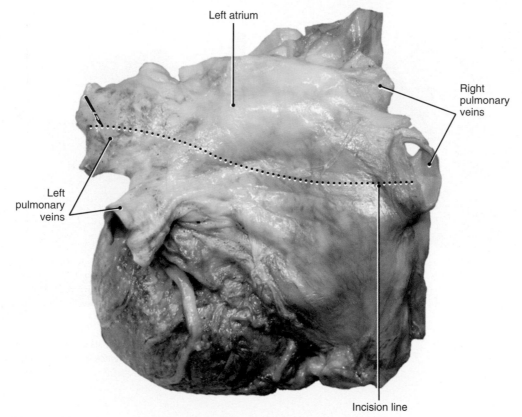

Left atrium

Right pulmonary veins

Left pulmonary veins

Incision line

Fig. 6.26 Base of heart with outline used for making incision to see contents of the left atrium.

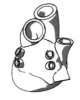

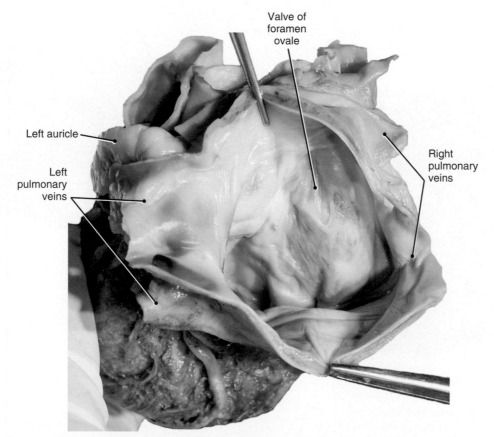

Valve of foramen ovale

Left auricle

Left pulmonary veins

Right pulmonary veins

Fig. 6.27 Left atrium incised superiorly, revealing internal structures.

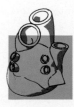

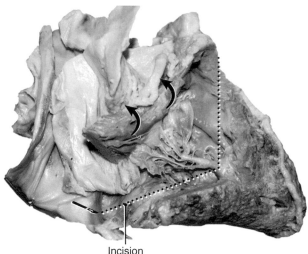

Incision

Fig. 6.28 Deep dissection of right ventricle using V-shaped incisions revealing internal structures.

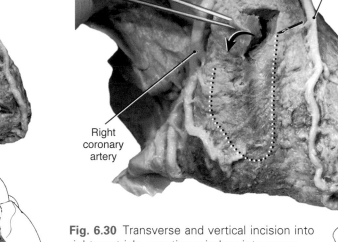

Aorta

Subpulmonary infundibulum (conus arteriosus)

Anterior interventricular artery

Right coronary artery

Fig. 6.30 Transverse and vertical incision into right ventricle, creating window into conus arteriosus; *dotted line* shows continuation of incision.

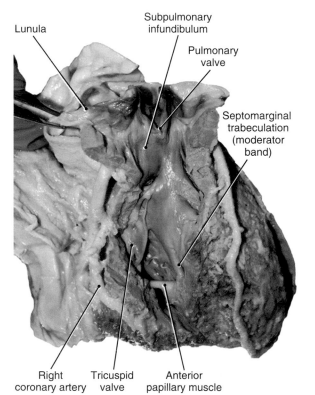

Lunula

Subpulmonary infundibulum

Pulmonary valve

Septomarginal trabeculation (moderator band)

Right coronary artery

Tricuspid valve

Anterior papillary muscle

Fig. 6.29 Right ventricle reflected away from apex and in line with pulmonary valve; anterior interventricular artery.

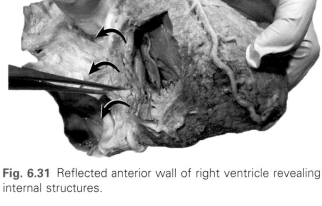

Fig. 6.31 Reflected anterior wall of right ventricle revealing internal structures.

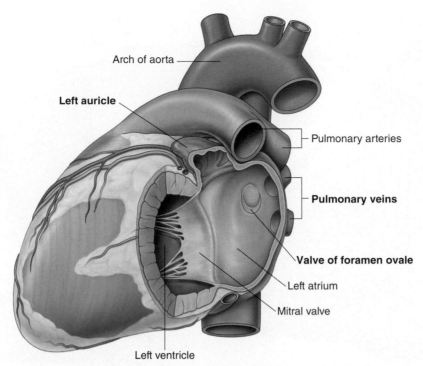

Arch of aorta

Left auricle

Pulmonary arteries

Pulmonary veins

Valve of foramen ovale

Left atrium

Mitral valve

Left ventricle

Plate 6.2 A view of the structures of the left atrium.

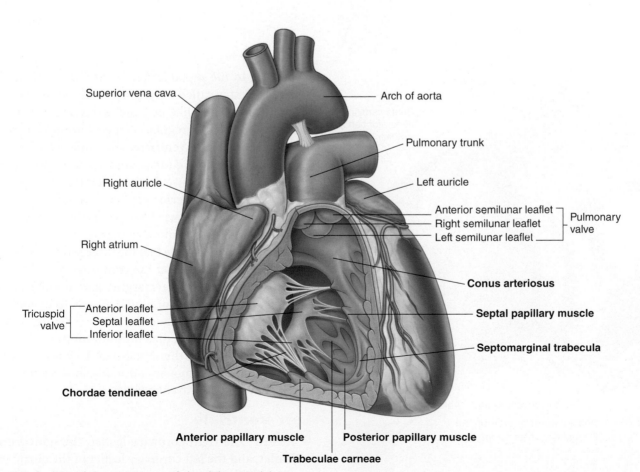

Superior vena cava

Arch of aorta

Pulmonary trunk

Right auricle

Left auricle

Anterior semilunar leaflet
Right semilunar leaflet
Left semilunar leaflet
Pulmonary valve

Right atrium

Conus arteriosus

Tricuspid valve
Anterior leaflet
Septal leaflet
Inferior leaflet

Septal papillary muscle

Septomarginal trabecula

Chordae tendineae

Anterior papillary muscle

Posterior papillary muscle

Trabeculae carneae

Plate 6.3 A view of the structures of the right ventricle.

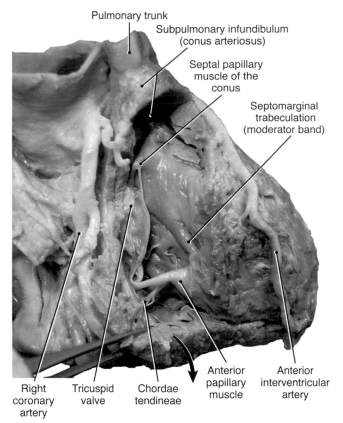

Fig. 6.32 Reflected anterior wall of right ventricle revealing internal structures.

Labels (Fig. 6.32): Pulmonary trunk; Subpulmonary infundibulum (conus arteriosus); Septal papillary muscle of the conus; Septomarginal trabeculation (moderator band); Right coronary artery; Tricuspid valve; Chordae tendineae; Anterior papillary muscle; Anterior interventricular artery

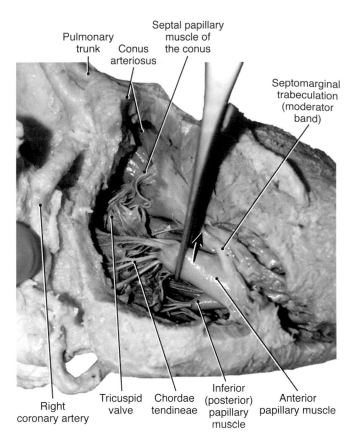

Fig. 6.34 Reflected anterior wall of right ventricle revealing internal structures.

Labels (Fig. 6.34): Pulmonary trunk; Conus arteriosus; Septal papillary muscle of the conus; Septomarginal trabeculation (moderator band); Right coronary artery; Tricuspid valve; Chordae tendineae; Inferior (posterior) papillary muscle; Anterior papillary muscle

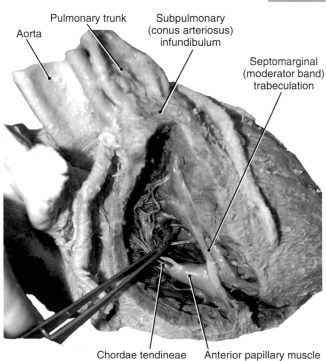

Labels (Fig. 6.33): Aorta; Pulmonary trunk; Subpulmonary (conus arteriosus) infundibulum; Septomarginal (moderator band) trabeculation; Chordae tendineae; Anterior papillary muscle

Fig. 6.33 Reflected anterior wall of the right ventricle revealing internal structures.

passing to the septal leaflet of the valve. The highest and largest is called the septal papillary muscle of the conus, or of Luschka or Lancisi (see Fig. 6.34).

○ Note the thick, irregular-shaped bundles of muscle within the right ventricle, the *trabeculae carneae*. The *moderator band* (or septomarginal trabeculation) passes from the muscular interventricular septum to the base of the anterior papillary muscle.

○ If Technique 2 was used to open right ventricle, now cut through the pulmonary trunk.

○ Refer to Fig. 6.29. Note that the three semilunar-shaped leaflets join together at the commissures.

○ Note the *lunula* (free margin) and nodule of each leaflet. Observe the horizontal muscle tissue in which the pulmonary (pulmonic) valve sits; this is the subpulmonary muscular infundibulum.

○ The area between the septal papillary muscle of the conus and subpulmonary infundibulum is demarcated by the crista supraventricularis.

Left Ventricle

○ Identify the right coronary leaflet, the noncoronary leaflet, and the left coronary leaflet of the aortic valve (Fig. 6.35).

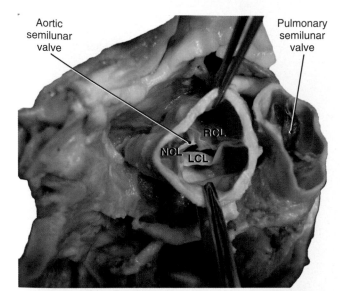

Aortic semilunar valve

Pulmonary semilunar valve

RCL.

NCL LCL

Fig. 6.35 Aorta and pulmonary vessels transected superior to base of heart revealing their valves, respectively. *LCL*, left coronary leaflet; *NCL*, noncoronary leaflet; *RCL*, right coronary leaflet.

- O Make a parallel incision from the anterior interventricular artery to the bifurcation of the left coronary artery into left anterior interventricular and coronary circumflex arteries (Figs. 6.36 and 6.37).
- O With your fingers or a retractor, open the left ventricle and observe the muscular ridges, the trabeculae carneae (Fig. 6.38).
- O Identify the mitral valve (left AV valve) with its two leaflets, an anterior and a posterior leaflet attaching by chordae tendineae to two papillary muscles, the inferomedial (posteromedial) papillary muscle (closer to intraventricular septum, *septophilic*) and the anterolateral papillary muscle (farther away from the intraventricular septum, *septophobic*) (see Fig. 6.38).
- O Make a vertical incision toward the aorta and cut through the aortic valve (Fig. 6.39).
- O Identify the leaflets of the aortic valve and the lunula (free margin) and nodule of each leaflet. Identify the ostia of the coronary arteries and the depressions in the wall of the aorta, the "aortic sinuses of Valsalva."
- O Beneath the noncoronary leaflet of the aorta, identify the membranous portion of the interventricular septum (Fig. 6.40).

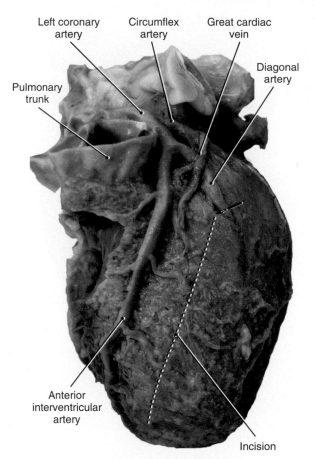

Left coronary artery

Circumflex artery

Great cardiac vein

Diagonal artery

Pulmonary trunk

Anterior interventricular artery

Incision

Fig. 6.36 Lateral view with vertical tilt revealing the left coronary artery and dominant branches, with tracing *(dotted line)* for incision into the left ventricle.

- O Observe the leaflets of the mitral valve and the aortic-mitral valve continuity (Fig. 6.40).
- O Notice the layer of lighter-colored tissue, which appears to travel inferiorly down the interventricular septum, between the coronary leaflet and the noncoronary leaflet of the aorta. This tissue forms the left bundle branch of the cardiac conduction system. Some of its fibers may be seen crossing the ventricular lumen freely as so-called false tendons (see Figs. 6.40 and 6.41 and Plate 6.4).

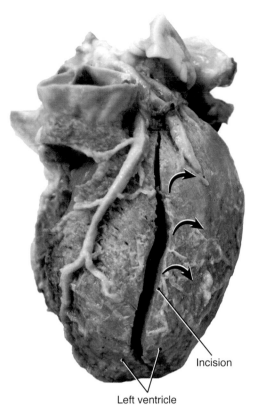

Incision

Left ventricle

Fig. 6.37 Lateral view with vertical tilt revealing the left coronary artery and dominant branches, with incision into the left ventricle.

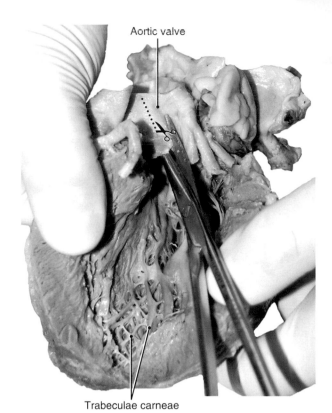

Aortic valve

Trabeculae carneae

Fig. 6.39 Opened left ventricle demonstrating internal structures and the scissors incising aortic valve.

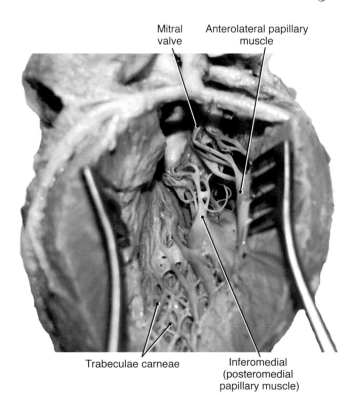

Mitral valve Anterolateral papillary muscle

Trabeculae carneae Inferomedial (posteromedial papillary muscle)

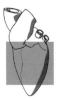

Fig. 6.38 Lateral view with vertical tilt revealing internal structures of the left ventricle.

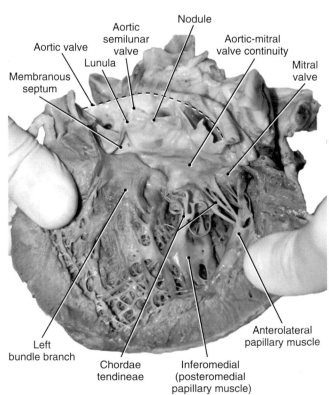

Nodule

Aortic semilunar valve Aortic-mitral valve continuity

Aortic valve Lunula Mitral valve

Membranous septum

Left bundle branch Chordae tendineae Inferomedial (posteromedial papillary muscle) Anterolateral papillary muscle

Fig. 6.40 Left ventricle reflected revealing internal structures, and highlighting the aortic and mitral valves.

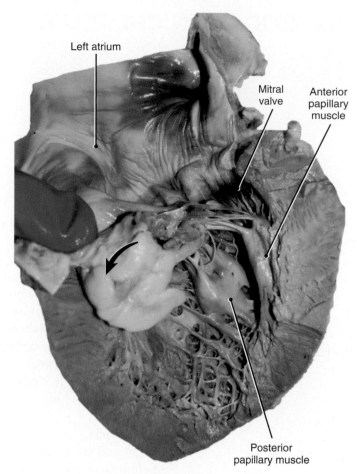

Left atrium

Mitral valve

Anterior papillary muscle

Posterior papillary muscle

Fig. 6.41 Left ventricle reflected open, revealing left atrioventricular valve and papillary muscles.

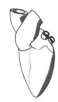

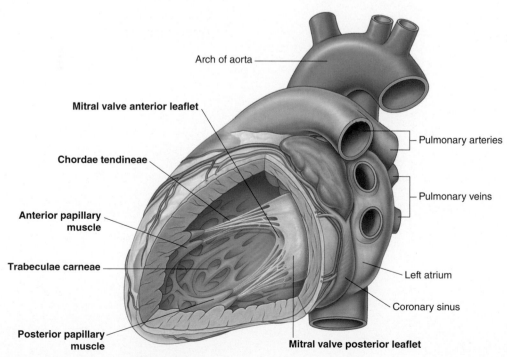

Arch of aorta

Mitral valve anterior leaflet

Chordae tendineae

Anterior papillary muscle

Trabeculae carneae

Posterior papillary muscle

Pulmonary arteries

Pulmonary veins

Left atrium

Coronary sinus

Mitral valve posterior leaflet

Plate 6.4 A view of the structures of the left ventricle.

LABORATORY IDENTIFICATION CHECKLIST

ARTERIES

- ☐ Aorta
- ☐ Common carotid
- ☐ Brachiocephalic trunk
- ☐ Pulmonary
- ☐ Left coronary
- ☐ Anterior interventricular
- ☐ Circumflex
- ☐ Interventricular septal branches
- ☐ Right coronary
- ☐ Marginal
- ☐ Sinu-atrial (SA) nodal
- ☐ Atrioventricular (AV) nodal
- ☐ Inferior (posterior) interventricular

VEINS

- ☐ Superior vena cava
- ☐ Inferior vena cava and eustachian valve
- ☐ Right and left pulmonary veins
- ☐ Coronary sinus and thebesian valve
- ☐ Great cardiac
- ☐ Middle cardiac
- ☐ Small cardiac

HEART

- ☐ Right atrium
  - ☐ Right auricle
  - ☐ Superior vena cava
  - ☐ Inferior vena cava
- ☐ Fossa ovalis
- ☐ Opening of coronary sinus
- ☐ Crista terminalis
- ☐ Pectinate muscle
- ☐ Sinus venosus region (smooth aspect)
- ☐ Right ventricle
  - ☐ Right atrioventricular (AV) valve, or tricuspid valve
  - ☐ Chordae tendineae
  - ☐ Anterior papillary muscle
  - ☐ Posterior papillary muscle
  - ☐ Septal papillary muscle
  - ☐ Septomarginal trabeculation (moderator band)
  - ☐ Interventricular septum
  - ☐ Trabeculae carneae
- ☐ Subpulmonary infundibulum (conus arteriosus)
  - ☐ Pulmonary (pulmonic) valve
- ☐ Left atrium
- ☐ Left auricle
- ☐ Right and left pulmonary veins
- ☐ Left atrioventricular (AV) valve, or bicuspid/mitral valve
- ☐ Left ventricle
- ☐ Aortic valve
  - ☐ Chordae tendineae
  - ☐ Anterolateral papillary muscle
  - ☐ Inferomedial (posteromedial) papillary muscle
  - ☐ Chordae tendineae
  - ☐ Trabeculae carneae

THORACENTESIS

Gray's Anatomy for Students: 62, 78
Netter: 197

Clinical Application

Introduce a needle or trocar into the intrathoracic cavity, creating a conduit to allow air (pneumothorax) to escape or to help remove fluid.

Anatomic Landmarks

- *Needle:* 2nd intercostal space at midclavicular line
  Skin
  Subcutaneous
  External intercostal fascia/muscle
  Internal intercostal fascia/muscle
  Parietal pleura
- *Tube:* 5th intercostal space at midaxillary line
  Skin
  Subcutaneous tissue
  Inferior angle of scapula
  Lateral pectoralis major border
  Lateral breast tissue
  Intercostal muscles
  Parietal pleura

Note: Needle placement for pneumothorax is 2nd intercostal space at midclavicular line; tube placement is at midaxillary line (Fig. III.1).

CENTRAL VENOUS LINE (CATHETERIZATION OF SUBCLAVIAN VEIN OR INTERNAL JUGULAR VEINS)

Gray's Anatomy for Students: 91, 114, 539
Netter: 38, 195

Clinical Application

Introduce a line (catheter) into the internal jugular vein above and behind the clavicle and medial to the sternocleidomastoid muscle for long-term infusion of fluids or medicines (Fig. III.2).

Anatomic Landmarks

- Skin
- Subcutaneous tissue
- Sternocleidomastoid muscle
- Clavicle
- Costoclavicular ligament
- Subclavian vein
- Anterior scalene, phenic nerve, lymphatic ducts
- Pleura

PERICARDIOCENTESIS

Gray's Anatomy for Students: 91, 92, 110
Netter: 215, 220

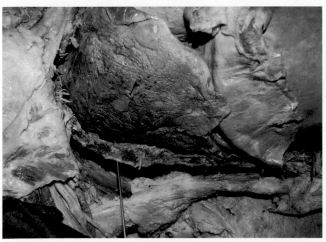

Fig. III.1

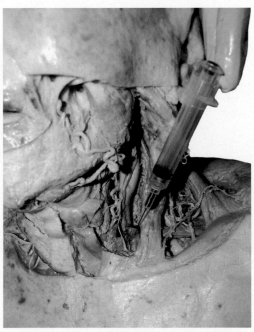

Fig. III.2

Clinical Application

Withdraw fluid from the pericardial space (Fig. III.3). *Note:* Liver, stomach, and internal thoracic artery may be in danger of injury (Fig. III.4).

Anatomic Landmarks

Subxiphoid Approach
- Xiphoid process of sternum
- Skin
- Subcutaneous tissue
- Rectus abdominis
- Pericardium
- Pericardial space

Parasternal Approach
- Left 5th intercostal space
- Left sternal border
- Skin
- Subcutaneous tissue
- External intercostal
- Internal intercostal
- Innermost intercostal
- Sternal space/pleura
- Pericardial space

OTHER LANDMARKS AND OBSERVATIONS

- Fig. III.5 shows an example of enlarged malignant lymph nodes in the axilla.
- The sternalis muscle is one of the most common variations found in the musculature of the anterior thoracic wall (Fig. III.6).
- Fig. III.7 shows a cadaver with a pacemaker.

- See Figs. III.8 to III.11 for examples of lungs with malignant lesions.
- The *myocardial bridge* is a muscular bridge that covers the anterior interventricular artery for a short distance within the myocardium. It is a common finding during dissection (Fig. III.12).
- Figs. III.13 and III.14 show the effects of myocardial infarction on the heart.

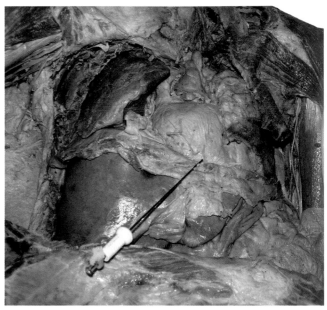

Fig. III.4

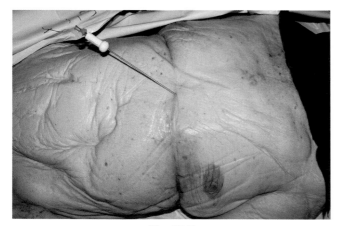

Fig. III.3

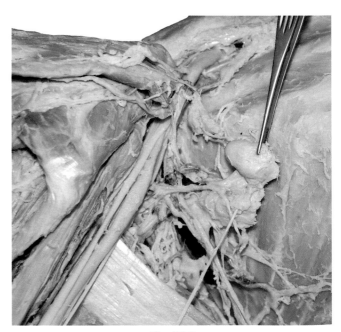

Fig. III.5

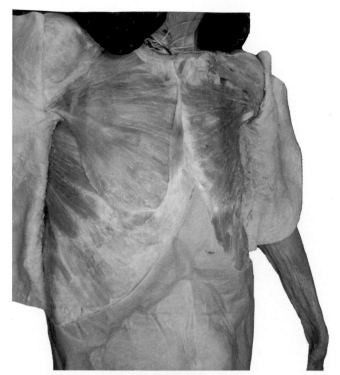

Fig. III.6

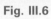

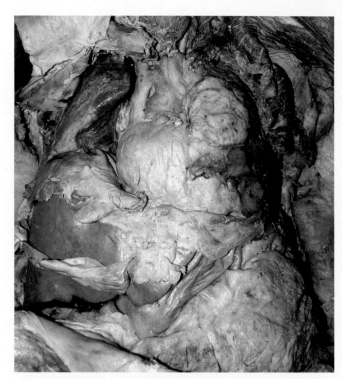

Fig. III.8

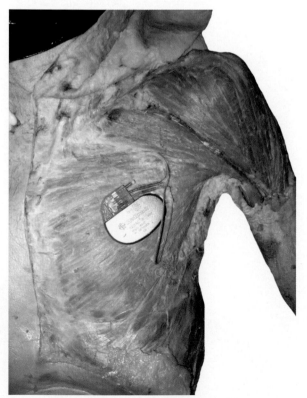

Fig. III.7

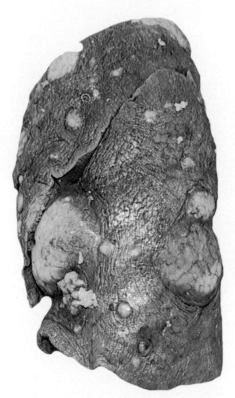

Fig. III.9

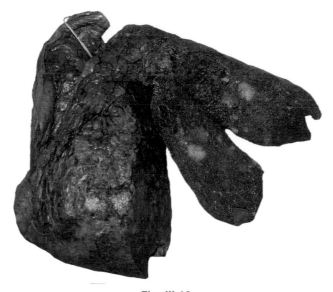

Fig. III.10

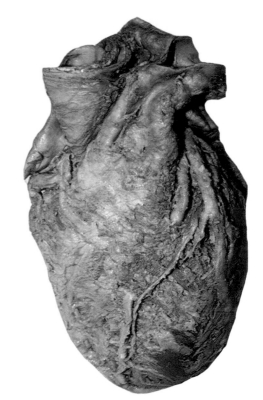

Fig. III.12

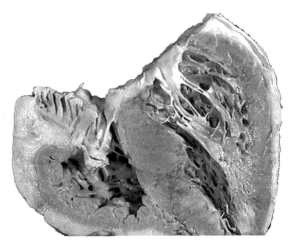

Fig. III.13

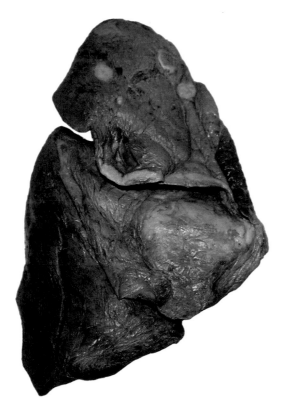

Fig. III.11

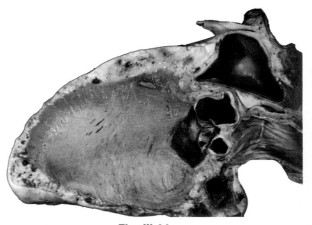

Fig. III.14

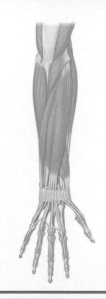

CHAPTER 7 | AXILLA AND ARM

ATLAS REFERENCES
Netter: 405, 414, 419–424
McMinn: 138–145
Gray's Atlas: 384–419

BEFORE YOU BEGIN
Axillary Borders

The pectoral region should have been dissected before the study of the axilla is begun. Refer to Chapter 4 for the regional anatomy of the pectoral region and breast. Review the following borders of the axilla:

- **Anterior wall:** Pectoralis major and minor muscles and clavipectoral fascia
- **Posterior wall:** Latissimus dorsi, teres major, and subscapularis muscles
- **Lateral wall:** Humerus, short head of biceps brachii muscle, and coracobrachialis muscle
- **Medial wall:** Upper five ribs, their intercostal muscles, and adjacent serratus anterior muscle
- **Base:** Axillary fascia
- **Apex** (*cervicoaxillary canal*): Superior border of scapula, 1st rib, and clavicle

DISSECTION STEPS
○ Make a skin incision from the shoulder distally to a point 2 to 3 inches (5 to 7.5 cm) above the elbow.
○ An encircling incision around the midportion of the arm allows for medial retraction of the skin from the upper arm.
○ Reflect the skin from the thorax, shoulders, axillae, and proximal portions of the arms medially to the axillary space (as shown previously in Fig. 4.4).
○ See Chapter 8 for the incisions used in the forearm.

○ Reflect the pectoralis muscles, better exposing the intercostobrachial and long thoracic nerves.
○ Identify the long thoracic nerve running over the serratus anterior muscle.
○ Note the intercostobrachial nerve emerging from the 2nd intercostal space.

ANATOMY **NOTE**

The intercostobrachial nerve emerging from the 2nd intercostal space is the lateral cutaneous branch of the 2nd thoracic (T2) nerve crossing over the long thoracic nerve, to supply the skin of the proximal, medial aspect of the arm and axilla (Fig. 7.1).

○ Preserve these two nerves.

DISSECTION **TIP**

Adipose tissue and lymphatics occupy most of the space in the axilla. Do not attempt to remove them at this stage. Push them away from the structures you identify, and remove them at a later stage.

○ Identify the fascia that invests the axillary artery, axillary vein, and the brachial plexus, called the *axillary sheath*.
○ Excise the axillary sheath between the axillary artery and the brachial plexus by gently pulling away the nerves (Fig. 7.2).
○ Remove the axillary sheath, and push the adipose tissue away from the brachial plexus (Fig. 7.3).
○ Identify and clean the axillary artery and vein (Fig. 7.4).

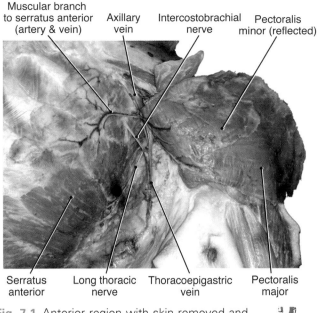

Muscular branch to serratus anterior (artery & vein)   Axillary vein   Intercostobrachial nerve   Pectoralis minor (reflected)

Serratus anterior   Long thoracic nerve   Thoracoepigastric vein   Pectoralis major

Fig. 7.1 Anterior region with skin removed and pectoralis muscles reflected, exposing intercostobrachial and long thoracic nerves.

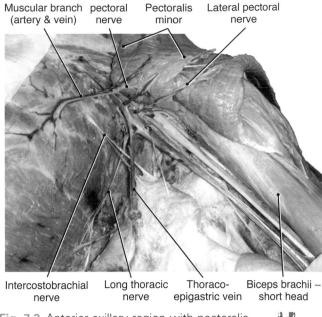

Muscular branch (artery & vein)   Medial pectoral nerve   Pectoralis minor   Lateral pectoral nerve

Intercostobrachial nerve   Long thoracic nerve   Thoraco-epigastric vein   Biceps brachii – short head

Fig. 7.3 Anterior axillary region with pectoralis muscles reflected and most of axillary sheath removed, revealing terminal branches of brachial plexus.

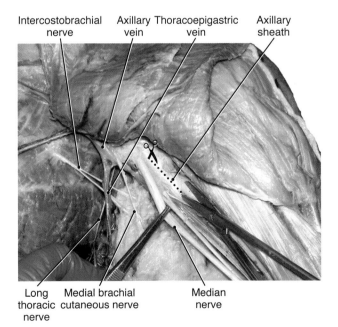

Intercostobrachial nerve   Axillary vein   Thoracoepigastric vein   Axillary sheath

Long thoracic nerve   Medial brachial cutaneous nerve   Median nerve

Fig. 7.2 Anterior axillary region with pectoralis muscles reflected, revealing excision of axillary sheath to expose terminal branches of brachial plexus.

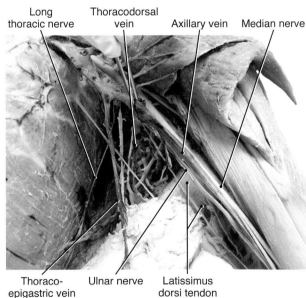

Long thoracic nerve   Thoracodorsal vein   Axillary vein   Median nerve

Thoraco-epigastric vein   Ulnar nerve   Latissimus dorsi tendon

Fig. 7.4 Anterior axillary view of deep dissection, revealing axillary vein and terminal branches of brachial plexus.

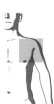

ANATOMY NOTE

The axillary vein is formed at the base of the axilla by the confluence of the venae comitantes of the brachial artery with the basilic vein. (Large arteries, such as the axillary or femoral, are accompanied by a single vein. Medium and smaller arteries, such as the brachial, have two or more accompanying veins, which are found on either side of the artery and are called *venae comitantes.*)

DISSECTION TIP

Do not attempt to identify any lymph nodes associated with the axillary vein and its tributaries. Nodes are evident and easily dissected only in cadavers with cancer. Similarly, do not attempt to identify the central axillary nodes within the fat of the central portion of the axilla. Smaller tributaries to the axillary vein that obscure the dissecting field can be removed.

○ Clean the adipose tissue between the pectoralis minor muscle and brachial plexus (see Fig. 7.4).

ANATOMY NOTE

The axillary artery extends from the lateral border of the 1st rib to the lower border of the teres major muscle. Just before it crosses the 1st rib, the artery is named the *subclavian artery.* Distal to the teres major, the name of the vessel changes to the *brachial artery.*

DISSECTION TIP

The arteries are named typically based on the structures they supply, not according to their origin.

○ Identify the axillary artery and its three divisions, demarcated with its relationship to the pectoralis minor muscle (Fig. 7.5).

○ Identify the superior thoracic artery arising from the 1st part of the axillary artery. To identify this vessel, look for an artery penetrating the musculature of the 1st or 2nd intercostal space.

○ From the 2nd part of the axillary artery (deep to pectoralis minor muscle), identify the thoracoacromial artery and the lateral thoracic artery (see Fig. 7.5).

○ Look for the pectoral branches of the thoracoacromial artery supplying the pectoralis major and minor muscles. Do not look for the remaining branches of the thoracoacromial artery (deltoid, acromial, and clavicular).

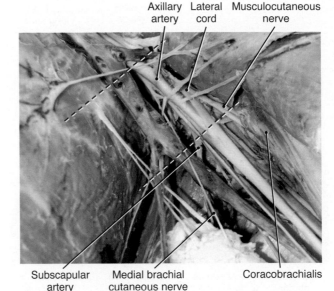

Axillary artery   Lateral cord   Musculocutaneous nerve

Subscapular artery   Medial brachial cutaneous nerve   Coracobrachialis

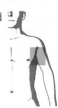

Fig. 7.5 Anterior axillary view revealing the second part of the axillary artery, thoracoacromial artery, and lateral cord. *Red dashed lines* represent the borders on the pectoralis minor muscle over the axillary artery, dividing its three portions.

DISSECTION TIP

The following anatomic landmarks may be helpful when identifying the branches of the axillary artery.

- **Superior thoracic artery:** 1st or 2nd intercostal spaces
- **Lateral thoracic artery:** Lateral border of pectoralis minor muscle. Often the lateral thoracic artery arises as a branch of the thoracoacromial artery.
- **Thoracoacromial artery:** 2nd part of axillary artery
- **Pectoral branches:** Look for these on the internal surface of the pectoralis major and minor muscles, and trace them backward to the axillary artery and thoracoacromial artery. The pectoral branches often originate directly from the 2nd part of the axillary artery.
- Separate the axillary artery from the branches of the brachial plexus, and remove fat from the latissimus dorsi muscle (Fig. 7.6).
- Do not remove fat deep to the axilla.
- Continue removing the axillary sheath from the brachial artery and vein, and expose the median nerve distally to the midportion of the arm (Fig. 7.7).

DISSECTION TIP

Exposing the branches of the brachial plexus to the midportion of the humerus allows greater mobility and facilitates the identification of structures deep in the axilla.

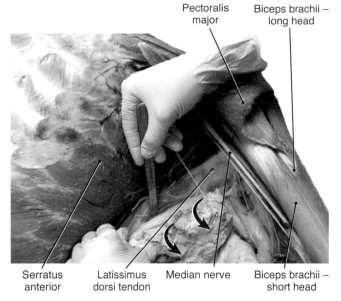

Pectoralis major — Biceps brachii – long head

Serratus anterior — Latissimus dorsi tendon — Median nerve — Biceps brachii – short head

Fig. 7.6 Anterior view revealing removal of the fat from the latissimus dorsi muscle.

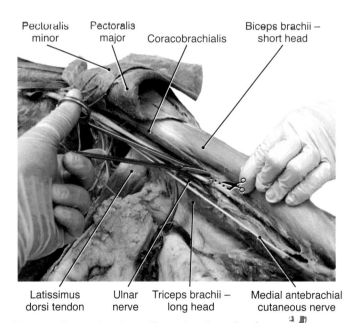

Pectoralis minor — Pectoralis major — Coracobrachialis — Biceps brachii – short head

Latissimus dorsi tendon — Ulnar nerve — Triceps brachii – long head — Medial antebrachial cutaneous nerve

Fig. 7.7 Removing the axillary sheath and soft tissue.

○ Cut the axillary vein at the point where the 1st part of the axillary artery originates, and reflect the vein and its tributaries toward the forearm.

○ Do not completely remove the vein from the cadaver.

○ Distal to the pectoralis minor muscle, from the 3rd portion of the axillary artery, identify the anterior

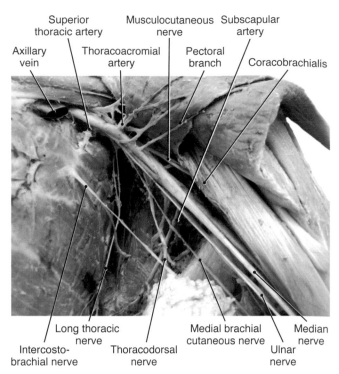

Superior thoracic artery — Musculocutaneous nerve — Subscapular artery

Axillary vein — Thoracoacromial artery — Pectoral branch — Coracobrachialis

Long thoracic nerve — Medial brachial cutaneous nerve — Median nerve

Intercosto-brachial nerve — Thoracodorsal nerve — Ulnar nerve

Fig. 7.8 Anterior axillary view with reflected pectoralis muscles, removed axillary vein, revealing the axillary artery and associated nerves.

circumflex humeral, posterior circumflex humeral, and subscapular arteries (Figs. 7.9 and 7.10).

ANATOMY **NOTE**

The subscapular artery runs vertically toward the latissimus dorsi and branches into the thoracodorsal artery, supplying the latissimus dorsi muscle, and the circumflex scapular artery, traveling posteriorly to the muscles of the posterior scapula (Figs. 7.8 and 7.9).

○ Identify the subscapular artery and thoracodorsal arteries.

○ Identify and clean the branches of the medial cord: the medial pectoral nerve, ulnar nerve, medial root of median nerve, medial brachial cutaneous nerve, and medial antebrachial cutaneous nerve.

○ Alongside the medial antebrachial cutaneous nerve, identify the basilic vein (formed at the medial aspect of the dorsal venous arch of the hand; see Chapters 8 and 9 for hand structures).

○ Trace and expose the median nerve to the elbow (see Fig. 7.9).

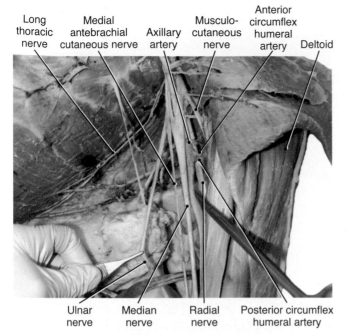

Long thoracic nerve | Medial antebrachial cutaneous nerve | Axillary artery | Musculo-cutaneous nerve | Anterior circumflex humeral artery | Deltoid

Ulnar nerve | Median nerve | Radial nerve | Posterior circumflex humeral artery

Fig. 7.9 Axillary artery and ulnar and median nerves are pulled medially to expose radial nerve and anterior and posterior circumflex humeral arteries.

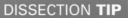

DISSECTION **TIP**

ANATOMIC LANDMARKS

- **Subscapular artery:** Arises from the 3rd part of the axillary artery (pull the medial cord upward to expose it) and runs vertically down between the latissimus dorsi and subscapularis muscles.
- **Thoracodorsal artery:** Arises from the subscapular artery and continues to run downward to supply the latissimus dorsi muscle. This artery is found on the surface of the latissimus dorsi accompanied by the middle subscapular nerve (trace the artery backward to its origin).

ANATOMY **NOTE**

The brachial plexus is divided into rami, trunks, divisions, cords, and terminal branches. The rami, trunks, and divisions are identified later in the root of the neck dissection. In this dissection, you will be able to identify the cords and terminal branches of the brachial plexus. The cords are named in respect to their positions in relationship to the axillary artery. As a result, the *lateral cord* is situated lateral to the axillary artery, the *medial cord* medial to the axillary artery, and the *posterior cord* posterior (deep) to the axillary artery. The lateral cord gives off two branches: the lateral pectoral nerve supplies the pectoralis major muscle, and the musculocutaneous nerve supplies the biceps brachii, coracobrachialis, and brachialis muscles (see Fig. 7.8) (Plate 7.1).

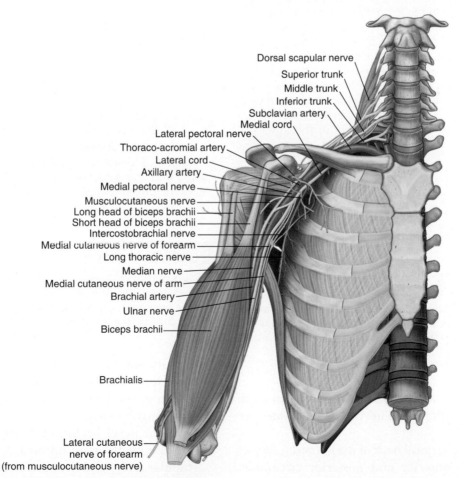

Dorsal scapular nerve
Superior trunk
Middle trunk
Inferior trunk
Subclavian artery
Medial cord
Lateral pectoral nerve
Thoraco-acromial artery
Lateral cord
Axillary artery
Medial pectoral nerve
Musculocutaneous nerve
Long head of biceps brachii
Short head of biceps brachii
Intercostobrachial nerve
Medial cutaneous nerve of forearm
Long thoracic nerve
Median nerve
Medial cutaneous nerve of arm
Brachial artery
Ulnar nerve
Biceps brachii
Brachialis
Lateral cutaneous nerve of forearm (from musculocutaneous nerve)

Plate 7.1 Lateral and medial cords of the brachial plexus.

DISSECTION TIP

A landmark for identifying the musculocutaneous nerve is that the nerve pierces the proximal portion of the coracobrachialis muscle.

DISSECTION TIP

ANATOMIC LANDMARKS

- **Ulnar nerve:** Look for the nerve traveling along the medial aspect of the arm, not providing any branches to the arm, and crossing posterior to the medial epicondyle.
- **Median nerve:** Look for the nerve traveling along the medial aspect of the arm without giving off any branches to the arm. It is found easily as it travels underneath the bicipital aponeurosis.
- **Medial brachial cutaneous nerve:** Runs parallel for a short distance in the arm with the medial antebrachial cutaneous nerve and is distributed to the skin of the arm. This nerve is often cut when the skin of the arm is reflected.
- **Medial antebrachial cutaneous nerve:** Runs parallel and superficial to the ulnar nerve and is distributed to the skin of the forearm. The basilic vein runs together with this nerve.

DISSECTION TIP

The medial brachial cutaneous nerve (medial cutaneous nerve to the arm) often is severed during the removal of the skin over the brachium. The medial antebrachial cutaneous nerve (medial cutaneous nerve to the forearm) runs parallel to the ulnar nerve. The landmark for identifying the ulnar nerve is to trace it as it crosses posterior to the medial epicondyle of the humerus. In contrast, the medial antebrachial cutaneous nerve runs more superficially and terminates in the skin of the forearm (see Fig. 7.14).

ANATOMY **NOTE**

The posterior cord gives rise to the following branches: upper, middle thoracodorsal, and lower subscapular nerves; axillary nerve; and radial nerve.

DISSECTION TIP

To identify the posterior cord, pull the medial cord and the axillary artery, laterally, away from the coracobrachialis muscle (Figs. 7.8 to 7.10). Look posteriorly and deep to it for the posterior cord.

○ Deep to the axillary artery, identify the posterior cord.
○ Identify and trace the radial nerve as it penetrates the triceps brachii.
○ At the level of the surgical neck of the humerus, dissect and expose the anterior and posterior circumflex humeral arteries (see Fig. 7.10).

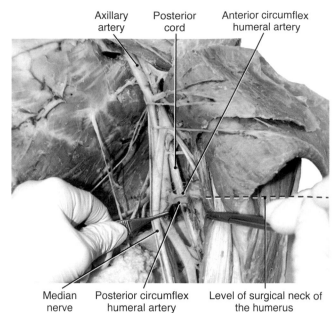

Axillary artery   Posterior cord   Anterior circumflex humeral artery

Median nerve   Posterior circumflex humeral artery   Level of surgical neck of the humerus

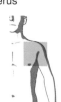

Fig. 7.10 Anterior axillary view with reflected pectoralis muscles, traction from axillary artery, revealing lateral cord, posterior cord, and musculocutaneous nerve. *Red dashed line* shows level of the surgical neck of the humerus.

DISSECTION TIP

ANATOMIC LANDMARKS

Radial nerve: Look at the medial surface of the arm for the nerve innervating the triceps brachii muscle (see Fig. 7.15). Trace the nerve backward to the axilla and posterior cord.

DISSECTION TIP

ANATOMIC LANDMARKS

Posterior circumflex humeral artery: Pull the axillary artery away from the coracobrachialis at the level of the surgical neck of the humerus, and identify the artery. It runs alongside the axillary nerve.

DISSECTION TIP

The posterior circumflex humeral artery is typically much larger than the anterior circumflex humeral artery. In some specimens, the posterior humeral artery may arise from the subscapular artery.

○ Identify the axillary nerve running alongside the posterior circumflex humeral artery passing posterior to the surgical neck of the humerus to reach the quadrangular space.
○ Trace the nerve backward to the posterior cord.
○ Pull the medial cord upward, and observe the subscapular artery and the posterior cord of the brachial plexus (Fig. 7.11).

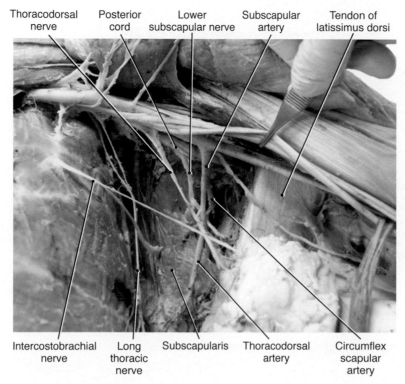

Thoracodorsal nerve | Posterior cord | Lower subscapular nerve | Subscapular artery | Tendon of latissimus dorsi

Intercostobrachial nerve | Long thoracic nerve | Subscapularis | Thoracodorsal artery | Circumflex scapular artery

Fig. 7.11 Anterior view revealing posterior structures.

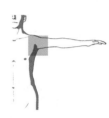

- Identify the thoracodorsal nerve that supplies the latissimus dorsi muscle and runs alongside the thoracodorsal artery, which also supplies the latissimus dorsi (see Figs. 7.11 and 7.12).
- Distal to the origin of the thoracodorsal nerve, identify the lower subscapular nerve running at the lateral border of subscapularis with the scapular circumflex artery.
- Identify the scapular circumflex artery.
- Clean out the subscapularis muscle and at its deeper portion, identify the upper subscapular nerve supplying the subscapularis muscle (Figs. 7.12 and 7.13).

DISSECTION TIP

ANATOMIC LANDMARKS
Thoracodorsal nerve: Found on the surface of the latissimus dorsi muscle running alongside the thoracodorsal artery.

ANATOMY NOTE

The lower subscapular nerve supplies part of the subscapularis and the entire teres major muscle.

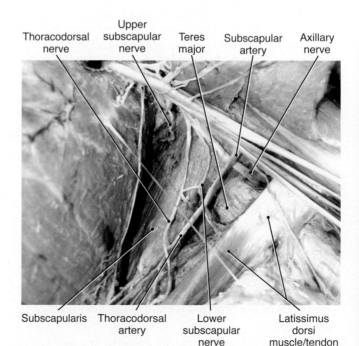

Thoracodorsal nerve | Upper subscapular nerve | Teres major | Subscapular artery | Axillary nerve

Subscapularis | Thoracodorsal artery | Lower subscapular nerve | Latissimus dorsi muscle/tendon

Fig. 7.12 Deep anterior axillary view revealing upper, middle (thoracodorsal), and lower subscapular nerves.

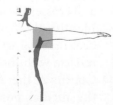

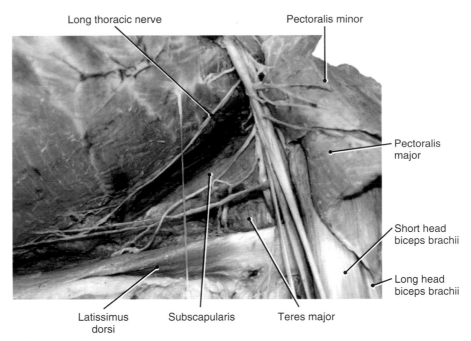

Fig. 7.13 Deep anterior view revealing posterior nerve structures.

DISSECTION **TIP**

ANATOMIC LANDMARKS
- **Scapular circumflex artery:** Arises from the subscapular artery and turns around to enter the gap between the lateral border of the subscapularis and latissimus dorsi muscles alongside the lower subscapular nerve (trace the nerve proximally to its origin from the posterior cord).
- **Lower subscapular nerve:** It runs with the scapular circumflex artery in the gap between the lateral border of the subscapularis and latissimus dorsi muscles.

DISSECTION **TIP**

ANATOMIC LANDMARKS
Upper subscapular nerve: Look deep in the axilla for the nerve that penetrates the subscapularis muscle. It is located deep and medial to the subscapularis muscle.

○ Continue the dissection by exposing the terminal branches of the brachial plexus in the arm (Figs. 7.14 and 7.15).

○ The *axillary* artery changes its name to *brachial* artery as it crosses the lower border of the teres major tendon.

○ Identify the first branch of the brachial artery, the *deep* brachial artery running deep to the triceps brachii muscle with the radial nerve.

○ Continue the dissection, reflecting the skin over the medial portion of the triceps brachii muscle,

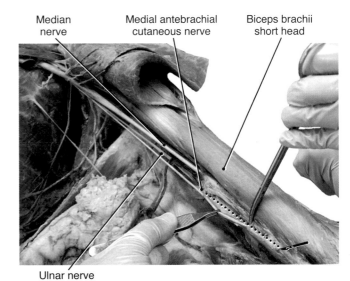

Fig. 7.14 Complete exposure of median, ulnar, and medial antebrachial cutaneous nerves in the arm.

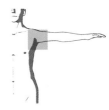

and expose all the branches of the radial nerve (Fig. 7.16).

○ Reflect the skin medially over the biceps brachii muscle (Figs. 7.16 and 7.17).

○ Identify the long and short heads of the biceps brachii.

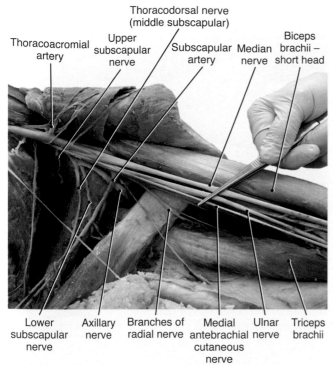

Thoracoacromial artery
Upper subscapular nerve
Thoracodorsal nerve (middle subscapular)
Subscapular artery
Median nerve
Biceps brachii – short head

Lower subscapular nerve
Axillary nerve
Branches of radial nerve
Medial antebrachial cutaneous nerve
Ulnar nerve
Triceps brachii

Fig. 7.15 Lower axillary and upper arm view with skin reflected, revealing muscles and nerves.

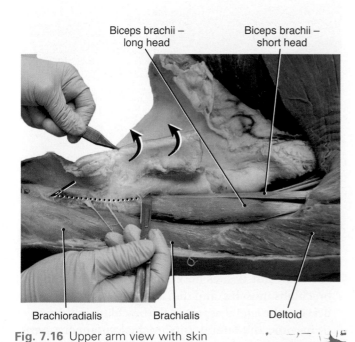

Biceps brachii – long head
Biceps brachii – short head

Brachioradialis
Brachialis
Deltoid

Fig. 7.16 Upper arm view with skin reflected, revealing biceps brachii, brachialis, and deltoid muscles.

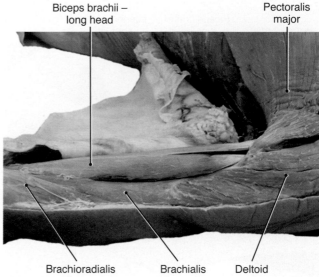

Biceps brachii – long head
Pectoralis major

Brachioradialis
Brachialis
Deltoid

Fig. 7.17 Upper arm view with skin reflected, revealing biceps brachii, brachialis, and deltoid muscles.

DISSECTION **TIP**

If time permits, expose the short head of the biceps brachii from its origin at the coracoid process of the scapula. The tendon of the long head of the biceps brachii lies lateral to the short head. You may expose the tendon of the long head of the biceps brachii muscle from the supraglenoid tubercle, just above the glenoid fossa of the scapula.

- Just inferior to the biceps brachii, identify the brachialis muscle (see Fig. 7.17).
- Identify the coracobrachialis muscle, noting the musculocutaneous nerve passing through the muscle.

ANATOMY **NOTE**

The brachialis muscle is innervated primarily by the musculocutaneous nerve; however, the radial nerve also may contribute to its innervation.

- Reflect the skin over the lateral aspect of the arm inferiorly (Fig. 7.18).
- Identify the posterior cutaneous nerve to the forearm (branch of radial nerve) emerging between the brachialis and triceps brachii muscles (Fig. 7.19).
- Trace the origin of the posterior cutaneous nerve to the forearm by separating the brachialis from the triceps brachii (Fig. 7.20).
- Lift the inferior portion of the deltoid muscle from the humeral surface.
- Reflect the fascia covering the triceps, and expose the lateral head of the triceps brachii muscle (Fig. 7.21).

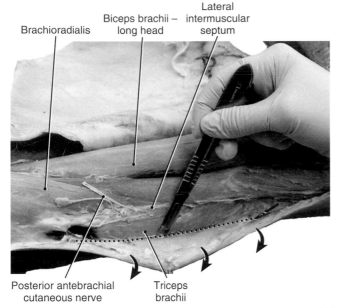

Brachioradialis

Biceps brachii – long head

Lateral intermuscular septum

Posterior antebrachial cutaneous nerve

Triceps brachii

Fig. 7.18 Dissection and reflection of skin over lateral head of triceps brachii, with exposure of posterior antebrachial cutaneous nerve.

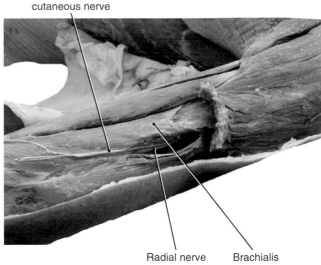

Posterior antebrachial cutaneous nerve

Radial nerve

Brachialis

Fig. 7.20 Reflection of deltoid muscle and exposure of the origin of the posterior antebrachial cutaneous nerve.

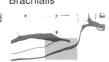

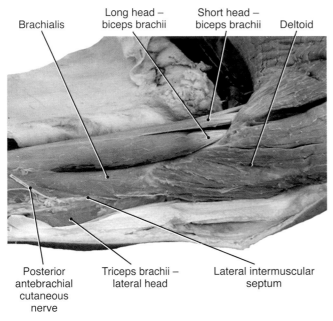

Brachialis

Long head – biceps brachii

Short head – biceps brachii

Deltoid

Posterior antebrachial cutaneous nerve

Triceps brachii – lateral head

Lateral intermuscular septum

Fig. 7.19 Upper arm view with skin reflected, revealing superficial musculature.

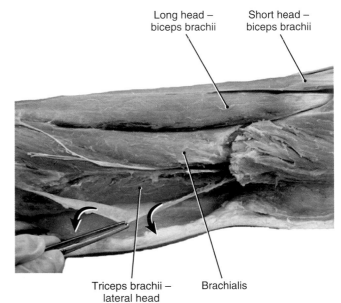

Long head – biceps brachii

Short head – biceps brachii

Triceps brachii – lateral head

Brachialis

Fig. 7.21 Reflection of deltoid and lateral head of triceps brachii, with exposure of posterior cutaneous nerve to the forearm.

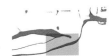

○ Trace the radial nerve to the radial groove of the humerus between the medial and long heads of the triceps brachii muscle (Fig. 7.22).

○ Trace the musculocutaneous nerve as it penetrates the coracobrachialis muscle; then lift the biceps brachii up and observe the course of the musculocutaneous nerve (Fig. 7.23).

○ Clean all soft tissues between the biceps brachii and brachialis muscles, and dissect the musculocutaneous nerve to the lateral aspect of the brachium as it emerges to become the lateral antebrachial cutaneous nerve (Fig. 7.24 and Plate 7.2).

○ Identify the three heads of the triceps brachii muscle.

The *lateral* head is the most inferior part of the triceps brachii muscle and is recognizable on the lateral surface of this muscle. The *medial* head arises from the posterior and medial surfaces of the humerus distal to the radial groove. The *long* head arises from the infraglenoid tubercle of the scapula and is located medial and proximal to the radial groove.

DISSECTION **TIP**

If time permits, trace the ascending branch of the deep brachial artery, and look for its anastomosis with the posterior circumflex humeral artery.

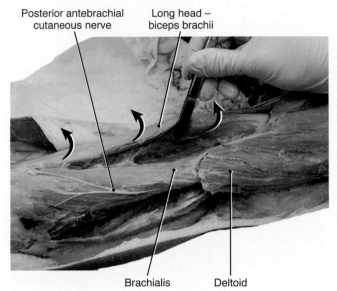

Posterior antebrachial cutaneous nerve

Long head – biceps brachii

Brachialis

Deltoid

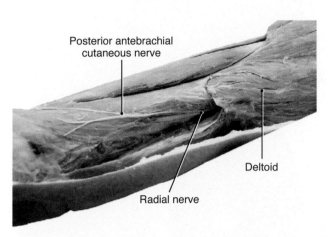

Posterior antebrachial cutaneous nerve

Deltoid

Radial nerve

Fig. 7.22 Reflection of deltoid and lateral head of triceps, with exposure of posterior cutaneous nerve to the forearm and radial nerve.

Fig. 7.23 Anterior arm view, with traction to biceps brachii revealing musculature and nerve.

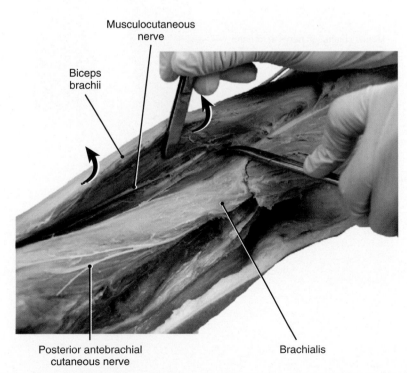

Musculocutaneous nerve

Biceps brachii

Posterior antebrachial cutaneous nerve

Brachialis

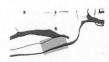

Fig. 7.24 Anterior view of the arm with elevation of the biceps brachii, demonstrating the underlying musculocutaneous nerve.

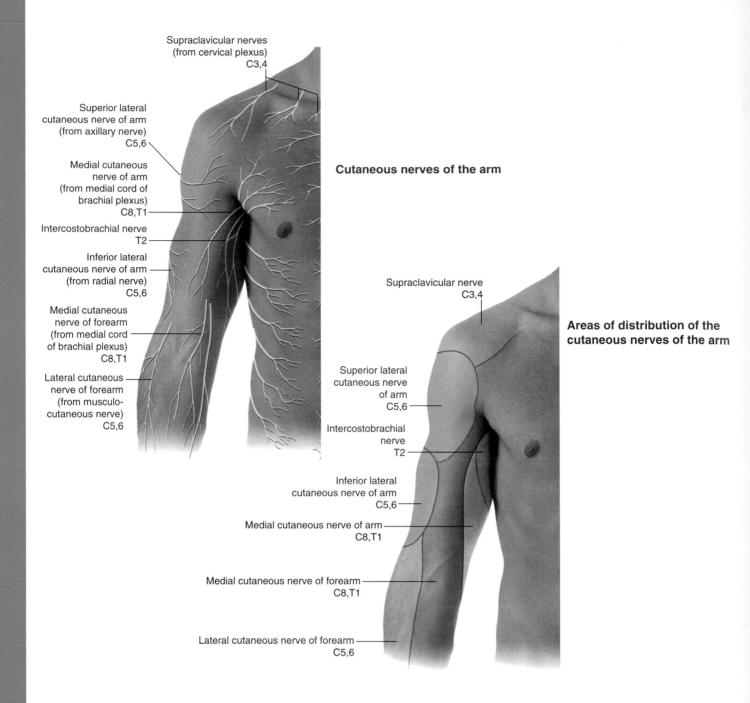

Cutaneous nerves of the arm

Supraclavicular nerves (from cervical plexus) C3,4

Superior lateral cutaneous nerve of arm (from axillary nerve) C5,6

Medial cutaneous nerve of arm (from medial cord of brachial plexus) C8,T1

Intercostobrachial nerve T2

Inferior lateral cutaneous nerve of arm (from radial nerve) C5,6

Medial cutaneous nerve of forearm (from medial cord of brachial plexus) C8,T1

Lateral cutaneous nerve of forearm (from musculo-cutaneous nerve) C5,6

Areas of distribution of the cutaneous nerves of the arm

Supraclavicular nerve C3,4

Superior lateral cutaneous nerve of arm C5,6

Intercostobrachial nerve T2

Inferior lateral cutaneous nerve of arm C5,6

Medial cutaneous nerve of arm C8,T1

Medial cutaneous nerve of forearm C8,T1

Lateral cutaneous nerve of forearm C5,6

Plate 7.2 Cutaneous innervation of the arm.

LABORATORY IDENTIFICATION CHECKLIST

NERVES

Lateral Cords
- ☐ Musculocutaneous
- ☐ Lateral pectoral

Medial Cords
- ☐ Medial pectoral
- ☐ Medial brachial cutaneous
- ☐ Medial antebrachial cutaneous
- ☐ Ulnar nerve

Posterior Cords
- ☐ Axillary
- ☐ Upper subscapular
- ☐ Lower subscapular
- ☐ Thoracodorsal
- ☐ Radial

ARTERIES
- ☐ Axillary
- ☐ Superior thoracic
- ☐ Thoracoacromial
- ☐ Pectoral
- ☐ Lateral thoracic
- ☐ Subscapular
- ☐ Thoracodorsal
- ☐ Circumflex scapular
- ☐ Anterior circumflex humeral
- ☐ Posterior circumflex humeral

VEINS
- ☐ Axillary
- ☐ Thoracoepigastric
- ☐ Cephalic
- ☐ Brachial
- ☐ Venae comitantes

LYMPH NODES (IF EVIDENT IN YOUR CADAVER)
- ☐ Infraclavicular
- ☐ Apical
- ☐ Lateral
- ☐ Central
- ☐ Subscapular
- ☐ Pectoral

MUSCLES
- ☐ Short head of biceps brachii
- ☐ Long head of biceps brachii
- ☐ Long head of triceps brachii
- ☐ Lateral head of triceps brachii
- ☐ Latissimus dorsi
- ☐ Pectoralis major
- ☐ Pectoralis minor
- ☐ Serratus anterior
- ☐ Subclavius
- ☐ Deltoid
- ☐ Subscapularis
- ☐ Teres major
- ☐ Teres minor

FASCIA
- ☐ Clavipectoral fascia

BONES
- ☐ Clavicle
- ☐ Humerus
- ☐ Scapula

ATLAS REFERENCES

Netter: 430–440, 463–469
McMinn: 148–153
Gray's Atlas: 424, 430–439, 457–459

BEFORE YOU BEGIN

Palpate the following bony landmarks on the cadaver or on yourself:

- Lateral and medial epicondyles of the humerus
- Styloid process of the radius
- Head, styloid process, olecranon, and shaft of the ulna
- Carpal bones

GETTING STARTED

- Continue the incision from the lateral side of the shoulder with a vertical incision across the length of the forearm toward the wrist.
- Make an encircling incision around the wrist (Fig. 8.1).
- Reflect the skin medially from the anterior compartment of the forearm, and expose the antebrachial fascia and the extensor retinaculum (Fig. 8.2).

- Identify the posterior cutaneous nerve of the forearm (posterior antebrachial nerve) (see Fig. 8.2).
- Identify the lateral cutaneous nerve to the forearm (lateral antebrachial cutaneous nerve), and medial cutaneous nerve to the forearm (medial antebrachial cutaneous nerve) (Fig. 8.3).

DISSECTION TIP

Preserve as many of the cutaneous nerve branches as possible. Typically, the posterior cutaneous nerve to the forearm emerges between the triceps brachii and brachialis muscles; the lateral cutaneous nerve to the forearm emerges lateral to the bicipital aponeurosis between the biceps brachii and brachioradialis muscles; and the medial cutaneous nerve to the forearm can be traced proximally to the medial cord of the brachial plexus.

CUBITAL FOSSA

- Reflect the skin over the bicipital aponeurosis, and expose the cubital fossa. The biceps brachii tendon enters the cubital fossa as an aponeurotic expansion.

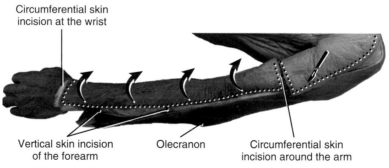

Fig. 8.1 Skin incisions for arm and forearm dissections.

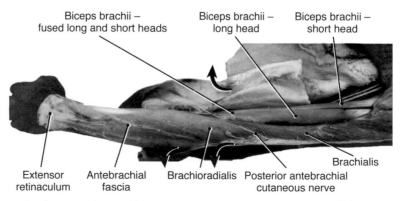

Fig. 8.2 Lateral arm and posterior forearm view with skin reflected, demonstrating superficial structures.

- Remove the deep fascia and the fat on the anterior surface of the cubital fossa, preserving the bicipital aponeurosis.
- Observe how the lateral and medial cutaneous nerves to the forearm relate to the bicipital aponeurosis (Fig. 8.4).
- Lateral to the tendon of the biceps brachii, separate the brachioradialis muscle from the brachialis muscle, and identify the **radial nerve** as it enters the forearm.
- Reflect the bicipital aponeurosis laterally, and identify the **brachial artery**, just deep to the veins of the cubital fossa.
- Retract the brachial artery laterally, and on its medial side, identify the **median nerve**.

LATERAL ARM AND EXTENSOR COMPARTMENT

- Continue the dissection by reflecting the skin over the extensor compartment of the forearm, and identify the distribution of the medial and lateral cutaneous nerves to the forearm (Fig. 8.5).
- Identify the **superficial branch of the radial nerve** just proximal to the lateral side of the wrist (Fig. 8.6).
- With a pair of scissors, make a small incision into the antebrachial fascia (deep fascia) near the lateral epicondyle (Fig. 8.7).
- Reflect the antebrachial fascia, and expose the underlying musculature of the extensor compartment of the forearm (Figs. 8.8 to 8.10).
- Remove all remnants of deep fascia covering the extensor surface.

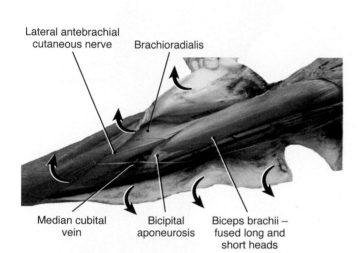

Fig. 8.3 Lateral arm view with skin reflected, demonstrating superficial structures.

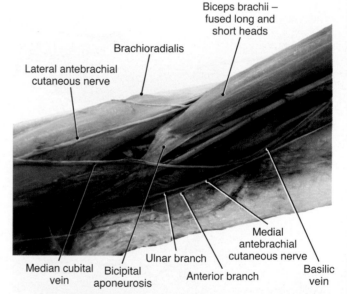

Fig. 8.4 Cubital region with skin reflected, showing superficial structures.

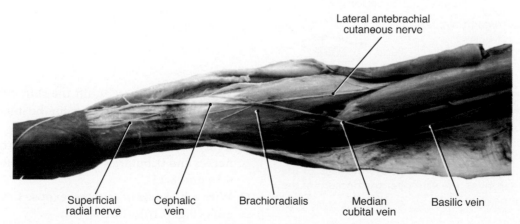

Fig. 8.5 Anterior arm and forearm view with skin reflected, demonstrating superficial structures.

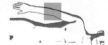

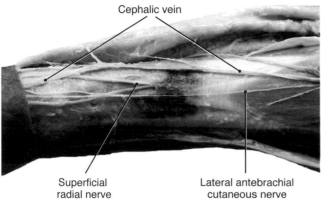

Cephalic vein

Superficial radial nerve

Lateral antebrachial cutaneous nerve

Fig. 8.6 Cubital fossa view with skin reflected, showing superficial structures.

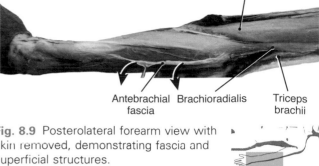

Biceps brachii – fused long and short heads

Antebrachial fascia   Brachioradialis   Triceps brachii

Fig. 8.9 Posterolateral forearm view with skin removed, demonstrating fascia and superficial structures.

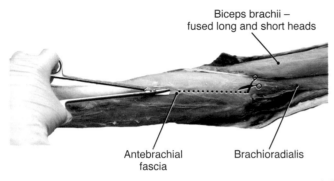

Biceps brachii – fused long and short heads

Antebrachial fascia

Brachioradialis

Fig. 8.7 Anterior forearm and cubital fossa view with skin removed, demonstrating fascia.

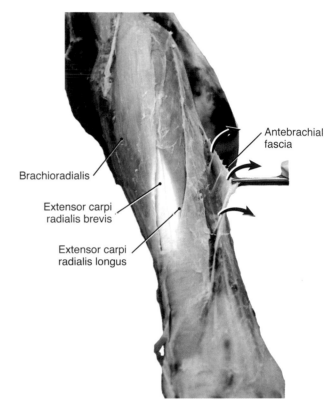

Antebrachial fascia

Brachioradialis

Extensor carpi radialis brevis

Extensor carpi radialis longus

Fig. 8.10 Posterior forearm view with skin reflected, showing fascia and superficial structures.

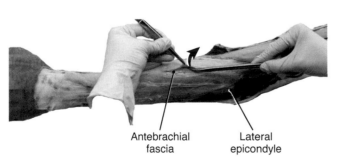

Antebrachial fascia

Lateral epicondyle

Fig. 8.8 Posterior forearm with skin removed, showing fascia.

DISSECTION TIP

Take special care when the deep fascia is removed. In the majority of cases, the deep fascia adheres tightly to the muscles of the extensor compartment (Fig. 8.11). To identify the tendinous insertions of the muscles of the extensor compartment, the skin over the dorsum of the hand also is removed.

○ Make a vertical incision at the midpoint of the wrist to the midline of the 3rd digit (Fig. 8.12).

○ With a pair of forceps, lift the skin over the dorsum of the hand, and detach it from the underlying dermis (Fig. 8.13).

○ Reflect the skin laterally without cutting any of the nerves and tributaries of the **dorsal venous arch** (Figs. 8.14 and 8.15).

○ With a fine pair of scissors, expose the dorsal venous arch (Fig. 8.16).

○ As the subcutaneous tissue is removed, pay special attention to identifying the cutaneous nerves running alongside the dorsal venous arch (Fig. 8.17).

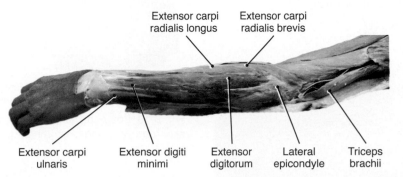

Extensor carpi radialis longus · Extensor carpi radialis brevis

Extensor carpi ulnaris · Extensor digiti minimi · Extensor digitorum · Lateral epicondyle · Triceps brachii

Fig. 8.11 Posterior arm and forearm view with skin removed, demonstrating fascia.

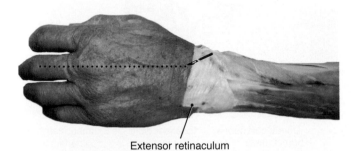

Extensor retinaculum

Fig. 8.12 Posterior wrist view with skin removed, showing extensor retinaculum.

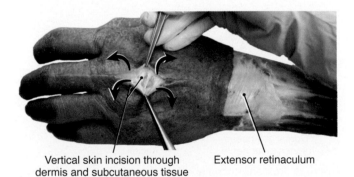

Vertical skin incision through dermis and subcutaneous tissue · Extensor retinaculum

Fig. 8.13 Posterior wrist view with skin removed, demonstrating extensor retinaculum.

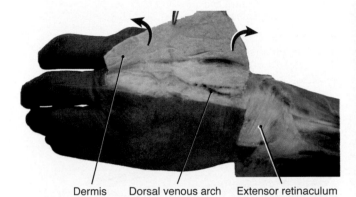

Dermis · Dorsal venous arch · Extensor retinaculum

Fig. 8.14 Posterior hand view after skin reflection.

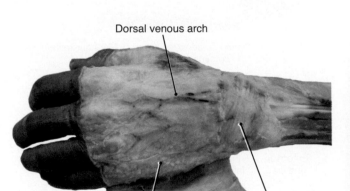

Dorsal venous arch

Dermis and subcutaneous tissue · Extensor retinaculum

Fig. 8.15 Posterior hand and wrist view with skin reflected, demonstrating superficial structures.

DISSECTION TIP

Exposing the dorsal venous arch and the cutaneous nerves on the dorsum of the hand can take some time (see Fig. 8.17). If time does not permit, skip this step and remove the subcutaneous tissue, dorsal venous arch, and cutaneous branches en bloc.

○ Continue the reflection of the skin over the 3rd digit (Fig. 8.18).
○ Identify the *extensor retinaculum,* a thick fibrous band of the antebrachial fascia that holds the tendons of the extensor compartment in place (Fig. 8.19).

○ Place a probe or scissors underneath the extensor retinaculum (Fig. 8.20), and release it from the underlying tendons.
○ Make a vertical incision, and retract the retinaculum laterally to expose the tendons of the extensor compartment (Fig. 8.21).
○ Identify the extensor digitorum muscle (see Fig. 8.21).
○ Lift its tendons and clean away its tendinous sheath (Fig. 8.22).

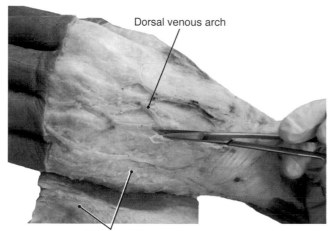

Dorsal venous arch

Dermis and subcutaneous tissue

Fig. 8.16 Posterior hand and wrist view with skin reflected, showing venous arch.

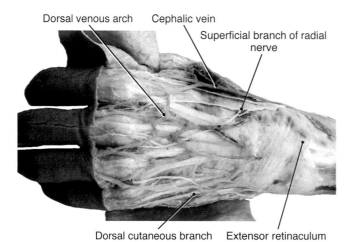

Dorsal venous arch   Cephalic vein

Superficial branch of radial nerve

Dorsal cutaneous branch of ulnar nerve   Extensor retinaculum

Fig. 8.17 Posterior hand and wrist view with skin reflected, highlighting superficial nerves and veins.

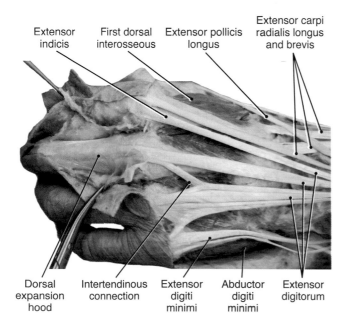

Extensor indicis   First dorsal interosseous   Extensor pollicis longus   Extensor carpi radialis longus and brevis

Dorsal expansion hood   Intertendinous connection   Extensor digiti minimi   Abductor digiti minimi   Extensor digitorum

Fig. 8.18 Posterior hand and wrist with skin reflected, exposing extensor tendons.

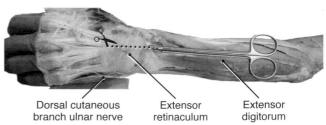

Dorsal cutaneous branch ulnar nerve   Extensor retinaculum   Extensor digitorum

Fig. 8.19 Posterior hand and forearm with skin removed, demonstrating superficial structures.

Extensor retinaculum

Extensor digitorum

Dorsal cutaneous branch ulnar nerve   Extensor digiti minimi   Extensor carpi ulnaris

Fig. 8.20 Posterior hand and forearm view with skin removed, showing superficial structures.

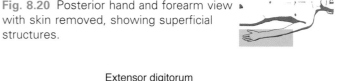

Extensor digitorum

Dorsal cutaneous branch ulnar nerve   Extensor digiti minimi

Fig. 8.21 Posterior hand and forearm with skin removed, highlighting superficial structures.

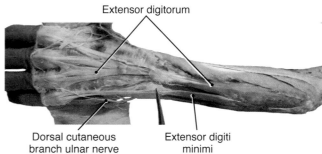

Tendinous sheath   Extensor pollicis brevis   Abductor pollicis longus

Dorsal cutaneous branch ulnar nerve   Extensor digiti minimi   Extensor carpi ulnaris   Extensor digitorum

Fig. 8.22 Posterior hand and forearm with skin reflected, demonstrating musculotendinous structures.

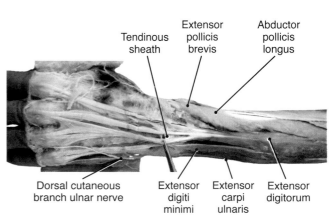

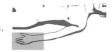
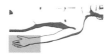
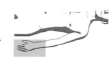
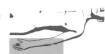
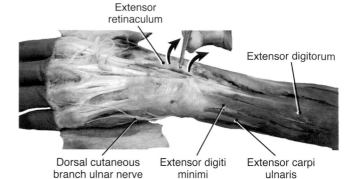

- On the radial side of the extensor digitorum muscle, identify the tendons of the **abductor pollicis longus**, **extensor pollicis brevis**, and **extensor pollicis longus** muscles (see Fig. 8.22).
- On its ulnar side, identify the **extensor digiti minimi** muscle, which is seen traveling to the 5th digit. In the majority of specimens, this muscle belly is fused with the extensor digitorum muscle (Fig. 8.23).

DISSECTION **TIP**

In the majority of specimens, the muscle bellies of the abductor pollicis longus and extensor pollicis brevis muscles are fused. Use your scissors to separate them (see Fig. 8.23).

- Lift the extensor digitorum muscle, and identify the **extensor indicis** muscle deep to it (Fig. 8.24). The extensor indicis typically runs along the ulnar side of the tendon from the extensor digitorum to the 2nd digit.
- At the distal third of the forearm, lift the extensor pollicis longus and extensor pollicis brevis muscles, and

underneath them, identify the **extensor carpi radialis longus and brevis** muscles (Figs. 8.25 and 8.26).
- Medial to the extensor carpi radialis brevis muscle, palpate Lister's (dorsal radial) tubercle (Fig. 8.27).
- On the ulnar side of the extensor digitorum, identify the extensor digiti minimi and the extensor carpi ulnaris muscles (Fig. 8.28).

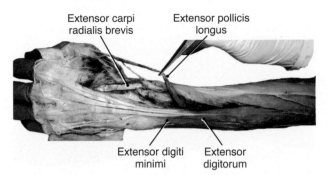

Fig. 8.25 Posterior hand and forearm view with skin reflected.

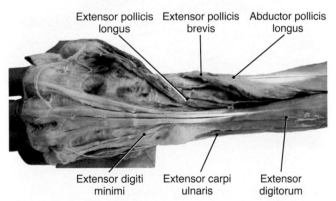

Fig. 8.23 Posterior hand and forearm with skin reflected, highlighting musculotendinous structures.

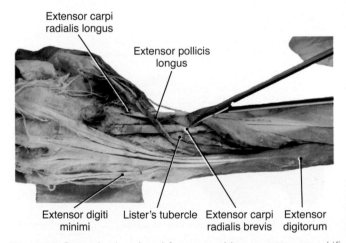

Fig. 8.26 Posterior hand and forearm with skin reflected.

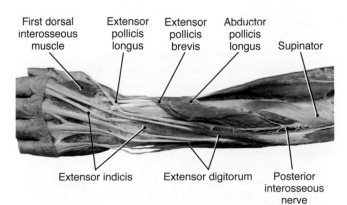

Fig. 8.24 Posterior forearm view with brachioradialis muscle reflected, demonstrating muscles and tendons.

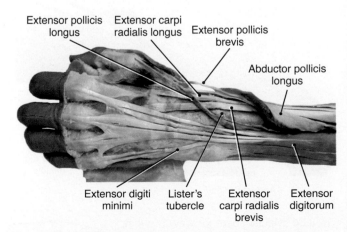

Fig. 8.27 Posterior hand and forearm with skin reflected.

- Follow the extensor carpi ulnaris to the wrist. Cut the extensor retinaculum (Fig. 8.29), and release the tendons underneath it (Fig. 8.30).
- Retract the extensor carpi ulnaris muscle, and separate it from the adjacent extensor digiti minimi muscle (Figs. 8.31 and 8.32).
- On the radial aspect of the proximal part of the forearm, identify and separate the **brachioradialis**, **extensor carpi radialis longus, extensor carpi radialis brevis, and extensor digitorum muscles** (Fig. 8.33).
- Lift the brachioradialis from the underlying extensor carpi radialis longus muscle. Use a probe or scissors to complete the separation of these two muscles (Figs. 8.34 and 8.35).
- Reflect or lift the brachioradialis muscle anteriorly, and identify the **radial nerve** (Fig. 8.36). Lift the brachioradialis muscle to allow maximum exposure of the radial nerve.
- Clean the radial nerve and identify its division into **superficial and deep branches.** The superficial branch runs beneath the brachioradialis to reach the dorsum of the hand. The deep branch of the radial nerve runs through the **supinator muscle.**
- With a pair of scissors, cut between the fibers of the extensor carpi radialis brevis and extensor digitorum muscles, and expose the supinator muscle lying underneath (Fig. 8.37).

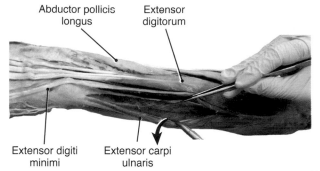

Abductor pollicis longus
Extensor digitorum
Extensor digiti minimi
Extensor carpi ulnaris

Fig. 8.28 Anteromedial forearm view, demonstrating ulnar artery and nerves.

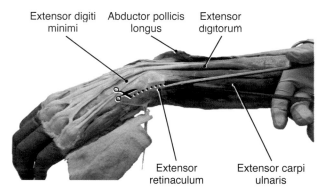

Extensor digiti minimi
Abductor pollicis longus
Extensor digitorum
Extensor retinaculum
Extensor carpi ulnaris

Fig. 8.29 Medial posterior view of wrist, demonstrating superficial structures.

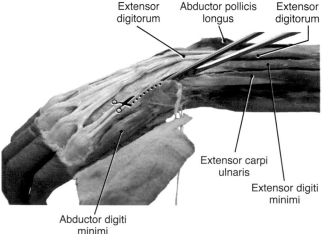

Extensor digitorum
Abductor pollicis longus
Extensor digitorum
Extensor carpi ulnaris
Extensor digiti minimi
Abductor digiti minimi

Fig. 8.30 Medial posterior view of wrist, demonstrating superficial structures.

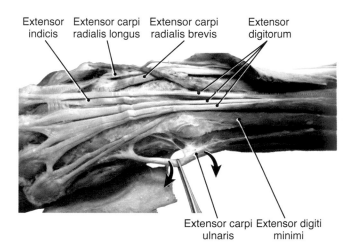

Extensor indicis
Extensor carpi radialis longus
Extensor carpi radialis brevis
Extensor digitorum
Extensor carpi ulnaris
Extensor digiti minimi

Fig. 8.31 Posteromedial view of wrist, showing muscle tendons.

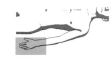

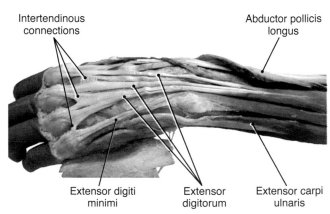

Intertendinous connections
Abductor pollicis longus
Extensor digiti minimi
Extensor digitorum
Extensor carpi ulnaris

Fig. 8.32 Posteromedial view of wrist, exposing muscle tendons.

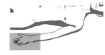

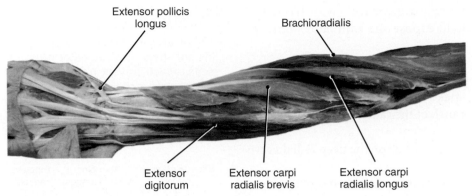

Extensor pollicis longus

Brachioradialis

Extensor digitorum

Extensor carpi radialis brevis

Extensor carpi radialis longus

Fig. 8.33 Posterior view of upper forearm, highlighting musculature.

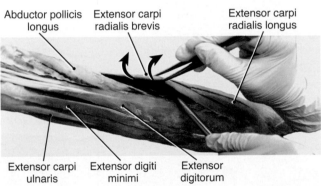

Abductor pollicis longus

Extensor carpi radialis brevis

Extensor carpi radialis longus

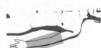

Extensor carpi ulnaris

Extensor digiti minimi

Extensor digitorum

Fig. 8.34 Posterior upper forearm view, demonstrating musculature.

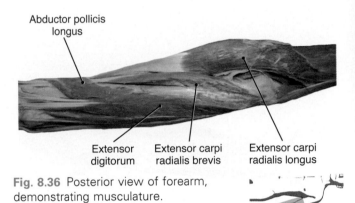

Abductor pollicis longus

Extensor digitorum

Extensor carpi radialis brevis

Extensor carpi radialis longus

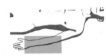

Fig. 8.36 Posterior view of forearm, demonstrating musculature.

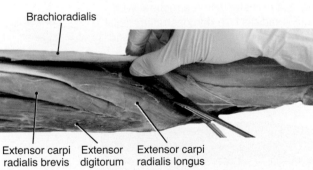

Brachioradialis

Extensor carpi radialis brevis

Extensor digitorum

Extensor carpi radialis longus

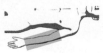

Fig. 8.35 Posterior upper forearm view, showing musculature.

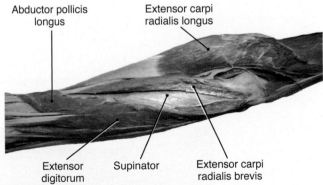

Abductor pollicis longus

Extensor carpi radialis longus

Extensor digitorum

Supinator

Extensor carpi radialis brevis

Fig. 8.37 Posterior view of forearm, showing musculature.

- Reflect the extensor digitorum away from the supinator muscle to expose the supinator's borders (Fig. 8.38).
- At the inferior border of the supinator, trace and expose the **deep radial nerve** (Fig. 8.39, Plate 8.1). With a scalpel, make an **incision in the supinator** where the deep branch of the radial nerve first enters it (Fig. 8.40).
- Reflect the supinator, and expose the deep radial nerve (Fig. 8.41, Plate 8.2).
- Make an incision on the posterior border of the ulna, and detach the extensor carpi ulnaris muscle. Look for the emergence of the **posterior interosseous artery** running parallel to the deep branch of the radial nerve between the radius and the ulna.

DISSECTION **TIP**

The recurrent interosseous artery can be found between the anconeus and supinator muscles. Remove the anconeus, which travels from the lateral epicondyle to the lateral aspect of the olecranon. Just beneath it, on the anterior surface of the supinator, identify the recurrent interosseous artery. This artery is usually small and often is cut during routine dissection.

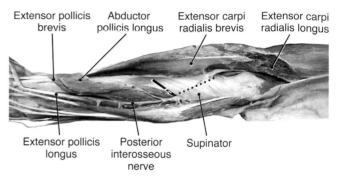
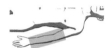

Fig. 8.40 Posterior view with brachioradialis cut, demonstrating supinator muscle.

Extensor pollicis brevis — Abductor pollicis longus — Extensor carpi radialis brevis — Extensor carpi radialis longus

Extensor pollicis longus — Posterior interosseous nerve — Supinator

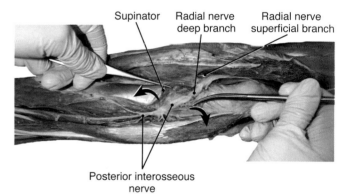
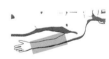

Fig. 8.41 Posterior forearm view with brachioradialis cut, demonstrating radial nerve branches, supinator muscle, and posterior interosseous nerve.

Supinator — Radial nerve deep branch — Radial nerve superficial branch

Posterior interosseous nerve

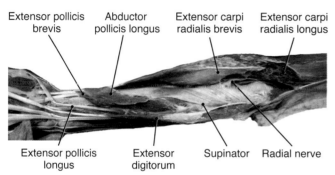

Extensor pollicis brevis — Abductor pollicis longus — Extensor carpi radialis brevis — Extensor carpi radialis longus

Extensor pollicis longus — Extensor digitorum — Supinator — Radial nerve

Fig. 8.38 Posterior view with brachioradialis muscle cut, demonstrating radial nerve and supinator muscle.

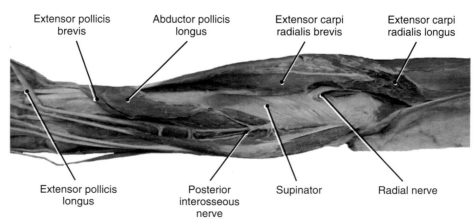

Extensor pollicis brevis — Abductor pollicis longus — Extensor carpi radialis brevis — Extensor carpi radialis longus

Extensor pollicis longus — Posterior interosseous nerve — Supinator — Radial nerve

Fig. 8.39 Posterior view with brachioradialis muscle cut, showing radial nerve and supinator muscle.

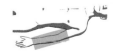

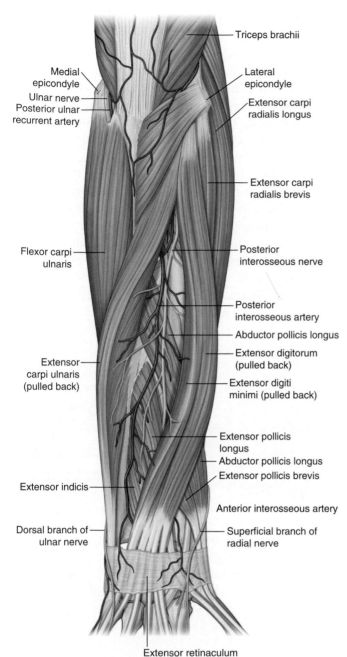

Triceps brachii

Medial epicondyle

Lateral epicondyle

Ulnar nerve

Extensor carpi radialis longus

Posterior ulnar recurrent artery

Extensor carpi radialis brevis

Flexor carpi ulnaris

Posterior interosseous nerve

Posterior interosseous artery

Abductor pollicis longus

Extensor digitorum (pulled back)

Extensor carpi ulnaris (pulled back)

Extensor digiti minimi (pulled back)

Extensor pollicis longus

Abductor pollicis longus

Extensor indicis

Extensor pollicis brevis

Anterior interosseous artery

Dorsal branch of ulnar nerve

Superficial branch of radial nerve

Extensor retinaculum

Plate 8.1 Arteries and nerves of the extensor compartment of the forearm.

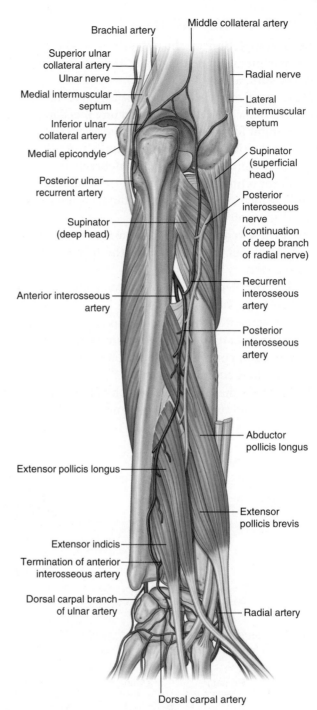

Brachial artery

Middle collateral artery

Superior ulnar collateral artery

Ulnar nerve

Radial nerve

Medial intermuscular septum

Lateral intermuscular septum

Inferior ulnar collateral artery

Medial epicondyle

Supinator (superficial head)

Posterior ulnar recurrent artery

Posterior interosseous nerve (continuation of deep branch of radial nerve)

Supinator (deep head)

Recurrent interosseous artery

Anterior interosseous artery

Posterior interosseous artery

Abductor pollicis longus

Extensor pollicis longus

Extensor pollicis brevis

Extensor indicis

Termination of anterior interosseous artery

Dorsal carpal branch of ulnar artery

Radial artery

Dorsal carpal artery

Plate 8.2 Arteries and nerves of the extensor compartment of the forearm (deeper dissection).

FLEXOR COMPARTMENT

- After completion of the dissection of the extensor compartment, rotate the upper limb and visualize the flexor compartment (Fig. 8.42).
- Make a vertical incision across the length of the forearm toward the wrist. Make an encircling incision around the cubital fossa and the wrist (see Fig. 8.42).
- Reflect the skin medially and laterally from the flexor compartment, and expose the antebrachial fascia and the flexor retinaculum (Fig. 8.43). Continue the vertical midline incision toward the 3rd digit. Chapter 9 details the dissection of the hand.
- Identify the venous network in the flexor compartment and in the cubital fossa. Trace the tributaries of the basilic vein.
- Identify the **median cubital vein** connecting the **basilic** and **cephalic veins** (Fig. 8.44).
- Once you identify the cephalic vein, trace it proximally to the arm. Lateral to the cephalic vein, identify the **lateral cutaneous nerve to the forearm, or lateral antebrachial cutaneous nerve.**
- This nerve is the cutaneous branch of **musculocutaneous nerve** and supplies the lateral aspect of the forearm (see Fig. 8.44).

- Notice the thick, flat connective tissue aponeurosis of the biceps brachii muscle, the *bicipital aponeurosis.*
- An easy way to identify the muscles of the forearm is to expose them from the wrist toward the cubital fossa.
- At the wrist, the tendons of each muscle are fairly evident and require minimal dissection.
- The following three muscles occupy the superficial layer of the muscles of the flexor compartment.
  - On the radial side of the forearm, identify the **flexor carpi radialis** muscle (Fig. 8.45). The flexor carpi radialis attaches to the second metacarpal bone, and some of its fibers may radiate to the adjacent 3rd metacarpal.
  - Medial to the flexor carpi radialis, note the **palmaris longus** muscle inserting into the palmar aponeurosis.
  - On the ulnar side of the forearm, identify the **flexor carpi ulnaris** muscle.

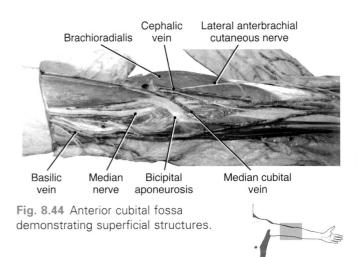

Fig. 8.44 Anterior cubital fossa demonstrating superficial structures.

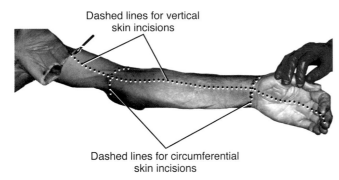

Fig. 8.42 Anterior view of arm, forearm, and hand, with dashed lines for incisions.

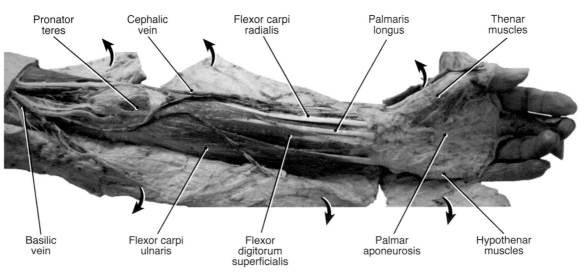

Fig. 8.43 Anterior view of forearm and hand with skin reflected, demonstrating superficial structures.

DISSECTION TIP

The palmaris longus muscle is absent in roughly 10% of the population.

○ Dissect out the deep fascia and the connective tissue over the tendons and the muscles of the flexor compartment (Figs. 8.46 and 8.47).

○ Expose the tendon insertions of the flexor carpi ulnaris and flexor carpi radialis muscles (Fig. 8.48).

○ Deep to the palmaris longus muscle, note the **flexor digitorum superficialis muscle.**

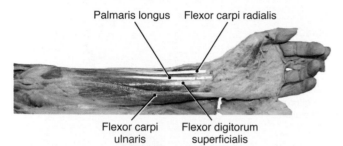

Fig. 8.45 Anterior view of forearm and hand showing muscle-tendon units.

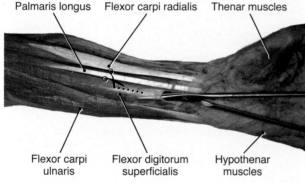
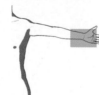

Fig. 8.46 Anterior forearm and hand demonstrating muscle-tendon units.

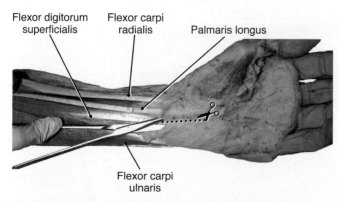

Fig. 8.47 Anterior forearm and hand, highlighting muscle-tendon units.

○ Retract the flexor carpi ulnaris, and in the space between it and the **flexor digitorum superficialis,** identify a thick bundle of connective tissue encircling the **ulnar artery and nerve** (Fig. 8.49).

○ With the aid of scissors, separate the connective tissue over the ulnar artery and nerve (Fig. 8.50).

○ Further retract the flexor digitorum superficialis muscle, and clean and expose the ulnar artery and nerve along the entire length of the forearm (Figs. 8.51 and 8.52).

○ Underneath the flexor digitorum superficialis, identify the **flexor digitorum profundus** muscle.

○ Clean the loose connective tissue over the flexor digitorum profundus (Fig. 8.53).

○ Identify the **radial artery** between the brachioradialis and flexor carpi radialis muscles (Fig. 8.54).

○ Further retract the brachioradialis muscle, and expose the radial artery in the forearm (Figs. 8.55 and 8.56).

○ Parallel to the radial artery, identify and expose the **superficial branch of the radial nerve** (Fig. 8.57).

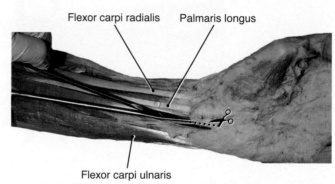

Fig. 8.48 Anterior view of forearm and hand showing muscle-tendon units.

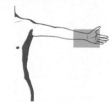

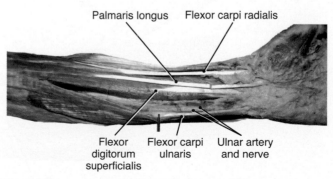

Fig. 8.49 Anterior forearm and hand view, demonstrating muscle-tendon units, with traction of flexor carpi ulnaris.

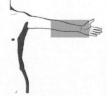

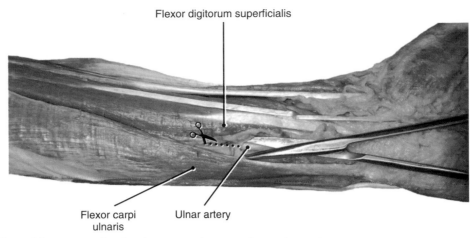

Flexor digitorum superficialis

Flexor carpi
ulnaris

Ulnar artery

Fig. 8.50 Anterior view of forearm and wrist demonstrating muscle-tendon units.

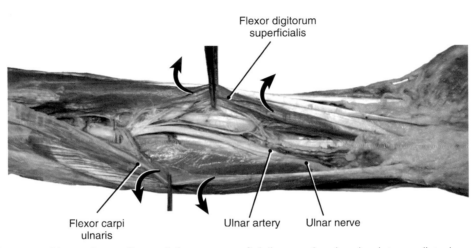

Flexor digitorum
superficialis

Flexor carpi
ulnaris

Ulnar artery

Ulnar nerve

Fig. 8.51 Anterior forearm with traction to flexor digitorum superficialis muscle, showing intermediate layer.

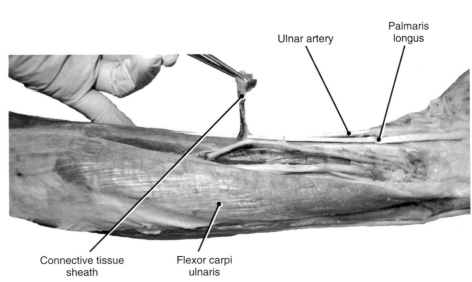

Ulnar artery

Palmaris
longus

Connective tissue
sheath

Flexor carpi
ulnaris

Fig. 8.52 Anterior forearm noting the flexor carpi ulnaris and palmaris longus muscles.

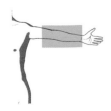

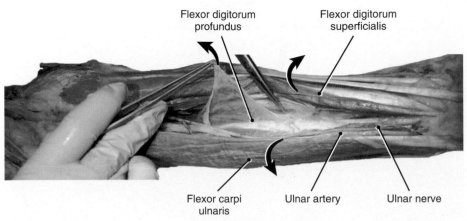

Fig. 8.53 Anterior forearm view with traction to flexor digitorum superficialis muscle, exposing the flexor digitorum profundus.

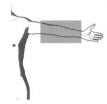

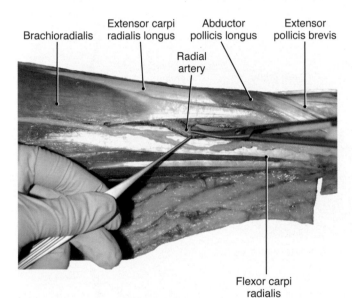

Fig. 8.54 Anterolateral view of distal forearm, demonstrating radial neurovascular bundle.

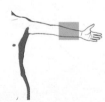

DISSECTION TIP

Note the following landmarks in the course of the radial artery:
- Passes superficial to the pronator teres muscle.
- Travels deep to the brachioradialis muscle.

At the wrist, the radial artery is found between the tendons of the flexor carpi radialis and the brachioradialis muscles. This point is used to feel the radial pulse or to perform arterial catheterization.

○ The flexor digitorum profundus muscle inserts onto the bases of the distal phalanx of each of the medial four digits.

DISSECTION TIP

A common variation of the flexor digitorum profundus is that its tendon to the 2nd digit may form an independent muscle. The flexor pollicis longus muscle inserts onto the distal phalanx of the 1st digit.

○ The flexor digitorum superficialis muscle inserts onto the base of the middle phalanx of digits 2 to 5. However, the tendon to the 5th digit may be absent.
○ Expose the radial artery (Fig. 8.58).

CUBITAL FOSSA AND FLEXOR COMPARTMENT

○ Cut the bicipital aponeurosis (Fig. 8.59) to trace the radial artery to its branch point from the brachial artery.
○ Coursing with the ulnar artery, identify the median nerve, and the vena comitans (Fig. 8.60).
○ Lift the brachial and radial arteries, and expose the ulnar artery with its branches (Fig. 8.61).
○ At this point, use a retractor between the brachioradialis and the flexor digitorum superficialis muscles to expose deeper structures (Fig. 8.62).
○ Follow the course of the ulnar and radial arteries, and identify the recurrent ulnar and recurrent radial arteries.
○ Identify the pronator teres and its two heads; the humeral (superficial) head is attached to the medial epicondyle and the ulnar (deep) head to the coronoid process of the ulna.
○ Trace the course of the medial nerve as it travels from the cubital fossa and then enters the forearm between the two heads of the pronator teres (see Fig. 8.62).
○ Note the ulnar artery entering the forearm deep to the ulnar (deep) head of the pronator teres muscle (see Fig. 8.62).

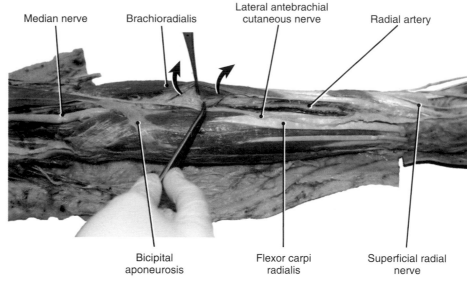

Median nerve　　Brachioradialis　　Lateral antebrachial cutaneous nerve　　Radial artery

Bicipital aponeurosis　　Flexor carpi radialis　　Superficial radial nerve

Fig. 8.55 Anteromedial view of forearm with skin reflected, demonstrating radial artery and vein.

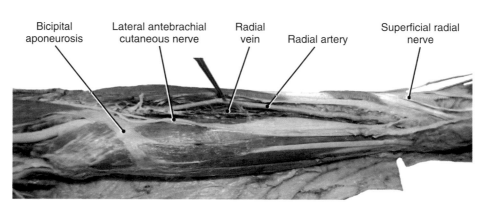

Bicipital aponeurosis　　Lateral antebrachial cutaneous nerve　　Radial vein　　Radial artery　　Superficial radial nerve

Fig. 8.56 Anterior forearm view with skin reflected, demonstrating radial artery and vein.

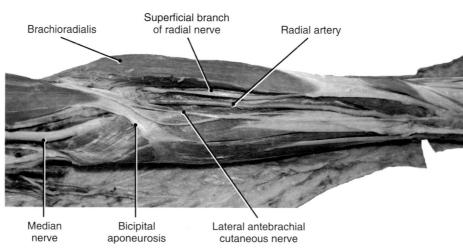

Brachioradialis　　Superficial branch of radial nerve　　Radial artery

Median nerve　　Bicipital aponeurosis　　Lateral antebrachial cutaneous nerve

Fig. 8.57 Anterior forearm view, showing radial artery, vein, and nerve.

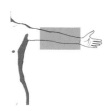

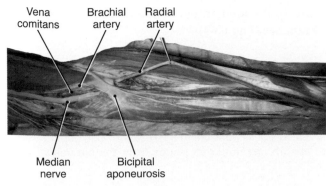

Vena comitans   Brachial artery   Radial artery

Median nerve   Bicipital aponeurosis

Fig. 8.58 Anterior forearm view with radial artery and traction, demonstrating musculature.

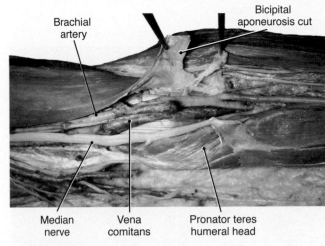

Brachial artery   Bicipital aponeurosis cut

Median nerve   Vena comitans   Pronator teres humeral head

Fig. 8.60 Anterior cubital fossa view with bicipital aponeurosis reflected, highlighting brachial artery and median nerve.

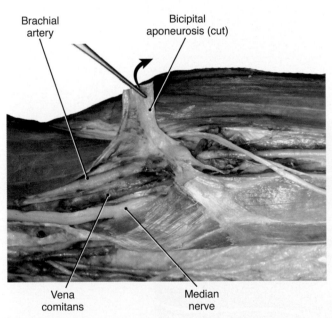

Brachial artery   Bicipital aponeurosis (cut)

Vena comitans   Median nerve

Fig. 8.59 Anterior view of cubital fossa with bicipital aponeurosis reflected, demonstrating brachial artery and median nerve.

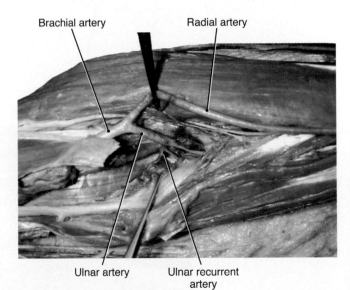

Brachial artery   Radial artery

Ulnar artery   Ulnar recurrent artery

Fig. 8.61 Anterior view of cubital fossa with bicipital aponeurosis cut, demonstrating the bifurcation of the brachial artery.

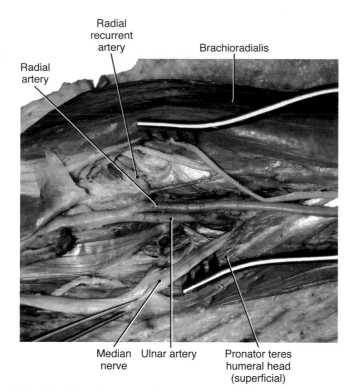

Fig. 8.62 Anterior cubital fossa view with bicipital aponeurosis reflected, exposing neurovascular structures.

○ Lift up the median nerve, and identify its muscular branches (Fig. 8.63).

DISSECTION TIP

To continue the dissection, the vena comitans must be removed (Fig. 8.64). Cut the veins in the cubital fossa and as distal as possible in the forearm. Use paper towels to absorb any fluid that issues from the cut veins.

○ Expose the borders of the pronator teres, and retract the radial artery (Fig. 8.65).
○ Carefully **split the humeral head of the pronator teres** (Fig. 8.66) from the underlying ulnar (deep) head and flexor digitorum superficialis muscle (Figs. 8.67 and 8.68).
○ Lift the median nerve and expose its course in the deep flexor compartment of the forearm (Fig. 8.69).
○ Dissect distally the **ulnar artery** and identify the common interosseous artery (Fig. 8.70).
○ The common interosseous artery arises from the ulnar artery and then divides into the anterior and posterior interosseous branches (Fig. 8.71).

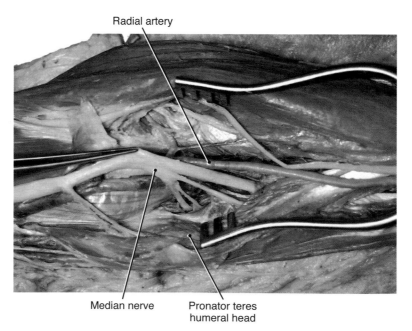

Fig. 8.63 Cubital fossa view with bicipital aponeurosis reflected, demonstrating neurovascular structures.

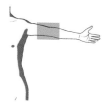

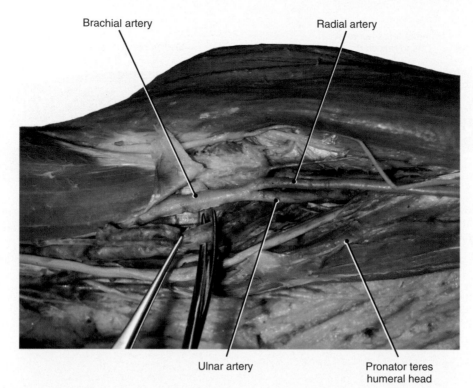

Brachial artery   Radial artery

Ulnar artery   Pronator teres
                humeral head

Fig. 8.64 Anterior view of cubital fossa with bicipital aponeurosis reflected, highlighting neurovascular structures.

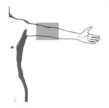

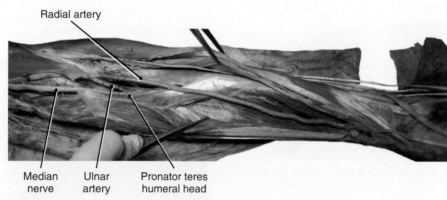

Radial artery

Median   Ulnar   Pronator teres
nerve   artery   humeral head

Fig. 8.65 Anterolateral forearm view with skin reflected, demonstrating radial artery and musculature.

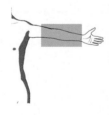

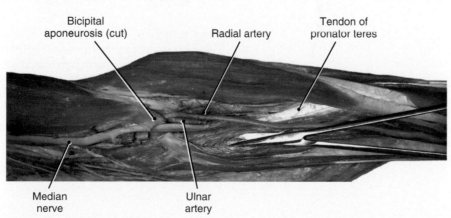

Bicipital   Radial artery   Tendon of
aponeurosis (cut)   pronator teres

Median   Ulnar
nerve   artery

Fig. 8.66 Anterior cubital fossa with bicipital aponeurosis cut, exposing median nerve, radial artery, and pronator teres muscle.

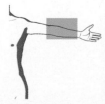

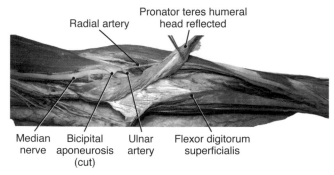

Radial artery

Pronator teres humeral
head reflected

Median
nerve

Bicipital
aponeurosis
(cut)

Ulnar
artery

Flexor digitorum
superficialis

Fig. 8.67 Anterior view of lateral cubital
fossa and forearm with reflected pronator
teres, demonstrating musculature.

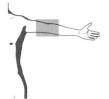

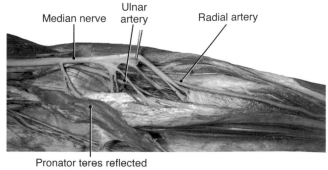

Median nerve

Ulnar
artery

Radial artery

Pronator teres reflected

Fig. 8.69 Anterior cubital fossa view with
superficial (humeral) head of pronator teres
muscle reflected, and median nerve
traction demonstrating deep (ulnar) head of
pronator teres.

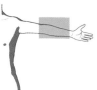

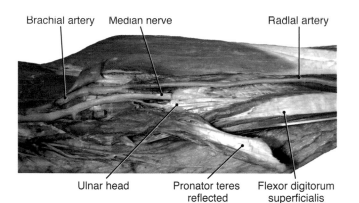

Brachial artery   Median nerve

Radial artery

Ulnar head

Pronator teres
reflected

Flexor digitorum
superficialis

Fig. 8.68 Anterior cubital fossa view with
pronator teres muscle reflected,
demonstrating deeper structures.

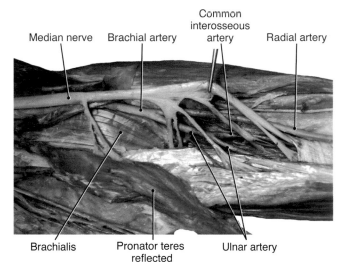

Median nerve   Brachial artery

Common
interosseous
artery

Radial artery

Brachialis

Pronator teres
reflected

Ulnar artery

Fig. 8.70 Anterior cubital fossa view with
superficial pronator teres head reflected,
and median nerve traction demonstrating
deep pronator teres head, and radial and
ulnar arteries.

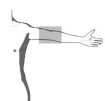

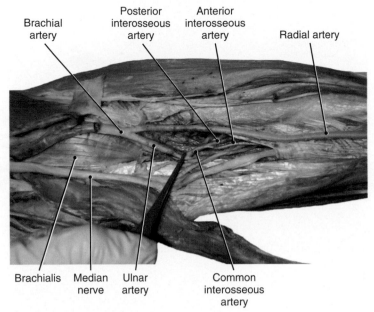

Brachial artery
Posterior interosseous artery
Anterior interosseous artery
Radial artery

Brachialis
Median nerve
Ulnar artery
Common interosseous artery

Fig. 8.71 Anterior cubital fossa view with superficial head of pronator teres reflected, and median nerve traction demonstrating deep head of pronator teres and radial and ulnar arteries.

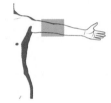

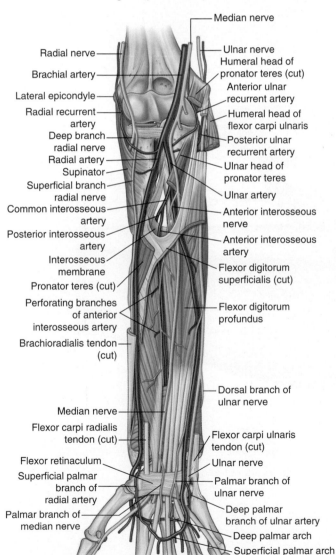

Median nerve

Radial nerve
Brachial artery
Lateral epicondyle
Radial recurrent artery
Deep branch radial nerve
Radial artery
Supinator
Superficial branch radial nerve
Common interosseous artery
Posterior interosseous artery
Interosseous membrane
Pronator teres (cut)
Perforating branches of anterior interosseous artery
Brachioradialis tendon (cut)

Median nerve
Flexor carpi radialis tendon (cut)
Flexor retinaculum
Superficial palmar branch of radial artery
Palmar branch of median nerve

Ulnar nerve
Humeral head of pronator teres (cut)
Anterior ulnar recurrent artery
Humeral head of flexor carpi ulnaris
Posterior ulnar recurrent artery
Ulnar head of pronator teres
Ulnar artery
Anterior interosseous nerve
Anterior interosseous artery
Flexor digitorum superficialis (cut)
Flexor digitorum profundus

Dorsal branch of ulnar nerve

Flexor carpi ulnaris tendon (cut)
Ulnar nerve
Palmar branch of ulnar nerve
Deep palmar branch of ulnar artery
Deep palmar arch
Superficial palmar arch

Plate 8.3 Arteries and nerve of the flexor compartment of the forearm.

○ The posterior interosseous artery passes through the interosseous membrane to reach the extensor compartment of the forearm.

○ As the median nerve is lifted, identify the anterior interosseous nerve, which arises from the median nerve just proximal to the pronator teres muscle (see Figs. 8.70 and 8.71, Plate 8.3).

DEEP FLEXOR COMPARTMENT

○ Cut the tendons of the flexor digitorum superficialis, or widely retract them, and identify the **flexor digitorum profundus** and **flexor pollicis longus** muscles (Fig. 8.72).

○ Finally, identify the **pronator quadratus**, which connects the distal portions of the ulna and radius (Fig. 8.73).

○ In the space between the flexor pollicis longus and flexor digitorum profundus muscles, trace the course of the anterior interosseous artery and anterior interosseous nerve, a branch of the median nerve (see Figs. 8.72 and 8.73).

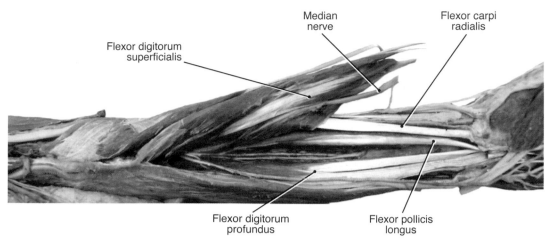

Flexor digitorum
superficialis

Median
nerve

Flexor carpi
radialis

Flexor digitorum
profundus

Flexor pollicis
longus

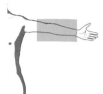

Fig. 8.72 Anterior forearm view with superficial and intermediate muscle layers cut and reflected, exposing deeper structures.

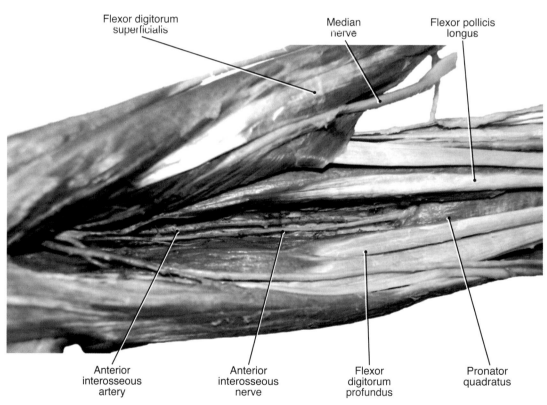

Flexor digitorum
superficialis

Median
nerve

Flexor pollicis
longus

Anterior
interosseous
artery

Anterior
interosseous
nerve

Flexor
digitorum
profundus

Pronator
quadratus

Fig. 8.73 Anterior view of forearm with superficial and intermediate muscle layers cut and reflected, demonstrating deeper structures.

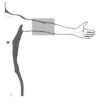

LABORATORY IDENTIFICATION CHECKLIST

NERVES
- [ ] Musculocutaneous
- [ ] Lateral antebrachial cutaneous
- [ ] Median
- [ ] Anterior interosseous
- [ ] Medial brachial cutaneous
- [ ] Medial antebrachial cutaneous
- [ ] Ulnar
- [ ] Radial
- [ ] Posterior interosseous

ARTERIES
- [ ] Brachial
- [ ] Radial
- [ ] Radial recurrent
- [ ] Interosseous recurrent
- [ ] Ulnar
- [ ] Common interosseous
- [ ] Anterior interosseous
- [ ] Posterior interosseous
- [ ] Ulnar anterior recurrent
- [ ] Ulnar posterior recurrent

VEINS
Superficial
- [ ] Cephalic
- [ ] Basilic
- [ ] Cubital

Deep
- [ ] Brachial
- [ ] Radial
- [ ] Ulnar

MUSCLES
Anterior Compartment of Arm
- [ ] Coracobrachialis
- [ ] Biceps brachii
  - [ ] Long head
  - [ ] Short head
- [ ] Brachialis

Posterior Compartment of Arm
- [ ] Triceps brachii
  - [ ] Long head
  - [ ] Lateral head
  - [ ] Medial head
- [ ] Anconeus

Anterior Compartment of Forearm
Superficial Layer
- [ ] Pronator teres
  - [ ] Humeral (superficial) head
  - [ ] Ulnar (deep) head
- [ ] Flexor carpi radialis
- [ ] Palmaris longus
- [ ] Flexor carpi ulnaris

Intermediate Layer
- [ ] Flexor digitorum superficialis

Deep Layer
- [ ] Flexor digitorum profundus
- [ ] Flexor pollicis longus
- [ ] Pronator quadratus

Posterior Compartment of Forearm
Superficial Layer
- [ ] Brachioradialis
- [ ] Extensor carpi radialis longus
- [ ] Extensor carpi radialis brevis
- [ ] Extensor digitorum
- [ ] Extensor digiti minimi
- [ ] Extensor carpi ulnaris

Deep Layer
- [ ] Supinator
- [ ] Abductor pollicis longus
- [ ] Extensor pollicis longus
- [ ] Extensor pollicis brevis
- [ ] Extensor indicis

LIGAMENTS
- [ ] Ulnar collateral
- [ ] Radial collateral
- [ ] Anular

CONNECTIVE TISSUE
- [ ] Bicipital aponeurosis
- [ ] Antebrachial fascia
- [ ] Flexor retinaculum
- [ ] Extensor retinaculum

BONES
- [ ] Scapula
- [ ] Humerus
- [ ] Radius
- [ ] Ulna
- [ ] Carpals
- [ ] Metacarpals
- [ ] Phalanges

ATLAS REFERENCES
Netter: 442–469
McMinn: 154–169
Gray's Atlas: 426–429, 440–456

BEFORE YOU BEGIN
Palpation

Flex and extend your digits, noting the movements of the tendons beneath the skin. On the dorsal side of your hand, identify the tendons of the extensor digitorum muscle. At the flexor aspect of the palm, note the distal skin crease (crease between wrist and forearm), marking the proximal edge of the flexor retinaculum (Fig. 9.1).

- At the ulnar side of the distal skin crease, palpate the pisiform bone. At the radial side of the distal skin crease, palpate the scaphoid bone. Immediately beneath the radial and ulnar sides of the distal skin crease, palpate the **radial** and **ulnar styloid processes**, respectively.
- By flexing the closed fist against resistance, you should be able to identify several tendons at the anterior wrist, from medial to lateral: the flexor carpi ulnaris, flexor digitorum superficialis, palmaris longus, and flexor carpi radialis. However, the most prominent tendons are those of the palmaris longus, lying at the midline, and the flexor carpi radialis, lying in the radial side. Lateral to the tendon of the flexor carpi radialis, you can palpate the radial artery. The pulsations of the ulnar artery are more difficult to detect but usually are felt about 3 cm proximal to the pisiform bone, lateral to the flexor carpi ulnaris muscle. Note the thenar and hypothenar eminences, which contain muscles of the 1st digit and the 5th digit, respectively.

On the dorsum surface of the hand, extend the 1st digit, noting the tendons of the abductor pollicis longus (to base of 1st metacarpal bone), the extensor pollicis brevis (to base of 1st phalanx), and the extensor pollicis longus muscles (to base of distal phalanx of 1st digit) forming the "anatomic snuffbox" (Fig. 9.2). This anatomic area is important because the radial artery lies on the scaphoid bone and passes to reach the dorsum of the 1st digit.

If the dorsum of the hand has not been dissected already on your cadaver as it was in Chapter 8, then refer to Chapter 8, Figs. 8.12 to 8.16 before proceeding to the palmar dissection (Fig. 9.3).

PALMAR HAND

○ Make a similar midline incision on the palmar surface, starting from the distal palmar crease to the base of

Metacarpo-phalangeal joint

Interphalangeal joints

Palmar creases

Thenar eminence

Hypothenar eminence

Distal wrist crease

Proximal wrist crease

Fig. 9.1 Anterior view of palmar surface of hand. Note positioning of interphalangeal and metacarpal phalangeal joints, palmar and wrist creases, and thenar and hypothenar eminences.

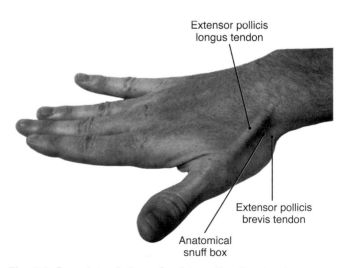

Extensor pollicis longus tendon

Extensor pollicis brevis tendon

Anatomical snuff box

Fig. 9.2 Dorsolateral view of wrist, noting "anatomic snuffbox," which is bordered by the underlying extensor pollicis longus and brevis tendons.

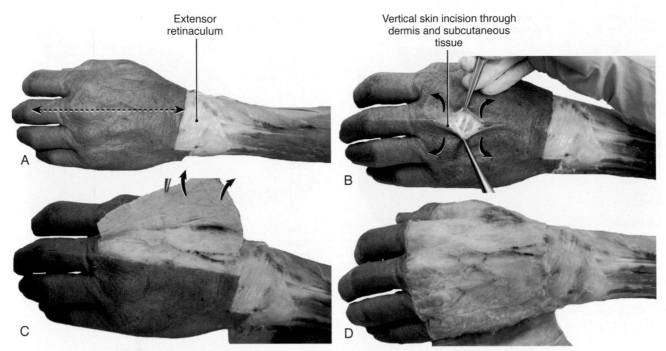

Fig. 9.3 Make a midline incision on the dorsal surface of the hand as indicated in Chapter 8 (Figs. 8.12 to 8.16).

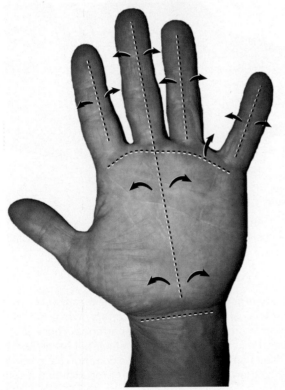

Fig. 9.4 Anterior view of palmar hand, with dashed lines showing skin incision sites.

DISSECTION TIP

The skin on the dorsum of the hand is very thin, whereas the skin on the palmar surface is thick and tightly bound to the underlying palmar aponeurosis. Make a shallow incision on the dorsum of the hand, and with the aid of dissecting scissors, separate the skin from the underlying tissues. Make a deeper incision on the palmar surface of the hand, using the palmaris longus muscle as a guide to remove the skin with sharp dissection.

- After removal of the skin on the palmar surface of the hand, trace the continuation of the palmaris longus muscle to the palmar aponeurosis (see Fig. 9.5).
- Note the **thenar eminence with the flexor pollicis brevis and abductor pollicis muscles** (Fig. 9.6).
- Lift the palmar aponeurosis (Fig. 9.7) and with the aid of dissecting scissors separate it from the underlying structures (Fig. 9.8).

ANATOMY NOTE

The *palmar aponeurosis* is composed of longitudinal and transversely oriented fibers of dense connective tissue. The longitudinal fibers form digital bands that attach to the bases of the proximal phalanges and become continuous with the fibrous digital sheaths (ligamentous tubes enclosing synovial sheaths).

the 3rd digit (Fig. 9.4). Make a second midline incision on the palmar surface of each digit. Join these with transverse incisions at the bases of the digits.
- With additional incisions as necessary, reflect and remove the skin from the hand (Fig. 9.5).

- With scissors, cut the attachments of the longitudinal bands from the bases of the proximal phalanges. Reflect the palmaris longus muscle and the palmar aponeurosis toward the forearm (Fig. 9.9).

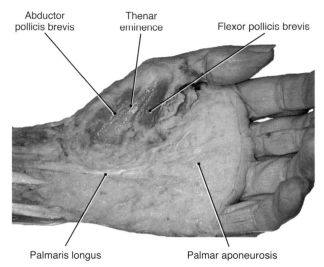

Fig. 9.5 Anterior view of hand with skin reflected, noting superficial structures, including muscles of thenar eminence and the palmar aponeurosis. Note palmaris longus muscle inserting into palmar aponeurosis.

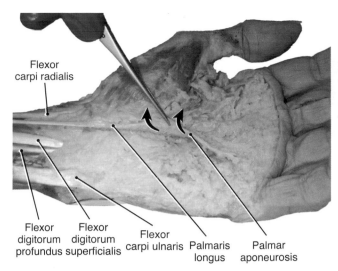

Fig. 9.7 Anterior hand with skin reflected and traction on the palmar aponeurosis. The aponeurosis will be reflected to reveal deeper structures.

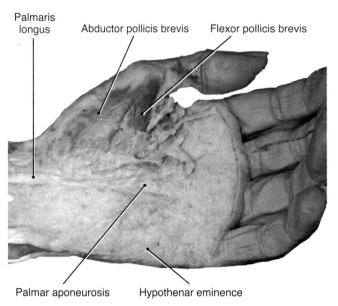

Fig. 9.6 Anterior view of hand with skin reflected, illustrating subcutaneous fat covering muscles that make up the hypothenar eminence.

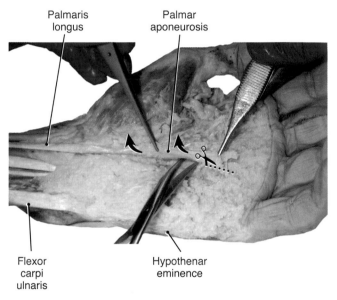

Fig. 9.8 Anterior hand with skin reflected, revealing palmar aponeurosis. Constant tension of the aponeurosis will allow scissors to be inserted deep to it.

ANATOMY **NOTE**

The *superficial palmar arch* is the termination of the superficial branch of the ulnar artery, which gives rise to three common palmar digital arteries. These arteries anastomose with the palmar metacarpal branches from the deep palmar arterial arch. The common palmar digital arteries then divide into a pair of proper digital arteries, supplying the adjacent sides of the 2nd to 4th digits.

DISSECTION **TIP**

The removal of the palmar aponeurosis takes time. Pay special attention to using the scalpel as little as possible so as not to injure the palmar digital nerves and the superficial palmar arch. These structures travel deep to the palmar aponeurosis.

○ After removal of the palmar aponeurosis, start exposing the **superficial palmar arch** (Figs. 9.10 and 9.11, Plate 9.1).

DISSECTION **TIP**

The superficial palmar arch is related to the superficial venous arch, as well as with common palmar digital branches of the median nerve. With scissors, separate the nerves from the superficial palmar arch (see Figs. 9.10 to 9.12). Also, remove any venous structures from this area.

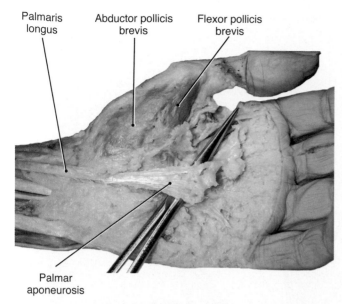

Palmaris longus   Abductor pollicis brevis   Flexor pollicis brevis

Palmar aponeurosis

Fig. 9.9 Anterior hand with skin reflected, revealing palmar aponeurosis. Once the aponeurosis is cut distally, it can be reflected to demonstrate deeper structures.

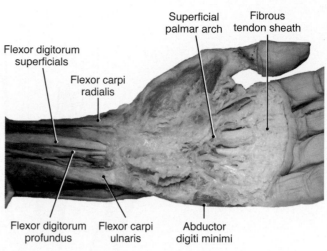

Flexor digitorum superficials   Flexor carpi radialis   Superficial palmar arch   Fibrous tendon sheath

Flexor digitorum profundus   Flexor carpi ulnaris   Abductor digiti minimi

Fig. 9.11 Anterior view of hand with skin and aponeurosis reflected, showing tendon sheaths and neurovascular structures such as superficial palmar arch.

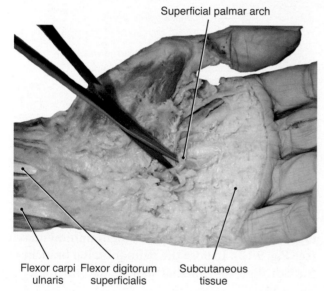

Superficial palmar arch

Flexor carpi ulnaris   Flexor digitorum superficialis   Subcutaneous tissue

Fig. 9.10 Anterior view of hand with skin and aponeurosis reflected, revealing deeper structures such as the superficial palmar arch.

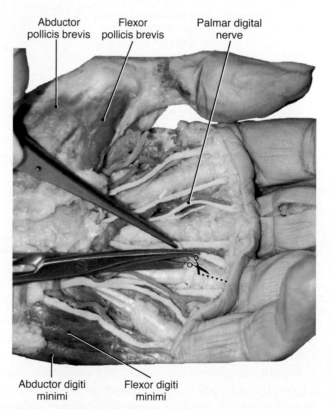

Abductor pollicis brevis   Flexor pollicis brevis   Palmar digital nerve

Abductor digiti minimi   Flexor digiti minimi

Fig. 9.12 Anterior view of hand with skin and aponeurosis reflected, revealing tendon sheaths and adjacent neurovascular structures.

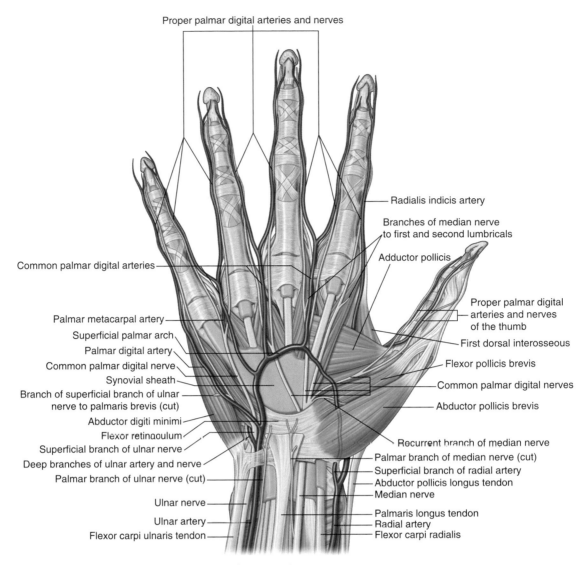

Proper palmar digital arteries and nerves

Radialis indicis artery

Branches of median nerve to first and second lumbricals

Adductor pollicis

Common palmar digital arteries

Proper palmar digital arteries and nerves of the thumb

First dorsal interosseous

Palmar metacarpal artery

Superficial palmar arch

Palmar digital artery

Common palmar digital nerve

Synovial sheath

Branch of superficial branch of ulnar nerve to palmaris brevis (cut)

Abductor digiti minimi

Flexor retinaculum

Superficial branch of ulnar nerve

Deep branches of ulnar artery and nerve

Palmar branch of ulnar nerve (cut)

Ulnar nerve

Ulnar artery

Flexor carpi ulnaris tendon

Flexor pollicis brevis

Common palmar digital nerves

Abductor pollicis brevis

Recurrent branch of median nerve

Palmar branch of median nerve (cut)

Superficial branch of radial artery

Abductor pollicis longus tendon

Median nerve

Palmaris longus tendon

Radial artery

Flexor carpi radialis

Plate 9.1 Superficial muscles, arteries, and nerves of the hand.

○ Immediately after its passage through the carpal tunnel, the **median nerve** gives rise to several smaller branches: the recurrent branch of the median nerve and the common palmar digital branches. At this point in the dissection, identify the **common palmar digital branches of the median nerve** running alongside the common palmar digital arteries (Fig. 9.13, Plate 9.2).

○ Continue the dissection toward the phalanges, and expose the separation of the common palmar digital branches of the median nerve into proper palmar digital nerves of the digits.

○ Similarly, expose the site at which the common palmar digital arteries give rise to palmar digital arteries (Fig. 9.14).

○ Clean away the fascia investing the **abductor and flexor digiti minimi muscles** over the hypothenar region.

○ Continue the removal of fat and remnants of the palmar aponeurosis at the medial aspect of the palm, the *hypothenar eminence* (see Fig. 9.8). Identify the flexor

digiti minimi and the abductor digiti minimi muscles (see Fig. 9.12). Expose the palmar digital branches to the 5th digit and medial half of the 4th digit (see Fig. 9.14).

DISSECTION **TIP**

The most superficially placed muscle in the hypothenar eminence is the *palmaris brevis*. This muscle is extremely thin and often blended with adipose tissue, arising from the palmar aponeurosis to insert into the skin. It is rather difficult to expose the palmaris brevis, because it is detached during removal of the palmar aponeurosis and skin.

DISSECTION **TIP**

In about 65% of hands, a communication between the ulnar and median nerves exists distal to the flexor retinaculum.

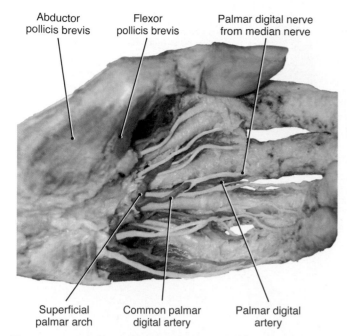

Fig. 9.13 labels: Abductor pollicis brevis · Flexor pollicis brevis · Palmar digital nerve from median nerve · Superficial palmar arch · Common palmar digital artery · Palmar digital artery

Fig. 9.13 Anterior view of hand with skin and aponeurosis reflected, highlighting tendon sheaths and neurovascular structures such as palmar digital nerves and arteries.

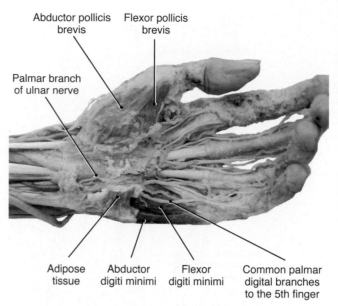

Fig. 9.15 labels: Abductor pollicis brevis · Flexor pollicis brevis · Palmar branch of ulnar nerve · Adipose tissue · Abductor digiti minimi · Flexor digiti minimi · Common palmar digital branches to the 5th finger

Fig. 9.15 Anterior hand with skin and aponeurosis reflected, revealing thenar and hypothenar muscles.

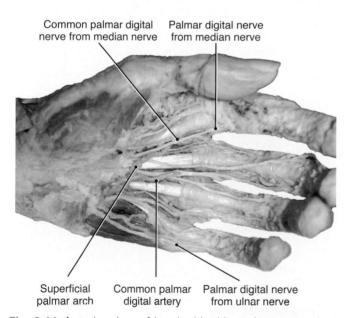

Fig. 9.14 labels: Common palmar digital nerve from median nerve · Palmar digital nerve from median nerve · Superficial palmar arch · Common palmar digital artery · Palmar digital nerve from ulnar nerve

Fig. 9.14 Anterior view of hand with skin and aponeurosis reflected, revealing tendon sheaths and neurovascular structures. Note common palmar arteries arising from superficial palmar arch.

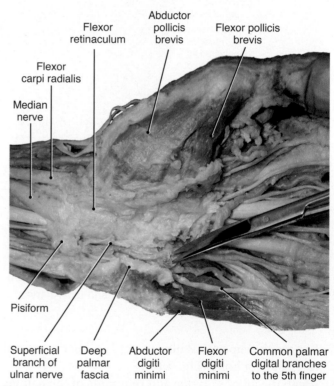

Fig. 9.16 labels: Flexor retinaculum · Abductor pollicis brevis · Flexor pollicis brevis · Flexor carpi radialis · Median nerve · Pisiform · Superficial branch of ulnar nerve · Deep palmar fascia · Abductor digiti minimi · Flexor digiti minimi · Common palmar digital branches to the 5th finger

Fig. 9.16 Anterior hand with skin and aponeurosis reflected, revealing thenar and hypothenar muscles. Note median nerve traveling deep to flexor retinaculum within the carpal tunnel.

- Trace the palmar digital branches to the 5th digit and medial half of the 4th digit toward their origin from the superficial branch of the ulnar nerve (Fig. 9.15).
- Remove the deep fascia at the ulnar side of the wrist, and using scissors (Fig. 9.16), expose the superficial branch of the ulnar nerve (Fig. 9.17). The ulnar artery and nerve travel lateral to the pisiform bone to enter the palm.

ANATOMY **NOTE**

This point is referred to as *Guyon's canal* (or tunnel) and is formed by the pisiform bone, the flexor retinaculum, and an extension of the deep fascia of the forearm (palmar carpal ligament).

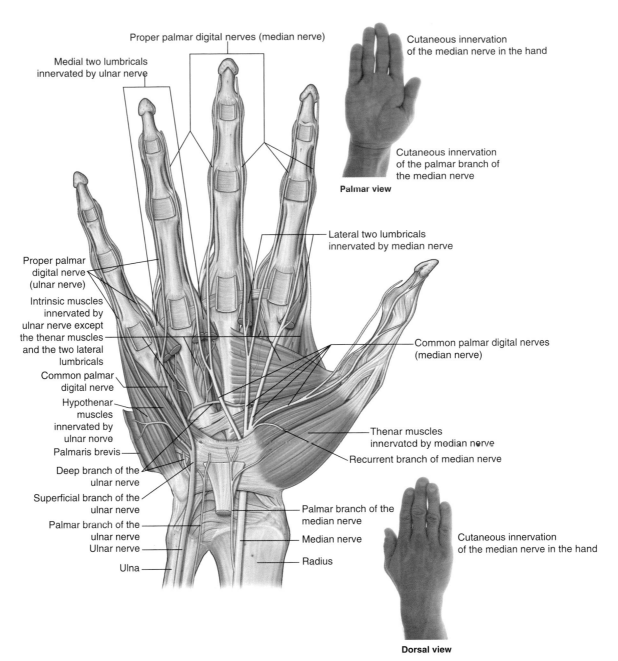

Plate 9.2 Innervation of the hand median and ulnar nerves.

Labels (clockwise):

Proper palmar digital nerves (median nerve)

Medial two lumbricals innervated by ulnar nerve

Cutaneous innervation of the median nerve in the hand

Cutaneous innervation of the palmar branch of the median nerve

Palmar view

Lateral two lumbricals innervated by median nerve

Proper palmar digital nerve (ulnar nerve)

Intrinsic muscles innervated by ulnar nerve except the thenar muscles and the two lateral lumbricals

Common palmar digital nerve

Hypothenar muscles innervated by ulnar nerve

Palmaris brevis

Deep branch of the ulnar nerve

Superficial branch of the ulnar nerve

Palmar branch of the ulnar nerve

Ulnar nerve

Ulna

Common palmar digital nerves (median nerve)

Thenar muscles innervated by median nerve

Recurrent branch of median nerve

Palmar branch of the median nerve

Median nerve

Radius

Cutaneous innervation of the median nerve in the hand

Dorsal view

○ Expose the superficial ulnar artery and nerve toward the pisiform bone (Fig. 9.18).

○ Clean the adipose tissue and remnants of the palmar aponeurosis surrounding the superficial palmar arch distally to the carpal tunnel and flexor retinaculum (see Fig. 9.18).

DISSECTION **TIP**

The tendons of the flexor digitorum superficialis and flexor digitorum profundus muscles are enclosed by a synovial sheath, the *ulnar bursa.* The tendon of the flexor pollicis longus is also enclosed by a synovial sheath, the *radial bursa.*

ANATOMY **NOTE**

The primary contributor to the superficial palmar arch is the ulnar artery.

○ Expose the ulnar artery and clean the surface of the flexor retinaculum (Fig. 9.19).

○ To free up the superficial palmar arch and nerve structures from the underlying long flexor tendons, use scissors to incise the fibrous tendinous sheaths longitudinally. Identify tendons of flexor digitorum superficialis and profundus muscles (Fig. 9.20).

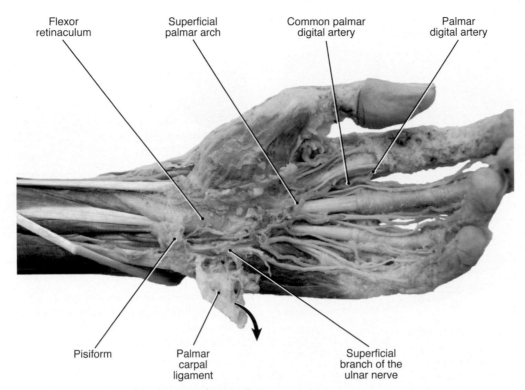

Flexor retinaculum

Superficial palmar arch

Common palmar digital artery

Palmar digital artery

Pisiform

Palmar carpal ligament

Superficial branch of the ulnar nerve

Fig. 9.17 Anterior hand with skin and aponeurosis reflected, revealing thenar and hypothenar muscles. Note the palmar carpal ligament that has been reflected to better illustrate the deeper flexor retinaculum.

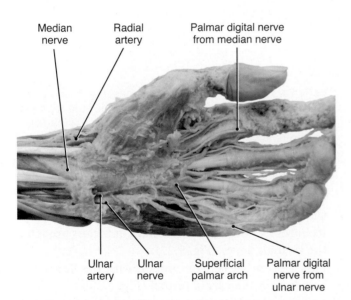

Median nerve

Radial artery

Palmar digital nerve from median nerve

Ulnar artery

Ulnar nerve

Superficial palmar arch

Palmar digital nerve from ulnar nerve

Fig. 9.18 Anterior hand with skin and aponeurosis removed, revealing superficial palmar arch.

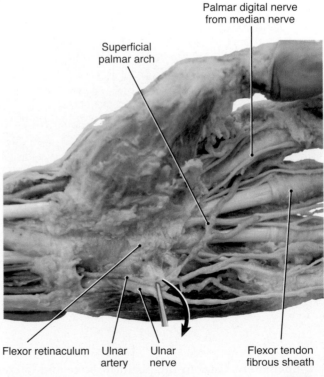

Superficial palmar arch

Palmar digital nerve from median nerve

Flexor retinaculum

Ulnar artery

Ulnar nerve

Flexor tendon fibrous sheath

Fig. 9.19 Anterior hand with skin and aponeurosis removed, revealing superficial palmar arterial arch and branches to the digits.

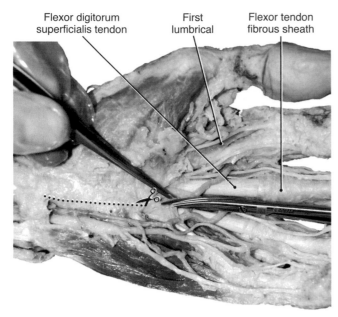

Flexor digitorum superficialis tendon — First lumbrical — Flexor tendon fibrous sheath

Fig. 9.20 Anterior hand with skin and aponeurosis removed. Use scissors to open the fibrous tendon sheaths to identify tendons of flexor digitorum superficialis and profundus muscles.

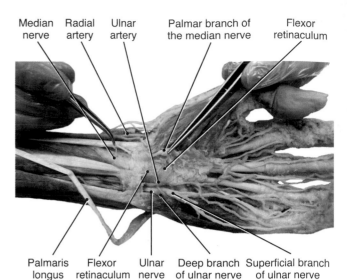

Median nerve — Radial artery — Ulnar artery — Palmar branch of the median nerve — Flexor retinaculum

Palmaris longus — Flexor retinaculum — Ulnar nerve — Deep branch of ulnar nerve — Superficial branch of ulnar nerve

Fig. 9.22 Anterior hand with skin and aponeurosis removed, revealing palmar cutaneous branch of median nerve, which passes superficial to the flexor retinaculum to supply skin over the thenar eminence.

DISSECTION **TIP**

The palmar cutaneous branch of the median nerve is often cut during routine dissection. The median nerve is seen at the distal forearm between the tendons of the palmaris longus and flexor carpi radialis and supplies the skin over the central portion of the palm.

ANATOMY **NOTE**

The *flexor retinaculum* is a dense connective tissue band that helps create a tunnel *(carpal tunnel)* for the tendons of the flexor digitorum superficialis, flexor digitorum profundus, flexor pollicis longus, and the median nerve to reach the palm.

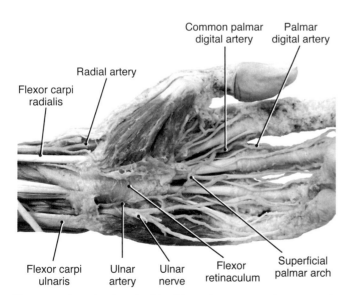

Common palmar digital artery — Palmar digital artery

Radial artery

Flexor carpi radialis

Flexor carpi ulnaris — Ulnar artery — Ulnar nerve — Flexor retinaculum — Superficial palmar arch

Fig. 9.21 Anterior hand with skin and aponeurosis removed, revealing digital arteries and nerves and superficial branches of ulnar nerve and artery (superficial palmar arch).

○ Immediately distal to the pisiform bone and lateral to the flexor retinaculum, expose the division of the ulnar artery and nerve into deep and superficial branches (Fig. 9.21).

○ The deep branches dive deeply between the abductor and flexor digiti minimi muscles of the 5th digit.

○ Carefully expose the flexor retinaculum and identify its borders. Look for the palmar cutaneous branch of the median nerve (Fig. 9.22).

○ Pass a probe or scissors underneath the flexor retinaculum in the carpal tunnel (Fig. 9.23).

○ Leave the probe within the carpal tunnel and with scissors divide the flexor retinaculum on top of the probe (Fig. 9.24). This retinaculum is transected by inserting the scissors into the carpal tunnel upwardly, cutting in a proximal-to-distal manner.

○ Remove the probe, and retract the flexor retinaculum to expose the median nerve and tendons of the flexor digitorum superficialis (Figs. 9.25 and 9.26).

○ Remove the connective tissue sheath over the median nerve and the underlying flexor digitorum superficialis muscle (Fig. 9.27).

○ Continue exposing the median nerve within the carpal tunnel. Identify the recurrent branch of the median nerve (Fig. 9.28). Finish the exposure of the common palmar digital branches of the median nerve.

DISSECTION **TIP**

The recurrent branch of the median nerve usually travels deep to the thenar muscles, and tracing its course anteriorly may be difficult. In such cases, gently retract the median nerve (within exposed carpal tunnel) laterally, and identify the recurrent branch of the median nerve. You also may dissect between the flexor pollicis brevis and the underlying adductor pollicis muscle to trace the recurrent branch of the median nerve.

DISSECTION **TIP**

In some cases, branches of the superficial palmar arch travel close to the common palmar digital branches or penetrate them. Use special care when you dissect these structures (Fig. 9.29).

○ With forceps, retract the abductor digiti minimi muscle laterally, and expose the flexor digiti minimi brevis and the opponens digiti minimi muscles (Fig. 9.30).
○ You may cut and reflect the abductor digiti minimi near its origin to expose the underlying opponens digiti minimi muscle.

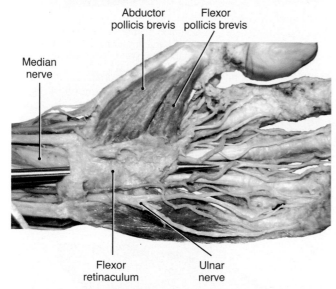

Fig. 9.23 Anterior hand with removed skin and aponeurosis showing flexor retinaculum. Note that the ulnar nerve and artery travel superficial to the flexor retinaculum but deep to the palmar carpal ligament.

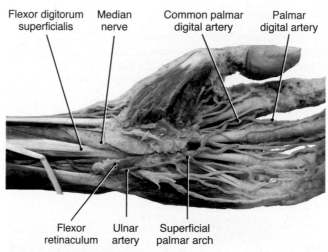

Fig. 9.25 Anterior hand with transection of the flexor retinaculum. Deeper dissection will reveal the nine tendons and one nerve that course through the carpal tunnel.

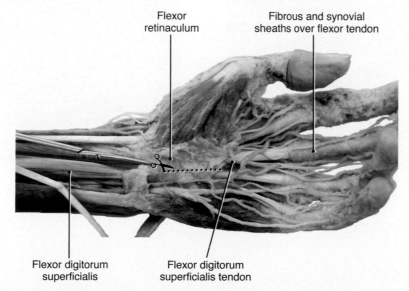

Fig. 9.24 Anterior hand with removed skin and aponeurosis revealing the flexor retinaculum.

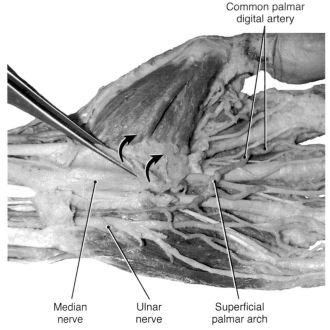

Common palmar
digital artery

Median
nerve   Ulnar
nerve   Superficial
palmar arch

Fig. 9.26 Anterior hand with flexor
retinaculum reflected. Median nerve can
be traced from distal forearm to the hand
through exposed carpal tunnel. Distal to
the flexor retinaculum, note branching
pattern of the median nerve.

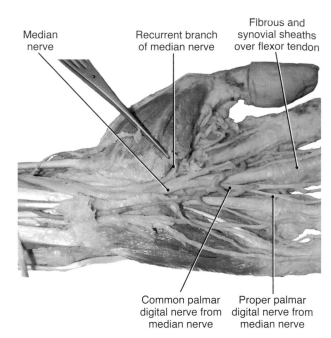

Median
nerve   Recurrent branch
of median nerve   Fibrous and
synovial sheaths
over flexor tendon

Common palmar
digital nerve from
median nerve   Proper palmar
digital nerve from
median nerve

Fig. 9.28 Anterior hand with cut flexor retinaculum revealing
the carpal tunnel. The median nerve can be traced through
the tunnel and its recurrent branch identified near the distal
end of the flexor retinaculum.

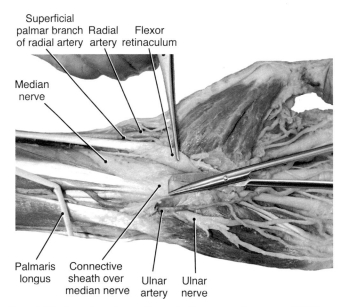

Superficial
palmar branch   Radial   Flexor
of radial artery   artery   retinaculum

Median
nerve

Palmaris   Connective
longus   sheath over   Ulnar   Ulnar
median nerve   artery   nerve

Fig. 9.27 Anterior view of hand after
transection of the flexor retinaculum,
revealing the carpal tunnel.

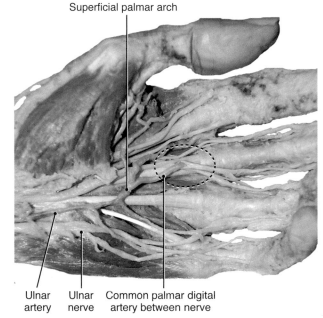

Superficial palmar arch

Ulnar   Ulnar   Common palmar digital
artery   nerve   artery between nerve

Fig. 9.29 Anterior hand with removed aponeurosis, cut flexor
retinaculum, and opened carpal tunnel. Note relationship
between common palmar digital arteries and nerves *(circled)*.

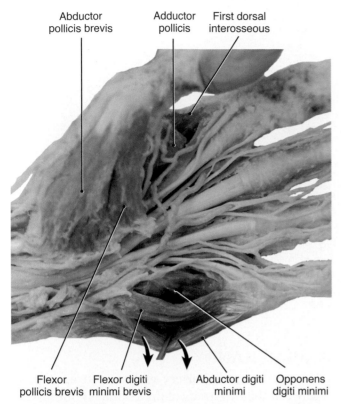

Abductor pollicis brevis   Adductor pollicis   First dorsal interosseous

Flexor pollicis brevis   Flexor digiti minimi brevis   Abductor digiti minimi   Opponens digiti minimi

Fig. 9.30 Anterior hand with removed skin and aponeurosis and cut flexor retinaculum revealing carpal tunnel. With separation, muscular components of hypothenar eminence are seen.

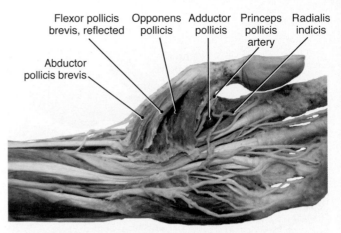

Flexor pollicis brevis, reflected   Opponens pollicis   Adductor pollicis   Princeps pollicis artery   Radialis indicis

Abductor pollicis brevis

Fig. 9.31 Anterior hand with removed skin and aponeurosis and cut flexor retinaculum revealing carpal tunnel. With separation, muscles of the thenar eminence are seen.

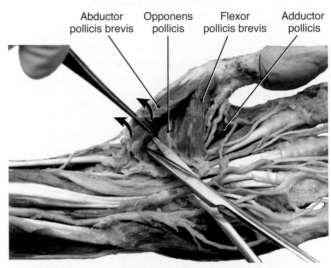

Abductor pollicis brevis   Opponens pollicis   Flexor pollicis brevis   Adductor pollicis

Fig. 9.32 Anterior hand with skin and aponeurosis removed and flexor reticulum cut revealing thenar muscles. Scissors are used to transect the origin of the abductor pollicis brevis muscle.

DISSECTION **TIP**

In the majority of the specimens, the flexor digiti minimi muscle is difficult to separate from the abductor digiti minimi muscle. Follow the deep branch of the ulnar nerve to the hypothenar muscles. This nerve runs between the flexor digiti minimi and abductor digiti minimi muscles, facilitating their identification. The deepest of the hypothenar muscles is the opponens digiti minimi muscle.

○ Trace the superficial palmar arch laterally in the space between the 1st digit and the 2nd digit.

DISSECTION **TIP**

There is usually an anastomosis between the superficial palmar arch and a branch of the radial artery, the *radialis indicis,* and a branch to the 1st digit, the *princeps pollicis* (Fig. 9.31).

○ Identify the *abductor pollicis brevis muscle,* lying at the lateral side of the base of the 1st phalanx of the 1st digit (see Fig. 9.31).
○ Medial and next to the abductor pollicis brevis muscle, identify the flexor pollicis brevis muscle, which is passing along the radial side of the tendon of the flexor pollicis longus muscle. Retract the abductor pollicis brevis muscle laterally from the flexor pollicis brevis muscle, and identify the opponens pollicis muscle (Fig. 9.32). Flexor pollicis brevis has two heads. Its deep head can be mistaken for the opponens pollicis brevis. Reflect both heads.
○ Finally, identify the adductor pollicis muscle, which can be seen between the base of the 2nd and 1st digits.

DISSECTION **TIP**

You may also transect the abductor pollicis brevis and identify the opponens pollicis muscle just underneath it (Fig. 9.33). Another way to distinguish the opponens pollicis brevis muscle from the abductor pollicis brevis and the flexor pollicis muscles is its insertion point. The opponens pollicis brevis muscle inserts alongside the 1st metacarpal.

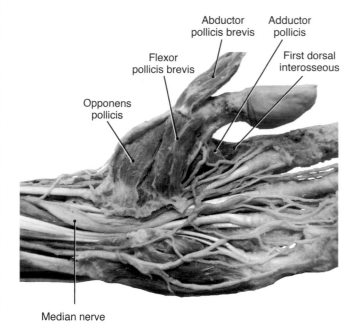

Abductor
pollicis brevis

Adductor
pollicis

Flexor
pollicis brevis

First dorsal
interosseous

Opponens
pollicis

Median nerve

Fig. 9.33 Anterior hand with skin and aponeurosis removed and flexor reticulum cut revealing thenar structures. With abductor pollicis brevis reflected, the deeper-lying opponens pollicis is visualized.

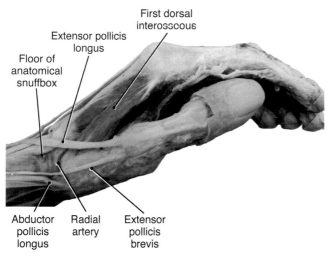

First dorsal
interosseous

Extensor pollicis
longus

Floor of
anatomical
snuffbox

Abductor
pollicis
longus

Radial
artery

Extensor
pollicis
brevis

Fig. 9.34 Region of "anatomic snuffbox," with borders and contents, including radial artery. Note 1st dorsal interosseous muscle between 1st and 2nd digits.

○ On the dorsum of the hand, clean and expose the tendinous insertions of abductor pollicis longus, the extensor pollicis brevis, and the extensor pollicis longus (Fig. 9.34).

ANATOMY NOTE

The tendons of these three muscles (abductor pollicis longus, the extensor pollicis brevis, and the extensor pollicis longus) form the boundaries of the anatomic snuffbox, through which the radial artery passes to reach the dorsum of the 1st digit.

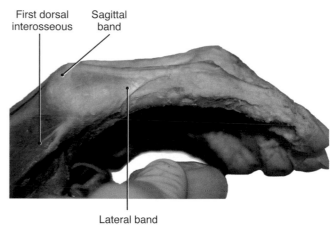

First dorsal
interosseous

Sagittal
band

Lateral band

Fig. 9.35 Dorsal view of 1st and 2nd digits with skin removed, revealing superficial structures. Note components of dorsal expansion, including sagittal and lateral bands.

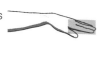

DORSAL HAND

○ Identify the radial artery and trace it as it passes between the two heads of the 1st dorsal interosseous muscle (see Fig. 9.34).
○ Observe the radial side of the 2nd digit. At the level of the proximal interphalangeal joint, note the extensor mechanism splitting into three parts. Note that one of these parts, the lateral bands, to which the extensor tendons contribute, eventually unite with the transverse metacarpal ligament (Fig. 9.35).
○ At the palmar side of the digits, observe the fibrous synovial sheaths surrounding the tendons of the long flexor muscles (Fig. 9.36).

DISSECTION TIP

These fibrous sheaths are thin at the interphalangeal joints (cruciate fibers) and thick over the phalanges (anular fibers/ligament).

RETURN TO PALMAR HAND AND ANTERIOR FOREARM

○ With a scalpel, cut at the midline the fibrous synovial sheath, and expose the tendon of the flexor digitorum superficialis and flexor digitorum profundus (Figs. 9.37 and 9.38).
○ Extend the distal interphalangeal joint. Observe the tendon of the flexor digitorum superficialis dividing before inserting at the base of the middle phalanx. In addition, the tendon of the flexor digitorum profundus passes through the divided tendon of the flexor digitorum superficialis to insert onto the distal phalanges (Figs. 9.39 and 9.40). Note the vinculum longum,

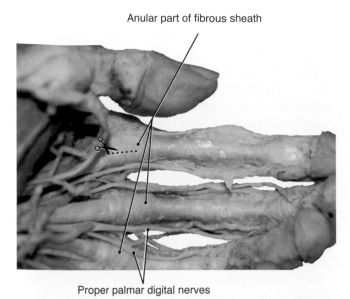

Anular part of fibrous sheath

Proper palmar digital nerves

Fig. 9.36 Anterior view of palm illustrating fibrous digital sheaths and related structures (e.g., palmar digital nerves).

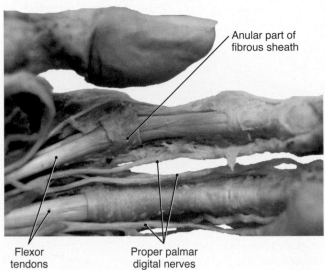

Anular part of fibrous sheath

Flexor tendons

Proper palmar digital nerves

Fig. 9.38 Anterior view of 1st to 3rd digits. Note anular component of fibrous digital sheath and deeper-lying flexor tendons.

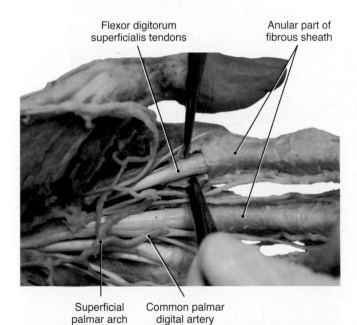

Flexor digitorum superficialis tendons

Anular part of fibrous sheath

Superficial palmar arch

Common palmar digital artery

Fig. 9.37 Anterior view of palm after partial opening of flexor digital sheaths of the 2nd and 3rd digits. Note anular components of fibrous sheaths and internally located flexor tendons.

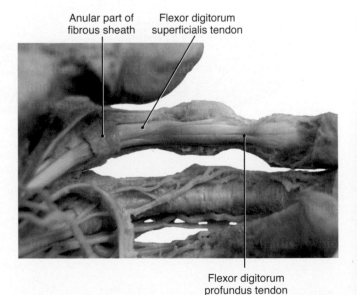

Anular part of fibrous sheath

Flexor digitorum superficialis tendon

Flexor digitorum profundus tendon

Fig. 9.39 Anterior view of 1st to 4th digits with portions of fibrous digital sheaths removed. Note the deeper-lying flexor tendons of flexor digitorum superficialis and profundus muscles.

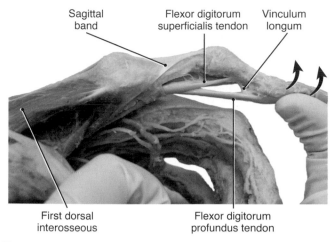

Sagittal band   Flexor digitorum superficialis tendon   Vinculum longum

First dorsal interosseous   Flexor digitorum profundus tendon

Fig. 9.40 Lateral view of interspace between 1st and 2nd digits. Note the flexor digitorum profundus tendon passing through the split tendon of flexor digitorum superficialis muscle.

a thin ligament that adds support for the attachments of the flexor digitorum superficialis and flexor digitorum profundus.

- Once all muscles, nerves, and arteries of the hand have been identified (Fig. 9.41), pass a probe or a pair of scissors underneath the flexor digitorum superficialis tendons (Fig. 9.42), and transect them at the level of the carpal tunnel (Fig. 9.43).
- Lift the flexor digitorum superficialis and expose the median nerve. Clean the median nerve and its surrounding muscles from any loose connective tissue (Figs. 9.44 and 9.45).
- Transect the median, ulnar, and radial nerves, as well as the ulnar artery at the same level (Fig. 9.46).
- Retract the neurovascular bundles distally to expose the tendons of the flexor digitorum superficialis. Lift the tendons of the flexor digitorum superficialis and expose all four lumbrical muscles (Fig. 9.47).

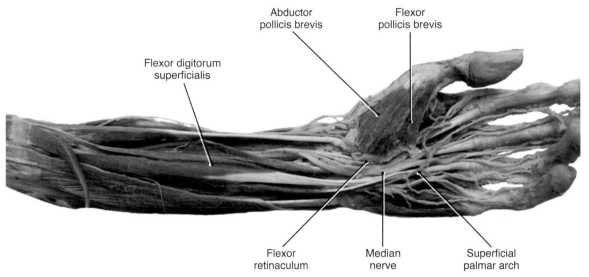

Abductor pollicis brevis   Flexor pollicis brevis

Flexor digitorum superficialis

Flexor retinaculum   Median nerve   Superficial palmar arch

Fig. 9.41 Anterior forearm and hand view with aponeurosis removed, revealing superficial and intermediate musculature.

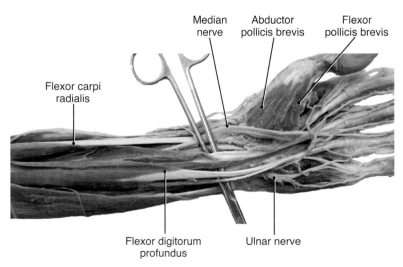

Median nerve   Abductor pollicis brevis   Flexor pollicis brevis

Flexor carpi radialis

Flexor digitorum profundus   Ulnar nerve

Fig. 9.42 Anterior view of forearm and hand with aponeurosis removed, revealing superficial and intermediate musculature. The median nerve is pulled from between flexor digitorum superficialis and profundus muscles; these muscles are pulled forward and scissors placed deep to them.

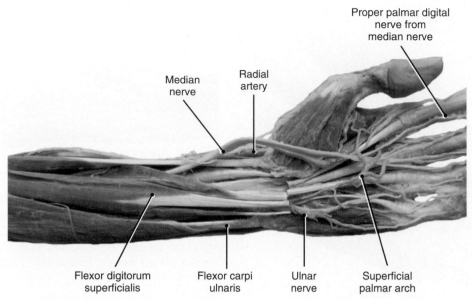

Fig. 9.43 Anterior forearm and hand with skin and aponeurosis removed; superficial and intermediate muscles are cut at the wrist. The median nerve is retracted.

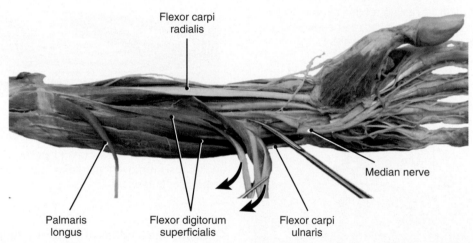

Fig. 9.44 Anterior forearm and hand with skin and aponeurosis removed and superficial and intermediate muscles reflected, revealing neurovascular structures.

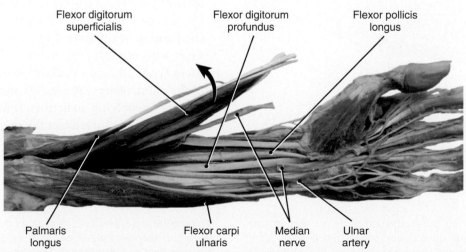

Fig. 9.45 Anterior hand with skin and aponeurosis removed and flexor retinaculum cut, revealing tendons and muscles. The median nerve has been transected in the distal forearm.

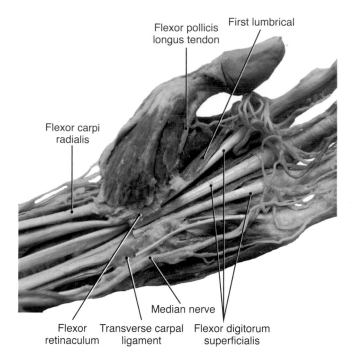

Fig. 9.46 Anterior hand with skin and aponeurosis removed and flexor retinaculum cut, revealing tendons and muscles. Flexor pollicis longus tendon is exposed, and superficial neurovascular structures are reflected distally.

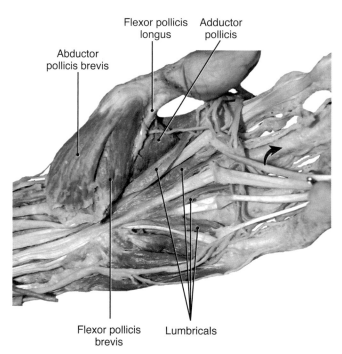

Fig. 9.47 Anterior hand with skin and aponeurosis removed, revealing deeper muscles (e.g., adductor pollicis, lumbricals).

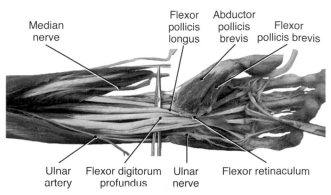

Fig. 9.48 Anterior forearm and hand with skin and aponeurosis removed; superficial and intermediate muscles reflected, revealing deep muscles. Tendon of flexor pollicis longus can be seen entering and exiting carpal tunnel. Scissors placed deep to nine tendons that travel through the carpal tunnel.

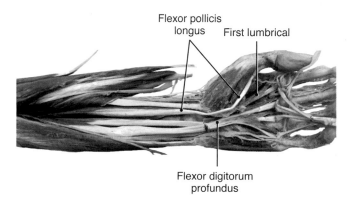

Fig. 9.49 Anterior view of hand and wrist with skin and aponeurosis removed and flexor retinaculum cut, revealing carpal tunnel tendons.

- Clamp the tendons of the flexor digitorum superficialis with a hemostat and retract the tendons distally.
- Pass a probe or scissors underneath the flexor digitorum profundus (Fig. 9.48) and transect it at the level of the carpal tunnel (Fig. 9.49).
- Lift this part of the flexor digitorum profundus within the palm, and separate it from the underlying structures with scissors (Fig. 9.50).
- Identify the adductor pollicis muscle, and at the center of the palm, observe the loose connective tissue covering the underlying structures (Fig. 9.51).
- With sharp scissors, clean the connective tissue, and expose the deep palmar arch and the deep branch of the ulnar nerve (Fig. 9.52).

ANATOMY NOTE

The lumbricals arise from the tendons of the flexor digitorum profundus muscle and travel to the radial side of the medial four digits to insert into the extensor expansion of each digit.

ANATOMY NOTE

The radial artery enters the deep portion of the hand between the two heads of the first dorsal interosseous muscle and anastomoses with the deep branch of the ulnar artery.

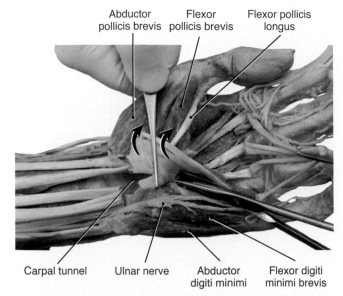

Abductor pollicis brevis | Flexor pollicis brevis | Flexor pollicis longus

Carpal tunnel | Ulnar nerve | Abductor digiti minimi | Flexor digiti minimi brevis

Fig. 9.50 Anterior hand with skin and aponeurosis removed; superficial and deep tendons cut and reflected, revealing carpal tunnel and its contents. Tendons of flexor digitorum superficialis and profundus are cut and reflected.

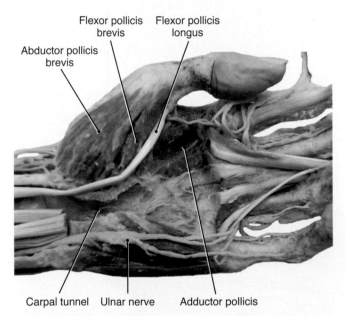

Flexor pollicis brevis | Flexor pollicis longus

Abductor pollicis brevis

Carpal tunnel | Ulnar nerve | Adductor pollicis

Fig. 9.51 Anterior hand with skin and aponeurosis removed; tendons reflected from carpal tunnel revealing thenar and palmar muscles.

○ Continue exposing the deep palmar arch and the ulnar nerve and identify the interossei muscles. Identify four dorsal and three palmar interossei muscles (Fig. 9.53).

○ Reflect the flexor digitorum profundus and superficialis, and note the pronator quadratus muscle. This muscle requires no dissection (Fig. 9.54).

○ At the end of the dissection, place all structures back in their original anatomic position (Fig. 9.55). By following this dissection technique, you will be able to examine the specimen with all the structures in their original position.

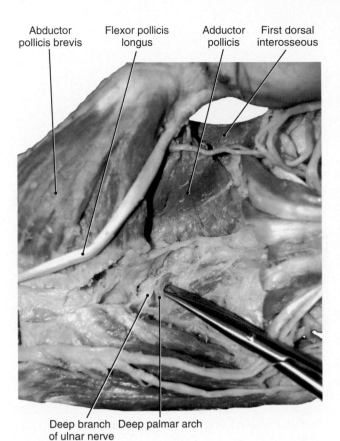

Abductor pollicis brevis | Flexor pollicis longus | Adductor pollicis | First dorsal interosseous

Deep branch of ulnar nerve | Deep palmar arch

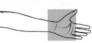

Fig. 9.52 Anterior hand with skin and aponeurosis removed; tendons cut and reflected to reveal the deep palmar arch, with its blood flow contributed to primarily by the radial artery.

DISSECTION TIP

The dorsal and palmar interossei muscles insert partially on the base of the 1st phalanx of each of the medial four digits and into their extensor expansions:
- 1st dorsal interosseous muscle inserts on radial side of 2nd digit.
- 2nd and 3rd dorsal interossei insert on either side of 3rd digit.
- 4th dorsal interosseous muscle inserts on ulnar side of 4th digit.
- 1st palmar interosseous muscle inserts on ulnar side of 2nd digit.
- 2nd palmar interosseous muscle inserts on radial side of 4th digit.
- 3rd palmar interosseous muscle inserts on radial side of 5th digit.

DISSECTION TIP

The palmar fascial spaces are **potential spaces**, which are clinically important as routes of infection spread. These are not dissected in routine dissection.

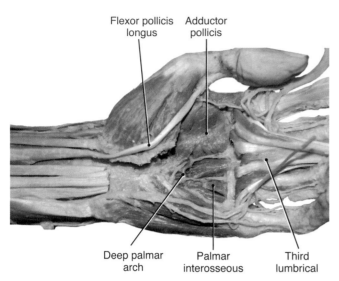

Flexor pollicis longus   Adductor pollicis

Deep palmar arch   Palmar interosseous   Third lumbrical

Fig. 9.53 Anterior forearm and hand with skin and aponeurosis removed; superficial and intermediate muscles reflected, revealing deep structures, including deep palmar arch and interosseous muscles.

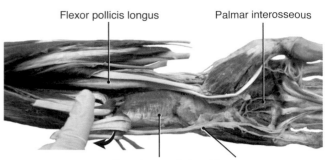

Flexor pollicis longus   Palmar interosseous

Pronator quadratus   Ulnar nerve

Fig. 9.54 Anterior hand and wrist with skin and aponeurosis removed and tendons cut, revealing deeper structures such as pronator quadratus muscle.

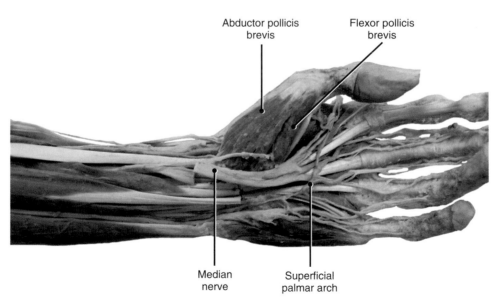

Abductor pollicis brevis   Flexor pollicis brevis

Median nerve   Superficial palmar arch

Fig. 9.55 Anterior view of hand and wrist with skin and aponeurosis removed. Median nerve is transected in distal anterior forearm. Note palmar cutaneous branch of median nerve crossing superficial to flexor retinaculum.

LABORATORY IDENTIFICATION CHECKLIST

NERVES
- [ ] Median
  - [ ] Superficial branch
  - [ ] Recurrent branch
- [ ] Common palmar digital
  - [ ] Palmar digital
- [ ] Ulnar
  - [ ] Superficial branch
- [ ] Common palmar digital
  - [ ] Palmar digital
  - [ ] Dorsal branch
  - [ ] Dorsal digital
- [ ] Radial
  - [ ] Superficial branch
  - [ ] Dorsal digital branches

ARTERIES
- [ ] Ulnar
  - [ ] Superficial palmar arch
    - [ ] Common palmar digital
    - [ ] Palmar digital
- [ ] Radial
  - [ ] Deep arch
- [ ] Princeps pollicis
- [ ] Radialis indicis
- [ ] Palmar metacarpal
  - [ ] Palmar digital
  - [ ] Dorsal arterial arch
- [ ] Dorsal metacarpal
  - [ ] Dorsal digital

VEINS
- [ ] Dorsal digital
- [ ] Dorsal metacarpal
- [ ] Dorsal venous arch
  - [ ] Cephalic
  - [ ] Basilic
- [ ] Palmar digital

MUSCLES
Thenar Muscles
- [ ] Abductor pollicis brevis
- [ ] Flexor pollicis brevis
- [ ] Opponens pollicis brevis

Hypothenar Muscles
- [ ] Abductor digiti minimi brevis
- [ ] Flexor digiti minimi
- [ ] Opponens digiti minimi
- [ ] Palmaris brevis

Palmar Muscles
- [ ] Adductor pollicis
- [ ] Palmar interosseous
- [ ] Dorsal interosseous
- [ ] Lumbricals

LIGAMENTS
- [ ] Ulnar collateral
- [ ] Radial collateral
- [ ] Palmar carpal

CONNECTIVE TISSUE
- [ ] Digital fibrous sheath with anular and cruciate regions
- [ ] Palmar aponeurosis
- [ ] Flexor retinaculum
- [ ] Extensor retinaculum
- [ ] Vinculum longum

BONES
Carpal Bones
- [ ] Scaphoid
- [ ] Lunate
- [ ] Triquetrum
- [ ] Hamate
- [ ] Capitate
- [ ] Trapezium
- [ ] Trapezoid
- [ ] Pisiform
- [ ] Metacarpals
- [ ] Phalanges
  - [ ] Proximal
  - [ ] Middle
  - [ ] Distal

CLINICAL APPLICATIONS

SUBACROMIAL BURSITIS INJECTION

Gray's Anatomy for Students: 64, 392
Netter: 192, 193

Clinical Application

Provides relief for frequently inflamed bursa lying beneath the acromion near the supraspinatus tendon.

Anatomic Landmarks (Fig. IV.1)

- Anterior acromion
- Lateral acromion
- Posterior acromion
- Scapular spine
- Humeral head

ACROMIOCLAVICULAR JOINT INSPECTION

Gray's Anatomy for Students: 35, 388, 398
Netter: 192, 193

Clinical Application

Relieve pain from acromioclavicular joint irritation.

Anatomic Landmarks

- Anterior acromion
- Lateral acromion
- Acromioclavicular joint

GLENOHUMERAL JOINT INJECTION

Gray's Anatomy for Students: 390–392, 399
Netter: 192, 193

Clinical Application

Relieve pain from glenohumeral joint irritation.

Anatomic Landmarks (Figs. IV.2 and IV.3) (Posterior Approach)

- Skin
- Subcutaneous tissue
- Infraspinatus
- Joint capsule
- Glenoid cavity
- Humeral head
- Posterior cord of brachial plexus and its branches

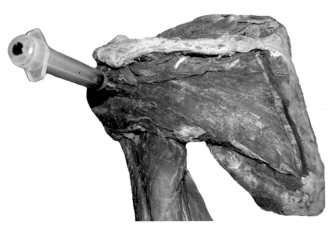

Fig. IV.2

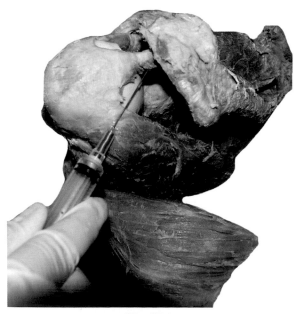

Fig. IV.1

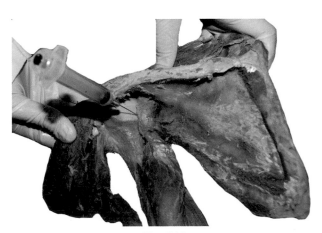

Fig. IV.3

STERNOCLAVICULAR JOINT INJECTION

Gray's Anatomy for Students: 62, 386, 388
Netter: 192, 193

Clinical Application

Relieve pain from sternoclavicular joint irritation.

Anatomic Landmarks

- Skin
- Subcutaneous tissue
- Anterior sternoclavicular ligament
- Articular disc
- Medial clavicle
- Manubrium
- Brachiocephalic vein
- Subclavian artery

BICIPITAL TENOSYNOVITIS INJECTION

Gray's Anatomy for Students: 396
Netter: 412, 421

Clinical Application

Acute trauma or chronic overuse of the biceps brachii tendon (usually long head); relieves pain and may prevent further shoulder pathology.

Anatomic Landmarks (Fig. IV.4)

- Supinated upper limb
- Inferior border of pectoralis major
- Biceps brachii long head
- Humerus

ULNAR NERVE BLOCK FOR CUBITAL TUNNEL SYNDROME

Gray's Anatomy for Students: 414, 424
Netter: 437

Clinical Application

For relief of pain caused by irritation of the ulnar nerve.

Anatomic Landmarks

- Externally rotated upper limb
- Medial epicondyle
- Ulnar sulcus
- Olecranon
- Flexor carpi ulnaris
- Tendinous arch connecting two heads of flexor carpi ulnaris
  Needle is advanced parallel to the ulnar nerve.

MEDIAN NERVE BLOCK (INJECTION AT WRIST)

Gray's Anatomy for Students: 448, 449
Netter: 436, 437, 450

Clinical Application

Median nerve block anesthetizes the lateral palmar 3½ digits.

Anatomic Landmarks (Figs. IV.5 and IV.6)

- Skin
- Proximal palmar skin crease
- Subcutaneous tissue
- Flexor retinaculum
- Palmaris longus muscle (absent in approximately 20%)

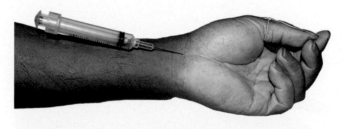

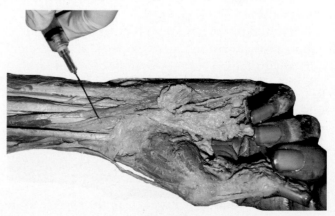

Fig. IV.5

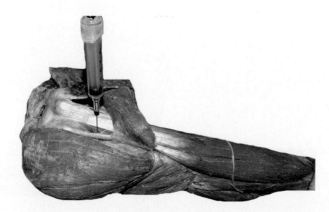

Fig. IV.4

Fig. IV.6

- Flexor carpi radialis muscle
- Median nerve

DE QUERVAIN DISEASE INJECTION

Gray's Anatomy for Students: 452, 453
Netter: 457

Clinical Application

Relieve pain associated with stenosing tenosynovitis of the extensor pollicis brevis muscle.

Anatomic Landmarks (Figs. IV.7 and IV.8)

- Skin
- Subcutaneous tissue
- 1st dorsal compartment retinaculum
- Cephalic vein
- Radial artery branches
- 1st metacarpal base
- 1st metacarpophalangeal joint
- Extensor pollicis brevis

MEDIAL EPICONDYLITIS INJECTION

Gray's Anatomy for Students: 410
Netter: 438, 464

Clinical Application

Relief of pain caused by strain to the attachment of the forearm flexors at the medial epicondyle region.

Anatomic Landmarks

- Skin
- Subcutaneous tissue
- Common flexor tendon
- Medial epicondyle

LATERAL EPICONDYLITIS INJECTION

Gray's Anatomy for Students: 432–434
Netter: 438, 464

CLINICAL APPLICATION

Relief of pain caused by strain to the attachment of the forearm flexors at the lateral epicondyle region.

Anatomic Landmarks (Figs. IV.9 and IV.10)

- Skin
- Subcutaneous tissue
- Common extensor tendon
- Lateral epicondyle

DIGITAL NERVE BLOCK (HAND)

Gray's Anatomy for Students: 488
Netter: 456–458

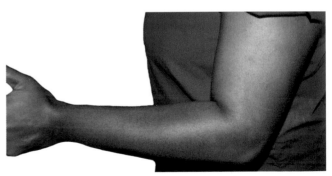

Fig. IV.9

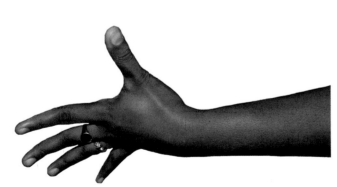

Fig. IV.7

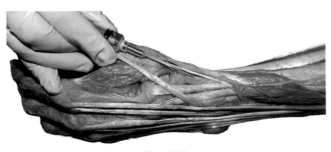

Fig. IV.8

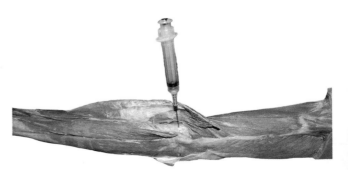

Fig. IV.10

Clinical Application

Anesthetize the palmar or dorsal side of a single or multiple digits to perform invasive procedures.

Anatomic Landmarks (Figs. IV.11 and IV.12)

- Skin
- Subcutaneous tissue
- Common digital nerves/arteries

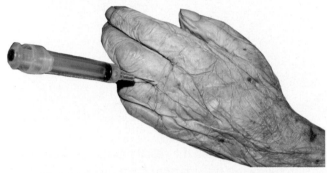

Fig. IV.11

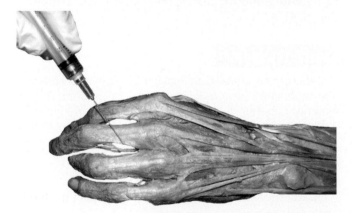

Fig. IV.12

- Palmar digital nerves/arteries
- Dorsal digital nerves/arteries
- Metacarpophalangeal joints
- Proximal interphalangeal joints

VENIPUNCTURE OR PHLEBOTOMY

Gray's Anatomy for Students: 457
Netter: 406, 407

Clinical Application

To withdraw venous blood through needle penetration, or to insert intravenous (IV) cannula.

Anatomic Landmarks (Fig. IV.13)

- Skin
- Subcutaneous tissue
  Elbow: Antecubital vein
  Forearm: Cephalic vein
           Basilic vein
  Hand dorsum: Cephalic vein
           Basilic vein
           Dorsal venous arch
           Metacarpal veins

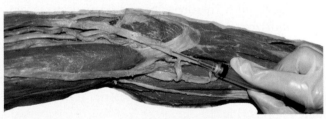

Fig. IV.13

SECTION V

ABDOMEN

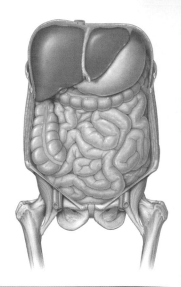

ATLAS REFERENCES
Netter: 249–264, 389, 390
McMinn: 217–225, 253
Gray's Atlas: 134–146, 148–150

BEFORE YOU BEGIN
In general, the abdomen can be divided into right and left superior (upper) quadrants and right and left inferior (lower) quadrants. This division in based on drawing vertical and horizontal lines through the umbilicus (Fig. 10.1).

More specifically, the anterior abdominal wall can be divided into regions: the right and left *hypochondriac* regions; the right and left *lateral* regions; the right and left *inguinal* regions; and the epigastric, umbilical, and pubic regions (Fig. 10.2).

Identify and palpate the following:
- Xiphoid process
- The lower costal margins, which form the subcostal plane
- The umbilicus (typically located at the level of 4th lumbar vertebra)
- Anterior superior iliac spines
- Pubic symphysis
- Pubic crests
- Iliac crests
- Tubercles of the iliac crests, which form the intertubercular plane when connected. This plane is located at the L5 level just inferior to the bifurcation of the abdominal aorta

SKIN AND SUPERFICIAL FASCIA
From the xiphoid process make a midline vertical skin incision from the xiphoid process to the pubic symphysis. Do not cut through the umbilicus; make a circumferential

incision around it. From the costal margins make a second incision following this margin, from the midaxillary line to the xiphoid process. Finally, make an incision from the anterior superior iliac spine to the pubic symphysis (Fig. 10.3).

DISSECTION TIP
An alternate method is to make a vertical incision from the midaxillary line to 2 inches (5 cm) inferior to the anterior superior iliac spine. Make a transverse incision inferior to the inguinal ligament. Reflect the skin inferiorly to the level of the anterior superior iliac spine to expose the inguinal region.

○ Dissect the skin from the midline and reflect it laterally (Fig. 10.4).
○ Expose the superficial fascia (fatty layer) beneath the skin (Fig. 10.5).

ANATOMY NOTE
The fatty layer (fatty) of the superficial fascia is also known as *Camper's fascia,* whereas the membranous layer is known as *Scarpa's fascia.*

○ As the superficial fascia is reflected (Fig. 10.6), note a superficial fatty layer and a deeper membranous layer.
○ Reflect the superficial fatty layer similar to the previously made skin incision.
○ Make a shallow incision with the scalpel and place your index finger into the incision so that lateral traction can be applied and reflection performed.
○ Continue with blunt dissection to identify the deep membranous fascia over the abdominal muscles.
○ Once this is achieved, continue the dissection using a scalpel.

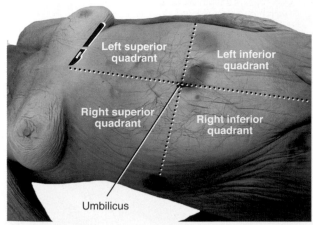

Fig. 10.1 Anterior view of abdomen showing simplified division into quadrants.

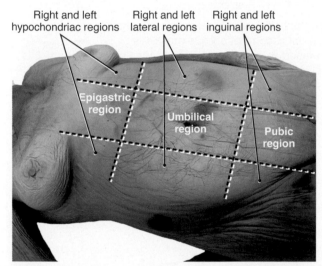

Fig. 10.2 Anterior view of abdomen showing division into regions.

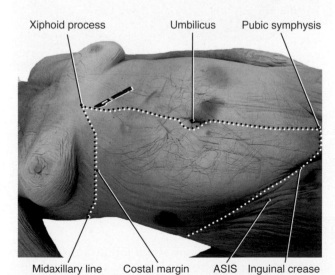

Fig. 10.3 Anterior view of abdomen showing the skin incisions *(dashed lines)* used to begin dissection. *ASIS,* anterior superior iliac spine.

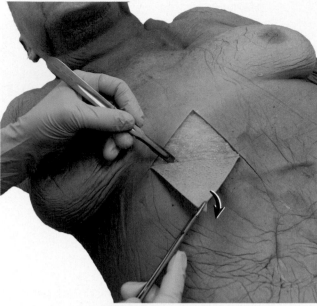

Fig. 10.4 Method used to reflect skin from underlying fascia. Note tension placed on corner of skin flap as scalpel liberates this layer from underlying fascia.

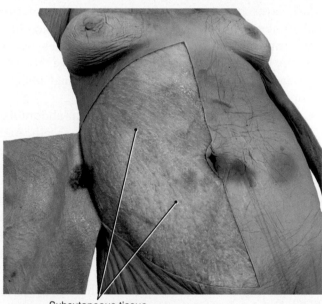

Subcutaneous tissue
(superficial fascia of abdomen)

Fig. 10.5 Anterior view of abdomen showing skin reflection with underlying subcutaneous tissues.

MUSCLES OF THE ANTERIOR ABDOMINAL WALL

ANATOMY **NOTE**

The three flat muscles of the anterolateral abdominal wall—external abdominal oblique, internal abdominal oblique, and transversus abdominis—are covered by a superficial fascia and a deep fascia. The outermost fascia covering the external abdominal oblique muscle (deep) is called the *fascia of Gallaudet.*

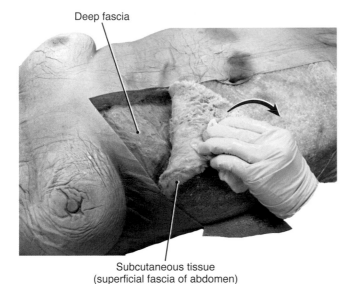

Deep fascia

Subcutaneous tissue
(superficial fascia of abdomen)

Fig. 10.6 Anterior view of abdomen with skin and fascia reflected from the midline on right side.

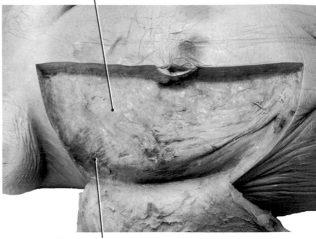

Outer rectus sheath covered
with membranous layer of
superficial fascia

External abdominal
oblique

Fig. 10.7 With additional dissection, the external abdominal oblique muscle is identified with its contribution to the outer rectus sheath.

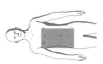

- O Continue the dissection by reflecting the superficial fatty layer and exposing the muscles of the anterior abdomen (covered with deep fascia) and the outer layer of the rectus sheath (anterior lamina) (Fig. 10.7).
- O At the level of the midaxillary line, remove the deep fascia and expose the external abdominal oblique muscle (Fig. 10.8).
- O Clean the deep fascia over the external abdominal oblique and outer layer of the rectus sheath, and identify the linea alba, and linea semilunaris (at the lateral border of the rectus sheath) and inguinal ligament (Figs. 10.9 and 10.10).
- O Once the external abdominal oblique muscle is exposed at the midabdomen on both sides, continue the reflection of the deep fascia over the pubic symphysis and inguinal ligament to further expose the external abdominal oblique muscle (Fig. 10.11).
- O With forceps, lift the outer layer of the rectus sheath (anterior lamina) at the level of the xiphoid process.
- O With scissors, make a small incision into the rectus sheath (anterior lamina) (Fig. 10.12).
- O Lift the rectus sheath upward and identify the rectus abdominis muscle underneath it (Fig. 10.13).
- O With your scalpel, detach the outer layer of the rectus sheath (anterior lamina) alongside its border with the external abdominal oblique muscle (Fig. 10.14).

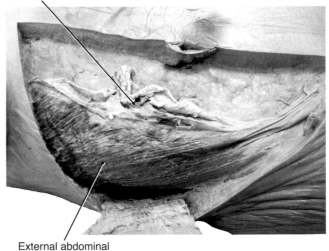

Outer rectus
sheath

External abdominal
oblique

Fig. 10.8 Anterior view of abdomen noting exposed external abdominal oblique muscle and contributions medially into outer rectus sheath.

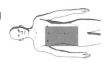

DISSECTION **TIP**

An alternative method is to make a vertical incision at the midline and reflect the outer layer of the rectus sheath laterally from the linea alba.

DISSECTION **TIP**

The tendinous intersections attach firmly to the anterior lamina of the rectus sheath. Employ sharp dissection when necessary to remove the anterior lamina. Observe the linea alba becoming wider and thicker above the umbilicus.

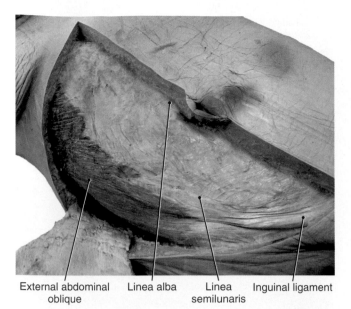

External abdominal oblique | Linea alba | Linea semilunaris | Inguinal ligament

Fig. 10.9 Anterior view of abdomen noting exposed external abdominal oblique muscle and contributions medially into outer rectus sheath.

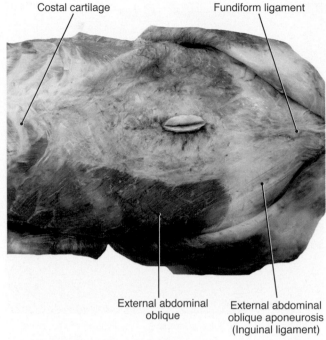

Costal cartilage | Fundiform ligament

External abdominal oblique | External abdominal oblique aponeurosis (Inguinal ligament)

Fig. 10.11 Anterior view of abdomen noting upper attachments of external abdominal oblique muscle along costal margin and inferiorly with specialization of its aponeurosis, the inguinal ligament.

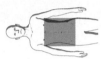

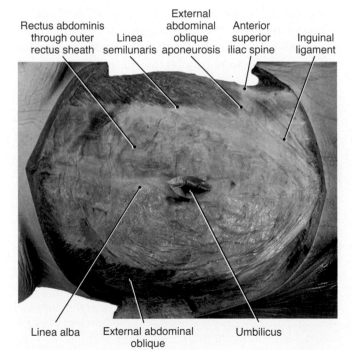

Rectus abdominis through outer rectus sheath | Linea semilunaris | External abdominal oblique aponeurosis | Anterior superior iliac spine | Inguinal ligament

Linea alba | External abdominal oblique | Umbilicus

Fig. 10.10 Anterior view of full abdominal exposure showing anatomic landmarks. Note linea alba traveling in the midline with interposed umbilicus.

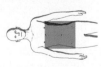

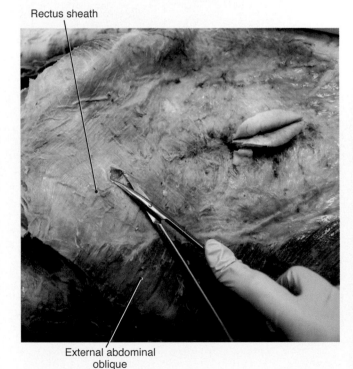

Rectus sheath

External abdominal oblique

Fig. 10.12 Anterior view of abdomen showing expansion of outer rectus fascia.

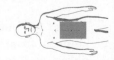

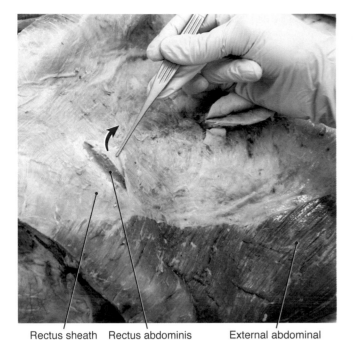

Fig. 10.13 Anterior view of abdomen noting continued opening of outer rectus sheath.

Rectus sheath   Rectus abdominis   External abdominal oblique

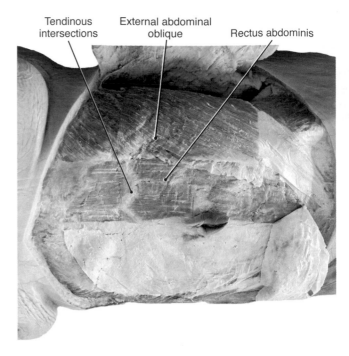

Tendinous intersections   External abdominal oblique   Rectus abdominis

Fig. 10.15 Rectus abdominis muscle is exposed more or less along its entirety.

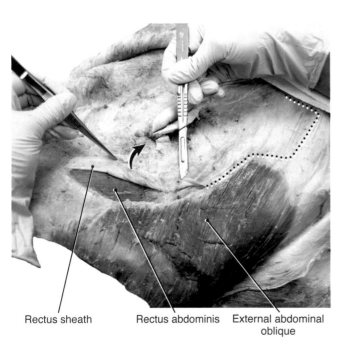

Rectus sheath   Rectus abdominis   External abdominal oblique

Fig. 10.14 Outer sheath is exposed along lateral edge of the junction of external abdominal oblique muscle with its aponeurosis.

○ Reflect the outer layer of the rectus sheath (anterior lamina) from the xiphoid process to pubic symphysis and completely expose the rectus abdominis muscle. Leave a small part of the rectus sheath intact (Fig. 10.15).

○ Identify the tendinous intersections, formed by the tendinous inscriptions of the rectus abdominis muscle and its segmentation, and the *linea alba,* the avascular fusion point of the aponeuroses of the muscles of the anterior abdominal wall at the midline extending from the xiphoid process to the pubic symphysis. (Fig. 10.16).

○ At the inferior portion of the rectus abdominis muscle and anterior to it, identify the pyramidalis muscle (see Fig. 10.16).

DISSECTION TIP

The pyramidalis muscle is absent in about 20% of cases.

DISSECTION TIP

During the dissection of the anterior abdominal wall, note the anterior primary rami of the 7th to 12th thoracic nerves (T7 to T12) supplying the muscles of the anterior abdominal wall. Below are five important nerves in this region and some anatomic landmarks:

1. T7, usually found just inferior to xiphoid process.
2. T10, at the level of the umbilicus.
3. T12, at the level just above the pubis.
4. Ilioinguinal nerve, at the level of the anterior superior iliac spine, underneath the external abdominal oblique muscle.

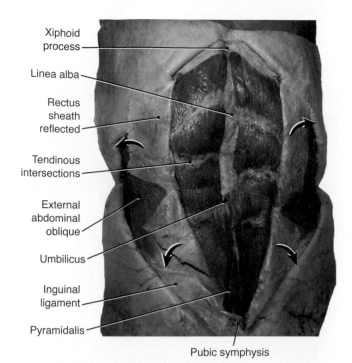

Xiphoid process
Linea alba
Rectus sheath reflected
Tendinous intersections
External abdominal oblique
Umbilicus
Inguinal ligament
Pyramidalis
Pubic symphysis

Fig. 10.16 Continued exposure of outer rectus sheath.

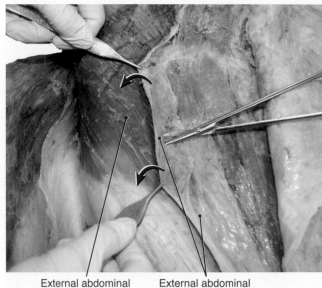

External abdominal oblique
External abdominal oblique aponeurosis

Fig. 10.17 Continued exposure of outer rectus sheath.

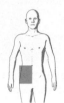

5. Iliohypogastric nerve, 3 to 4 cm above the ilioinguinal nerve at the level of the anterior superior iliac spine.

○ At the level of the linea semilunaris, make a small incision between the external abdominal oblique and rectus abdominis muscles (Fig. 10.17).

○ Retract the external abdominal oblique muscle laterally, and expose the fibers of the underlying internal abdominal oblique muscle (Fig. 10.18).

○ Similarly, cut the internal abdominal oblique muscle at the level of the linea semilunaris, and expose the underlying transversus abdominis muscle (Fig. 10.19).

○ Note the difference in the muscle fiber orientation among the external abdominal oblique, internal abdominal oblique, and transversus abdominis muscles.

○ Cut the transversus abdominis muscle and reflect it to expose the underlying transversalis fascia (Fig. 10.20).

○ Between the internal oblique and transversus abdominis muscles, identify anterior primary rami from T7 to T12 (see Fig. 10.20).

○ Note the fascia that lies deep to the transversus abdominis (at its deepest surface) is the *transversalis fascia* (see Fig. 10.20).

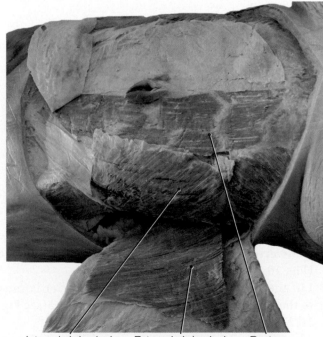

Internal abdominal oblique
External abdominal oblique
Rectus abdominis

Fig. 10.18 After reflecting part of the external abdominal oblique muscle, the deeper layer composed of the internal abdominal oblique muscle is visualized.

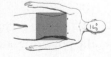

Rectus abdominis | Transversus abdominis | Internal abdominal oblique | Anterior primary rami

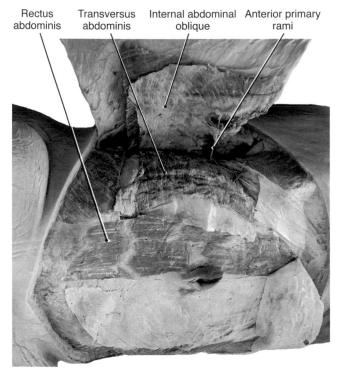

Fig. 10.19 After part of the internal abdominal oblique is reflected, the deeper transversus abdominis muscle is visible.

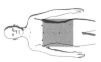

Transversalis fascia | Transversus abdominis | Anterior primary rami

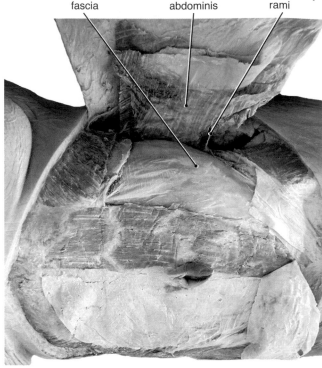

Fig. 10.20 After reflecting part of the transversus abdominis muscle, the deeper transversalis fascia is observed.

DISSECTION **TIP**

An alternate method is to make a vertical incision at the external abdominal oblique muscle on the midaxillary line, where the underlying internal abdominal oblique and transversus abdominis muscles are usually the thickest. Reflect the external abdominal oblique muscle, and identify the internal abdominal oblique muscle. Continue the same process with the internal abdominal oblique, and identify the transversus abdominis muscle (Figs. 10.21 and 10.22).

○ At the level of the xiphoid process, make a shallow transverse incision at the rectus abdominis muscle (Fig. 10.23).

○ Lift the rectus abdominis from its posterior lamina of the rectus sheath, and reflect it downward (see Fig. 10.23 and Plate 10.1).

○ Identify the primary ventral rami of T7 to T12 penetrating the posterior lamina of the rectus sheath (Fig. 10.24).

○ Reflect the rectus abdominis muscle superiorly from the posterior lamina of the rectus sheath, and identify, on its deep surface, the superior and inferior epigastric arteries (Fig. 10.25).

External abdominal oblique | Rectus abdominis

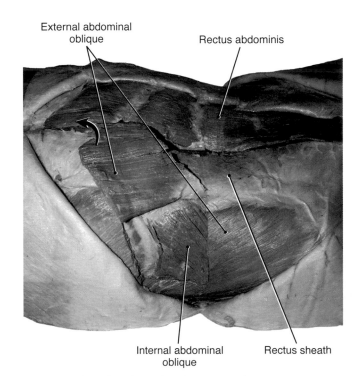

Internal abdominal oblique | Rectus sheath

Fig. 10.21 Anterior view showing external abdominal oblique and rectus abdominis muscles.

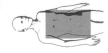

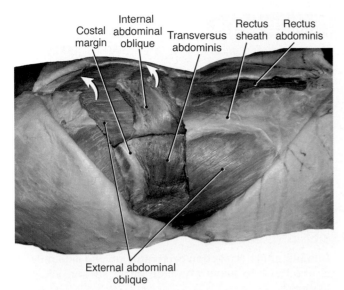

Costal margin — Internal abdominal oblique — Transversus abdominis — Rectus sheath — Rectus abdominis

External abdominal oblique

Fig. 10.22 Additional view after muscular flap cuts showing outermost external abdominal oblique muscle and reflected, deeper-lying internal abdominal oblique muscle. Deep to reflected internal abdominal oblique, the transversus abdominis muscle is seen.

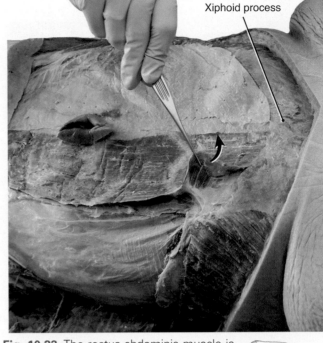

Xiphoid process

Fig. 10.23 The rectus abdominis muscle is reflected inferiorly.

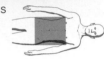

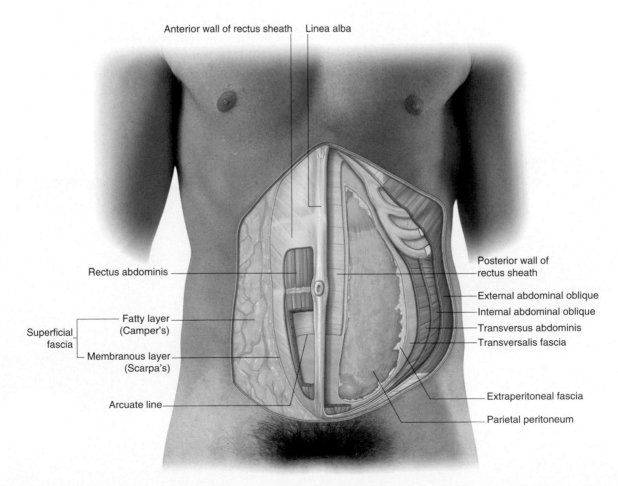

Anterior wall of rectus sheath — Linea alba

Rectus abdominis

Superficial fascia — Fatty layer (Camper's)

Membranous layer (Scarpa's)

Arcuate line

Posterior wall of rectus sheath

External abdominal oblique
Internal abdominal oblique
Transversus abdominis
Transversalis fascia

Extraperitoneal fascia

Parietal peritoneum

Plate 10.1 Layers of the anterior abdominal wall.

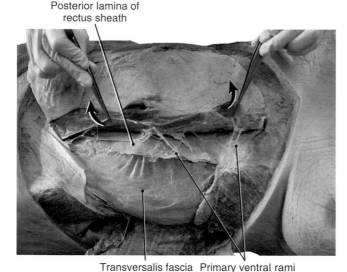

Posterior lamina of
rectus sheath

Transversalis fascia   Primary ventral rami
of T7-T12

Fig. 10.24 With reflection of the rectus abdominis muscle, the segmental nerves of this region are appreciated.

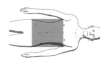

DISSECTION **TIP**

The superior epigastric artery may be difficult to identify.

○ Just inferior to the umbilicus, identify the arcuate line of the rectus sheath, where the posterior lamina of the sheath is formed only by transversalis fascia (Figs. 10.26, 10.27, and 10.28).

INGUINAL REGION

DISSECTION **TIP**

Complete this dissection preferably on one side only! It is important to leave one side intact so that you can compare.

○ Identify the inferior edge of the aponeurosis of the external abdominal oblique muscle, the *inguinal ligament* (Fig. 10.28, Plate 10.2).
○ Reflect part of the skin over the superior portion of the thigh, and identify the great saphenous vein (Fig. 10.29).
○ Extend the skin flap medially and expose the inferior border of the inguinal ligament (Fig. 10.30).
○ Cut the skin covering the spermatic cord inferiorly toward the testis (Fig. 10.31).
○ Clean the adipose tissue and identify the superficial (external) inguinal ring and the spermatic cord covered

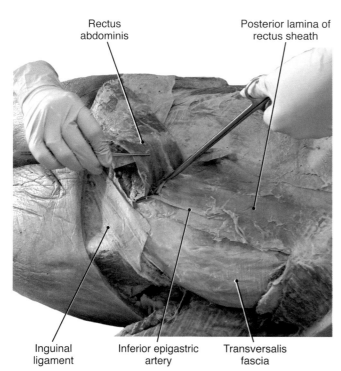

Rectus
abdominis

Posterior lamina of
rectus sheath

Inguinal
ligament

Inferior epigastric
artery

Transversalis
fascia

Fig. 10.25 With continued reflection of the rectus abdominis muscle, the inferior epigastric vessels are seen.

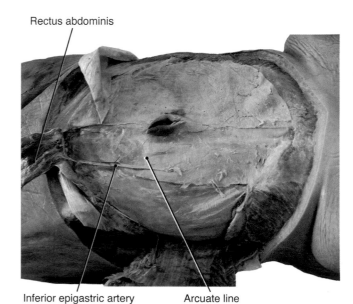

Rectus abdominis

Inferior epigastric artery   Arcuate line

Fig. 10.26 Rectus abdominis muscle is reflected superiorly, and inferior epigastric vessels are seen. Note the arcuate line.

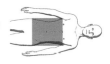

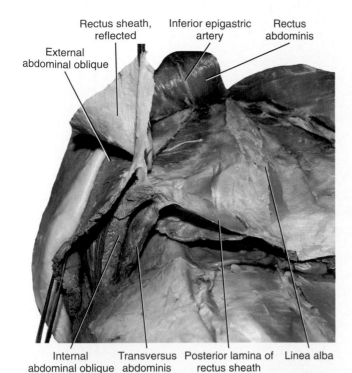

External abdominal oblique — Rectus sheath, reflected — Inferior epigastric artery — Rectus abdominis

Internal abdominal oblique — Transversus abdominis — Posterior lamina of rectus sheath — Linea alba

Fig. 10.27 Anterior view of the left abdominal wall muscles. Note that rectus abdominis muscles are reflected inferiorly and shown laterally are the external and internal oblique and transversus abdominis muscles.

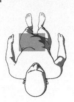

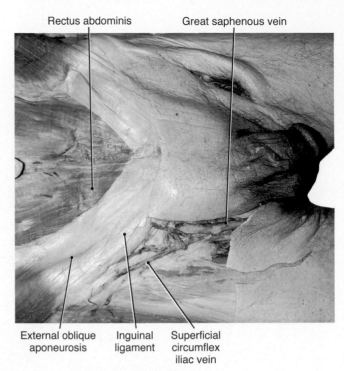

Rectus abdominis — Great saphenous vein

External oblique aponeurosis — Inguinal ligament — Superficial circumflex iliac vein

Fig. 10.29 Anterior view of the inguinal region in the male.

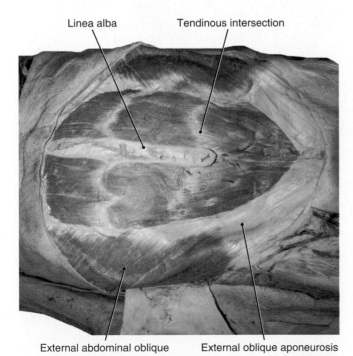

Linea alba — Tendinous intersection

External abdominal oblique — External oblique aponeurosis

Fig. 10.28 Anterior view of anterior abdominal wall. With muscles intact, note the linea alba and external abdominal oblique muscle and its aponeurosis.

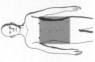

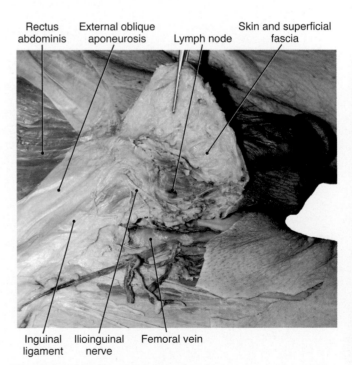

Rectus abdominis — External oblique aponeurosis — Lymph node — Skin and superficial fascia

Inguinal ligament — Ilioinguinal nerve — Femoral vein

Fig. 10.30 Anterior view of the inguinal region in the male showing the ilioinguinal nerve.

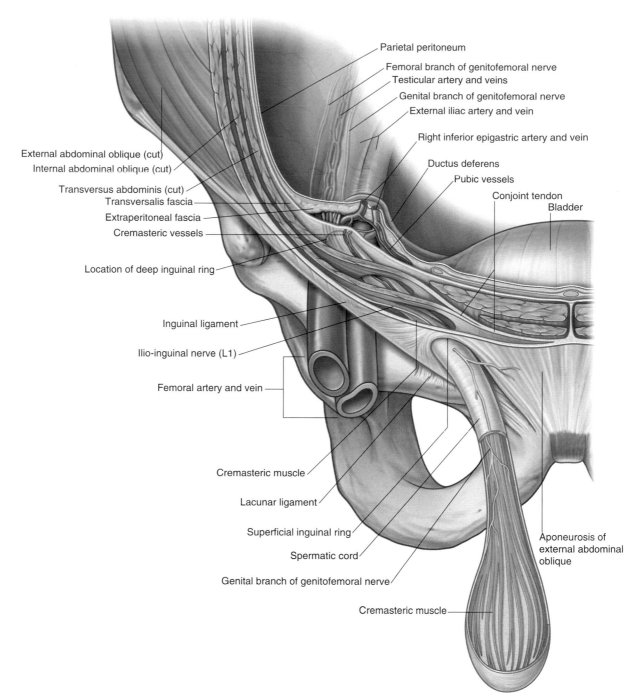

Parietal peritoneum

Femoral branch of genitofemoral nerve

Testicular artery and veins

Genital branch of genitofemoral nerve

External iliac artery and vein

Right inferior epigastric artery and vein

Ductus deferens

Pubic vessels

Conjoint tendon

Bladder

External abdominal oblique (cut)

Internal abdominal oblique (cut)

Transversus abdominis (cut)

Transversalis fascia

Extraperitoneal fascia

Cremasteric vessels

Location of deep inguinal ring

Inguinal ligament

Ilio-inguinal nerve (L1)

Femoral artery and vein

Cremasteric muscle

Lacunar ligament

Superficial inguinal ring

Spermatic cord

Genital branch of genitofemoral nerve

Cremasteric muscle

Aponeurosis of external abdominal oblique

Plate 10.2 Inguinal canal and spermatic cord.

by the external spermatic fascia (see Figs. 10.31 and 10.32).

○ Identify the superomedial part of the inguinal ligament, the *superior crus,* and the inferolateral part, the *inferior crus* (Fig. 10.33).

○ Just superior and anterior to the superior crus, identify the ilioinguinal nerve.

○ Look for the genital branch of the genitofemoral nerve as it travels through the internal and the external inguinal rings within the spermatic cord.

○ Retract the testis laterally (see Fig. 10.33).

○ With scissors, cut the aponeurosis of the external oblique muscle between the two crura at the external inguinal ring (Fig. 10.34).

○ Place the scissors underneath the external spermatic fascia, and make a small incision (Fig. 10.35) to expose the contents of the spermatic cord (Fig. 10.36).

DISSECTION **TIP**

Place your index finger in the opening of the superficial ring to appreciate the oblique course of the *spermatic cord* through the body wall toward the internal ring.

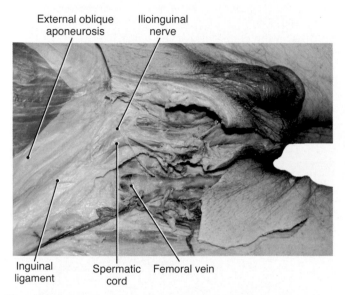

Fig. 10.31 Anterior view of the inguinal region in the male.

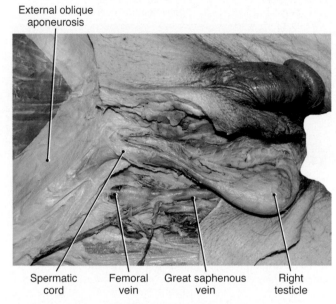

Fig. 10.33 Inguinal region, noting superficial ring of inguinal canal and spermatic cord and right testicle.

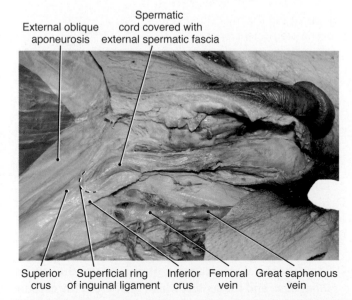

Fig. 10.32 The inguinal region noting the inguinal ligament.

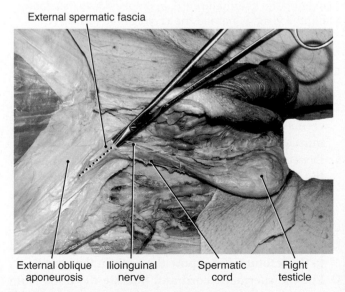

Fig. 10.34 Inguinal and proximal femoral regions.

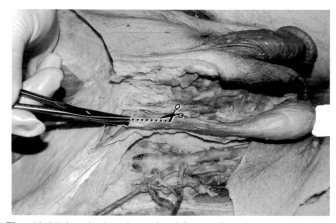

Fig. 10.35 Inguinal and proximal femoral regions.

Ilioinguinal nerve   Genital branch of genitofemoral nerve

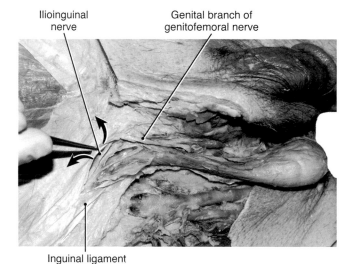

Inguinal ligament

Fig. 10.36 Inguinal region. Note the genital branch of the genitofemoral nerve.

ANATOMY **NOTE**

In the female, the *round ligament* of the uterus replaces the spermatic cord in the inguinal canal. The fascia covering the spermatic cord, and specifically its supero-lateral aspect, is named the *cremasteric fascia*.

○ Incise the external spermatic fascia, formed by the external abdominal oblique muscle.

○ Trace the pampiniform venous plexus, and incise the cremasteric fascia, derived from the internal oblique muscle.

○ Dissect the deepest fascial layer of the spermatic cord, the *internal spermatic fascia,* formed from the fascia of the transversus abdominis muscle, and identify the ductus deferens (Fig. 10.37, Plate 10.3).

○ Identify the cremasteric artery (Fig. 10.38).

○ Continue the incision of the external spermatic fascia to the scrotum and expose the testis in the scrotal sac.

○ Lift the spermatic cord and liberate the testis from the scrotum (Fig. 10.39).

Ductus deferens

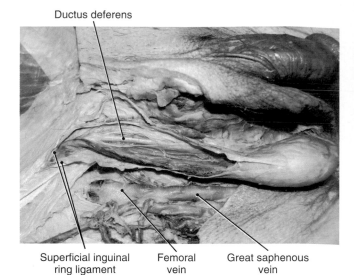

Superficial inguinal ring ligament   Femoral vein   Great saphenous vein

Fig. 10.37 With deeper dissection within spermatic cord, note the ductus deferens.

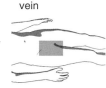

Ductus deferens

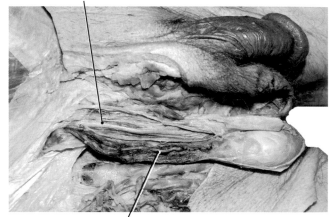

Cremasteric artery

Fig. 10.38 Inguinal region in the male showing cremasteric artery.

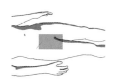

○ Note the outermost layer, called the parietal layer, and the inner, visceral layer of the tunica vaginalis, connecting the epididymis to the testis (with a distinct fold).

○ Identify the epididymis, and note its head, body, and tail (see Fig. 10.39).

○ Hold the testis and with a scalpel make a longitudinal incision to open (Fig. 10.40).

○ Identify the dense capsule of the testis, the *tunica albuginea,* and the septae, which arise from the capsule and divide the testis into several compartments.

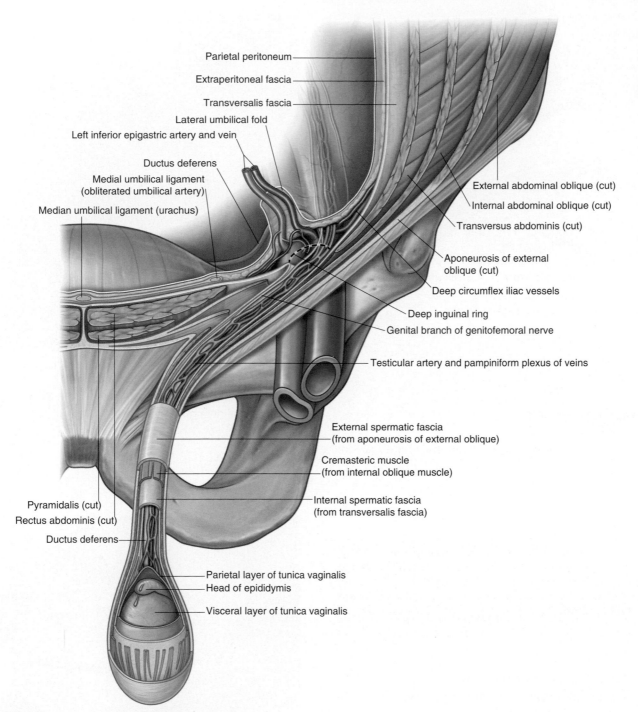

Parietal peritoneum

Extraperitoneal fascia

Transversalis fascia

Lateral umbilical fold

Left inferior epigastric artery and vein

Ductus deferens

Medial umbilical ligament (obliterated umbilical artery)

Median umbilical ligament (urachus)

External abdominal oblique (cut)

Internal abdominal oblique (cut)

Transversus abdominis (cut)

Aponeurosis of external oblique (cut)

Deep circumflex iliac vessels

Deep inguinal ring

Genital branch of genitofemoral nerve

Testicular artery and pampiniform plexus of veins

External spermatic fascia (from aponeurosis of external oblique)

Cremasteric muscle (from internal oblique muscle)

Internal spermatic fascia (from transversalis fascia)

Pyramidalis (cut)

Rectus abdominis (cut)

Ductus deferens

Parietal layer of tunica vaginalis

Head of epididymis

Visceral layer of tunica vaginalis

Plate 10.3 Inguinal canal and contents of spermatic cord.

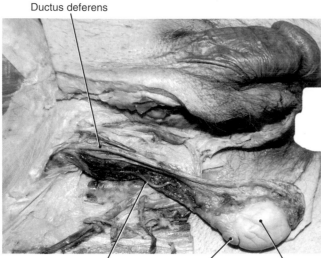

Ductus deferens

Cremasteric artery   Epididymis   Testicle

Fig. 10.39 Inguinal region showing epididymis and its relationship to ductus deferens.

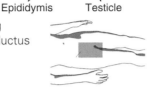

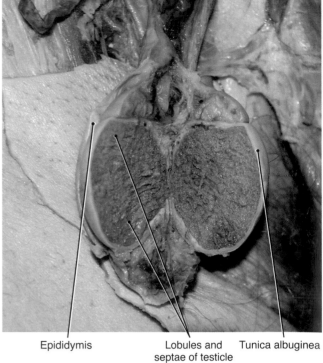

Epididymis   Lobules and septae of testicle   Tunica albuginea

Fig. 10.40 Coronal section through proximal testis noting its layers and components.

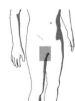

DISSECTION TIP

If you dissect a female cadaver, identify the round ligament of the uterus.

ANATOMY NOTE

The round ligament (ligamentum teres) of the uterus is a fibrous cord traveling from the uterus through the inguinal canal to attach to the labia majora. Identify the round ligament at the superficial ring, and follow it toward the labia majora.

○ Cut the skin covering the penis.

○ Continue to remove fat and skin over the pubic symphysis and the penis.

○ Identify the superficial dorsal vein of the penis embedded in the superficial fascia of the penis (Fig. 10.41).

○ Dissect out and reflect the superficial fascia of the penis laterally (Fig. 10.42).

○ Notice the deep fascia, *Buck's fascia,* of the penis deep to the superficial fascia.

○ On the dorsal surface of the penis, note the separation between the superficial and deep dorsal veins of the penis by Buck's fascia (Fig. 10.43).

○ Separate Buck's fascia and identify the dorsal artery of the penis, which is located bilaterally on the dorsum of the penis medial to the dorsal nerves of the penis (Fig. 10.44).

Superficial dorsal vein of penis

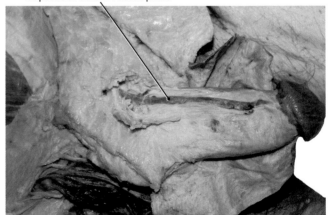

Fig. 10.41 Deeper dissection of dorsal penis shows superficial dorsal vein of penis.

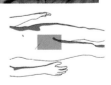

○ Continue the removal of the fat toward the pubic symphysis and expose the fundiform ligament of the penis arising from the superficial fascia (Fig. 10.45).

○ Insert scissors or a probe into the superficial ring just underneath the tendon of the external abdominal oblique muscle, directed toward the anterior superior iliac spine (Fig. 10.46).

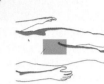

Superficial penile fascia

Fig. 10.42 Dorsal view of penis and its related fascia.

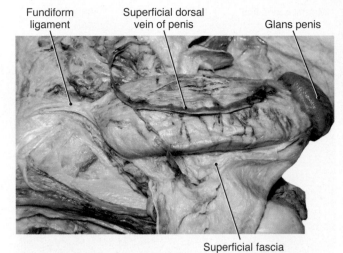

Fundiform ligament   Superficial dorsal vein of penis   Glans penis

Superficial fascia

Fig. 10.45 Dorsal view of penis showing relationship between fundiform ligament and penis.

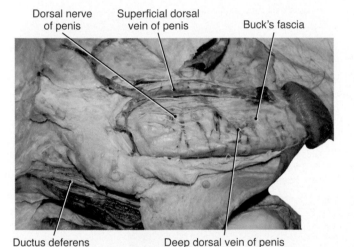

Dorsal nerve of penis   Superficial dorsal vein of penis   Buck's fascia

Ductus deferens   Deep dorsal vein of penis

Fig. 10.43 Dorsal view of penis showing relationship between superficial and deep fasciae. Note position of superficial dorsal vein of penis.

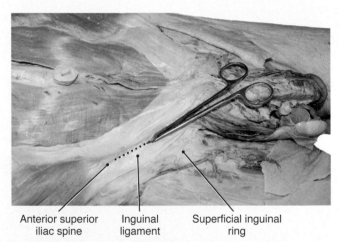

Anterior superior iliac spine   Inguinal ligament   Superficial inguinal ring

Fig. 10.46 The superficial inguinal ring is opened, revealing deeper structures of the inguinal canal.

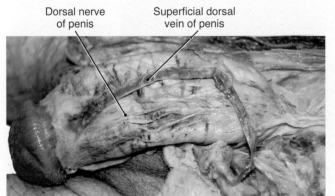

Dorsal nerve of penis   Superficial dorsal vein of penis

Fig. 10.44 Dorsal view of penis with deeper dissection, showing underlying dorsal nerve of penis and its branches.

○ Incise the inguinal ligament over the probe or scissors that was previously inserted, and reflect its borders laterally (Fig. 10.47).

○ Pull the spermatic cord laterally and expose the lacunar ligament (Gimbernat's ligament), which represents the medial triangular expansion of the inguinal ligament to the pectineal line of the pubis (Figs. 10.48 and 10.49).

○ Locate the pectineal ligament (Cooper's ligament), which is a strong fibrous band that extends laterally from the lacunar ligament along the pectineal line of the pubis (see Figs. 10.48 and 10.49).

Internal abdominal oblique | Ilioinguinal nerve | Medial crus

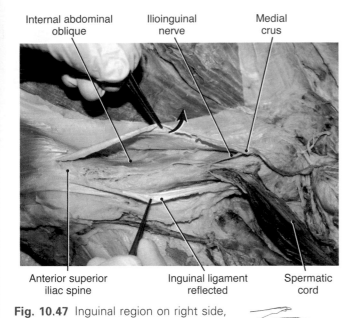

Anterior superior iliac spine | Inguinal ligament reflected | Spermatic cord

Fig. 10.47 Inguinal region on right side, showing exposed inguinal canal and its contents.

Internal abdominal oblique reflected | Lacunar ligament | Medial crus | Pectineal ligament

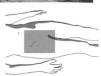

Fig. 10.49 Inguinal region on right side, showing specializations of inguinal ligament, the lacunar and pectineal ligaments.

Internal abdominal oblique | Ilioinguinal nerve | Medial crus | Pectineal ligament | Lacunar ligament

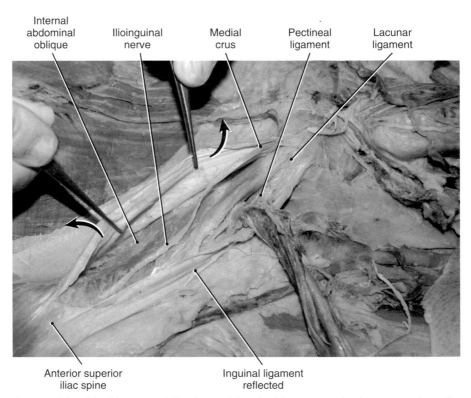

Anterior superior iliac spine | Inguinal ligament reflected

Fig. 10.48 Inguinal region on right side. Note specializations of inguinal ligament—the lacunar and pectineal ligaments.

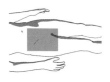

LABORATORY IDENTIFICATION CHECKLIST

NERVES
- ☐ Iliohypogastric
- ☐ Ilioinguinal
- ☐ Genitofemoral
  - ☐ Genital branch
  - ☐ Femoral branch
- ☐ Dorsal, of penis
- ☐ Femoral

ARTERY
- ☐ Cremasteric
- ☐ Inferior epigastric

VEINS
- ☐ Inferior epigastric
- ☐ Superficial external pudendal
- ☐ Superficial dorsal, of penis
- ☐ Femoral
- ☐ Great saphenous

MUSCLES
- ☐ External abdominal oblique
  - ☐ External oblique aponeurosis
- ☐ Internal oblique
- ☐ Cremasteric
- ☐ Transversus abdominis
- ☐ Rectus abdominis
  - ☐ Tendinous intersections
  - ☐ Linea alba

BONES
- ☐ Pubis
  - ☐ Pubic tubercle
  - ☐ Pubic crest
- ☐ Ischium
- ☐ Ilium
  - ☐ Anterior superior iliac spine

LIGAMENTS
- ☐ Inguinal
  - ☐ Superficial ring
  - ☐ Deep ring
- ☐ Lacunar
- ☐ Pectineal
- ☐ Fundiform

FASCIA
- ☐ Superficial
  - ☐ Fatty or Camper's layer
  - ☐ Membranous or Scarpa's layer
- ☐ External spermatic
- ☐ Cremasteric
- ☐ Superficial, of penis
- ☐ Deep, of penis

OTHER STRUCTURES
- ☐ Spermatic cord
- ☐ Testes
  - ☐ Lobules
  - ☐ Septae
- ☐ Epididymis
- ☐ Ductus deferens
- ☐ Tunica vaginalis
- ☐ Tunica albuginea

THREE DIFFERENT TECHNIQUES FOR OPENING THE PERITONEAL CAVITY

DISSECTION TIP

All cuts with the scalpel should be made carefully to avoid cutting too deeply into the peritoneal cavity and underlying viscera.

Technique 1

○ After removal of the skin over the anterior abdominal wall, palpate the most inferior costal cartilages and the xiphoid process (Fig. 11.1).

○ With scissors or a scalpel, cut the attachments of the rectus abdominis and external abdominal oblique muscles over the right and left hypochondriac areas (Fig. 11.2).

○ Continue the incision of the muscles from the xiphoid process toward the midaxillary line on both sides of the cadaver (Fig. 11.3).

○ Reflect the rectus abdominis and abdominal oblique muscles inferiorly (Fig. 11.4).

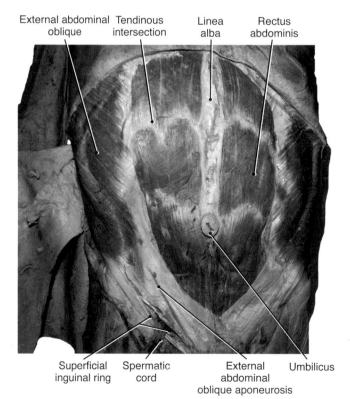

Fig. 11.1 Anterior abdomen with skin and subcutaneous tissue reflected revealing rectus abdominis and external oblique muscles.

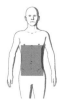

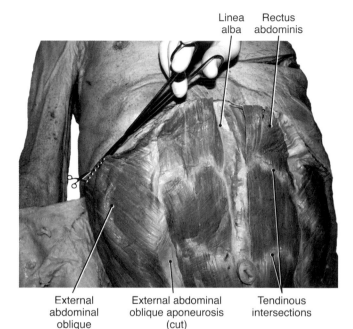

Fig. 11.2 Attachments of rectus abdominis and external oblique muscles incised over right and left hypochondriac areas.

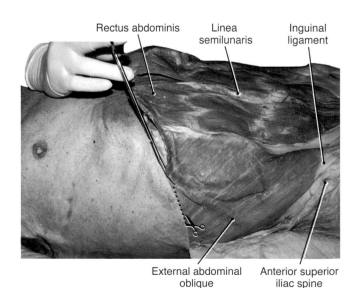

Fig. 11.3 Incision of the muscles from xiphoid process to midaxillary line on both sides.

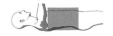

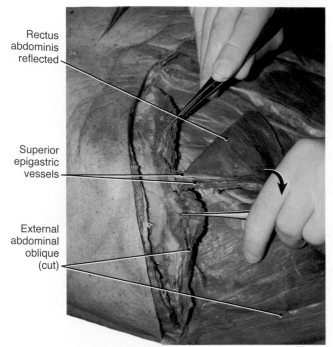

Fig. 11.4 Rectus abdominis and abdominal oblique muscles reflected inferiorly.

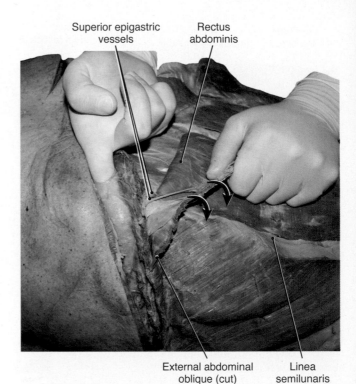

Fig. 11.5 Blunt dissection to expose peritoneal cavity.

○ When necessary, use blunt dissection to expose the peritoneal cavity (Fig. 11.5).

○ Cut the attachments of the diaphragm, falciform ligament, and ligamentum teres (round ligament) of the liver to the abdominal wall.

○ Reflect the anterior abdominal wall toward the pubic symphysis, and observe the contents of the abdominal cavity (Figs. 11.6 and 11.7).

Technique 2

○ Reflect the rectus sheath and expose the rectus abdominis muscle and the posterior lamina of the rectus sheath (Figs. 11.8 and 11.9).

○ Make a midline vertical incision at the linea alba from the xiphoid process to the pubic symphysis.

○ Make a second horizontal incision from the xiphoid process to the midaxillary line, and reflect the muscle flap laterally (Fig. 11.10).

○ Use the same technique on the contralateral side, and expose the peritoneal cavity (Fig. 11.11).

Technique 3

○ Make a midline vertical incision on the linea alba from the xiphoid process to the pubic symphysis.

○ Make a second horizontal incision from the right to the left midaxillary line, passing through the umbilicus, and laterally reflect the four muscle flaps (Fig. 11.12).

○ Identify and cut the falciform and round ligaments on the anterior surface of the liver.

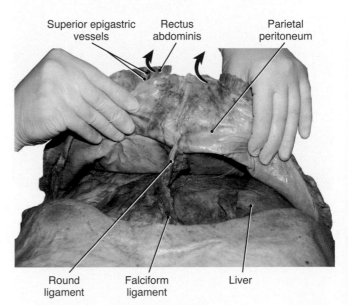

Fig. 11.6 Attachments of the diaphragm, falciform ligament, and round ligament of the liver incised at abdominal wall, with anterior abdominal wall reflected toward pubic symphysis.

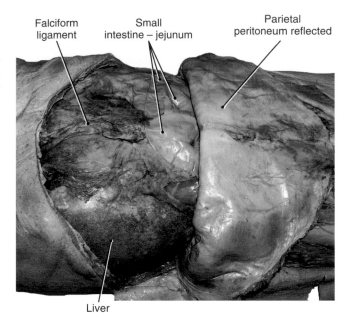

Falciform ligament
Small intestine – jejunum
Parietal peritoneum reflected

Liver

Fig. 11.7 Parietal peritoneum reflected, showing contents of abdomen and anterior abdominal wall.

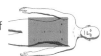

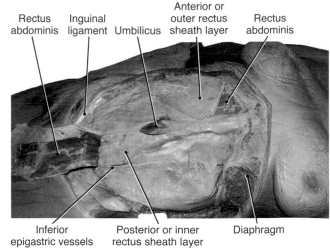

Rectus abdominis
Inguinal ligament
Umbilicus
Anterior or outer rectus sheath layer
Rectus abdominis

Inferior epigastric vessels
Posterior or inner rectus sheath layer
Diaphragm

Fig. 11.9 Observe exposed rectus abdominis muscles and posterior lamina of rectus sheath.

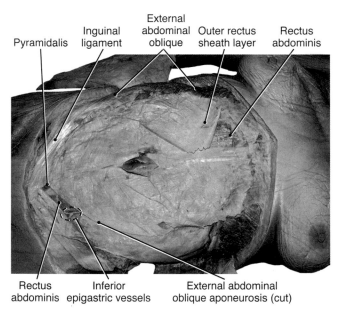

Pyramidalis
Inguinal ligament
External abdominal oblique
Outer rectus sheath layer
Rectus abdominis

Rectus abdominis
Inferior epigastric vessels
External abdominal oblique aponeurosis (cut)

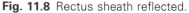

Fig. 11.8 Rectus sheath reflected.

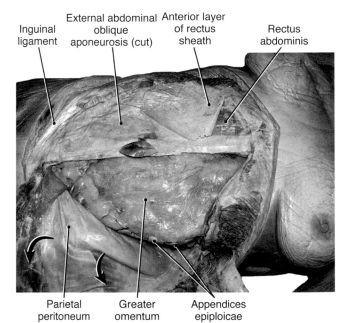

Inguinal ligament
External abdominal oblique aponeurosis (cut)
Anterior layer of rectus sheath
Rectus abdominis

Parietal peritoneum
Greater omentum
Appendices epiploicae

Fig. 11.10 Xiphoid process to pubic symphysis incision.

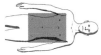

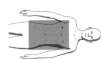

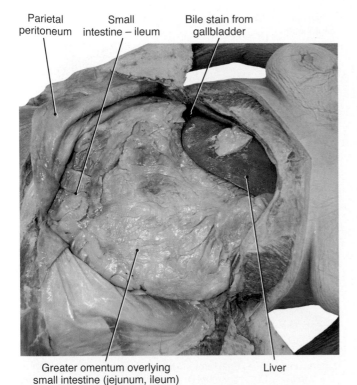

Parietal peritoneum | Small intestine – ileum | Bile stain from gallbladder

Greater omentum overlying small intestine (jejunum, ileum) | Liver

Fig. 11.11 Second horizontal incision from xiphoid process to midaxillary line on both sides with laterally reflected muscle flap.

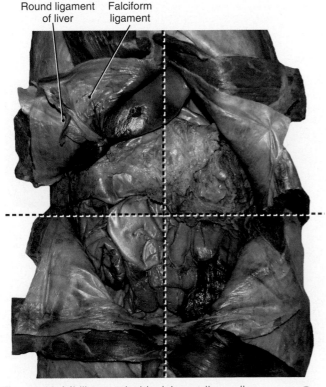

Round ligament of liver | Falciform ligament

Fig. 11.12 Midline vertical incision at linea alba from xiphoid process to pubic symphysis, with second horizontal incision from right to left midaxillary lines through umbilicus, with four muscle flaps reflected laterally.

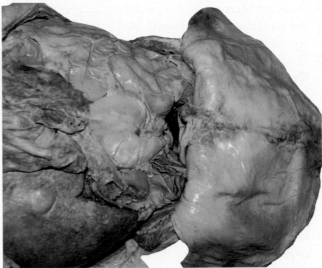

Fig. 11.13 Five peritoneal folds at internal surface of anterior abdominal wall: two lateral folds, two medial folds, and one median umbilical fold.

DISSECTION **TIP**

In some specimens the peritoneal cavity is small. To expose it further, with a saw, cut the ribs in the midaxillary line on both sides of the cadaver. You also may extend the cuts with those made previously to expose the thoracic cavity.

In some cadavers, you will be able to separate the parietal peritoneum from the transversalis fascia. In most, however, these two layers are tightly adherent.

PERITONEAL STRUCTURES

O Trace the round ligament of the liver along its pathway from the anterior surface of the liver to the median aspect of the anterior abdominal wall to the umbilicus.

O At the internal (posterior) surface of the anterior abdominal wall, identify five notable peritoneal folds: the lateral (right and left), the medial (right and left), and the single median umbilical folds (Fig. 11.13).

ANATOMY **NOTE**

The peritoneal fold covering the inferior epigastric artery and vein is the lateral umbilical peritoneal fold. The medial umbilical folds are formed by an elevation of the peritoneum over the obliterated umbilical arteries. Similarly, the median umbilical fold is an elevation of the peritoneum over the remnants of the urachus (intraabdominal part of allantois). The space between the medial umbilical fold and median umbilical fold is termed the *supravesical fossa*. The depressed region between the medial umbilical fold and the lateral umbilical fold is termed the *medial inguinal fossa*. The lateral inguinal fossa is the area lateral to the lateral inguinal fold.

- Make an incision at the posterior layer of the rectus sheath (and peritoneum) and expose the rectus abdominis muscle (Fig. 11.14).
- Trace the course of the inferior epigastric artery and identify its origin from the external iliac artery (Figs. 11.15 to 11.17).

DISSECTION **TIP**

In approximately 30% of cadavers, the inferior epigastric artery will give rise to the obturator artery, which travels medially over the pelvic brim.

- Remove the peritoneum covering the inferior epigastric artery and the base of the rectus abdominis muscle, and identify the inguinal ligament (Fig. 11.18).

ANATOMY **NOTE**

Notice the triangle of Hesselbach formed by the lateral border of the rectus abdominis muscle, the inguinal ligament, and the inferior epigastric vessels.

- Laterally to the inferior epigastric artery and vein, identify the deep inguinal ring and the ductus deferens (round ligament in females) passing within it.

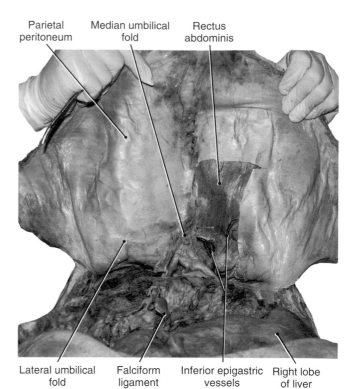

Parietal peritoneum · Median umbilical fold · Rectus abdominis

Lateral umbilical fold · Falciform ligament · Inferior epigastric vessels · Right lobe of liver

Fig. 11.15 Appreciate the inferior epigastric artery and vein, as well as medial and lateral umbilical peritoneal folds.

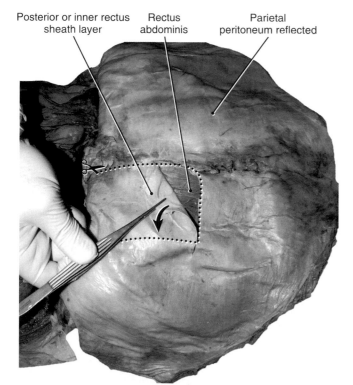

Posterior or inner rectus sheath layer · Rectus abdominis · Parietal peritoneum reflected

Fig. 11.14 Posterior layer of rectus sheath cut exposing rectus abdominis muscle.

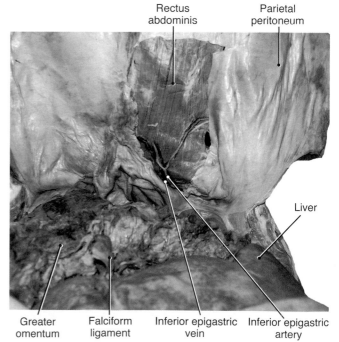

Rectus abdominis · Parietal peritoneum

Liver

Greater omentum · Falciform ligament · Inferior epigastric vein · Inferior epigastric artery

Fig. 11.16 Dissect the inferior epigastric artery and vein.

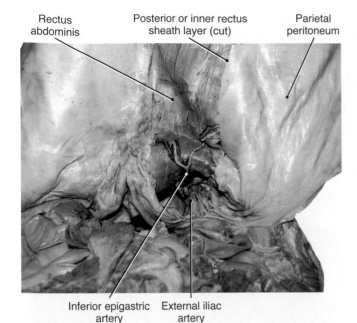

Rectus abdominis — Posterior or inner rectus sheath layer (cut) — Parietal peritoneum

Inferior epigastric artery — External iliac artery

Fig. 11.17 Dissect the inferior epigastric artery where it arises from the external iliac artery.

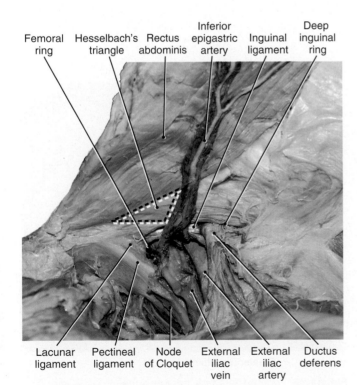

Femoral ring — Hesselbach's triangle — Rectus abdominis — Inferior epigastric artery — Inguinal ligament — Deep inguinal ring

Lacunar ligament — Pectineal ligament — Node of Cloquet — External iliac vein — External iliac artery — Ductus deferens

Fig. 11.18 Dissect the peritoneum covering the inferior epigastric artery and base of the rectus abdominis muscle and identify the inguinal ligament. Continue the dissection by locating the pubic tubercle, and lateral to it, identify the pectineal ligament.

- Continue the dissection by identifying the pubic tubercle and, lateral to it, a strong ligamentous band running over the periosteum of the pectineal line, the *pectineal ligament* (Cooper's ligament) (see Fig. 11.18).
- Note the medial one third of the inguinal ligament forming an aponeurotic expansion attaching to the pectineal line of the pubis and pectineal ligament, the *lacunar ligament* (Gimbernat's ligament) (see Fig. 11.18).
- Lateral to the lacunar ligament, expose the femoral vessels, and identify the *femoral ring* (lying medial to the femoral vein), the opening to the femoral canal.

DISSECTION **TIP**

Clean the adipose tissue and look for a large lymph node, the *node of Cloquet*.

- Retract the femoral vein medially and note a fascial partition under the inguinal ligament between the femoral vein and the iliopsoas muscle. This partition between the vascular portion (lacuna vasorum) and the muscular portion (lacuna musculorum) is called the *iliopectineal ligament* (see Fig. 11.18).
- Inspect the contents of the peritoneal cavity, and identify the liver, stomach (with its greater and lesser curvatures), small and large intestines, and greater omentum (Fig. 11.19).

ANATOMY **NOTE**

The peritoneal cavity is traditionally divided into two parts, the greater and lesser sacs, or into supracolic and infracolic compartments. The *greater sac* is the entire area of the peritoneal cavity with the exception of the area extending behind the stomach to the diaphragm at the left side, which is the *lesser sac* (omental bursa). Similarly, the *supracolic compartment* is the area of the peritoneal cavity that extends from the transverse mesocolon to the diaphragm. The *infracolic compartment* is the area of the peritoneal cavity extending from the transverse mesocolon below to the pelvic brim.

- Identify the greater curvature of the stomach, and lift the greater omentum (Fig. 11.20).
- Expose the transverse colon with its transverse mesocolon, and identify the ileum, jejunum, cecum, ascending colon, transverse colon, and descending sigmoid colon (Fig. 11.21).
- Observe the space between the liver and the stomach and identify the gallbladder and lesser omentum (Fig. 11.22).
- With blunt dissection using your fingertips, separate any adhesions between the stomach and the liver (Fig. 11.23).

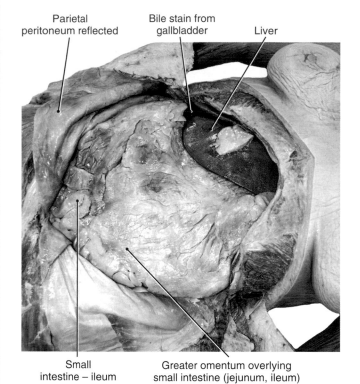

Parietal peritoneum reflected   Bile stain from gallbladder   Liver

Small intestine – ileum   Greater omentum overlying small intestine (jejunum, ileum)

Fig. 11.19 Appreciate the liver, stomach, small and large intestines, and greater omentum.

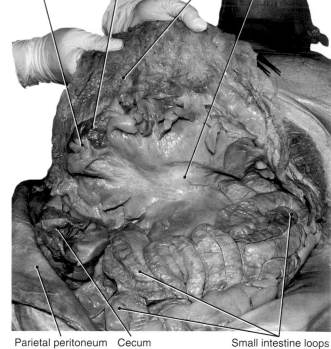

Appendices epiploicae   Right colic flexure of transverse colon   Greater omentum   Transverse mesocolon

Parietal peritoneum   Cecum   Small intestine loops

Fig. 11.21 Expose and locate the transverse colon and mesocolon.

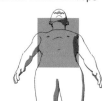

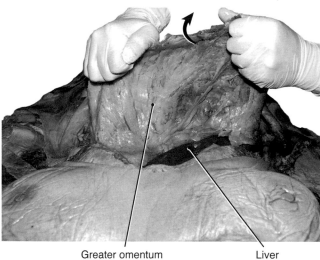

Greater omentum   Liver

Fig. 11.20 Lift the greater omentum at the greater curvature of stomach.

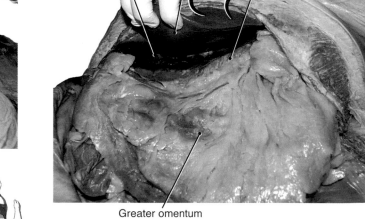

Gallbladder   Liver   Stomach

Greater omentum

Fig. 11.22 Locate the space between the liver and stomach and identify the gallbladder and lesser omentum.

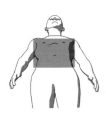

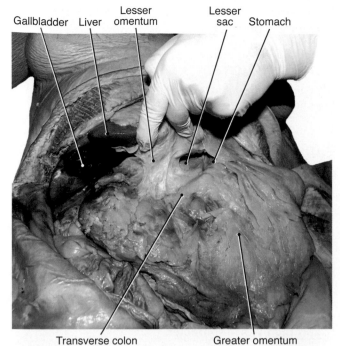

Gallbladder | Liver | Lesser omentum | Lesser sac | Stomach

Transverse colon | Greater omentum

Fig. 11.23 Continue the blunt dissection with your fingers.

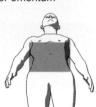

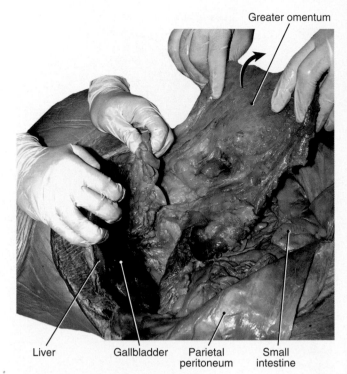

Greater omentum

Liver | Gallbladder | Parietal peritoneum | Small intestine

Fig. 11.24 Cut the greater omentum approximately 3 cm from the greater curvature of stomach, but do *not* cut its connection with the transverse colon.

DISSECTION **TIP**

Often you will find several adhesions between the contents of the peritoneal cavity. Take some time and separate these adhesions to restore the normal anatomy and position of the organs.

○ Cut the greater omentum 3 to 4 cm away from the greater curvature, and leave its attachments to the transverse colon (Fig. 11.24).

○ Pull the stomach away from the transverse colon, and note the area of the lesser sac. Also notice the pancreas lying directly behind the stomach (Fig. 11.25).

○ Continue the dissection by pulling the stomach inferiorly from the liver, and note the *epiploic foramen* (of Winslow) (Fig. 11.26).

○ Pass a probe or scissors underneath the lesser omentum through the epiploic foramen (Fig. 11.27 and Plate 11.1).

PALPATION AND IDENTIFICATION OF STRUCTURES (WITHOUT DISSECTION)

1. Lesser omentum
2. Epiploic foramen
3. Stomach
4. Gallbladder

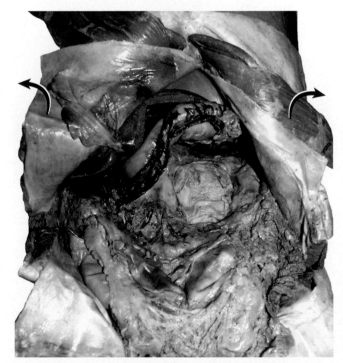

Fig. 11.25 Pull the stomach from the transverse colon to appreciate the lesser sac and pancreas.

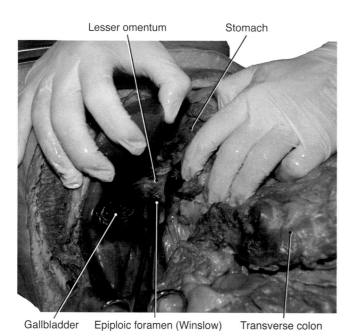

Liver   Lesser omentum   Stomach

Gallbladder   Epiploic foramen (of Winslow)   Transverse colon

Fig. 11.26 Pull the stomach inferiorly from the liver and locate the epiploic foramen.

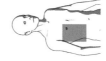

Lesser omentum   Stomach

Gallbladder   Epiploic foramen (Winslow)   Transverse colon

Fig. 11.27 Pass a probe or scissors posterior to the lesser omentum via the epiploic foramen.

5. Spleen
6. Liver
7. Small intestine
8. Large intestine

Lesser Omentum

○ The *lesser omentum* includes the hepatogastric and hepatoduodenal ligaments. To distinguish them, note that the *hepatogastric* ligament connects the liver to

the stomach, whereas the *hepatoduodenal* ligament connects the liver to the duodenum.

ANATOMY **NOTE**

The hepatoduodenal ligament contains the bile duct, the hepatic artery, and the hepatic portal vein.

Epiploic Foramen

○ Place your thumb at the *epiploic foramen* and index finger on top of the hepatoduodenal ligament, and feel for these structures. This is called the *Pringle maneuver* and is useful for controlling hemorrhage from the hepatic artery when accidentally injured.

Stomach

○ Palpate the anterior surface of the *stomach* and notice the greater and lesser curvatures, the body, the fundus, and the pyloric sphincter.

DISSECTION **TIP**

Note on neighboring cadavers the variable stomach shapes and sizes, which is a normal feature.

Gallbladder

○ Identify the *gallbladder* (if present) at the internal surface of the liver.

DISSECTION **TIP**

A surgical landmark to identify the gallbladder is the point of intersection between the 9th costal cartilage and the linea semilunaris.

Spleen

○ Lift the stomach and pass your fingers posterior to it to reach the spleen. Feel the *gastrosplenic ligament* connecting the greater curvature of the stomach to the spleen.
○ Palpate the *spleen*, and with your palm, try to feel the posterior surface of the spleen up against the body wall.

DISSECTION **TIP**

While attempting this maneuver, your palm will come up against the *splenorenal ligament,* which connects the spleen to the body wall. Similarly, if you try to reach the diaphragm, moving your fingertips upward from the spleen, you will feel the *phrenicocolic ligament* connecting the spleen to the diaphragm.

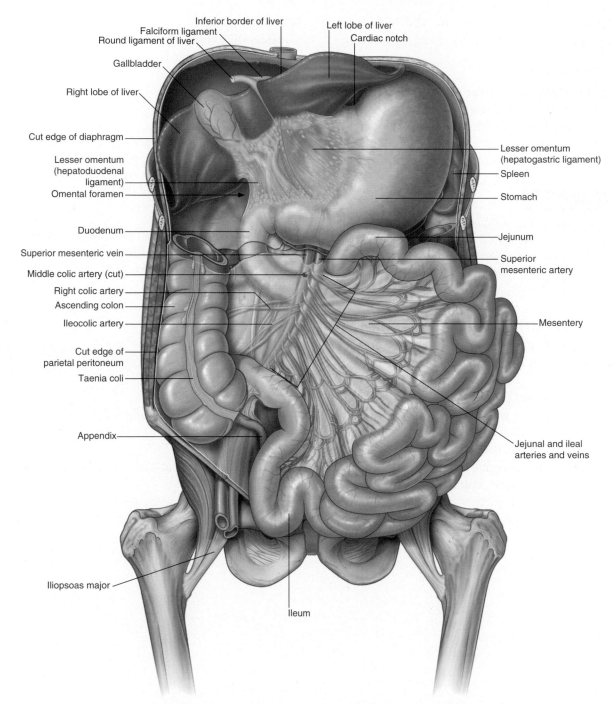

Small intestine displaced to show superior mesenteric vessels

Plate 11.1 Lesser omentum.

Liver

O With your fingertips, palpate the *liver,* and identify the falciform, round, and coronary ligaments.

Small Intestine

O Palpate the pyloric sphincter and distal to it, feel for the much softer, 1st portion of the duodenum.

O Lift the greater omentum, and identify the transverse colon with its mesentery, the *transverse mesocolon.*

O Just behind the transverse mesocolon, the 2nd part of the duodenum passes vertically on the right side of the cadaver.

O Identify the mesentery of the ileum and jejunum.

O The mesentery of the ileum and jejunum covers the 3rd (horizontal) part of the duodenum.

O Identify the final, 4th part, of the duodenum *duodenojejunal flexure.*

O At the duodenojejunal flexure feel for a connective tissue band, the "suspensory ligament of the duodenum" (ligament of Treitz).

- Continue palpating the *jejunum,* which makes up approximately two-fifths of the small intestine.

Large Intestine

- Palpate the distal part of the *ileum* and, in the right lower quadrant of the abdominal cavity, identify the *cecum* and the ileocecal junction.
- Explore the cecum for an attached *appendix.* Notice that the appendix has its own mesentery, the *mesoappendix.*

DISSECTION TIP

In most cadavers the appendix originates from the posterior part of the cecum. This is termed a *retrocecal appendix.* In addition, the appendix often has been surgically removed; look for the original location of the appendix, if possible.

- Continue identifying the ascending, transverse, descending, and sigmoid parts of the colon. The rectum and anus will not be identified during this part of dissection.
- Palpate the proximal part of the ascending colon, the *ileocecal junction,* as well as its distal part the right colic or hepatic flexure at the level of the liver.
- At the hepatic flexure, the ascending colon turns left and becomes the transverse colon.
- Similarly, the transverse colon reaches the splenic flexure or left colic flexure, which turns to the right (inferiorly) to become descending colon.

- At the lower lever of the left lower quadrant, the descending colon becomes the sigmoid colon, exhibiting a characteristic S shape. Notice its mesentery, the *sigmoid mesocolon.*

DISSECTION TIP

It is difficult to appreciate the entire length of the sigmoid mesocolon and sigmoid colon, because most of it is located within the pelvic cavity. This portion will be identified during a later dissection.

- With your hands, lift and medially pull up the ascending colon and descending colon, and identify the longitudinal depressions; they rest in the right and left paracolic gutters.

DISSECTION TIP

The large intestine exhibits some characteristic morphologic features:

- *Teniae coli* are three narrow muscular bands of the external longitudinal muscle layer of the large intestine.
- *Haustra,* or sacculations, are pouches produced by the teniae coli.
- *Appendices epiploicae* are peritoneum-covered fat-filled sacs, attached in rows along the teniae coli.

LABORATORY IDENTIFICATION CHECKLIST

LIGAMENTS

- ☐ Gastrosplenic
- ☐ Hepatogastric
- ☐ Hepatoduodenal
- ☐ Inguinal (Poupart's)
- ☐ Lacunar (Gimbernat's)
- ☐ Pectineal (Cooper's)
- ☐ Median arcuate
- ☐ Medial arcuate
- ☐ Lateral arcuate
- ☐ Median umbilical (urachus)
- ☐ Medial umbilical

LIVER

- ☐ Falciform
- ☐ Round (ligamentum teres)
- ☐ Right triangular
- ☐ Left triangular
- ☐ Coronary
- ☐ Suspensory ligament of duodenum (of Treitz)

OTHER CONNECTIVE TISSUES

- ☐ Greater omentum
- ☐ Lesser omentum
- ☐ External oblique aponeurosis
- ☐ Linea alba
- ☐ Anterior sheath of rectus abdominis
- ☐ Posterior sheath of rectus abdominis
- ☐ Greater omentum
- ☐ Lesser omentum
- ☐ Transverse mesocolon
- ☐ Sigmoid mesentery
- ☐ Appendicular mesentery
- ☐ Dorsal root mesentery
- ☐ Appendices epiploicae
- ☐ Teniae coli

ORGANS

- ☐ Esophagus
- ☐ Liver
  - ☐ Left lobe
  - ☐ Right lobe
  - ☐ Caudate
  - ☐ Quadrate
- ☐ Gallbladder
  - ☐ Fundus
  - ☐ Body
  - ☐ Neck
- ☐ Pancreas

- ☐ Spleen
- ☐ Stomach
  - ☐ Fundus
  - ☐ Body
  - ☐ Cardia
  - ☐ Pylorus
  - ☐ Greater curvature
  - ☐ Lesser curvature
- ☐ Small intestine
  - ☐ Duodenum
  - ☐ Jejunum
  - ☐ Ileum
- ☐ Large intestine
  - ☐ Cecum
  - ☐ Appendix
  - ☐ Ileocecal junction
    - ☐ Ascending colon
    - ☐ Transverse colon
    - ☐ Descending colon
    - ☐ Sigmoid colon
  - ☐ Hepatic flexure
  - ☐ Splenic flexure

MUSCLES

- ☐ External abdominal oblique
- ☐ Internal abdominal oblique
- ☐ Transversus abdominis
- ☐ Rectus abdominis
- ☐ Pyramidalis
- ☐ Psoas major

BONES

- ☐ Ribs 9–11
- ☐ Xiphoid process of sternum
- ☐ Sacrum
- ☐ Iliac crest of ilium

SPACES

- ☐ Omental foramen (of Winslow)
- ☐ Omental bursa
- ☐ Peritoneal cavity

VESSELS

- ☐ Inferior epigastric artery
- ☐ Inferior epigastric vein
- ☐ Superior epigastric artery
- ☐ Superior epigastric vein
- ☐ External iliac vein
- ☐ External iliac artery

ATLAS REFERENCES

Netter: 273–299, 301–305
McMinn: 234–252
Gray's Atlas: 157–182

In most cadavers, the liver occupies a significant portion of the peritoneal cavity. The gallbladder may be difficult to see at this point, but look for its fundus.

DISSECTION **TIP**

The gallbladder, if not surgically removed, will become visible as the dissection proceeds.

DISSECTION STEPS

○ With a scalpel, make a horizontal incision at the lower edge of the liver, removing 3 to 4 cm (1½ inches) of liver parenchyma (Fig. 12.1).
○ Pull the stomach downward and fully expose the gallbladder and the hepatoduodenal ligament (Figs. 12.2 and 12.3).

DISSECTION **TIP**

Stripping away the hepatoduodenal ligament, you will see several nerves running along the bile duct and proper hepatic artery. These nerves are part of the autonomic nervous system and are primarily sympathetic fibers (Fig. 12.4).

○ With scissors or a probe, carefully strip away the hepatoduodenal ligament and expose the bile duct, proper hepatic artery, and hepatic portal vein (see Figs. 12.4 and 12.5).
○ Note the relationships among these three structures: within the hepatoduodenal ligament, the portal vein

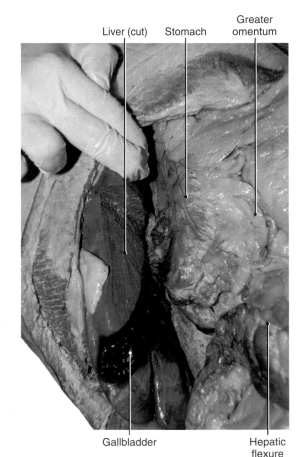

Liver (cut) Stomach Greater omentum

Gallbladder Hepatic flexure

Fig. 12.2 Identify the gallbladder.

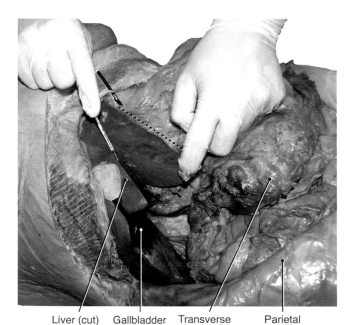

Liver (cut) Gallbladder Transverse colon Parietal peritoneum

Fig. 12.1 Horizontal incision at lower edge of the liver.

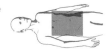

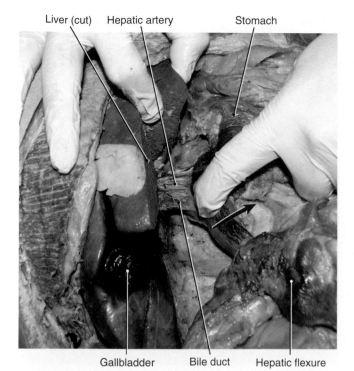

Liver (cut) Hepatic artery Stomach

Gallbladder Bile duct Hepatic flexure

Fig. 12.3 Pull the stomach downward to expose the gallbladder and hepatoduodenal ligament.

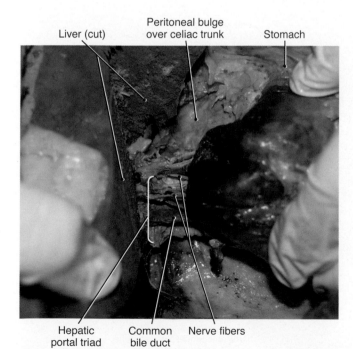

Liver (cut) Peritoneal bulge over celiac trunk Stomach

Hepatic portal triad Common bile duct Nerve fibers

Fig. 12.4 Cut the hepatoduodenal ligament to expose the bile duct, proper hepatic artery, portal vein, hepatic portal triad, and autonomic nerve fibers.

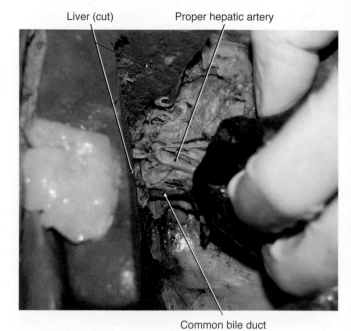

Liver (cut) Proper hepatic artery

Common bile duct

Fig. 12.5 View shows relationship of proper hepatic artery and bile duct.

is located posteriorly, deep to the bile duct and proper hepatic artery (Fig. 12.6).

○ Clean the proper hepatic artery toward the liver, and identify the right and left hepatic arteries.

○ Look for the *cystic artery* supplying the gallbladder.

○ The cystic artery usually arises from the right hepatic artery or the proper hepatic artery.

○ Dissect out the cystic duct from the gallbladder toward its junction with the common hepatic duct to form the bile duct (Fig. 12.7).

○ Once these structures are cleaned and identified, observe the *hepatocystic triangle* formed by the common hepatic duct, the cystic duct, and the liver.

○ In most cases, the cystic artery is identified within this triangular region (Plate 12.1).

DISSECTION **TIP**

In about 65% of cases, the cystic artery arises from the right hepatic artery. If you are not able to identify the cystic artery in its typical location, lift the cystic duct and look inferior to it.

○ To expose the celiac trunk and its branches, with blunt dissection, release the transverse and the descending colon from the gastrocolic ligament (Figs. 12.8 and 12.9).

○ With scissors, cut the gastrocolic ligament at the superior border of the transverse colon and release it from the stomach (Fig. 12.10).

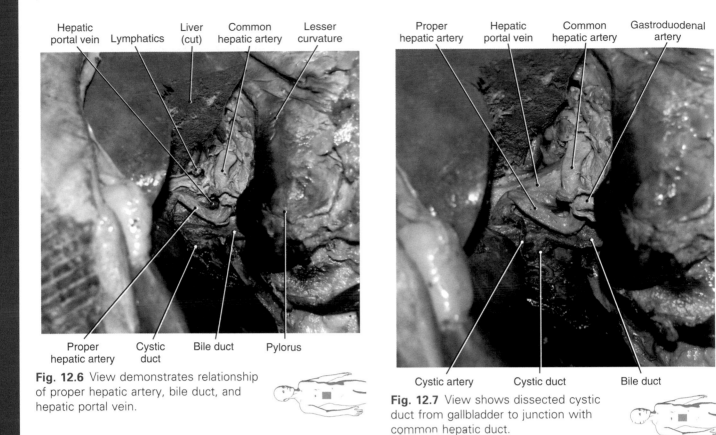

Hepatic portal vein Lymphatics Liver (cut) Common hepatic artery Lesser curvature

Proper hepatic artery Cystic duct Bile duct Pylorus

Fig. 12.6 View demonstrates relationship of proper hepatic artery, bile duct, and hepatic portal vein.

Proper hepatic artery Hepatic portal vein Common hepatic artery Gastroduodenal artery

Cystic artery Cystic duct Bile duct

Fig. 12.7 View shows dissected cystic duct from gallbladder to junction with common hepatic duct.

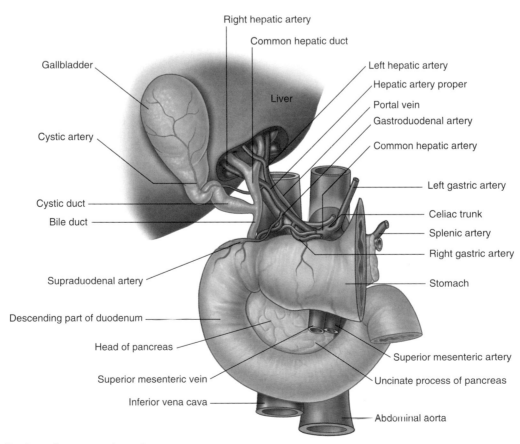

Right hepatic artery

Common hepatic duct

Gallblader

Liver

Left hepatic artery

Hepatic artery proper

Portal vein

Gastroduodenal artery

Common hepatic artery

Cystic artery

Cystic duct

Bile duct

Left gastric artery

Celiac trunk

Splenic artery

Right gastric artery

Supraduodenal artery

Stomach

Descending part of duodenum

Head of pancreas

Superior mesenteric vein

Inferior vena cava

Superior mesenteric artery

Uncinate process of pancreas

Abdominal aorta

Plate 12.1 Distribution of common hepatic artery.

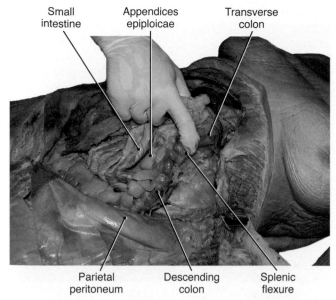

Fig. 12.8 Identify the transverse colon and descending colon.

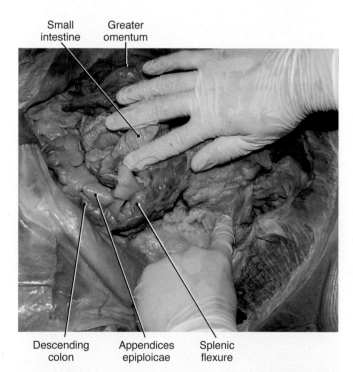

Fig. 12.9 Blunt dissection of transverse and descending colon from the gastrocolic ligament.

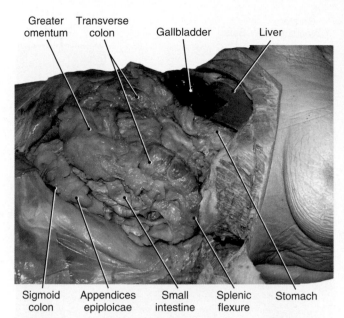

Fig. 12.10 Cut the gastrocolic ligament at superior border of the transverse colon to release the colon from stomach.

DISSECTION **TIP**

The spleen rests on an abundance of adipose tissue. Once the adipose tissue is cleaned away, the spleen will drop inferiorly and posteriorly, and its vessels will be stressed and possibly broken. Place some folded paper towels posterior to the spleen to keep it at the same level as the pancreas. In addition, the paper towels will absorb any embalming fluid that accumulates in this space.

○ Clean the fat and the gastrosplenic and splenorenal ligaments, and expose the splenic pedicle receiving the splenic artery and vein (Fig. 12.13).
○ Continue the exposure of the splenic artery and vein and identify the splenic hilum (Fig. 12.14).
○ Identify the short gastric arteries, which pass to the greater curvature of the stomach.
○ Note the relationship of the spleen with the stomach and the pancreas.
○ Identify the left gastroepiploic artery, which typically derives from the most inferior splenic artery hilar branch (Fig. 12.15).
○ Pull the stomach upward and expose the tail of the pancreas (see Fig. 12.15).
○ Continue the dissection of the splenic artery and vein from the hilum of the spleen toward the celiac trunk.
○ The splenic artery is tortuous and lies hidden at the upper border of the tail and body of the pancreas (Fig. 12.16).
○ Lift the stomach upward and expose the body and tail of the pancreas (Fig. 12.17).
○ Clean out the splenic artery and vein from the adjacent pancreas (Fig. 12.18).

○ To expose the splenic artery and spleen, cut the inferior edge of the costal cartilages with a saw to expose fully the area anterior to the spleen. Place paper towels underneath the costal cartilages (Fig. 12.11).
○ Identify the inferior border of the spleen, hidden by the gastrosplenic and splenorenal ligaments and, usually, abundant fat (Fig. 12.12).

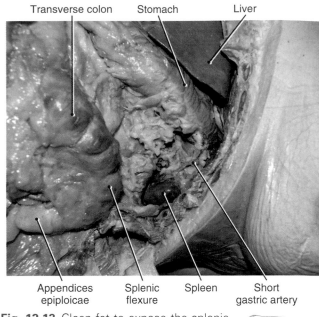

Transverse colon   Stomach   Liver

Appendices | Splenic | Spleen | Short
epiploicae | flexure | | gastric artery

Fig. 12.13 Clean fat to expose the splenic pedicle.

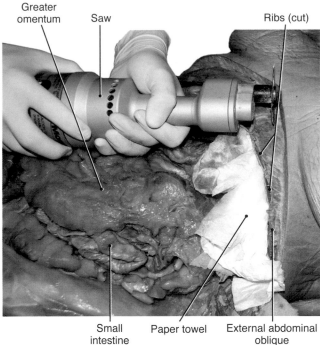

Small | Transverse | Gallbladder | Liver
intestine | colon

Splenic | Stomach | Spleen | Gastrosplenic
flexure | | | ligament

Fig. 12.12 Identify the inferior borders of the spleen.

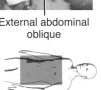

Greater | Saw | Ribs (cut)
omentum

Small | Paper towel | External abdominal
intestine | | oblique

Fig. 12.11 Saw the inferior edge of the costal cartilage.

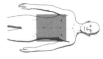

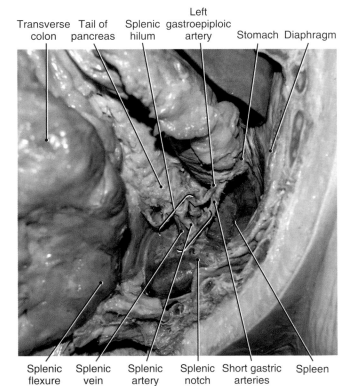

Transverse | Tail of | Splenic | Left gastroepiploic | Stomach | Diaphragm
colon | pancreas | hilum | artery

Splenic | Splenic | Splenic | Splenic | Short gastric | Spleen
flexure | vein | artery | notch | arteries

Fig. 12.14 Expose the splenic artery and vein and identify the splenic hilum.

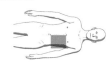

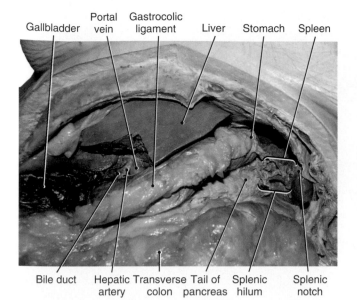

Gallbladder | Portal vein | Gastrocolic ligament | Liver | Stomach | Spleen

Bile duct | Hepatic artery | Transverse colon | Tail of pancreas | Splenic hilum | Splenic notch

Fig. 12.15 Identify the left gastroepiploic artery, and pull the stomach upward to expose tail of the pancreas.

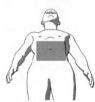

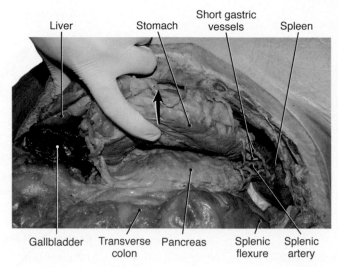

Liver | Stomach | Short gastric vessels | Spleen

Gallbladder | Transverse colon | Pancreas | Splenic flexure | Splenic artery

Fig. 12.17 Lift the stomach upward to expose the body and tail of the pancreas.

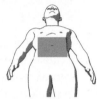

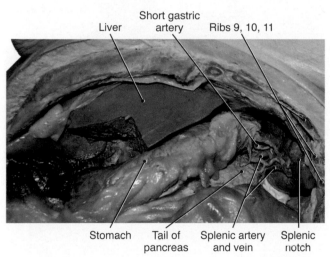

Liver | Short gastric artery | Ribs 9, 10, 11

Stomach | Tail of pancreas | Splenic artery and vein | Splenic notch

Fig. 12.16 Identify the splenic artery.

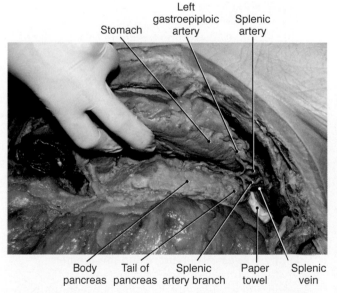

Stomach | Left gastroepiploic artery | Splenic artery

Body pancreas | Tail of pancreas | Splenic artery branch | Paper towel | Splenic vein

Fig. 12.18 Clean out splenic artery and vein from adjacent pancreas.

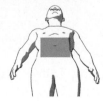

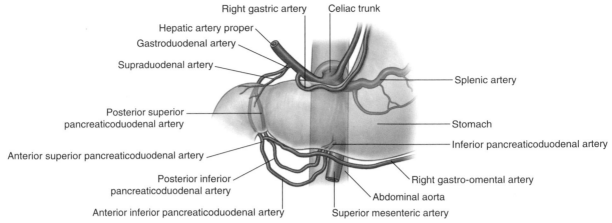

Right gastric artery   Celiac trunk

Hepatic artery proper

Gastroduodenal artery

Supraduodenal artery

Splenic artery

Posterior superior
pancreaticoduodenal artery

Stomach

Anterior superior pancreaticoduodenal artery

Inferior pancreaticoduodenal artery

Posterior inferior
pancreaticoduodenal artery

Right gastro-omental artery

Abdominal aorta

Anterior inferior pancreaticoduodenal artery

Superior mesenteric artery

Branches of the gastroduodenal artery

Plate 12.2 Branches of celiac trunk and gastroduodenal artery.

○ Do *not* pull the splenic artery away from the pancreas, because most of its branches are short and can be injured easily.

○ To visualize the area of the celiac trunk, it is necessary to lift the stomach upward and expose the pancreas. Palpate the upper border of the pancreas, and with your fingers, feel the celiac artery as a prominent bulge covered by the overlying peritoneum (Plate 12.2).

DISSECTION **TIP**

The reason for not dissecting the entire celiac trunk from the right side, at this time, is that the view from the gallbladder offers only limited exposure of the area. It is simpler to release the stomach from the gastrocolic ligament and greater omentum, identify the splenic artery at the splenic hilum, and then dissect the middle portion of the celiac trunk.

IDENTIFICATION OF DIFFERENT PARTS OF THE STOMACH

ANATOMY **NOTE**

The stomach is divided into four main regions: the cardia, fundus, body, and pylorus.
- Identify the *lesser curvature* and the *greater curvature* of the stomach.
- Identify the *angular notch*, found between the body and pyloric part of the stomach.
- Look for the cardia and the *cardiac notch* between the esophagus and fundus.

ANATOMY **NOTE**

The *fundus* is the portion of the stomach above the cardiac notch. The pylorus is divided further into the pyloric antrum and pyloric canal.

○ Return to the exposed proper hepatic artery, and dissect backward toward its origin from the common hepatic artery (Figs. 12.19 and 12.20).

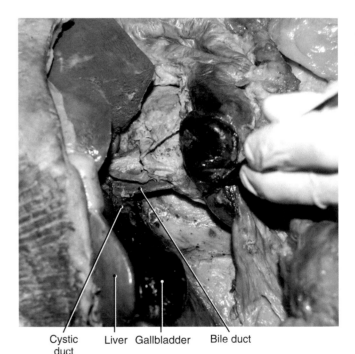

Cystic   Liver Gallbladder   Bile duct
duct

Fig. 12.19 Identify the bile duct and cystic duct.

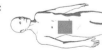

○ Identify and expose the other branch of the common hepatic artery, the gastroduodenal artery (see Fig. 12.20).

○ Dissect out the right side of the lesser curvature of the stomach and identify the *right gastric artery*, a branch of the proper hepatic artery.

○ Next to the right gastric artery, identify the right gastric vein and its connection to the right gastroepiploic vein via the prepyloric vein of Mayo.

○ On the left side of the lesser curvature of the stomach, identify and clean the left gastric artery; then trace it back from its origin from the celiac trunk (Fig. 12.21).

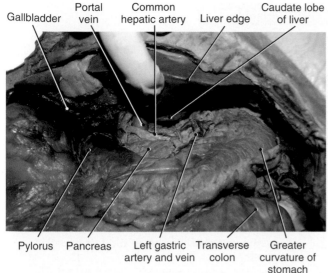

Gallbladder | Portal vein | Common hepatic artery | Liver edge | Caudate lobe of liver

Pylorus | Pancreas | Left gastric artery and vein | Transverse colon | Greater curvature of stomach

Fig. 12.20 Dissect the proper hepatic artery backward, toward its origin from the common hepatic artery.

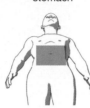

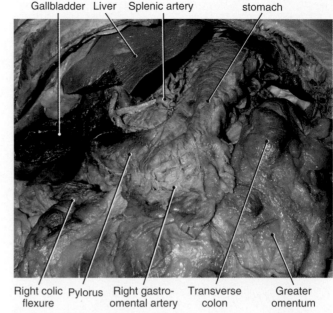

Gallbladder | Liver | Splenic artery | Greater curvature stomach

Right colic flexure | Pylorus | Right gastro-omental artery | Transverse colon | Greater omentum

Fig. 12.22 Identify the greater curvature of the stomach.

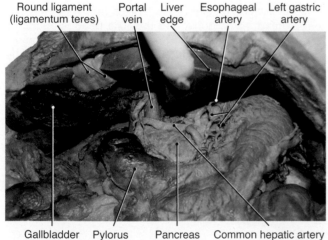

Round ligament (ligamentum teres) | Portal vein | Liver edge | Esophageal artery | Left gastric artery

Gallbladder | Pylorus | Pancreas | Common hepatic artery

Fig. 12.21 Identify and clean the left gastric artery.

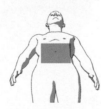

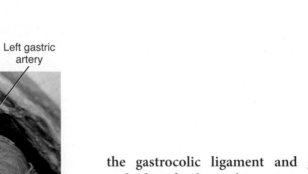

the gastrocolic ligament and greater omentum, and identify the right gastroepiploic artery (also known as right gastro-omental artery) (Figs. 12.22 and 12.23).

○ Similarly, dissect between the left side of the greater curvature of the stomach and spleen and identify the left gastroepiploic artery.

○ After identifying the right and left gastroepiploic arteries, with scissors, cut along the line marking the junction between the body of the stomach and the pyloric antrum, 4 to 5 cm (~2 inches) proximal to the pylorus (Fig. 12.24).

○ Retract the two parts of the transected stomach laterally and expose the celiac trunk and pancreas (Fig. 12.25).

○ Lift the splenic artery from the upper border of the pancreas and dissect it out (Fig. 12.26).

○ Once the splenic artery is fully exposed, notice its tortuosity (Fig. 12.27).

○ Place the left side of the stomach in such a position that you can visualize all the branches of the celiac trunk and identify the origins and distributions of these branches (Figs. 12.28 and 12.29).

○ Note the esophageal arterial branches of the left gastric artery ascending toward the esophagus.

○ The left gastric artery is accompanied by the left gastric vein. Trace out any esophageal tributaries to the left gastric vein.

○ In the area between the greater curvature of the stomach and the pylorus, dissect out the fat within

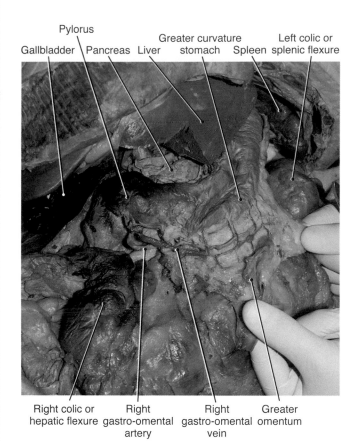

Pylorus

Gallblader | Pancreas Liver | Greater curvature stomach | Spleen | Left colic or splenic flexure

Right colic or hepatic flexure | Right gastro-omental artery | Right gastro-omental vein | Greater omentum

Fig. 12.23 Dissect out the fat within the gastrocolic ligament and greater omentum and identify the right gastroepiploic artery.

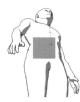

DISSECTION TIP

Note the following common arterial variations of the celiac trunk:

- Celiac artery and superior mesenteric artery arising as a common trunk (celiomesenteric trunk, 2.5% of cases)
- Proper hepatic and superior mesenteric arteries arising as a common trunk (hepatomesenteric trunk)
- Splenic artery and left gastric artery arising as a common trunk (lienogastric [splenogastric] trunk, 5.5%)
- Left gastric and common hepatic artery arising as a common trunk (gastrohepatic or hepatogastric trunk, 1.5%)
- Left gastric artery arising from the left hepatic artery (25%)
- Right hepatic artery arising from the superior mesenteric artery (18%)
- Cystic artery arising from proper hepatic or left hepatic artery
- Aberrant left hepatic artery arising from the left hepatic artery (25%)

ANATOMY NOTE

The pancreas typically is subdivided into the following parts: head, neck, body, and tail. The head is encircled by the first three parts of the duodenum and contains the *uncinate process*, which is located posteroinferiorly to the superior mesenteric artery and vein. Its terminal part, the tail, is related to the hilum of the spleen and left.

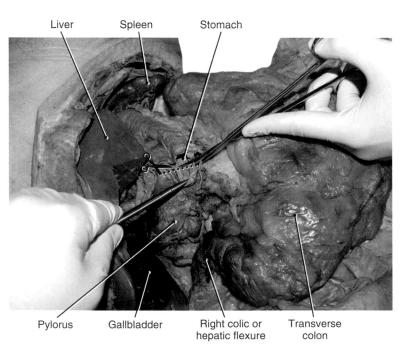

Liver | Spleen | Stomach

Pylorus | Gallbladder | Right colic or hepatic flexure | Transverse colon

Fig. 12.24 With scissors, cut along the junction between the body of the stomach and the pyloric antrum.

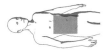

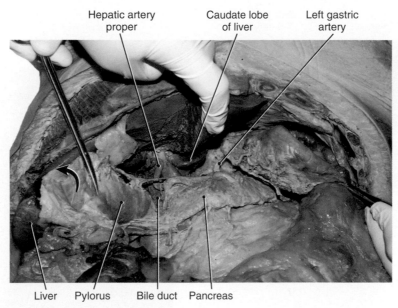

Hepatic artery proper Caudate lobe of liver Left gastric artery

Liver Pylorus Bile duct Pancreas

Fig. 12.25 Expose the celiac trunk and pancreas.

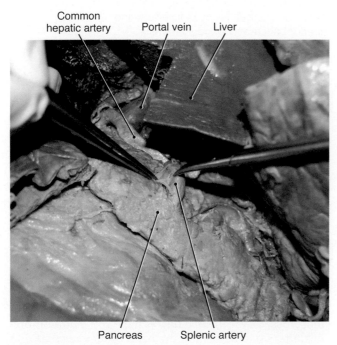

Common hepatic artery Portal vein Liver

Pancreas Splenic artery

Fig. 12.26 Dissect the splenic artery from the upper border of the pancreas.

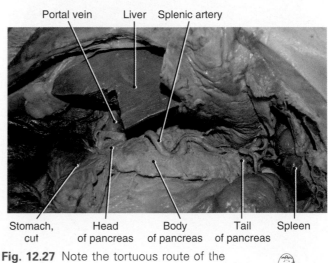

Portal vein Liver Splenic artery

Stomach, cut Head of pancreas Body of pancreas Tail of pancreas Spleen

Fig. 12.27 Note the tortuous route of the splenic artery.

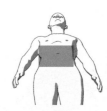

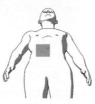

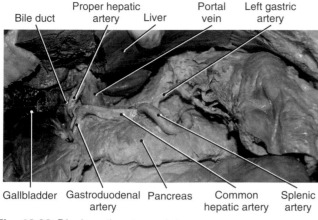

Fig. 12.28 Displace the stomach to visualize the branches of the celiac trunk.

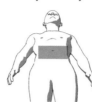

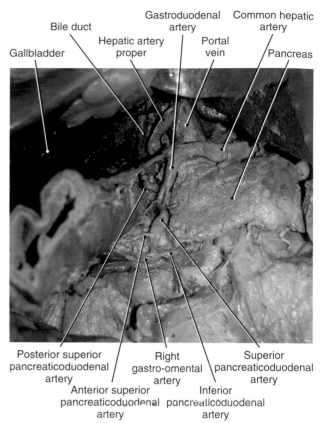

Fig. 12.30 Identify the origin of the two terminal branches of the gastroduodenal artery, the right gastroepiploic artery and superior pancreaticoduodenal artery.

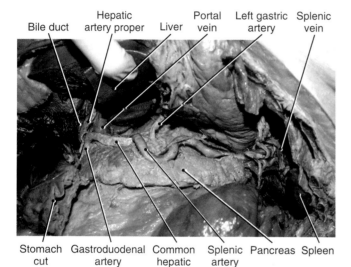

Fig. 12.29 Identify the origins and distributions of the branches of the celiac artery.

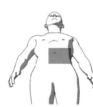

DISSECTION TIP

To expose the arterial branches, as well as the course of the bile duct down to the duodenum, reflect the stomach and duodenum to the left. Use your fingers to dissect the area underneath the duodenum and inferior vena cava; this is an avascular plane that is easily reflected to the left. This is called the *Kocher maneuver*, or "kocherizing" (Fig. 12.31).

DISSECTION TIP

A good way to trace and expose the posterior superior pancreaticoduodenal (PSPD) artery is to dissect out the bile duct from the lateral side (see Fig. 12.31). The artery that crosses over the bile duct is the PSPD. Furthermore, this artery passes behind the head of the pancreas and the 2nd part of the duodenum.

- On the right side of the cadaver, dissect out the branches of the gastroduodenal artery anteriorly.
- Around the head of the pancreas, look for the origin of the two terminal branches of the gastroduodenal artery, the right gastroepiploic and superior pancreaticoduodenal arteries (Fig. 12.30).
- The right gastroepiploic artery is typically found around the right side of the greater curvature of the stomach. Identify it.
- The superior pancreaticoduodenal artery divides into the posterior superior and anterior superior pancreaticoduodenal arteries supplying the head of the pancreas (see Fig. 12.30). Identify it.

- Follow the gastroduodenal artery posteriorly toward the 1st part of the duodenum and expose the origin of the PSPD artery (Figs. 12.32 and 12.33).
- Trace the course of the anterior superior pancreaticoduodenal artery (see Figs. 12.33 and 12.34), and expose its anastomosis with the inferior pancreaticoduodenal artery, a branch of the superior mesenteric artery.

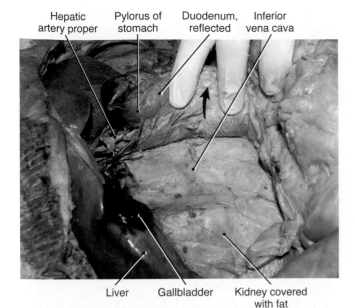

Hepatic artery proper | Pylorus of stomach | Duodenum, reflected | Inferior vena cava

Liver | Gallbladder | Kidney covered with fat

Fig. 12.31 Reflect the stomach and duodenum to the left, and bluntly dissect the area underneath the duodenum and inferior vena cava using the Kocher maneuver.

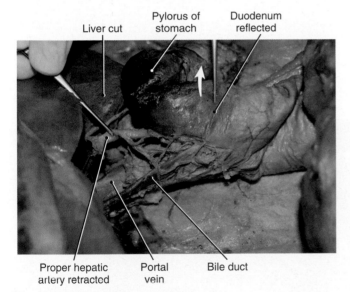

Liver cut | Pylorus of stomach | Duodenum reflected

Proper hepatic artery retracted | Portal vein | Bile duct

Fig. 12.32 Follow the gastroduodenal artery posteriorly toward the 1st part of the duodenum, and expose the origin of the posterior superior pancreaticoduodenal artery.

OPTIONAL DISSECTION OF BRANCHES OF SPLENIC ARTERY

○ Lift the splenic artery up and look for the origin of several branches. The following landmarks help identify these branches:

1. Lift the pancreas and look for the point where the portal vein crosses the pancreas posteriorly (neck of the pancreas). At this point, look for a branch from the splenic artery, the *dorsal pancreatic artery*.

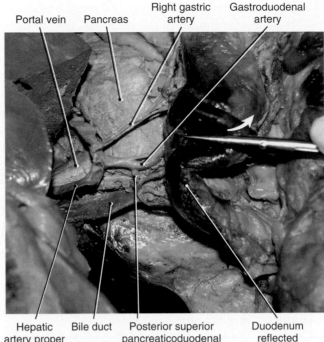

Portal vein | Pancreas | Right gastric artery | Gastroduodenal artery

Hepatic artery proper | Bile duct | Posterior superior pancreaticoduodenal artery | Duodenum reflected

Fig. 12.33 Trace the course of the anterior superior pancreaticoduodenal artery.

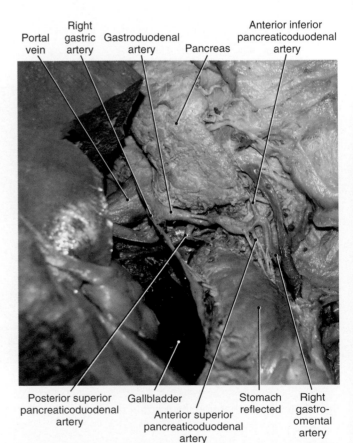

Portal vein | Right gastric artery | Gastroduodenal artery | Pancreas | Anterior inferior pancreaticoduodenal artery

Posterior superior pancreaticoduodenal artery | Gallbladder | Anterior superior pancreaticoduodenal artery | Stomach reflected | Right gastro-omental artery

Fig. 12.34 Expose the anterior superior pancreaticoduodenal artery's anastomosis with the inferior pancreaticoduodenal artery.

2. The splenic artery often gives off small branches at the superior border of the body and the tail of the pancreas, the *short pancreatic branches.*

3. The largest of these short pancreatic branches is the *great pancreatic artery,* which often is found at the distal one-third of the pancreas near its tail.

4. At the same point of the great pancreatic artery, look for a branch of the splenic artery traveling to the posterior part of the stomach supplying the gastric fundus, the *posterior gastric artery.*

5. Look 1 to 2 cm superior to the inferior border of the pancreas; embedded in its substance is the *transverse pancreatic artery.*

○ **Make a horizontal incision at the pyloric antrum, pylorus, and duodenum and observe the inner surface of these structures (Fig. 12.35).**

○ **Appreciate the gastric folds at the inner surface of the pyloric antrum and the circular muscle of the pyloric sphincter (Fig. 12.36).**

○ **Continue the incision at the 1st, 2nd, and 3rd parts of the duodenum, and note the circular folds of Kerckring (Figs. 12.37 and 12.38).**

○ **Cut the gastroduodenal artery and expose the course of the bile duct toward the duodenum (Fig. 12.39).**

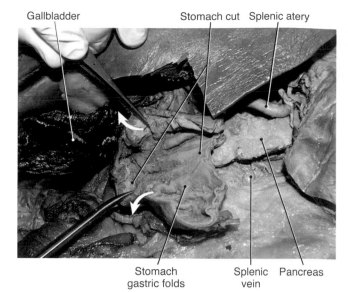

Gallbladder   Stomach cut   Splenic atery

Stomach gastric folds   Splenic vein   Pancreas

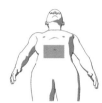

Fig. 12.36 Note gastric rugae at the inner surface of the pyloric antrum and circular muscle of the pyloric sphincter.

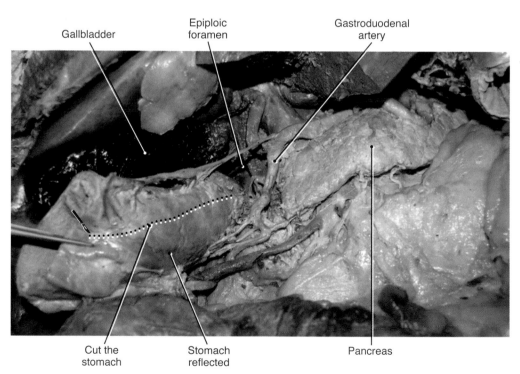

Gallbladder   Epiploic foramen   Gastroduodenal artery

Cut the stomach   Stomach reflected   Pancreas

Fig. 12.35 Make a horizontal cut at the pyloric antrum, pylorus, and duodenum.

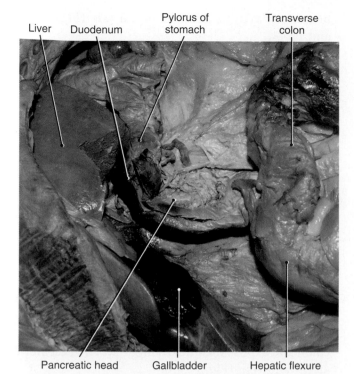

Fig. 12.37 Continue an incision through the 1st, 2nd, and 3rd parts of duodenum.

Liver | Duodenum | Pylorus of stomach | Transverse colon

Pancreatic head | Gallbladder | Hepatic flexure

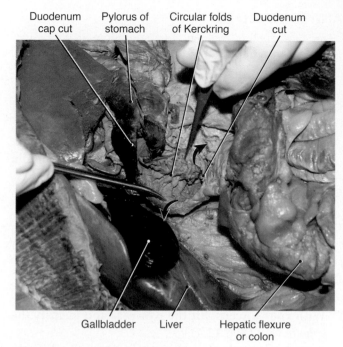

Fig. 12.38 Note the circular folds of Kerckring.

Duodenum cap cut | Pylorus of stomach | Circular folds of Kerckring | Duodenum cut

Gallbladder | Liver | Hepatic flexure or colon

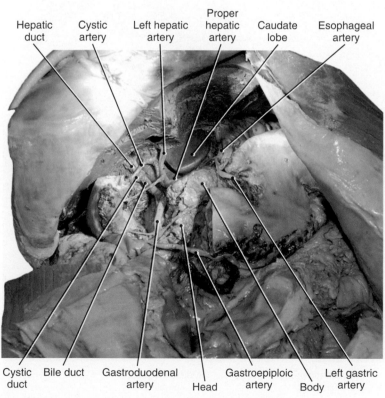

Fig. 12.39 Cut the gastroduodenal artery and expose the course of the bile duct.

Hepatic duct | Cystic artery | Left hepatic artery | Proper hepatic artery | Caudate lobe | Esophageal artery

Cystic duct | Bile duct | Gastroduodenal artery | Head | Gastroepiploic artery | Body | Left gastric artery

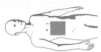

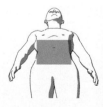

ANATOMY NOTE

The bile duct is divided into supraduodenal (above duodenum), retroduodenal (behind duodenum), and pancreatic parts (terminal part) (Fig. 12.40).

○ Open up the descending part of the duodenum and identify the intraduodenal portion of the bile duct; find its connection with the main pancreatic duct (of Wirsung), forming the hepatopancreatic ampulla (of Vater).

○ Identify the duodenal papilla, which contains the hepatopancreatic ampulla.

○ Expose the main pancreatic duct into the substance of the pancreas by removing pancreatic tissue with your forceps (see Fig. 12.40).

○ Look for an accessory pancreatic duct (of Santorini), if present.

○ With your forceps, lift the pancreas and identify the *splenic vein* (Fig. 12.41).

○ Expose the splenic vein along its entire length, and trace out its junction with the superior mesenteric vein to form the *portal vein* (Figs. 12.42 and 12.43).

○ Next to the superior mesenteric vein, look for the inferior mesenteric vein, usually draining into the splenic vein (Plate 12.3).

○ Continue exposing the tributaries of the superior mesenteric vein.

○ Next to its tributaries, expose the arterial branches of the *superior mesenteric artery* (Fig. 12.44).

DISSECTION TIP

The vast majority of tissue that must be removed to expose the branches of the superior mesenteric artery and vein is fat and dense autonomic nerve tissue.

○ Lift the transverse colon and observe the transverse *mesocolon* (Fig. 12.45).

○ With your fingertips, penetrate the transverse mesocolon and expose the underlying superior mesenteric artery and vein (Fig. 12.46).

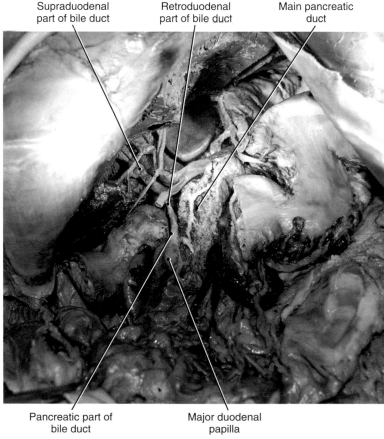

Supraduodenal part of bile duct

Retroduodenal part of bile duct

Main pancreatic duct

Pancreatic part of bile duct

Major duodenal papilla

Fig. 12.40 Note divisions of the bile duct: supraduodenal, retroduodenal, and pancreatic parts.

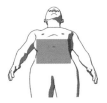

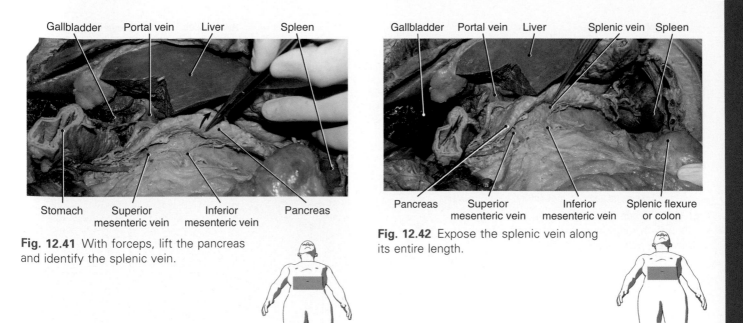

Fig. 12.41 With forceps, lift the pancreas and identify the splenic vein.

Fig. 12.42 Expose the splenic vein along its entire length.

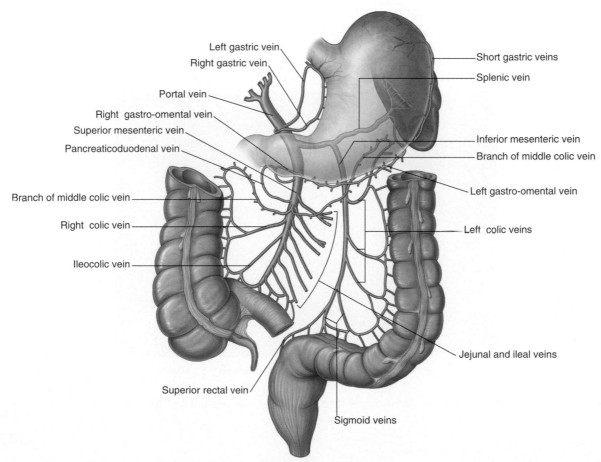

Plate 12.3 Venous drainage of the abdominal portion of the gastrointestinal tract.

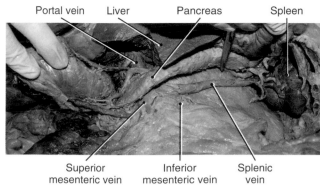

Portal vein Liver Pancreas Spleen

Superior
mesenteric vein Inferior
mesenteric vein Splenic
vein

Fig. 12.43 Trace the splenic vein to its junction with the superior mesenteric vein to form the portal vein.

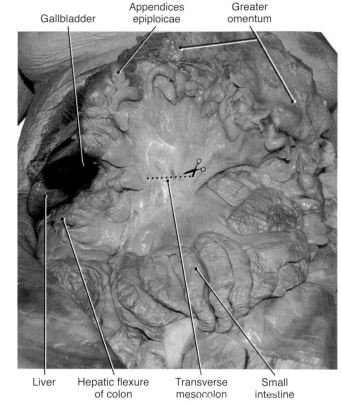

Gallbladder Appendices
epiploicae Greater
omentum

Liver Hepatic flexure
of colon Transverse
mesocolon Small
intestine

Fig. 12.45 Lift the transverse colon to see the transverse mesocolon.

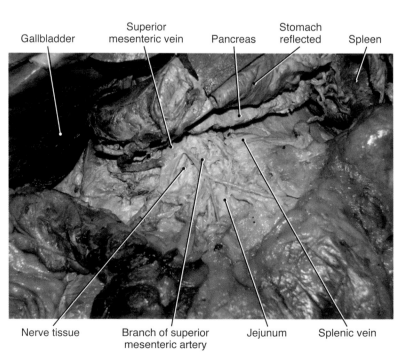

Gallbladder Superior
mesenteric vein Pancreas Stomach
reflected Spleen

Nerve tissue Branch of superior
mesenteric artery Jejunum Splenic vein

Fig. 12.44 Expose the tributaries of the superior mesenteric vein and arterial branches of the superior mesenteric artery.

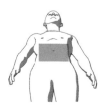

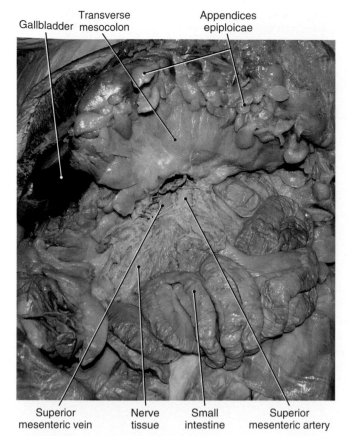

Fig. 12.46 With your fingertips, penetrate the transverse mesocolon and expose the underlying superior mesenteric artery and vein.

Gallbladder / Transverse mesocolon / Appendices epiploicae

Superior mesenteric vein / Nerve tissue / Small intestine / Superior mesenteric artery

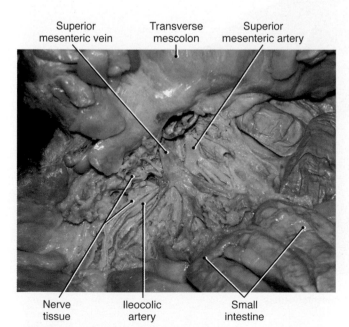

Superior mesenteric vein / Transverse mescolon / Superior mesenteric artery

Nerve tissue / Ileocolic artery / Small intestine

Fig. 12.47 Continue separating tributaries of the superior mesenteric vein and branches of the superior mesenteric artery from the fat and nerve tissue.

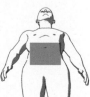

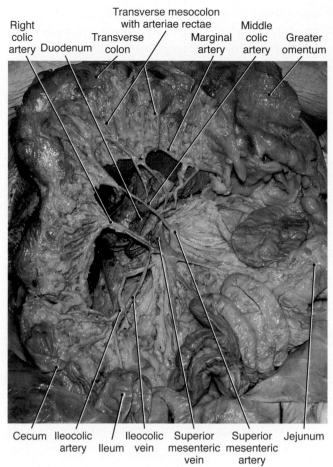

Right colic artery / Duodenum / Transverse colon / Transverse mesocolon with arteriae rectae / Marginal artery / Middle colic artery / Greater omentum

Cecum / Ileocolic artery / Ileum / Ileocolic vein / Superior mesenteric vein / Superior mesenteric artery / Jejunum

Fig. 12.48 Identify the ileocolic artery and trace it to the ileocecal junction.

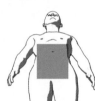

○ Continue cleaning the branches of the superior mesenteric artery and the tributaries of the superior mesenteric vein from fat and nerve tissue (Fig. 12.47).

DISSECTION **TIP**

The ileocolic artery is fairly constant and provides a good landmark for this dissection (Fig. 12.48).

ANATOMY **NOTE**

The ileocolic artery gives rise to the appendicular artery supplying the appendix in its own mesentery, the *mesoappendix.*

○ Identify the ileocolic artery and trace it to the *ileocecal junction,* between the ileum and the cecum.
○ Identify the middle and right colic arteries that supply the transverse and the ascending colon, respectively (see Fig. 12.48).
○ Look for a branch of the middle colic artery, the marginal artery (of Drummond), that supplies the

ascending, transverse, and descending colon, and anastomose with the left colic artery, a branch of the inferior mesenteric artery (see Fig. 12.52).

○ Once the main three arterial branches of the *superior mesenteric artery* (middle colic, right colic and ileo-colic) are identified, expose the ileal and jejunal arteries from their origin from the superior mesenteric artery to the margin of the ileum and jejunum.

DISSECTION **TIP**

Realize that the mesenteric fat is much more abundant in the ileal mesentery than in the jejunal mesentery.

○ Dissect out the vascular arcades, appreciating their greater number in the ileum than in the jejunum (Fig. 12.49).

○ Similarly, the vasa recti are shorter and more numerous in the ileum (Figs. 12.50 and 12.51).

○ Once the dissection of the superior mesenteric vessels is concluded, lift the transverse colon and review all dissected structures dissected out (Figs. 12.52 and 12.53).

○ Retract the small intestine to the right and expose the transverse, descending, and sigmoid colon (Fig. 12.54).

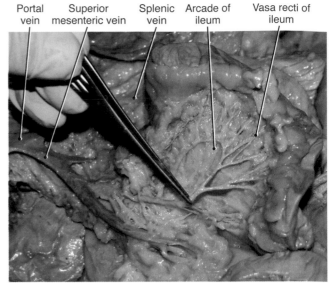

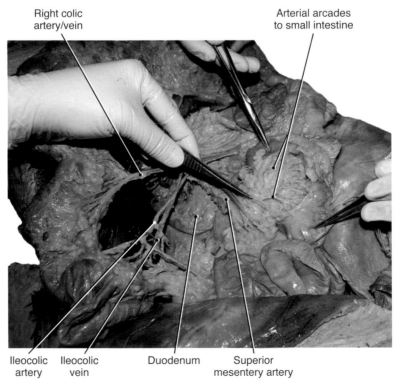

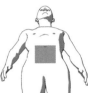

Fig. 12.50 Notice that the vasa recti are shorter and more numerous in the ileum than in the jejunum. Note the increased number of arcades in the ileum compared with the jejunum.

Fig. 12.49 Dissect out the vascular arcades.

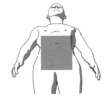

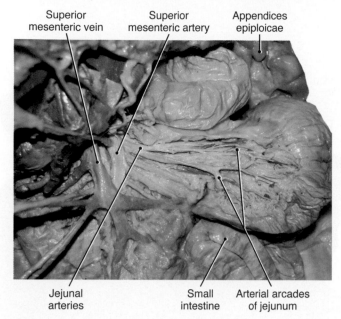

Superior mesenteric vein   Superior mesenteric artery   Appendices epiploicae

Jejunal arteries   Small intestine   Arterial arcades of jejunum

Fig. 12.51 Note the increased number of arcades in ileum compared with jejunum.

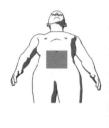

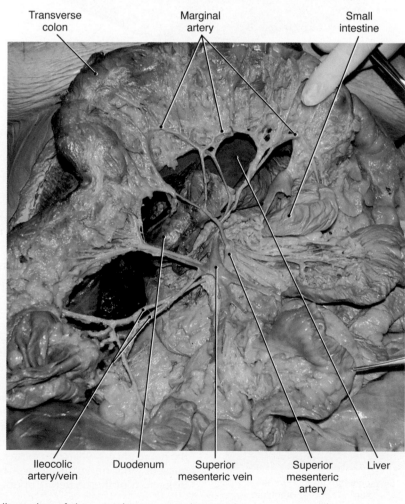

Transverse colon   Marginal artery   Small intestine

Ileocolic artery/vein   Duodenum   Superior mesenteric vein   Superior mesenteric artery   Liver

Fig. 12.52 Conclude the dissection of the superior mesenteric vessels.

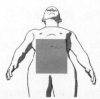

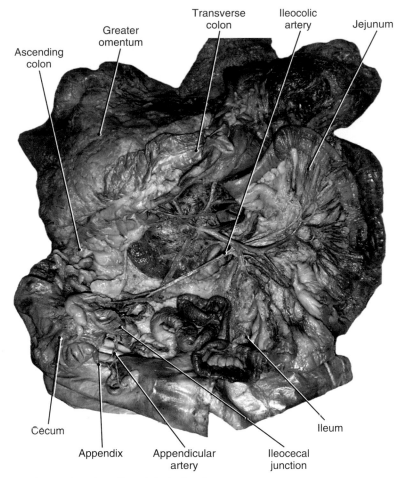

Fig. 12.53 Lift the transverse colon and review its related structures.

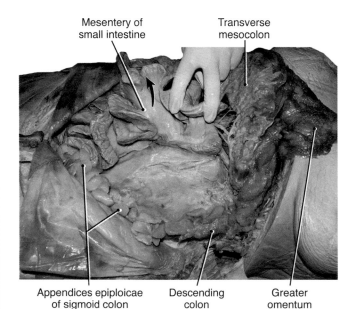

Fig. 12.54 Retract the small intestine to the right and expose the transverse, descending, and sigmoid colon.

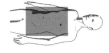

○ With scissors, continue the exposure of the inferior mesenteric vein (Fig. 12.55) toward the margins of the colon.

○ To the right or medial to the inferior mesenteric vein, identify the *inferior mesenteric artery* (Plate 12.4).

DISSECTION **TIP**

Both the inferior mesenteric artery and the inferior mesenteric vein require additional effort to expose because of the dense nerve plexuses covering them. To facilitate the dissection of the branches of the inferior mesenteric artery, make a shallow incision between the lateral wall of the descending colon and the body at the white line of Toldt (left paracolic gutter), and release the descending colon from the peritoneum. In addition, do *not* remove the nerve plexus when you expose the inferior mesenteric vessels. This nerve tissue will be examined in a later dissection of the posterior abdominal wall.

○ Identify the branches of the inferior mesenteric artery, the left colic artery and the sigmoid arteries and fully expose them (Fig. 12.56).

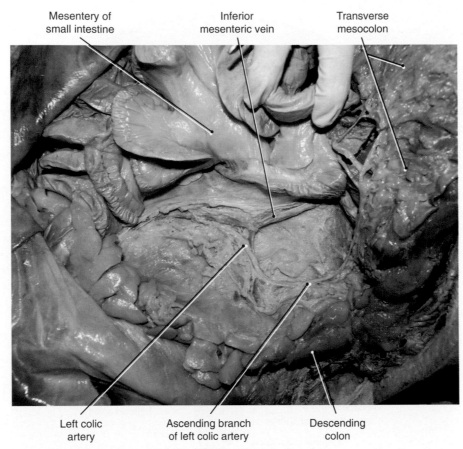

Mesentery of small intestine   Inferior mesenteric vein   Transverse mesocolon

Left colic artery   Ascending branch of left colic artery   Descending colon

Fig. 12.55 With scissors, continue the exposure of the inferior mesenteric vein.

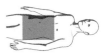

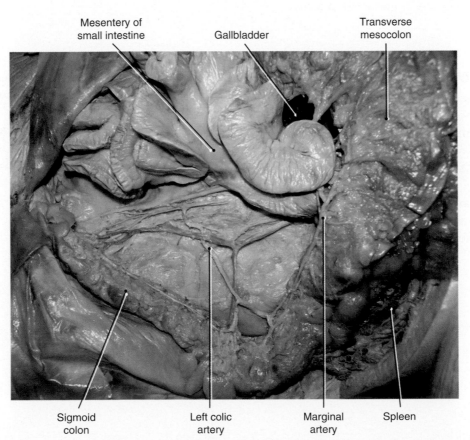

Mesentery of small intestine   Gallbladder   Transverse mesocolon

Sigmoid colon   Left colic artery   Marginal artery   Spleen

Fig. 12.56 Identify and fully expose the branches of inferior mesenteric artery, left colic artery, and sigmoid arteries.

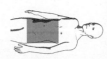

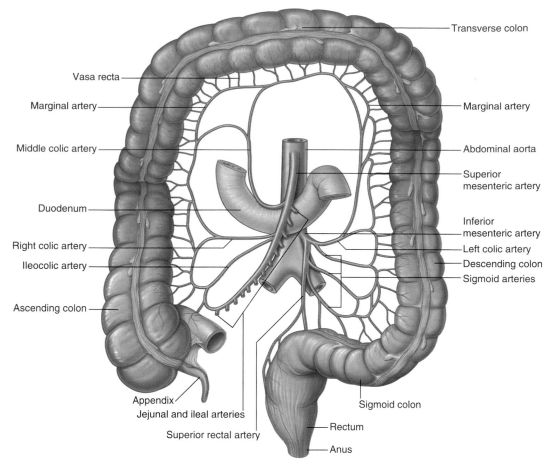

Transverse colon

Vasa recta

Marginal artery

Middle colic artery

Duodenum

Right colic artery

Ileocolic artery

Ascending colon

Appendix

Jejunal and ileal arteries

Superior rectal artery

Marginal artery

Abdominal aorta

Superior
mesenteric artery

Inferior
mesenteric artery

Left colic artery

Descending colon

Sigmoid arteries

Sigmoid colon

Rectum

Anus

Plate 12.4 Superior and inferior mesenteric arteries.

IF TIME PERMITS

○ Tie two strings close together around the proximal segment of the jejunum, and cut between them.

○ Perform the same technique along a distal portion of the ileum.

○ Clean the two segments and observe their internal morphology.

○ Note the increased number of plicae circulares and villi, as well as increased wall thickness in the jejunum compared to the ileum.

○ Similarly, place a ligature at the ileocecal junction and another ligature at the midportion of the ascending colon.

○ Remove this segment and examine its internal morphology.

○ Identify the ileocecal valve and the plicae semilunares coli.

LABORATORY IDENTIFICATION CHECKLIST

ARTERIES
- ☐ Abdominal aorta
- ☐ Celiac trunk
  - ☐ Common hepatic
  - ☐ Proper hepatic
  - ☐ Gastroduodenal
  - ☐ Right gastroepiploic
  - ☐ Right gastric
  - ☐ Splenic
  - ☐ Short gastrics
  - ☐ Left gastric
  - ☐ Left gastroepiploic
- ☐ Superior mesenteric artery
  - ☐ Ileocolic
  - ☐ Appendicular
  - ☐ Right colic
  - ☐ Middle colic
- ☐ Inferior mesenteric
  - ☐ Left colic
  - ☐ Sigmoid
  - ☐ Inferior rectal
- ☐ Marginal (formed between ileocolic [right, middle] and left colic arteries)
- ☐ Jejunal and ileal arteries (arcades) and recti branches

VEINS
- ☐ Inferior vena cava
  - ☐ Hepatic
- ☐ Portal
  - ☐ Superior mesenteric
  - ☐ Splenic
  - ☐ Inferior mesenteric

LYMPH NODES
- ☐ Mesenteric

MUSCLES
- ☐ External abdominal oblique
- ☐ Internal abdominal oblique
  - ☐ Cremaster
- ☐ Transversus abdominis
- ☐ Rectus abdominis
- ☐ Pyramidalis
- ☐ Crus (right and left) of diaphragm
- ☐ Psoas major
- ☐ Quadratus lumborum

CONNECTIVE TISSUE
- ☐ External oblique aponeurosis
- ☐ Greater omentum
- ☐ Lesser omentum
- ☐ Transverse mesocolon
- ☐ Sigmoid mesentery
- ☐ Appendicular mesentery
- ☐ Dorsal root mesentery

Liver
- ☐ Falciform ligament
- ☐ Ligamentum teres

VISCERA/ORGANS
Esophagus
- ☐ Abdominal esophagus

Stomach
- ☐ Fundus
- ☐ Body
- ☐ Cardia
- ☐ Pylorus
- ☐ Greater curvature
- ☐ Lesser curvature

Small Intestine
- ☐ Duodenum
- ☐ Jejunum
- ☐ Ileum

Large Intestine
- ☐ Cecum
- ☐ Appendix
- ☐ Ascending colon
- ☐ Transverse colon
- ☐ Descending colon
- ☐ Sigmoid colon
- ☐ Appendices epiploicae
- ☐ Teniae coli

Liver
- ☐ Left lobe
- ☐ Right lobe
- ☐ Caudate
- ☐ Quadrate

Gallbladder
- ☐ Fundus
- ☐ Body
- ☐ Neck

Pancreas
- ☐ Head
- ☐ Neck
- ☐ Body
- ☐ Tail
- ☐ Uncinate process

Spleen
- ☐ Splenic notch
- ☐ Hilum

ATLAS REFERENCES
Netter: 265–269, 300, 311–323
McMinn: 253–261
Gray's Atlas: 183–196, 198–199

EXPOSING THE KIDNEYS

○ Cut the white lines of Toldt (paracolic gutters) along the edges of the ascending and the descending colon, and reflect the large and small intestines to the left of the abdominal cavity (Fig. 13.1).

○ With your fingers, retract the duodenum and pancreas to the left, without disrupting their vascular supply (Fig. 13.2).

○ Palpate the abdominal aorta on the left and the *inferior vena cava* (IVC) on the right.

○ With scissors, cut the peritoneum of the posterior abdominal wall and expose the IVC (Fig. 13.3).

○ To the right of the IVC, dissect out the perirenal (renal) fascia (of Gerota), which is filled predominantly with abundant perirenal fat (Fig. 13.4).

○ Trace the right ureter; expose its course from the kidney to the pelvic brim and as it crosses over the iliac arteries.

○ Remove the fat posterior to the kidney, known as the *pararenal* fat (Fig. 13.5).

DISSECTION **TIP**
For the removal of the perirenal and pararenal fat, use scissors or a probe and scrape it from the kidney capsule.

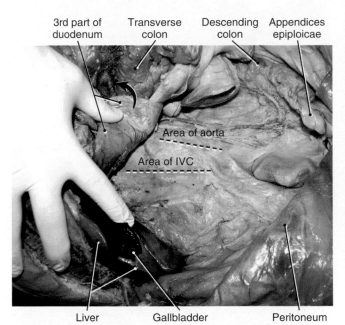

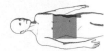

Fig. 13.2 Left duodenum and pancreas retracted. *IVC,* Inferior vena cava.

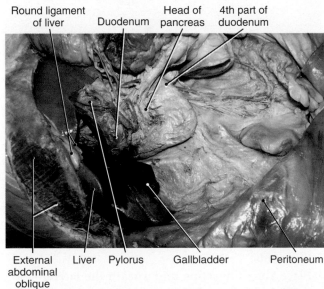

Fig. 13.1 Lines of Toldt cut along edges of ascending and descending colon with large and small intestines reflected to left of abdominal cavity.

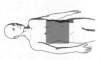

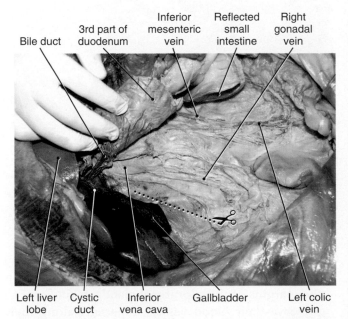

Fig. 13.3 Peritoneum of posterior abdominal wall incised to expose the inferior vena cava (IVC).

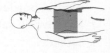

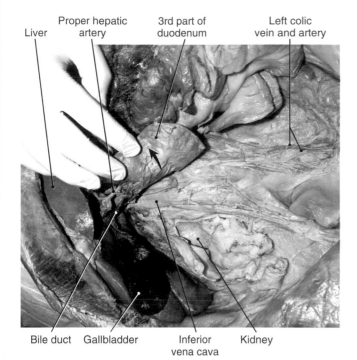

Liver · Proper hepatic artery · 3rd part of duodenum · Left colic vein and artery

Bile duct · Gallbladder · Inferior vena cava · Kidney

Fig. 13.4 Perirenal fascia (of Gerota) dissected to the right of the IVC.

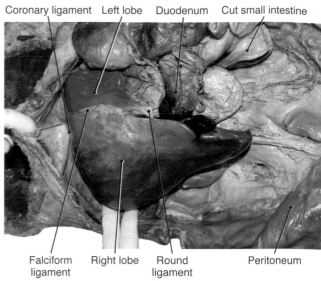

Coronary ligament · Left lobe · Duodenum · Cut small intestine

Falciform ligament · Right lobe · Round ligament · Peritoneum

Fig. 13.6 Falciform, left triangular, and coronary ligaments cut and right triangular ligament incised on lifting liver.

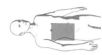

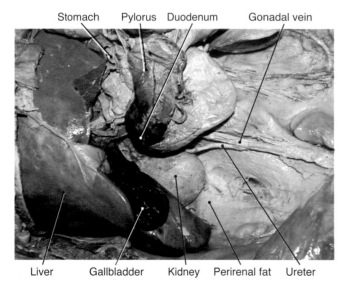

Stomach · Pylorus · Duodenum · Gonadal vein

Liver · Gallbladder · Kidney · Perirenal fat · Ureter

Fig. 13.5 Right ureter exposed as it leaves the right kidney, toward the pelvic brim and over the iliac arteries. Pararenal fat has been removed posterior to the kidney.

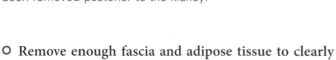

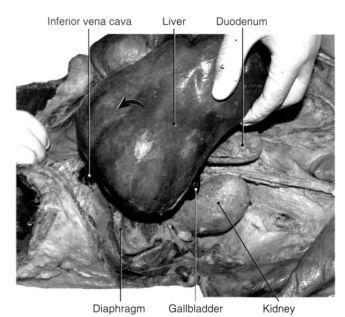

Inferior vena cava · Liver · Duodenum

Diaphragm · Gallbladder · Kidney

Fig. 13.7 With liver pulled inferiorly, cut the IVC in the space between superior aspect of the liver and the undersurface of the diaphragm.

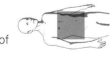

- Remove enough fascia and adipose tissue to clearly expose the kidneys and suprarenal glands. Free up the margins of the suprarenal glands, taking care to preserve their blood vessels, especially along their medial borders.
- Remove all fat from the posterior part of the kidney capsule.

LIVER

- Reflect the liver medially and expose the entire posterior abdominal wall.
- Cut the falciform, left triangular, and coronary ligaments.
- Place your fingertips underneath the lateral side of the liver, lift it up slightly, and cut the right triangular ligament (Fig. 13.6).
- Pull the liver inferiorly, and in the space between the diaphragm and the liver, cut the IVC (Fig. 13.7).

- Lift the liver upward and to the left; expose the infrahepatic portion of IVC away from the body wall (Fig. 13.8).
- Gently pull the liver to the left; otherwise, you will damage the right suprarenal vein as it enters the IVC.
- With a scalpel, make an incision through the IVC superior to the level of the renal veins and reflect the liver to the left (Fig. 13.9).
- The liver is attached to the abdominal cavity only by the portal vein, hepatic artery, and bile duct.
- On the reflected liver, identify the right and left lobes (divided by the falciform ligament), as well as the quadrate and caudate lobes of the right lobe.
- Identify the fissure for the ligamentum venosum and the ligamentum teres (round ligament) of the liver.
- Identify the round ligament, left triangular ligament, and coronary ligament (Fig. 13.10).
- To identify the ligamentum venosum, reflect the caudate lobe and clean the fissure for the ligament (Fig. 13.11).
- Reflect the inferior vena cava slightly inferiorly and expose the suprarenal gland and the bare area of the liver (Fig. 13.12).

KIDNEYS AND SUPRARENAL GLANDS

- Clean out the connective tissue and fat over the IVC and expose the right gonadal vein and right and left renal veins (Figs. 13.13 and 13.14).
- Continue the exposure of the left renal vein to the left and clean away the fat and connective tissue over the abdominal aorta (Fig. 13.15).

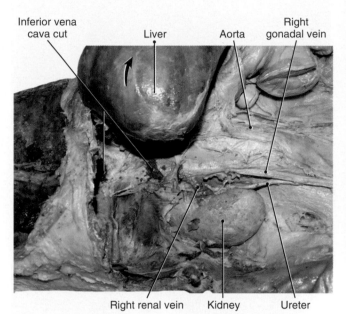

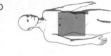

Fig. 13.9 Incision through IVC superior to level of renal veins, with liver reflected.

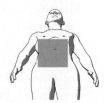

Fig. 13.8 Liver lifted upward and to the left exposing infrahepatic portion of IVC.

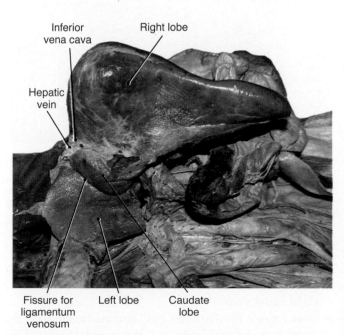

Fig. 13.10 Identify the right and left lobes of the liver. Trace the inferior vena cava and the hepatic vein. Identify the fissure for the ligamentum venosum between the left lobe of the liver and the caudate lobe.

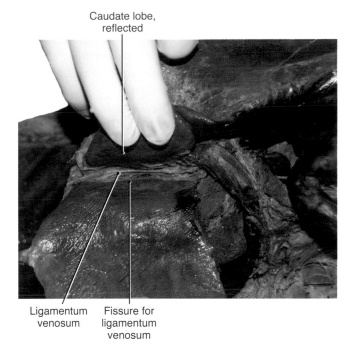

Fig. 13.11 Caudate lobe reflected and fissure cleaned to locate the ligamentum venosum.

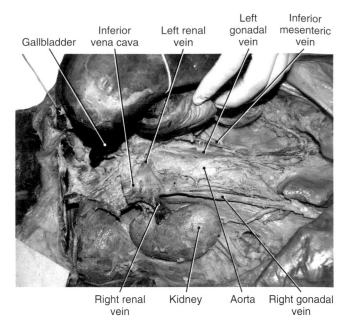

Fig. 13.13 Fat and connective tissue cleaned over IVC, exposing right gonadal vein and right renal vein.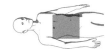

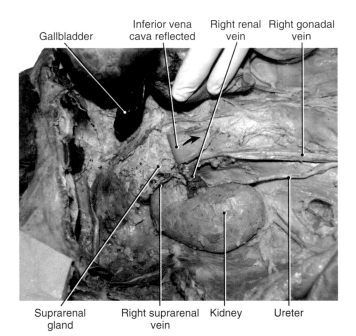

Fig. 13.12 Suprarenal gland and bare area of liver exposed by reflecting the IVC slightly inferiorly.

○ Paying special attention, identify the gonadal artery arising from the aorta just inferior to the level of the right renal vein.
○ In the space between the IVC and aorta, identify the right lymphatic trunk and the sympathetic fibers ascending from the superior hypogastric plexus. This plexus is located just anterior to the promontory of the sacrum (Fig. 13.16).

○ Complete the dissection by exposing the branches of the *inferior mesenteric artery* (Figs. 13.17 and 13.18).
○ Identify and expose the renal arteries and veins.

ANATOMY **NOTE**

The left renal vein crosses over the aorta, inferior to the origin of the superior mesenteric artery, to reach the IVC. In contrast, the right renal artery passes posterior to the IVC (Fig. 13.19).

DISSECTION **TIP**

Additional renal arteries are often seen arising from the aorta; these are normal variations.

○ Identify the right suprarenal gland with its connection between the right suprarenal vein and the IVC (see Fig. 13.12). This vein is very short.
○ Dissect out the right superior, middle, and inferior suprarenal arteries, typically arising from the inferior phrenic artery, aorta, and renal artery, respectively (Fig. 13.20).
○ Notice the drainage of the right gonadal vein directly into the IVC (Plate 13.1).
○ Identify the left suprarenal gland, and expose the left suprarenal vein and left gonadal vein draining into the left renal vein.
○ With a scalpel, make a coronal incision and expose the outer cortex, as well as the inner medulla, of the suprarenal gland.

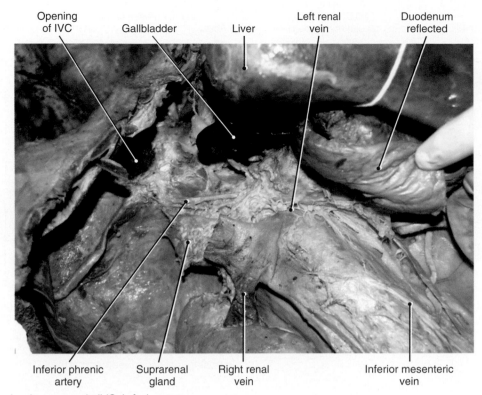

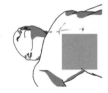

Fig. 13.14 Left renal vein exposed. *IVC*, Inferior vena cava.

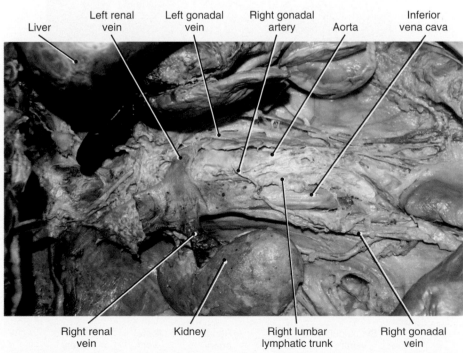

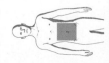

Fig. 13.15 Left renal vein exposed, showing left gonadal vein, with gonadal artery from aorta just inferior to right renal vein.

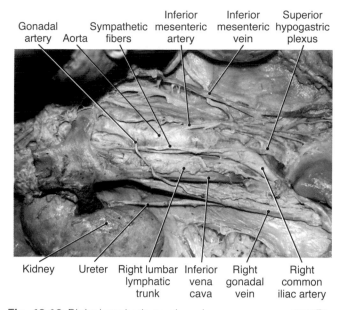

Gonadal artery — Aorta — Sympathetic fibers — Inferior mesenteric artery — Inferior mesenteric vein — Superior hypogastric plexus

Kidney — Ureter — Right lumbar lymphatic trunk — Inferior vena cava — Right gonadal vein — Right common iliac artery

Fig. 13.16 Right lymphatic trunk and sympathetic fibers ascending from superior hypogastric plexus.

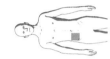

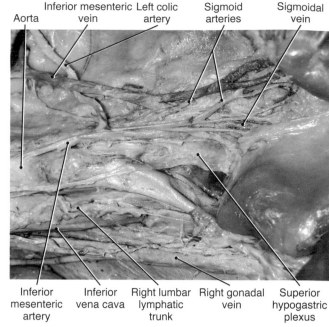

Aorta — Inferior mesenteric vein — Left colic artery — Sigmoid arteries — Sigmoidal vein

Inferior mesenteric artery — Inferior vena cava — Right lumbar lymphatic trunk — Right gonadal vein — Superior hypogastric plexus

Fig. 13.17 Dissection completed by exposing inferior mesenteric artery.

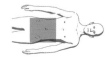

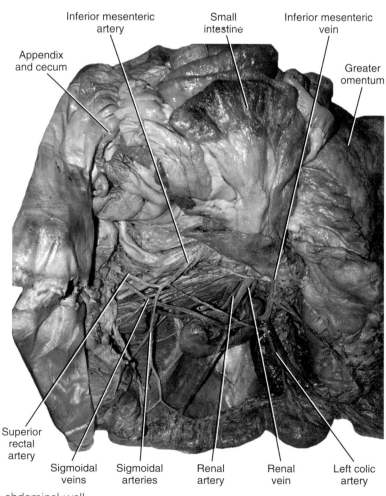

Inferior mesenteric artery — Small intestine — Inferior mesenteric vein

Appendix and cecum — Greater omentum

Superior rectal artery — Sigmoidal veins — Sigmoidal arteries — Renal artery — Renal vein — Left colic artery

Fig. 13.18 Structures of the abdominal wall.

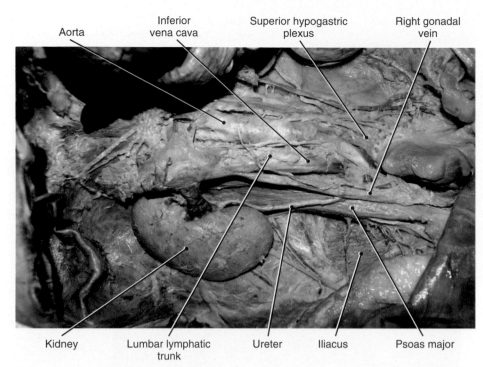

Fig. 13.19 Locate and expose the renal arteries and veins.

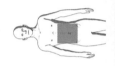

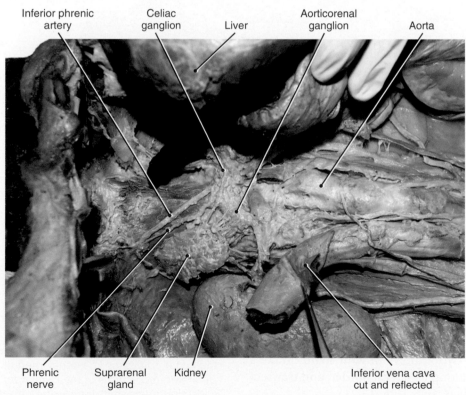

Fig. 13.20 Dissect the right superior, middle, and inferior suprarenal arteries typically arising from the inferior phrenic artery, aorta, and renal artery, respectively.

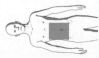

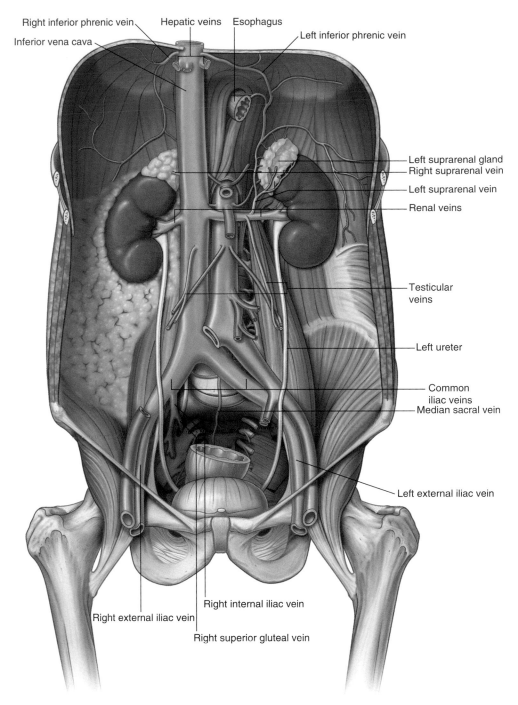

Right inferior phrenic vein
Hepatic veins
Esophagus
Inferior vena cava
Left inferior phrenic vein
Left suprarenal gland
Right suprarenal vein
Left suprarenal vein
Renal veins
Testicular veins
Left ureter
Common iliac veins
Median sacral vein
Left external iliac vein
Right internal iliac vein
Right external iliac vein
Right superior gluteal vein

Plate 13.1 Inferior vena cava and tributaries.

- Hold one of the two kidneys in your hand. Make a vertical incision along its lateral border, and transect the kidney into two parts (Fig. 13.21).
- Open and inspect the inner part of the kidney.
- Identify the outer layer, the renal cortex, and the inner layer, the *renal medulla* (Plate 13.2).

ANATOMY **NOTE**

Realize that the cortex sends extensions into the medulla, the *renal columns*. The renal medulla is composed of *pyramids,* projections of the renal *papillae,* which contain collecting ducts that drain urine into the minor *calyces.* About 10 minor calyces combine to form three major calyces; all major calyces combine to form the *renal pelvis,* located at the hilum of the kidney (Fig. 13.22).

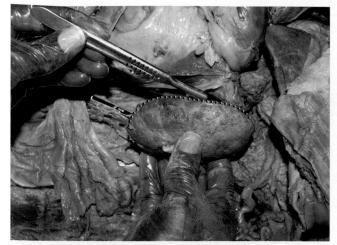

Fig. 13.21 An incision into the kidney along its border allows access to its internal structures.

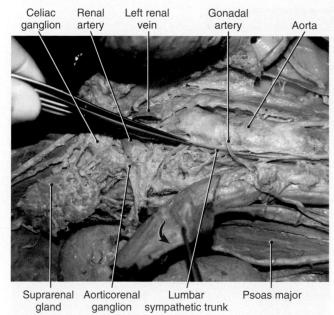

Celiac ganglion Renal artery Left renal vein Gonadal artery Aorta

Suprarenal gland Aorticorenal ganglion Lumbar sympathetic trunk Psoas major

Fig. 13.23 Right sympathetic trunk between the IVC and abdominal aorta.

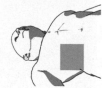

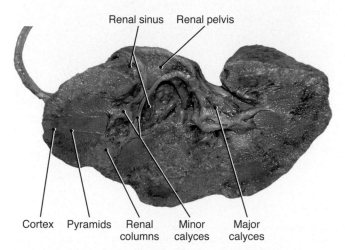

Renal sinus Renal pelvis

Cortex Pyramids Renal columns Minor calyces Major calyces

Fig. 13.22 Inside the kidney, note the cortex, medulla, calyces, pyramids, and columns.

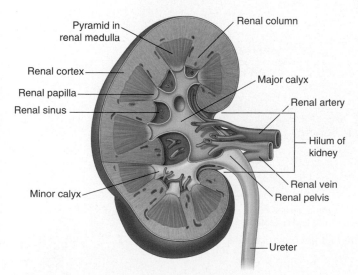

Pyramid in renal medulla

Renal column

Renal cortex

Renal papilla

Renal sinus

Major calyx

Renal artery

Hilum of kidney

Renal vein
Renal pelvis

Minor calyx

Ureter

Plate 13.2 Internal structure of the kidney.

○ Between the inferior vena cava and the abdominal aorta, at the level of the right renal vein, locate the right sympathetic trunk (Fig. 13.23).

○ You also can trace the sympathetic trunk just underneath the IVC, between the psoas major muscle and the vertebral column (Figs. 13.24 and 13.25). The sympathetic trunk contributes lumbar splanchnic nerves to the superior hypogastric plexus (see Fig. 13.24).

○ The right and left renal arteries are surrounded by a dense network of neural fibers (see Fig. 13.22). Identify the *aorticorenal ganglion*.

ANATOMY **NOTE**

This ganglion further connects with the celiac ganglion, occupying the area over the celiac trunk (see Fig. 13.22). Preganglionic sympathetic fibers reach the celiac, aorti-corenal, and superior mesenteric ganglia by way of the greater, lesser, and least splanchnic nerves, respectively. These fibers synapse in the ganglia, and postganglionic fibers travel along the arteries of the abdomen.

○ Lift the kidney upward, and clean out the posterior surface of the renal hilum (Fig. 13.26).

○ Identify the psoas major muscle, and remove the fascia over the right crus of the diaphragm and psoas major muscle (Fig. 13.27).

NERVES

○ At the opening of the IVC, look for the inferior phrenic artery, and trace it to its origin from the aorta.

DISSECTION **TIP**

In some cases, the inferior phrenic artery originates from the celiac trunk.

○ Next to the inferior phrenic artery, dissect out the continuation of the phrenic nerve into the abdominal cavity (see Fig. 13.27). The phrenic nerve accompanies the inferior phrenic artery and is related to the phrenic ganglion.

○ Lift the kidney upward, and look between the supero-medial border of the psoas major and the right crus of the diaphragm for the greater, lesser, and least splanchnic nerves (Figs. 13.28 and 13.29).

DISSECTION **TIP**

You also may pull the celiac ganglion upward and look for the greater splanchnic nerve underneath.

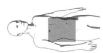

Inferior phrenic artery Aorta Lumbar splanchnic nerve Lumbar sympathetic ganglion

Phrenic nerve Suprarenal gland Inferior vena cava Lumbar sympathetic trunk Ureter Superior hypogastric plexus

Fig. 13.24 The sympathetic trunk is shown giving rise to lumbar splanchnic nerves that contribute to the pancreatic and superior hypogastric plexuses.

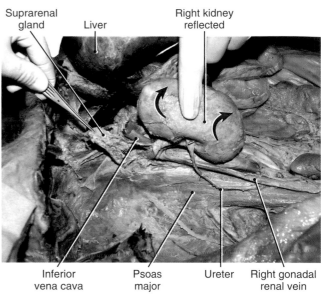

Suprarenal gland Liver Right kidney reflected

Inferior vena cava Psoas major Ureter Right gonadal renal vein

Fig. 13.26 Right kidney lifted upward to clean out posterior surface of renal hilum.

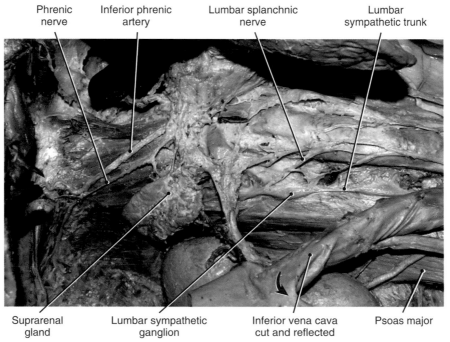

Phrenic nerve Inferior phrenic artery Lumbar splanchnic nerve Lumbar sympathetic trunk

Suprarenal gland Lumbar sympathetic ganglion Inferior vena cava cut and reflected Psoas major

Fig. 13.25 Sympathetic trunk courses underneath the IVC between psoas major muscle and vertebral column.

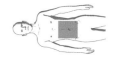

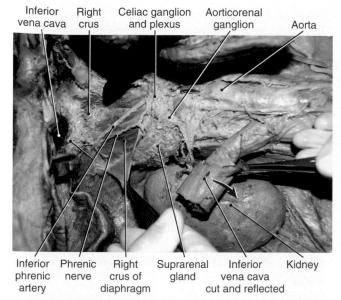

Inferior vena cava · Right crus · Celiac ganglion and plexus · Aorticorenal ganglion · Aorta

Inferior phrenic artery · Phrenic nerve · Right crus of diaphragm · Suprarenal gland · Inferior vena cava cut and reflected · Kidney

Fig. 13.27 Fascia removed over right crus of diaphragm and psoas major muscle.

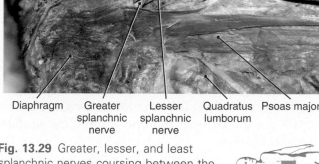

Inferior phrenic arteries · Suprarenal gland · Least splanchnic nerve · Right renal artery · Kidney · Inferior vena cava

Diaphragm · Greater splanchnic nerve · Lesser splanchnic nerve · Quadratus lumborum · Psoas major

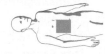

Fig. 13.29 Greater, lesser, and least splanchnic nerves coursing between the superomedial border of the psoas major muscle and the right crus of diaphragm.

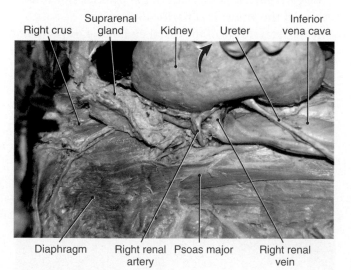

Right crus · Suprarenal gland · Kidney · Ureter · Inferior vena cava

Diaphragm · Right renal artery · Psoas major · Right renal vein

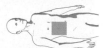

Fig. 13.28 Appreciate underlying structures with kidney lifted.

Right crus

Cisterna chyli · Right crus · IVC

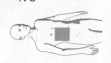

Fig. 13.30 Vertical incision at right crus of diaphragm exposes cisterna chyli. *IVC,* Inferior vena cava.

○ Trace these nerves to their terminations at the celiac ganglion (for the greater), aorticorenal ganglion (for the lesser), and superior mesenteric ganglion (for the least).

○ Between the abdominal aorta and the IVC and at the left side of the aorta, identify the right and left lumbar lymph trunks, respectively.

○ These lymph trunks eventually join the intestinal lymph trunk and form the *cisterna chyli.* Make a vertical incision at the right crus of the diaphragm, and expose the cisterna chyli (Fig. 13.30).

○ Open up the thoracic cavity and identify the anterior and posterior vagal trunks around the lower part of the esophagus.

○ Place slight traction on the anterior vagal trunk, which originates primarily from the left vagus nerve, and look anterior to the cardioesophageal junction for a mobile structure.

○ Locate the anterior vagal trunk and expose its branches.

○ Similarly, place slight traction on the posterior vagal trunk in the thorax (primarily right vagus nerve) and find the medial side of the *esophageal hiatus,* or the right side of the esophagus, for identification of the posterior vagal trunk (Fig. 13.31).

INSPECTION OF POSTERIOR ABDOMINAL STRUCTURES

○ Observe the thoracic and abdominal surfaces of the diaphragm. Note the central tendinous portion of the diaphragm, the *central tendon*.
○ Lateral to the esophagus, identify the *right and left crura*, the two muscular extensions of the diaphragm arising from the central tendon to insert onto the 2nd or 3rd lumbar (L2 or L3) vertebrae.
○ Fibers from the right and left crura intermix to encircle the esophagus as it passes through the diaphragm. Just superior to the celiac trunk, the right and left crura are united by a midline tendon, the *median arcuate ligament*.
○ Laterally, the diaphragm attaches to the ribs and inferolaterally it attaches to the psoas major forming a thickened connective tissue band, the *medial arcuate ligament*.
○ More laterally, the diaphragm arches over the quadratus lumborum to attach to the 12th rib, forming another thickened connective tissue band over the quadratus lumborum, the *lateral arcuate ligament* (see Fig. 13.31).

○ Remove any remaining fat inferior to the right and left kidneys to expose the lumbar plexus and the underlying muscles (Fig. 13.32).
○ Identify the psoas major muscle and, lateral to it, the quadratus lumborum muscle.

DISSECTION **TIP**

In about 50% of cadaveric donors, the psoas minor muscle is evident on the anterior surface of the psoas major.

○ Inferior to the quadratus lumborum, identify the iliacus muscle, which lies in the iliac fossa. Palpate the 12th rib and at its inferior border, expose the *subcostal nerve*.
○ On the lateral side of the psoas major muscle, identify the *genitofemoral nerve* as it travels on its anterior surface.
○ A few centimeters below the origin of the *iliohypogastric nerve*, identify the *ilioinguinal nerve*, which travels from the lateral side of the psoas major muscle toward the anterior superior iliac spine.
○ At the lateral side of the distal end of the psoas major muscle in the abdominal cavity, identify the *femoral nerve* and, lateral to it, the much smaller *lateral femoral cutaneous nerve*.
○ Medial to the psoas major muscle, place a probe or a pair of scissors and separate the psoas major

Anterior vagal trunk   Esophageal branch of left gastric artery   Stomach   Spleen

Right crus   Posterior vagal trunk   Cisterna chyli   Left gastric artery   Pancreas

Fig. 13.31 Thoracic cavity opened and anterior and posterior vagal trunks around lower esophagus used to locate anterior and posterior trunks in the abdominal cavity.

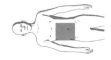

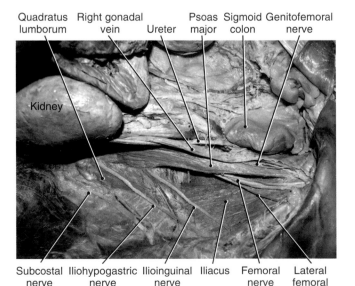

Quadratus lumborum   Right gonadal vein   Ureter   Psoas major   Sigmoid colon   Genitofemoral nerve

Kidney

Subcostal nerve   Iliohypogastric nerve   Ilioinguinal nerve   Iliacus   Femoral nerve   Lateral femoral cutaneous nerve

Fig. 13.32 Removal of fat inferior to right and left kidneys exposes branches of the lumbar plexus and underlying muscles.

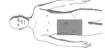

from the adjacent external iliac artery and vein (Fig. 13.33).

○ Deep and medial to the psoas major muscle, identify the *obturator nerve* (Fig. 13.34).

○ Once all branches of the lumbar plexus are identified, on one side of the cadaver, carefully remove the psoas major muscle in a piecemeal fashion, and expose the origin of the nerves of the lumbar plexus (Fig. 13.35 and Plate 13.3).

DISSECTION TIP

In most cadavers, the lumbar plexus exhibits great variation.
• The most common variation is that the ilioinguinal and iliohypogastric nerves fuse and split into their terminal branches just proximal to the *anterior superior iliac spine.*
• Similarly, the subcostal and iliohypogastric nerves can be fused and split more distally.

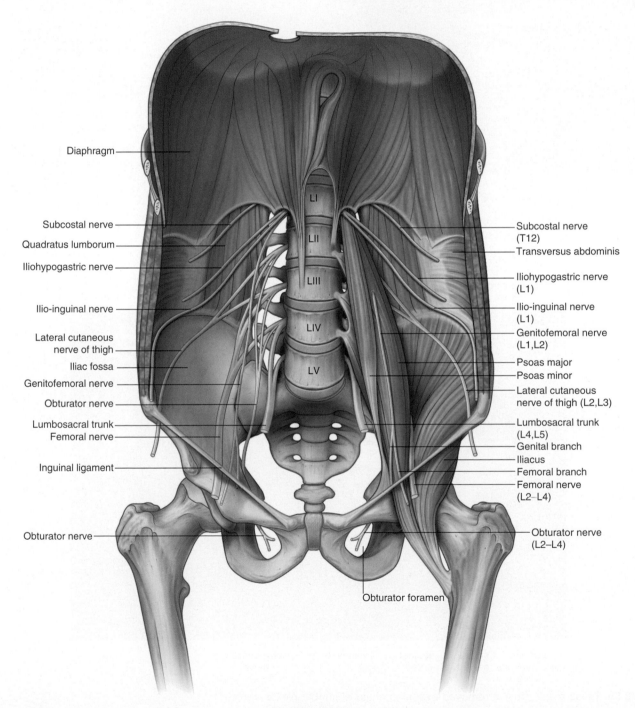

Lumbar plexus

Plate 13.3 The lumbar plexus.

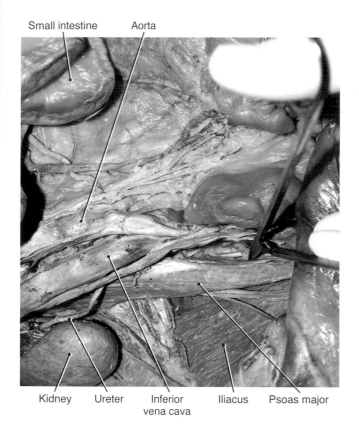

Small intestine   Aorta

Kidney   Ureter   Inferior   Iliacus   Psoas major
                    vena cava

Fig. 13.33 Psoas major muscle separated from adjacent external iliac artery and vein.

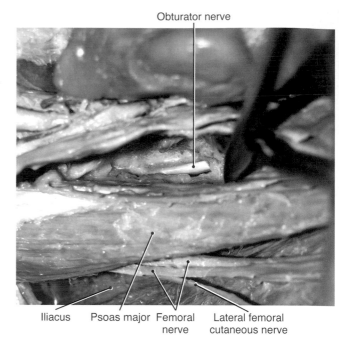

Obturator nerve

Iliacus   Psoas major   Femoral   Lateral femoral
                          nerve   cutaneous nerve

Fig. 13.34 Obturator nerve lies deep and medial to the psoas major muscle.

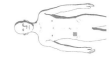

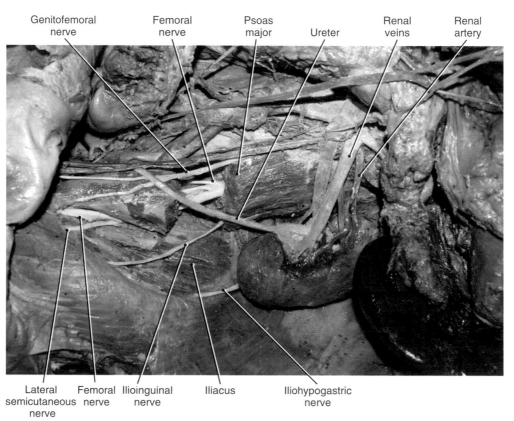

Genitofemoral   Femoral   Psoas   Ureter   Renal   Renal
nerve   nerve   major   veins   artery

Lateral   Femoral   Ilioinguinal   Iliacus   Iliohypogastric
semicutaneous   nerve   nerve   nerve
nerve

Fig. 13.35 Psoas major muscle removed exposing origin of lumbar plexus nerves.

LABORATORY IDENTIFICATION CHECKLIST

NERVES/CONNECTIVE TISSUE
- ☐ Iliohypogastric
- ☐ Ilioinguinal
- ☐ Genitofemoral
- ☐ Lateral femoral cutaneous
- ☐ Femoral
- ☐ Obturator
- ☐ Accessory obturator (variation)
- ☐ Lumbosacral trunk
- ☐ Sympathetic trunk
  - ☐ Gray/white rami communicantes
  - ☐ Sympathetic ganglion
  - ☐ Lumbar splanchnic
- ☐ Celiac ganglia
- ☐ Celiac plexus
- ☐ Suprarenal plexus
- ☐ Aorticorenal ganglion
- ☐ Superior mesenteric plexus
- ☐ Intermesenteric (aortic) plexus

ARTERIES
- ☐ Right and left inferior phrenic
- ☐ Superior suprarenal
- ☐ Middle suprarenal
- ☐ Inferior suprarenal
- ☐ Renal
- ☐ Gonadal
- ☐ Lumbar
- ☐ Subcostal
- ☐ Iliolumbar

VEINS
- ☐ Inferior vena cava (IVC)
- ☐ Inferior phrenic

- ☐ Suprarenal
- ☐ Renal
- ☐ Gonadal
- ☐ Lumbar
- ☐ Iliolumbar

LYMPH
- ☐ Cisterna chyli

MUSCLES/CONNECTIVE TISSUE
- ☐ Right crus
  - ☐ Ligament of Treitz
- ☐ Left crus
- ☐ Psoas major
- ☐ Psoas minor
- ☐ Quadratus lumborum
- ☐ Transversus abdominis
- ☐ Median arcuate ligament
- ☐ Medial arcuate ligament
- ☐ Lateral arcuate ligament

ORGANS
- ☐ Kidney
- ☐ Ureter
- ☐ Suprarenal gland

BONES
- ☐ Coxal, right and left
- ☐ Sacrum
- ☐ Vertebrae
  - ☐ 12th thoracic (T12)
  - ☐ 1st to 5th lumbar: (L1-L5)

PERITONEAL ASPIRATION/LAVAGE

Gray's Anatomy for Students: 135, 136
Netter: 252, 254

Clinical Application

Procedure introduces a trocar to withdraw fluid or to introduce saline into the peritoneal cavity for irrigation.

Anatomic Landmarks (Figs. V.1 and V.2)

- Infraumbilical region
- Skin
- Subcutaneous tissue
- Linea alba/rectus abdominis muscle
- Transversalis fascia

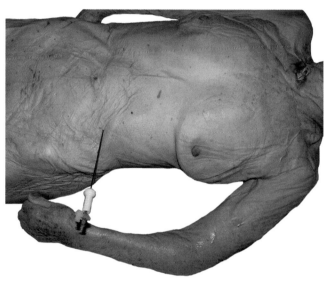

Fig. V.1

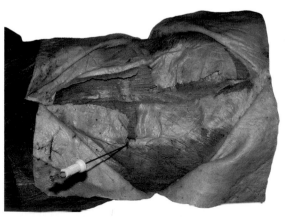

Fig. V.2

- Extraperitoneal fat
- Parietal peritoneum
- Umbilicus
- Anterior superior iliac spine (ASIS)

PARACENTESIS

Gray's Anatomy for Students: 135, 136
Netter: 252, 254

Clinical Application

Procedure withdraws fluid (e.g., ascites) from the peritoneal cavity.

Anatomic Landmarks

Infraumbilical Region

- Skin
- Subcutaneous tissue
- Linea alba
- Median umbilical fold/ligament
- Medial umbilical fold/ligament
- Transversalis fascia
- Extraperitoneal fat/space
- Peritoneal sac

About 5 cm Superior to ASIS

Layers traversed:

- Skin (lateral to rectus)
- Subcutaneous tissue
- External abdominal oblique aponeurosis
- Internal abdominal oblique muscle
- Transversus abdominis muscle
- Transversalis fascia
- Extraperitoneal fat/space
- Peritoneum

PUDENDAL NERVE BLOCK

Gray's Anatomy for Students: 267
Netter: 395

Clinical Application

Procedure places a bolus of local anesthetic into the pudendal canal, anesthetizing the pudendal nerve and its branches.

Anatomic Landmarks (Figs. V.3 and V.4)

- Vaginal introitus
- Lateral vagina wall and mucosa
- Vaginal mucosa
- Ischial spine

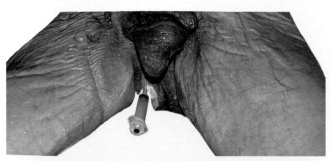

Fig. V.3

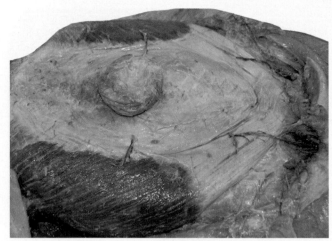

Fig. V.5

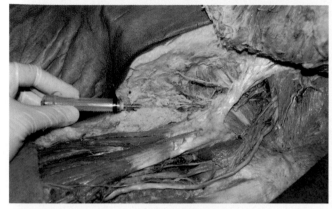

Fig. V.4

- Coccygeus
- Sacrospinous ligament (resistance)
- Pudendal canal (Alcock's canal)
- Pudendal nerve
- Internal pudendal artery
- Internal pudendal vein

HERNIATIONS AND OTHER PATHOLOGIES

The following cadavers exhibited marked herniations and other examples of abdominal and vascular abnormalities, including life-threatening aortic aneurysm.

- Umbilical hernia (Fig. V.5)
- Umbilical hernia and an indirect inguinal hernia (Figs. V.6 and V.7)
- Massive malignancies in the abdominal cavity and the liver (Fig. V.8)
- Multiple malignant nodules in a sagittal section of the liver (Fig. V.9)
- Example of hepatomegaly (Fig. V.10)
- Dissected liver with evident hepatic arteries and veins (Fig. V.11)
- Example of splenomegaly (Fig. V.12)
- Examples of kidneys with cysts (Figs. V.13, V.14, and V.15)
- Abdominal aortic aneurysm; large Gore-tex tube placed at site is visible (Fig. V.16)
- Large abdominal aortic aneurysm (Fig. V.17)

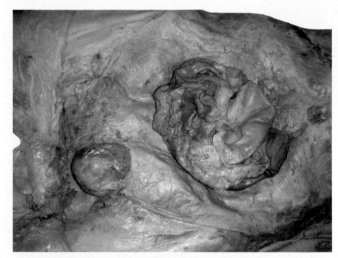

Fig. V.6

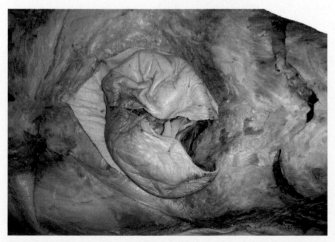

Fig. V.7

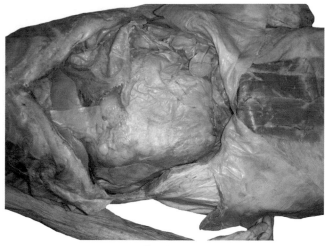

Fig. V.8

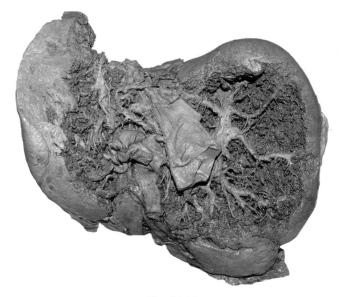

Fig. V.11

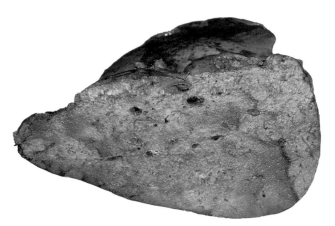

Fig. V.9

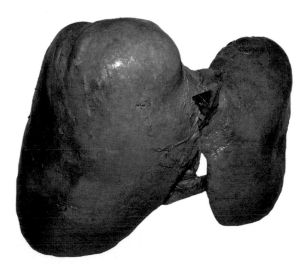

Fig. V.10

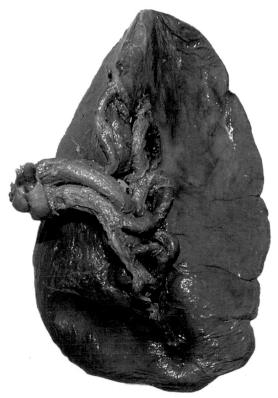

Fig. V.12

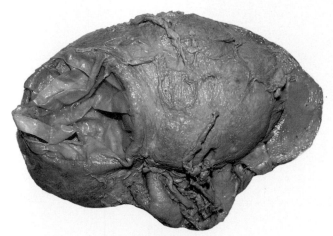

Fig. V.13

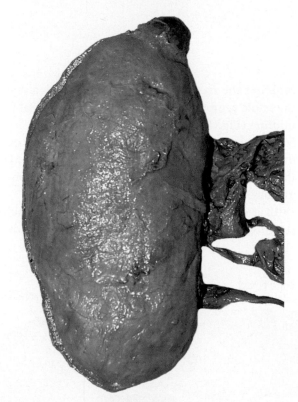

Fig. V.14

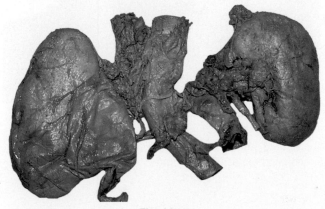

Fig. V.15

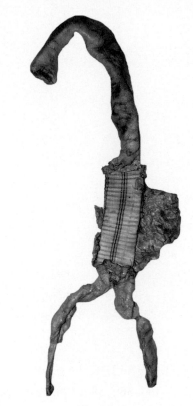

Fig. V.16

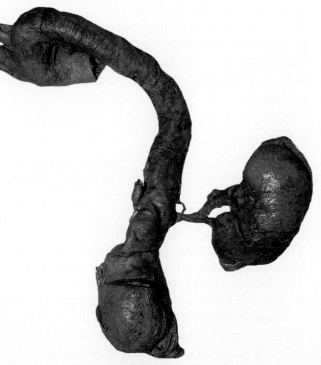

Fig. V.17

PELVIS AND PERINEUM

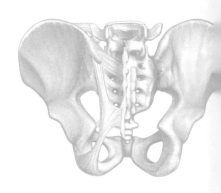

CHAPTER 14 PELVIS

ATLAS REFERENCES
Netter: 333–357, 366, 369, 380–385, 388, 390–392
McMinn: 261–275
Gray's Atlas: 212–254, 264–265

Several techniques are used for dissection of the pelvis. This chapter describes the traditional midline hemipelvectomy.

MIDLINE HEMIPELVECTOMY (MALE)

○ Identify the rectosigmoid junction and expose the rectum (Fig. 14.1). Posterior to the pubic symphysis, palpate the urinary bladder.

○ With a probe or scissors, dissect out and reflect the peritoneum from the posterior surface of the urinary bladder (Figs. 14.2 and 14.3). Notice the median umbilical ligament connecting to the urinary bladder (urachus).

ANATOMY NOTE

The adipose tissue between the posterior surface of the urinary bladder and the peritoneum is termed *preperitoneal fat.*

○ Place your fingertips, using blunt dissection, between the urinary bladder and the pubic symphysis into the retropubic space of Retzius (Fig. 14.4).

○ Pull on the fascia attached to the lateral sides of the median umbilical ligament and at the superior part of the urinary bladder, the *vesicoumbilical fascia,* and reflect it posteriorly. With this maneuver, observe the expansion of the retropubic space of Retzius.

○ Mobilize the rectum and the bladder. With a saw, cut the pubic symphysis vertically 2 to 3 cm lateral to the midline (Fig. 14.5).

○ Mobilize the rectum laterally, and with a scalpel, extend the incision from the pubic symphysis backward toward the sacrum and pelvis (Fig. 14.6). Cut the peritoneum, urinary bladder, aorta, and all soft tissues.

○ With a scalpel, make a second horizontal incision starting from the aorta, at the level of the kidneys,

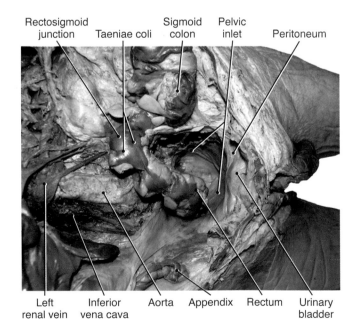

Rectosigmoid junction Sigmoid colon Pelvic inlet

Taeniae coli Peritoneum

Left renal vein Inferior vena cava Aorta Appendix Rectum Urinary bladder

Fig. 14.1 Identification of rectosigmoid junction and exposure of rectum.

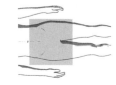

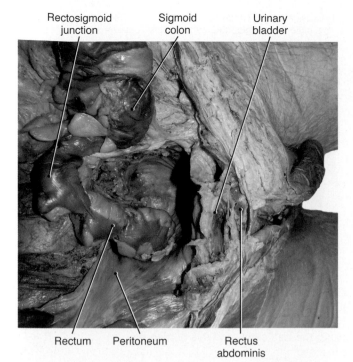

Fig. 14.2 Urinary bladder posterior to pubic symphysis.

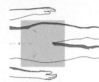

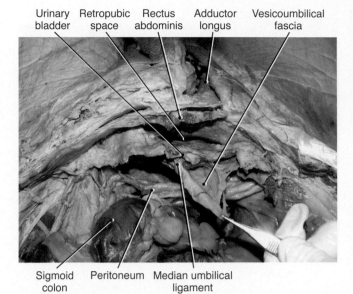

Fig. 14.4 Blunt dissection between urinary bladder and pubic symphysis into retropubic space.

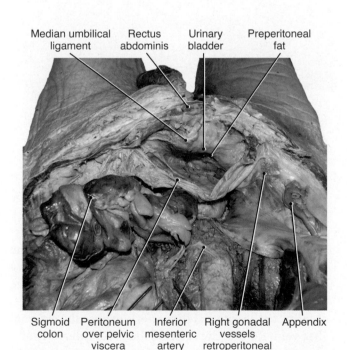

Fig. 14.3 Peritoneum reflected from posterior surface of urinary bladder.

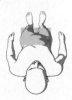

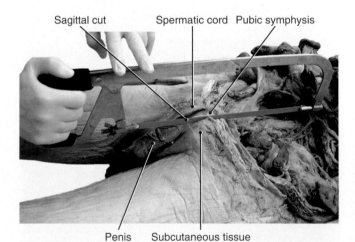

Fig. 14.5 Pubic symphysis cut vertically about 1 inch (2 to 3 cm) lateral to midline.

and extending laterally along the borders of the iliac crest (Fig. 14.7).

○ With the cadaver on its side, and using a saw, cut the sacrum through its promontory, up through the 4th lumbar vertebra. Saw through the pubic symphysis and make a horizontal incision along the iliac crest (as previously described) and detach this portion of the body (Figs. 14.7 and 14.8).

DISSECTION TIP

For the hemipelvectomy, you will need the help of your colleagues to lift and turn the cadaver on its side.

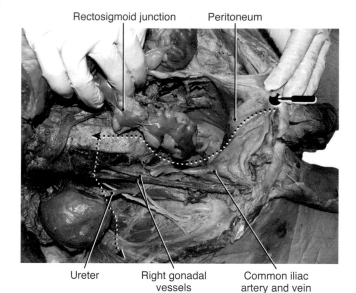

Rectosigmoid junction   Peritoneum

Ureter   Right gonadal   Common iliac
                 vessels   artery and vein

Fig. 14.6 Incision extended from pubic symphysis back toward sacrum and pelvis *(dashed line with arrowheads).*

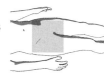

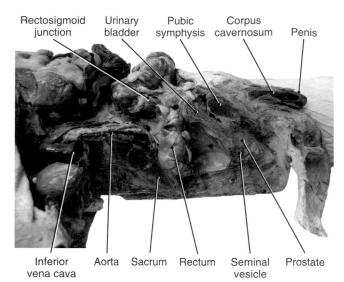

Rectosigmoid   Urinary   Pubic   Corpus
junction   bladder symphysis cavernosum   Penis

Inferior   Aorta   Sacrum   Rectum   Seminal   Prostate
vena cava   vesicle

Fig. 14.8 After the cadaver is turned on its side, the saw is passed through the open pubic symphysis. A horizontal cut is made along the iliac crest, and this portion is detached.

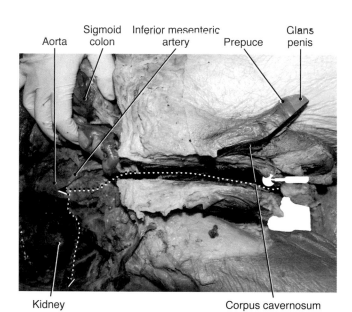

        Sigmoid   Inferior mesenteric   Glans
Aorta   colon   artery   Prepuce   penis

Kidney   Corpus cavernosum

Fig. 14.7 Second horizontal incision from aorta extends laterally along iliac crest.

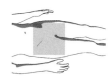

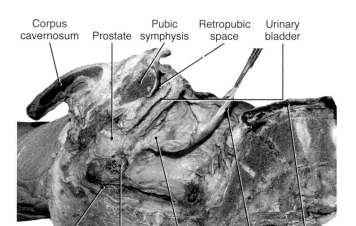

Corpus   Pubic   Retropubic   Urinary
cavernosum Prostate symphysis   space   bladder

Rectum   Seminal   Retrovesical Peritoneum Aorta
          vesicle   space

Fig. 14.9 The peritoneum is reflected upward.

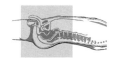

- With scissors, reflect the parietal peritoneum upward (Fig. 14.9).
- Start cleaning the soft tissues and adipose tissue around larger structures (Fig. 14.10).
- Identify the aorta and expose the external iliac artery (Fig. 14.11).

- Trace the ductus deferens and expose it toward the prostate. On surface of the external iliac artery, identify the ureter. Trace and expose the ureter to its entrance to the urinary bladder (Fig. 14.12).
- Inferior to the external iliac artery, expose the external iliac vein. Retract the external iliac vein inferiorly and clean the adipose tissue superior to it. Just inferior to the course of the external iliac vein, identify the obturator nerve and trace it to the obturator foramen (Fig. 14.13).
- Identify the internal iliac artery and expose its anterior and posterior divisions.

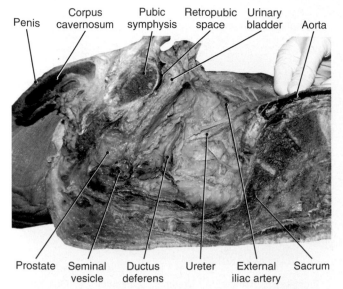

Fig. 14.10 Soft tissue and adipose tissue cleaned around large structures.

Penis | Corpus cavernosum | Pubic symphysis | Retropubic space | Urinary bladder | Aorta

Prostate | Seminal vesicle | Ductus deferens | Ureter | External iliac artery | Sacrum

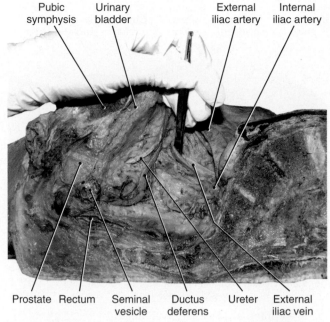

Fig. 14.12 External iliac vein retracted inferiorly. Ductus deferens and ureter exposed.

Pubic symphysis | Urinary bladder | External iliac artery | Internal iliac artery

Prostate | Rectum | Seminal vesicle | Ductus deferens | Ureter | External iliac vein

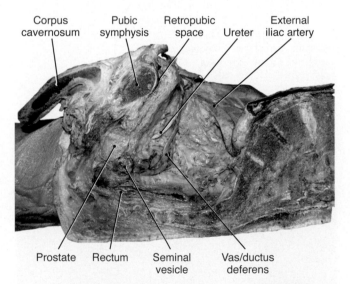

Fig. 14.11 Exposure of external iliac artery, with ductus deferens exposed toward prostate and ureter to its entrance.

Corpus cavernosum | Pubic symphysis | Retropubic space | Ureter | External iliac artery

Prostate | Rectum | Seminal vesicle | Vas/ductus deferens

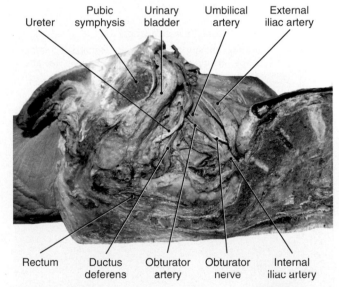

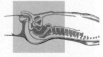

Fig. 14.13 Obturator nerve traced to obturator foramen.

Ureter | Pubic symphysis | Urinary bladder | Umbilical artery | External iliac artery

Rectum | Ductus deferens | Obturator artery | Obturator nerve | Internal iliac artery

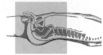

DISSECTION **TIP**

The branches of the internal iliac artery are very variable. An easy way to avoid confusion is to rely on landmarks (discussed in dissection tips below), and always name the artery based on its distribution, not its origin.

○ Identify the internal iliac artery and expose its anterior and posterior divisions. Expose the branches of the anterior division of the internal iliac artery. These branches are the umbilical, obturator, inferior gluteal, internal pudendal, middle rectal, inferior vesical, and uterine arteries (Figs. 14.14 to 14.23). These arteries are discussed in the following dissection tips and figures.

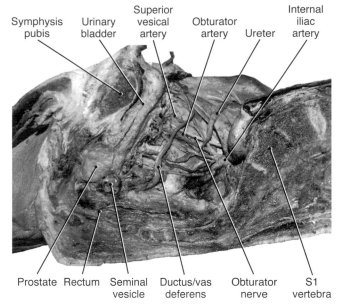

Symphysis pubis | Urinary bladder | Superior vesical artery | Obturator artery | Ureter | Internal iliac artery

Prostate | Rectum | Seminal vesicle | Ductus/vas deferens | Obturator nerve | S1 vertebra

Fig. 14.14 Internal iliac artery with anterior and posterior divisions.

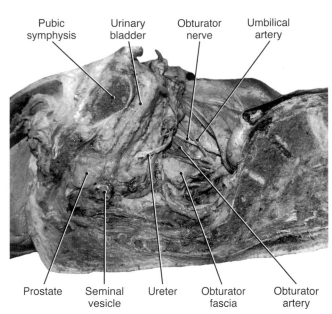

Pubic symphysis | Urinary bladder | Obturator nerve | Umbilical artery

Prostate | Seminal vesicle | Ureter | Obturator fascia | Obturator artery

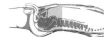

Fig. 14.16 Appreciate major landmarks of pelvis in relation to branches of the internal iliac artery.

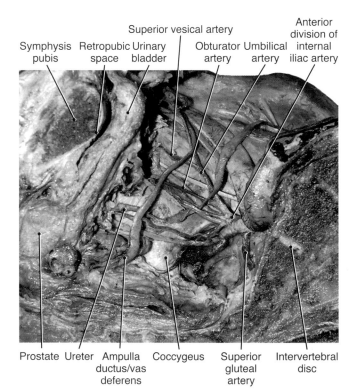

Superior vesical artery

Symphysis pubis | Retropubic space | Urinary bladder | Obturator artery | Umbilical artery | Anterior division of internal iliac artery

Prostate | Ureter | Ampulla ductus/vas deferens | Coccygeus | Superior gluteal artery | Intervertebral disc

Fig. 14.15 Branches of anterior division of internal iliac artery.

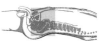

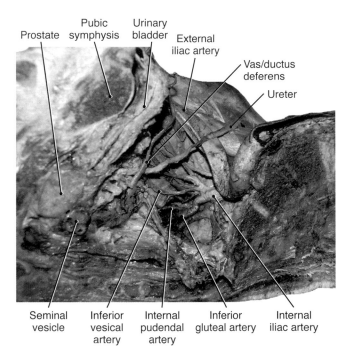

Prostate | Pubic symphysis | Urinary bladder | External iliac artery | Vas/ductus deferens | Ureter

Seminal vesicle | Inferior vesical artery | Internal pudendal artery | Inferior gluteal artery | Internal iliac artery

Fig. 14.17 Appreciate branches of the anterior division of the internal iliac artery.

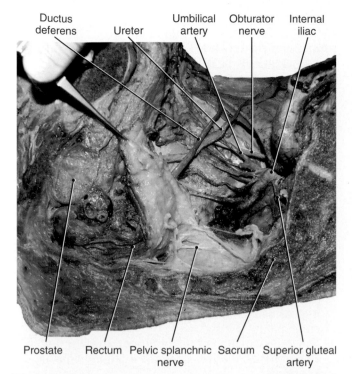

Ductus deferens · Ureter · Umbilical artery · Obturator nerve · Internal iliac

Prostate · Rectum · Pelvic splanchnic nerve · Sacrum · Superior gluteal artery

Fig. 14.18 Sympathetic trunk exposed in pelvis with gray communicating rami passing lateral to nerves of sacral plexus.

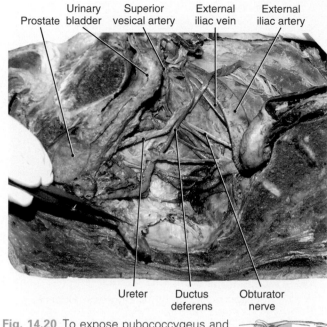

Prostate · Urinary bladder · Superior vesical artery · External iliac vein · External iliac artery

Ureter · Ductus deferens · Obturator nerve

Fig. 14.20 To expose pubococcygeus and iliococcygeus muscles, clean all the pelvic fascia and adipose tissue over the levator ani inferior to the prostate gland.

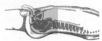

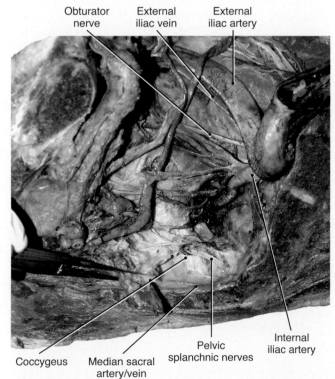

Obturator nerve · External iliac vein · External iliac artery

Coccygeus · Median sacral artery/vein · Pelvic splanchnic nerves · Internal iliac artery

Fig. 14.19 To expose pelvic splanchnic nerves fully, lift the rectum and anal canal superiorly.

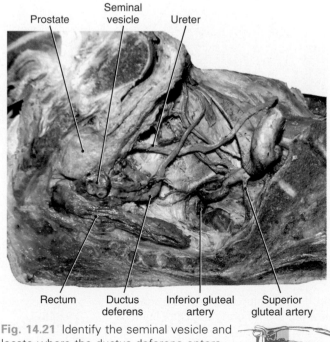

Prostate · Seminal vesicle · Ureter

Rectum · Ductus deferens · Inferior gluteal artery · Superior gluteal artery

Fig. 14.21 Identify the seminal vesicle and locate where the ductus deferens enters seminal vesicles.

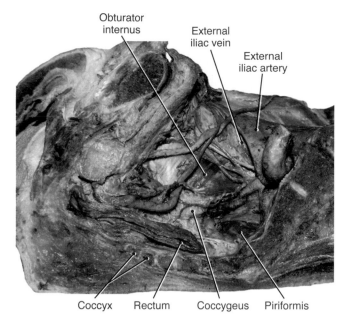

Fig. 14.22 Locate coccygeus muscle that arises from ischial spine and sacrospinous ligament and attaches to the coccyx and lower part of the sacrum.

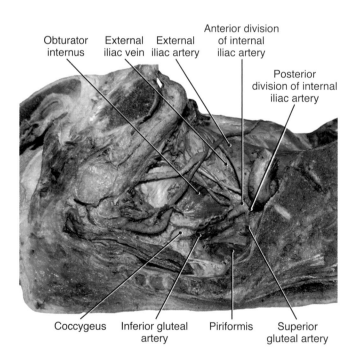

Fig. 14.23 Obturator internus fascia cleaned, exposing the obturator internus muscle.

DISSECTION TIPS

BRANCHES OF INTERNAL ILIAC ARTERY: ANTERIOR DIVISION (PLATE 14.1)

Umbilical artery: Usually the first branch of the anterior division. The umbilical artery courses upward and superior to the urinary bladder to become the median umbilical ligament (Figs. 14.13, 14.15, and 14.16). The umbilical artery often gives off the superior vesical branches that supply the superior portion of the urinary bladder; in 75% of cases, there are two or three superior vesical arteries.

Obturator artery: Usually arises parallel to the origin of the umbilical artery; travels with the obturator nerve to split into anterior and posterior branches in the obturator foramen (Figs. 14.14 and 14.15). The obturator artery travels anterior to the obturator internus and its fascia and is crossed medially by the ureter and the ductus deferens. It gives rise to small branches: iliac, vesical, and pubic.

The main variation of the obturator artery is that in 30% of cases, it arises from the inferior epigastric artery.

Inferior gluteal artery: Arises at the posterior side of the anterior division and is mainly distributed to the buttocks. The landmark for identifying the inferior gluteal artery is to look for the artery passing between the 1st and 2nd sacral nerves and between the piriformis and coccygeus muscles (Fig. 14.17).

Internal pudendal artery: The artery is more anterior in position than the inferior gluteal artery as these arteries leave the pelvis. The internal pudendal artery does not pass between S1 and S2 nerves but typically courses lower between the piriformis and coccygeus muscles (Fig. 14.17). It also accompanies the pudendal nerve to Alcock's canal. Several small branches arise from the internal pudendal artery: inferior rectal, perineal, artery of the bulb, urethral artery, deep artery of the penis or clitoris, and dorsal artery of the penis or clitoris.

Middle rectal: It arises with or from the internal pudendal, inferior vesical, or inferior gluteal arteries; mainly supplies the rectum.

Inferior vesical (vaginal in females): Usually arises from the internal pudendal artery. The inferior vesical artery supplies the fundus of the urinary bladder, the prostate, and the seminal vesicles.

Uterine: Usually arises from the medial surface of the anterior trunk. It runs medially on the levator ani and the broad ligament, and at about 2 cm at the cervix of the uterus, it crosses in front of the ureter to anastomose with the ovarian artery. The uterine artery typically gives off a *superior* branch, supplying the body and fundus of the uterus, and a *vaginal* branch, supplying the cervix and vagina.

○ Expose the branches of the posterior division of the internal iliac artery: These branches are the iliolumbar, lateral sacral, and the superior gluteal arteries.

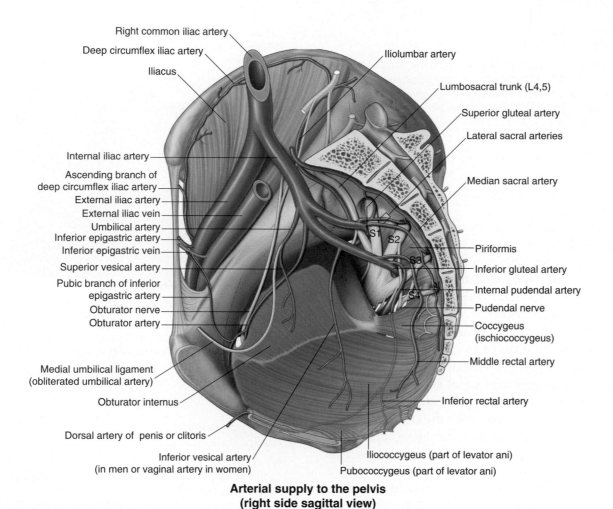

Right common iliac artery

Deep circumflex iliac artery

Iliacus

Iliolumbar artery

Lumbosacral trunk (L4,5)

Superior gluteal artery

Lateral sacral arteries

Internal iliac artery

Ascending branch of deep circumflex iliac artery

External iliac artery

External iliac vein

Umbilical artery

Inferior epigastric artery

Inferior epigastric vein

Superior vesical artery

Pubic branch of inferior epigastric artery

Obturator nerve

Obturator artery

Median sacral artery

S1 S2

S3

Piriformis

Inferior gluteal artery

S4

Internal pudendal artery

Pudendal nerve

Coccygeus (ischiococcygeus)

Middle rectal artery

Medial umbilical ligament (obliterated umbilical artery)

Obturator internus

Inferior rectal artery

Dorsal artery of penis or clitoris

Inferior vesical artery (in men or vaginal artery in women)

Iliococcygeus (part of levator ani)

Pubococcygeus (part of levator ani)

**Arterial supply to the pelvis
(right side sagittal view)**

Plate 14.1 Arteries of the pelvis.

DISSECTION **TIPS**

BRANCHES OF INTERNAL ILIAC ARTERY: POSTERIOR DIVISION (SEE PLATE 14.1)

Iliolumbar: This artery typically is found between the lumbosacral trunk and the obturator nerve. It then ascends superolaterally to the iliac fossa, finally to reach the psoas major muscle. The iliolumbar artery gives off an iliac and a lumbar branch.

Lateral sacral: Usually, two lateral sacral arteries are present, superior and inferior. The *superior* lateral sacral artery usually enters the 1st or 2nd sacral foramina. The *inferior* lateral sacral artery runs obliquely across the piriformis muscle to the medial side of the sacral foramina. It anastomoses with the middle sacral artery.

Superior gluteal: Largest branch of the posterior trunk and a direct continuation of its posterior trunk. The superior gluteal artery runs backward between the lumbosacral trunk and the 1st sacral nerve (Figs. 14.15 and 14.18). It divides into superficial and deep branches in the buttock.

○ Behind the internal and external iliac arteries, identify the obturator internus muscle covered with the obturator fascia (a part of the endopelvic fascia).

○ Expose the inferior part of the obturator fascia and note its white, thickened band of fibers, the *tendinous arch of the levator ani* (arcus tendineus levator ani).

ANATOMY **NOTE**

The tendinous arch runs from the obturator internus to the posterior part of the pubic bone and serves as an attachment site for the fibers of the levator ani muscle (Fig. 14.29). The tendinous arch is continuous with the obturator internus fascia.

The floor of the pelvis is mainly composed of the levator ani (anteriorly) and the coccygeus (posteriorly) muscles, forming the *pelvic diaphragm* (Fig. 14.19).

The levator ani consists mainly of the pubococcygeus muscle arising from the anterior/middle portion of the tendinous arch of levator ani and the iliococcygeus. It further divides into the puborectalis and pubovaginalis (in females) muscles and the levator prostatae (in males) muscles.

The iliococcygeus muscle arises mainly from the tendineus arch of the levator ani and attaches to the coccyx. The coccygeus muscle arises from the ischial spine and sacrospinous ligament and attaches to the coccyx and lower part of the sacrum (Fig. 14.22).

DISSECTION **TIP**

To expose the pubococcygeus and the iliococcygeus muscles, clean all the pelvic fascia and adipose tissue over the levator ani muscle inferior to the prostate gland (see Figs. 14.20 and 14.21). These muscles are often atrophied, and clear borders may be difficult to identify.

○ Clean the superior fascia of the pelvic diaphragm, which covers the levator ani. Note the continuity of the tendinous arch of the levator ani and the obturator internus fascia.

○ Clean the obturator internus fascia and expose the obturator internus muscle (Figs. 14.22 and 14.23).

○ Expose the sympathetic trunk in the pelvis, and observe the pelvic gray communicating rami passing lateral to nerves of the sacral plexus (there are no white communicating rami below the level of L2 or L3) and the origins of the pelvic splanchnic nerves (see Figs. 14.18 and 14.19; Plate 14.2).

○ To expose the pelvic splanchnic nerves completely, lift the rectum and anal canal superiorly. Note the pelvic splanchnic nerves penetrating the piriformis and coccygeus muscles to reach the lateral wall of the rectum. Trace the obturator nerve through the obturator foramen, and expose the lumbosacral trunk and the sacral nerves.

○ Expose the ductus deferens to the seminal vesicles. Expose the dilation of the ductus deferens near the seminal vesicle, the *ampulla.* Expose the seminal vesicles, and identify the ejaculatory duct formed by the union of the ductus deferens and the seminal vesicle.

○ Identify the prostate gland and expose its superior portion, the base, which is in contact with the urinary bladder. On either side of the prostate, palpate, if possible, the lateral lobes. Look for the wedge-shaped median lobe, located anterior to the ejaculatory ducts. Palpate the posterior lobe.

Dissection of the Female Pelvis

○ Identify the broad ligament with its different portions— the mesosalpinx, mesovarium, and mesometrium.

○ Identify the ovaries and the peritoneal fold covering the ovarian vessels, the suspensory ligament (infundibulopelvic) (Fig. 14.24).

○ Identify the proper ligament of the ovary.

DISSECTION **TIP**

This ovarian ligament connects to the body of the uterus and the round ligament of the uterus.

○ At the base of the broad ligament, look for a thickening of the endopelvic fascia, the cardinal ligament (ligament of Mackenrodt). Inferiorly, identify the uterosacral ligament connecting the uterus to the sacrum.

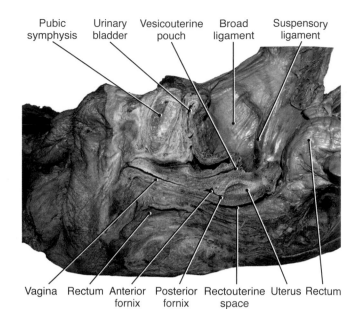

Fig. 14.24 Broad ligament of uterus and suspensory ligament of ovary; appreciate the relationship between the rectum and uterus forming the pouch of Douglas (retrovesical space).

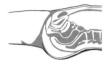

DISSECTION **TIP**

The cardinal and uterosacral ligaments may be difficult to identify in the cadaver. However, by pulling the uterus anteriorly toward the pubic symphysis and to the right, you may feel the left uterosacral ligament.

○ On the hemisected uterus, identify the fundus, body and cervix. Anterior to the cervix, identify the vagina. The deepest portion of the vagina behind the cervix is the posterior fornix (Figs. 14.24 and 14.25).

○ On the hemisected pelvis observe the most inferior portion of the abdomen, the pouch of Douglas (rectouterine space) (Fig. 14.24).

ANATOMY **NOTE**

A connective tissue septum extends inferiorly from the pouch of Douglas (retrovesical space) between the rectum and the vagina/uterus to attach to the perineal body, the rectovaginal septum (fascia of Denonvilliers). Its counterpart in the male is the rectoprostatic septum.

Ongoing Dissection of Male Pelvis

○ With a paper towel, clean the contents of the rectum and anal canal. Internally, identify the transverse folds of the rectum (valves of Houston), the anal columns (of Morgagni), and the pectinate line (Fig. 14.26).

○ Make a midsagittal incision through the prostate gland, and identify the three portions of the urethra: prostatic, membranous, and the spongy (Fig. 14.27). Within the prostatic urethra, identify an elevation, the *urethral crest,* and in the midline, the opening of the prostatic

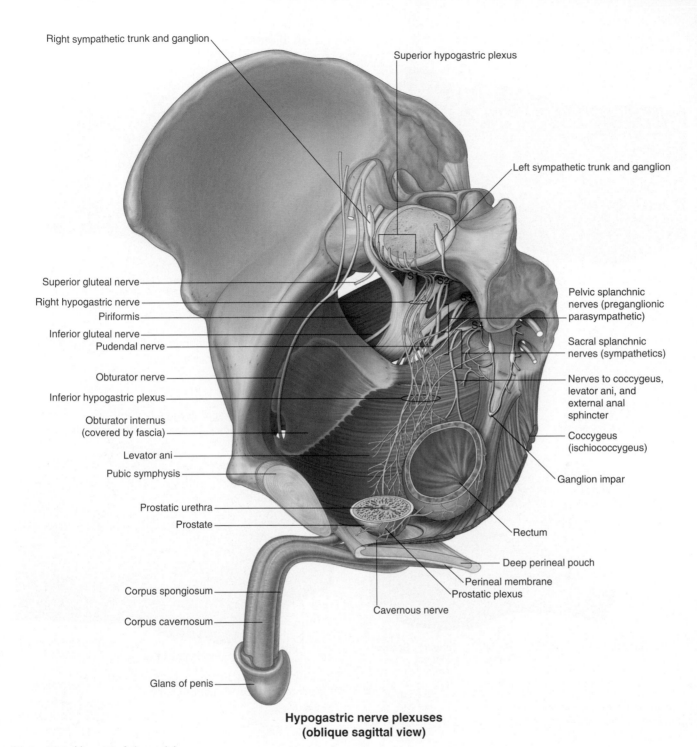

Right sympathetic trunk and ganglion

Superior hypogastric plexus

Left sympathetic trunk and ganglion

Superior gluteal nerve

Right hypogastric nerve

Piriformis

Inferior gluteal nerve

Pudendal nerve

Obturator nerve

Inferior hypogastric plexus

Obturator internus (covered by fascia)

Levator ani

Pubic symphysis

Prostatic urethra

Prostate

Corpus spongiosum

Corpus cavernosum

Glans of penis

S1 S2

S3

S4

Pelvic splanchnic nerves (preganglionic parasympathetic)

Sacral splanchnic nerves (sympathetics)

Nerves to coccygeus, levator ani, and external anal sphincter

Coccygeus (ischiococcygeus)

Ganglion impar

Rectum

Deep perineal pouch

Perineal membrane

Prostatic plexus

Cavernous nerve

**Hypogastric nerve plexuses
(oblique sagittal view)**

Plate 14.2 Nerves of the pelvis.

Internal iliac artery — Urinary bladder — Retropubic space — Pubic symphysis — Clitoris

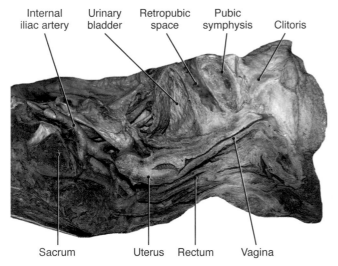

Sacrum — Uterus — Rectum — Vagina

Fig. 14.25 Vaginal canal with anterior and posterior fornices.

Urinary bladder — Prostate gland — Pubic symphysis — Penis

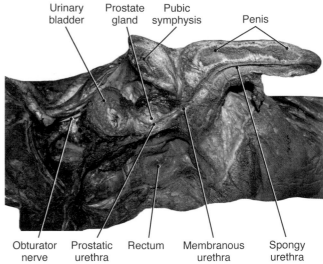

Obturator nerve — Prostatic urethra — Rectum — Membranous urethra — Spongy urethra

Fig. 14.27 In this hemisected pelvis, appreciate anatomic components of urethra (prostatic, membranous, and spongy parts).

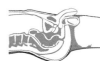

Pubic symphysis — Urinary bladder

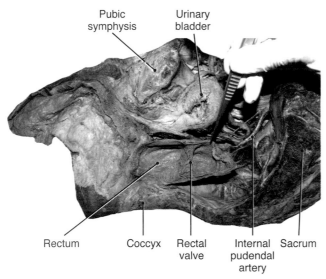

Rectum — Coccyx — Rectal valve — Internal pudendal artery — Sacrum

Fig. 14.26 In this specimen, note internal structures of rectum and anal canal (transverse folds, valves of Houston).

L5-S1 intervertebral disc — Obturator internus — Obturator nerve — Pubococcygeus — Penis

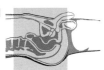

L5 — Sacrum — Piriformis — Coccygeus — Arcus tendineus levator ani

Fig. 14.28 Arteries and veins removed and musculature exposed; *L5,* 5th lumbar; *S1,* 1st sacral.

DISSECTION **TIP**

Trigone identification is difficult in the hemisected specimen because the incision plane usually transects it.

utricle. Lateral and distal to the prostatic utricle, identify the ejaculatory ducts. Lateral to the urethral crest, identify the openings of the prostatic ducts.

○ In Fig. 14.28 the arteries and veins have been removed and the underlying musculature has been exposed.

○ Pull the hemisected urinary bladder medially and posteriorly, and identify the puboprostatic ligaments (pubovesical in females) lying laterally between the pubic symphysis and the bladder (Fig. 14.29).

○ Identify the trigone of the urinary bladder.

○ Identify the ureteric orifice and the interureteric ridge or crest created by a muscular fold between the two ureteric orifices. The orifice of the urethra forms a muscular elevation, the *uvula.*

○ Lift the rectum upward, and expose the pelvic splanchnic nerves (Fig. 14.30).

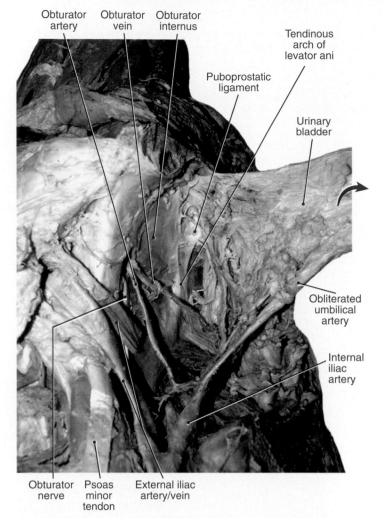

Fig. 14.29 Urinary bladder retracted medially and puboprostatic ligaments identified in the space between the obturator internus muscle and urinary bladder, just behind the pubic symphysis.

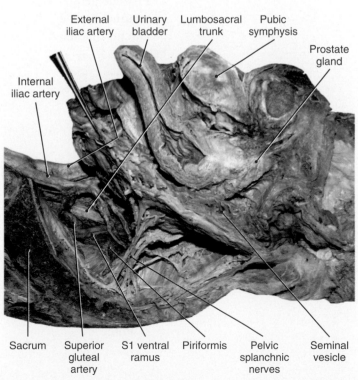
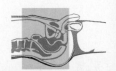

Fig. 14.30 Rectum lifted upward to expose pelvic splanchnic nerves. *S1,* 1st sacral vertebra.

LABORATORY IDENTIFICATION CHECKLIST

NERVES
- [ ] Pudendal
- [ ] Obturator
- [ ] Lumbosacral trunk
- [ ] S1 ventral rami
- [ ] S2 ventral rami
- [ ] S3 ventral rami
- [ ] S4 ventral rami
- [ ] Pelvic splanchnic
- [ ] Sacral sympathetic trunk/ganglia
- [ ] Superior hypogastric plexus
- [ ] Inferior hypogastric plexus
- [ ] Sacral splanchnic nerves

ARTERIES
- [ ] Aorta
- [ ] Middle sacral
- [ ] Common iliac
  - [ ] External iliac
  - [ ] Internal iliac
    - [ ] *Anterior division*
    - [ ] Umbilical
    - [ ] Superior vesical
    - [ ] Obturator
    - [ ] Uterine
    - [ ] Vaginal
    - [ ] Inferior gluteal
    - [ ] *Posterior division*
    - [ ] Lateral sacral
    - [ ] Iliolumbar
    - [ ] Superior gluteal
- [ ] Gonadal (testicular/ovarian)
- [ ] Internal pudendal
- [ ] Superior rectal

VEINS
- [ ] Inferior vena cava
- [ ] Common iliac
  - [ ] External iliac
  - [ ] Internal iliac

MUSCLES
- [ ] Piriformis
- [ ] Obturator internus
- [ ] Levator ani

- [ ] Coccygeus
- [ ] Pubococcygeus
- [ ] Iliococcygeus

CONNECTIVE TISSUE
- [ ] Pelvic fascia
- [ ] Obturator fascia

LIGAMENTS
- [ ] Sacrotuberous
- [ ] Sacrospinous
- [ ] Iliolumbar
- [ ] Broad
- [ ] Uterosacral
- [ ] Lateral (cardinal, Mackenrodt)

ORGANS/URINARY/REPRODUCTIVE
- [ ] Urinary bladder
- [ ] Ureter
- [ ] Sigmoid colon
- [ ] Rectosigmoid junction
- [ ] Rectum
- [ ] Anal canal

Male
- [ ] Prostate gland
- [ ] Seminal vesicle
- [ ] Ductus deferens

Female
- [ ] Uterus
- [ ] Fallopian tube
- [ ] Ovary

SPACES
- [ ] Retropubic
- [ ] Retrovesical (pouch of Douglas)
- [ ] Retrouterine

BONES
- [ ] Sacrum
- [ ] Coccyx
- [ ] Os coxae (hip bone)
  - [ ] Ilium
  - [ ] Ischium
  - [ ] Pubic

ATLAS REFERENCES

Netter: 358–365, 377, 378, 387, 389, 393, 395, 486–489
McMinn: 276–279
Gray's Atlas: 255–263, 266, 267, 270

BEFORE YOU BEGIN

Dissection of the male and female pelvis is discussed separately in this chapter.

DISSECTION **TIP**

To best dissect the perineum, first perform the gluteal region dissection, including the ischioanal fossae and thighs. This makes it much easier to expose and dissect the structures of the perineum.

DISSECTION OF THE MALE CADAVER

○ Place the cadaver in the supine position. Place a block under the sacrum and abduct the thighs as far as possible. A wooden block or rod is placed between the thighs at the level of the femoral condyles to maintain them in abduction (Fig. 15.1).

○ Identify the adductor longus and gracilis muscles. These muscles can be transected so that the thighs can be abducted more easily. In this specimen, it was not necessary to transect these muscles (Fig. 15.2).

○ Draw imaginary lines outlining the borders of the *urogenital triangle:* a line between the ischial tuberosities and two lines along the ischiopubic rami to the pubic symphysis (Fig. 15.3). At the midpoint of a line connecting the two ischial tuberosities, palpate a fibromuscular mass of tissue, the *perineal body.*

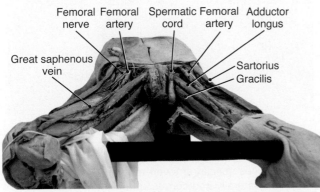

Fig. 15.1 Male cadaver in supine position with block under sacrum with thighs abducted.

ANATOMY **NOTE**

The perineal body is an important structure because the superficial and deep transverse perineus muscles, the bulbospongiosus muscle, the levator ani muscle, and the external anal sphincter muscles are attached to it.

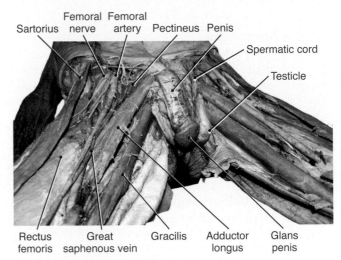

Fig. 15.2 Transecting the adductor longus and gracilis muscles to abduct thighs more easily was not necessary in this cadaver.

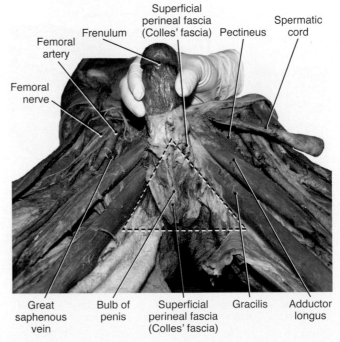

Fig. 15.3 Urogenital triangle *(dashed outline),* with line between ischial tuberosities and two lines along ischiopubic rami to pubic symphysis.

- Remove the skin of the urogenital region, including the scrotum. Reflect the testis toward the inguinal ligament, and expose the urogenital triangle. Lift the penis upward, and remove the adipose tissue and the rich venous network (Fig. 15.4).

ANATOMY **NOTE**

The fat that is removed here is located in the superficial perineal fascia (of Colles). This fascia is the continuation of Scarpa's fascia (membranous layer of anterior abdominal wall) into the perineum (Figs. 15.5 and 15.6). Camper's fascia (fatty layer of anterior abdominal wall) continues into the perineum (Plate 15.1).

DISSECTION **TIP**

The superficial perineal fascia is fairly thick and intermingled with the adipose tissue of the urogenital triangle. This fascia attaches laterally to the ischiopubic rami.

- Remove Colles' fascia, and identify the corpus cavernosum laterally and the corpus spongiosum medially (see Fig. 15.6).
- Expose the bulbospongiosus muscle covered with a fascial layer, the *deep perineal fascia* (Gallaudet's fascia).

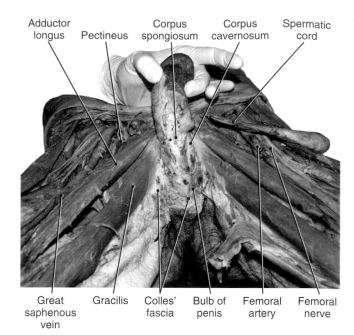

Fig. 15.5 Lift the penis upward and remove the adipose tissue and the rich venous network.

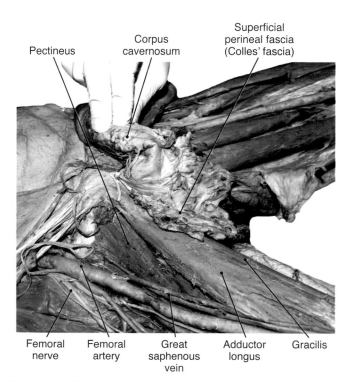

Fig. 15.4 Skin of urogenital region removed and testis reflected toward inguinal ligament, exposing urogenital triangle.

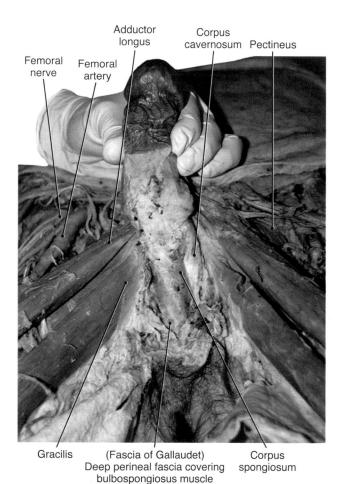

Fig. 15.6 Colles' fascia removed to identify corpus cavernosum laterally and corpus spongiosum medially. Bulbospongiosus muscle is covered with deep perineal fascia.

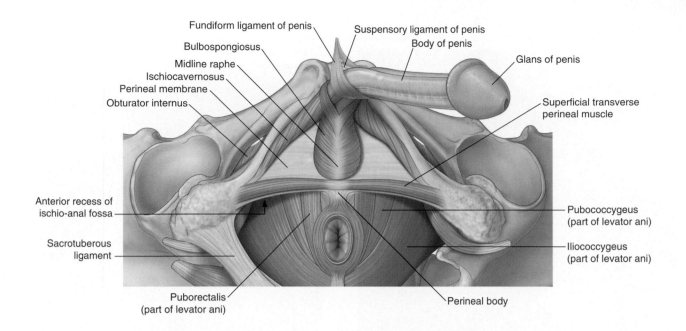

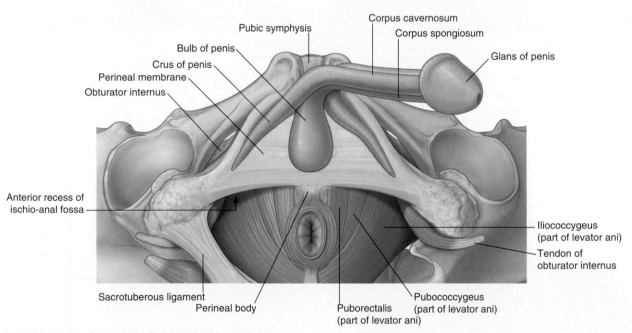

Plate 15.1 Muscles of the superficial perineal pouch in males.

ANATOMY **NOTE**

The deep perineal fascia invests the bulbospongiosus muscle, superficial transverse perineal muscles, and ischiocavernosus muscles.

○ Continue the exposure of the bulbospongiosus inferiorly, exposing the deep perineal fascia. The potential space between the superficial perineal fascia and deep perineal fascia is called the *superficial perineal cleft* (space between Colles' and Gallaudet's fasciae) (Figs. 15.7 and 15.8).

DISSECTION **TIP**

During the removal of the superficial perineal cleft, you may encounter branches of the posterior femoral cutaneous nerve, as well as scrotal vessels and nerves.

○ Dissect lateral to the bulbospongiosus muscle and identify the ischiocavernosus muscle arising from the ischiopubic rami (see Fig. 15.8). The ischiocavernosus surrounds the crus of the penis (corpora cavernosa), a bilateral collection of erectile tissue (Fig. 15.9).

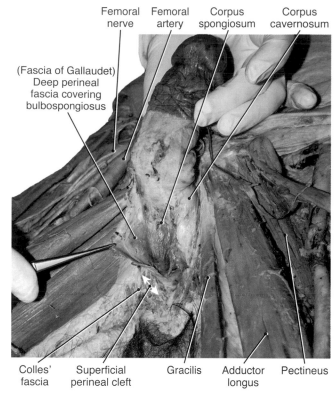

Femoral nerve | Femoral artery | Corpus spongiosum | Corpus cavernosum

(Fascia of Gallaudet) Deep perineal fascia covering bulbospongiosus

Colles' fascia | Superficial perineal cleft | Gracilis | Adductor longus | Pectineus

Fig. 15.7 Exposure of bulbospongiosus muscle continued inferiorly, further revealing the deep perineal fascia.

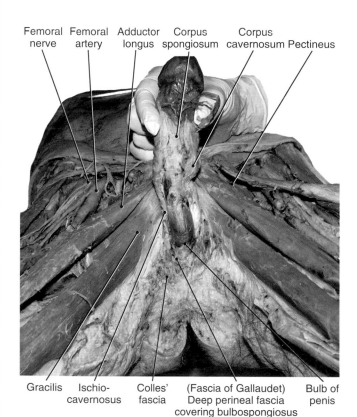

Femoral nerve | Femoral artery | Adductor longus | Corpus spongiosum | Corpus cavernosum | Pectineus

Gracilis | Ischio-cavernosus | Colles' fascia | (Fascia of Gallaudet) Deep perineal fascia covering bulbospongiosus | Bulb of penis

Fig. 15.8 Ischiocavernosus muscle arises from the ischiopubic rami.

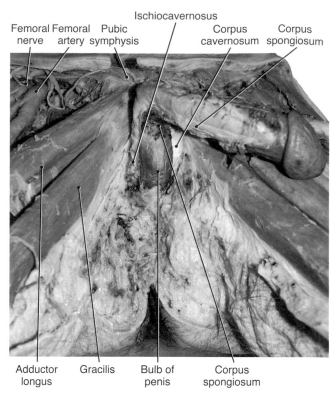

Ischiocavernosus

Femoral nerve | Femoral artery | Pubic symphysis | Corpus cavernosum | Corpus spongiosum

Adductor longus | Gracilis | Bulb of penis | Corpus spongiosum

Fig. 15.9 Crus of penis is surrounded by ischiocavernosus muscle.

○ The inferior portion of the corpus spongiosum becomes dilated, forming the bulb of the penis. At the level of the bulb, remove the superficial perineal fascia and identify the superficial perineal muscle laterally (Figs. 15.10 and 15.11).

DISSECTION TIP

The superficial transverse perineal muscle is absent in some cadavers. It also has been shown that these muscles atrophy with age.

○ Clean the superficial transverse perineal muscles, and superior to them, expose the perineal membrane (Fig. 15.12).
○ Inferior and lateral to the transverse perineal muscles, expose the perineal nerve and perineal artery, which are branches of the pudendal nerve and internal pudendal artery, respectively (see Figs. 15.11 and 15.12).
○ Expose the ischiocavernosus muscle along the ischiopubic rami (Fig. 15.13).
○ Lift the penis and expose the crus. Make an incision into the crus and expose its spongy matrix and its *tunica albuginea,* the outer covering of the corpus (Fig. 15.14). Observe the pubic symphysis for the *suspensory ligament* of the penis, arising from deep fascia of the anterior abdominal wall, and the *fundiform ligament,* arising from the membranous layer of the superficial fascia of the abdomen.

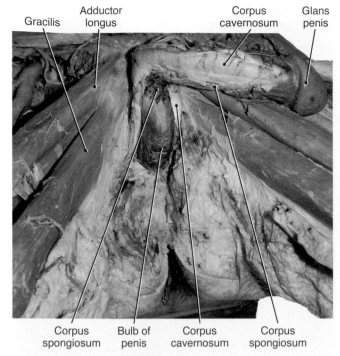

Gracilis — Adductor longus — Corpus cavernosum — Glans penis

Corpus spongiosum — Bulb of penis — Corpus cavernosum — Corpus spongiosum

Fig. 15.10 Dilated corpus spongiosum forms the bulb of penis.

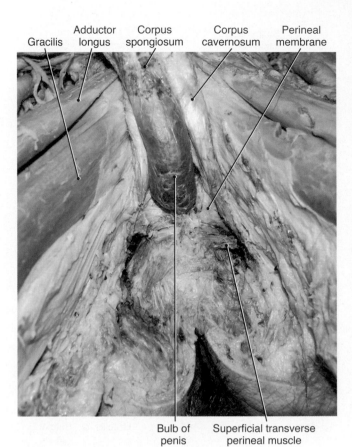

Gracilis — Adductor longus — Corpus spongiosum — Corpus cavernosum — Perineal membrane

Bulb of penis — Superficial transverse perineal muscle

Fig. 15.12 Superficial transverse perineal muscles cleaned, exposing perineal membrane. Perineal nerve and artery are inferior and lateral to the transverse perineal muscle.

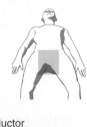

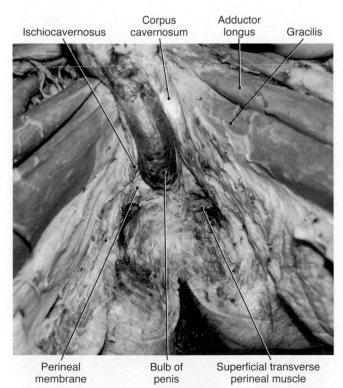

Ischiocavernosus — Corpus cavernosum — Adductor longus — Gracilis

Perineal membrane — Bulb of penis — Superficial transverse perineal muscle

Fig. 15.11 Superficial fascia removed at level of penile bulb to identify the superficial perineal muscle laterally.

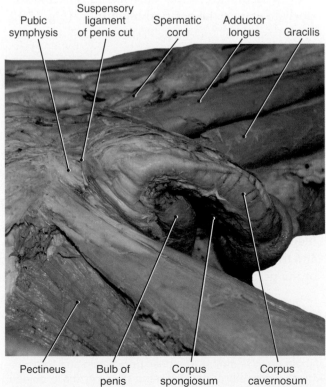

Pubic symphysis — Suspensory ligament of penis cut — Spermatic cord — Adductor longus — Gracilis

Pectineus — Bulb of penis — Corpus spongiosum — Corpus cavernosum

Fig. 15.13 Ischiocavernosus muscle along ischiopubic rami.

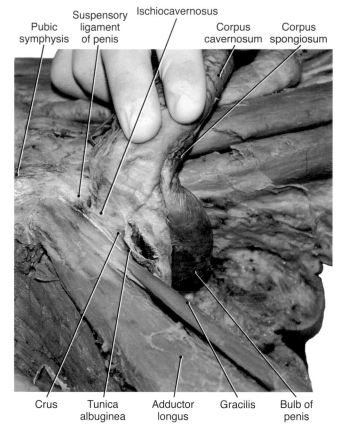

Fig. 15.14 Penis lifted to expose crus with incision revealing spongy matrix and tunica albuginea.

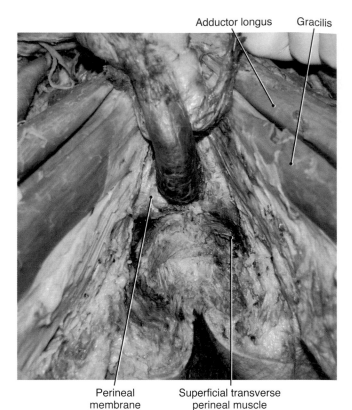

Fig. 15.15 Ischiocavernosus muscle reflected anteriorly to expose the perineal membrane.

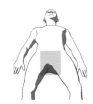

○ Cut the ischiocavernosus muscle and reflect it anteriorly to expose the perineal membrane (Fig. 15.15).

DISSECTION **TIP**

The bulbourethral gland in males may be difficult to find in the urogenital diaphragm.

○ Cut the suspensory and fundiform ligaments of the penis and push the penis downward (Fig. 15.16).
○ With a scalpel, cut through the bulb of the penis at the perineal membrane and remove the penis (Fig. 15.17).
○ Identify the deep dorsal vein of the penis, the urethra, and the perineal body, and appreciate the dimensions of the perineal membrane.

ANATOMY **NOTE**

The deep dorsal vein of the penis is a large vein located deep to Buck's fascia (of the penis) just inferior to the arcuate pubic ligament. The deep dorsal vein anastomoses with the internal pudendal veins through the prostatic venous plexus.

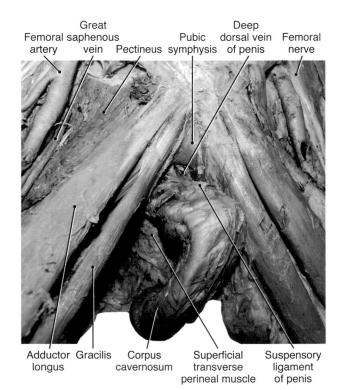

Fig. 15.16 Suspensory and fundiform ligaments cut and penis pushed downward.

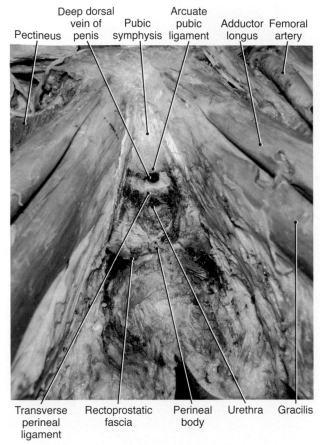

Pectineus — Deep dorsal vein of penis — Pubic symphysis — Arcuate pubic ligament — Adductor longus — Femoral artery

Transverse perineal ligament — Rectoprostatic fascia — Perineal body — Urethra — Gracilis

Fig. 15.17 Bulb cut from perineal membrane and penis removed revealing deep dorsal vein, urethra, and perineal body.

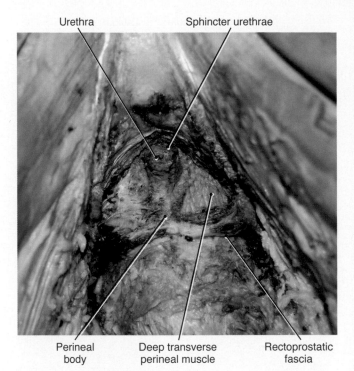

Urethra — Sphincter urethrae

Perineal body — Deep transverse perineal muscle — Rectoprostatic fascia

Fig. 15.18 Deep perineal membrane reflected, exposing underlying musculature, deep transverse perineal muscle, and sphincter urethrae.

○ Palpate the perineal membrane between the deep dorsal vein of the penis and the urethra, and note its thickening, the *transverse perineal ligament* (see Fig. 15.17).

DISSECTION TIP

Inferior and lateral to the superficial transverse perineal muscle, locate the perineal nerve and the perineal artery, tracing these toward the ischioanal fossa if time permits.

○ Reflect the deep perineal membrane, and expose the underlying musculature, the deep transverse perineal muscle and sphincter urethrae (Fig. 15.18).

DISSECTION TIP

If time permits, cut the external urethral orifice of the penis and open the corpus spongiosum to expose the urethra. Extend the incision throughout the entire course of the urethra.

DISSECTION OF THE FEMALE CADAVER

With the female cadaver in the supine position, identify the following structures (Figs. 15.19 and 15.20):

○ Anterior commissure of labia majora
○ Labia majora
○ Labia minora
○ Glans of clitoris
○ Vaginal orifice
○ Vestibular fossa
○ Posterior commissure of labia major
○ Make an incision into the skin around the vaginal orifice, leaving the labia minora and clitoris intact. Incise the skin following the medial surface of the labia majora to the anterior commissure of the labia majora. Reflect the skin laterally and detach along the medial thigh (Figs. 15.21 and 15.22).

ANATOMY NOTE

There are two layers that make up the superficial perineal fascia: a fatty superficial layer and a membranous deep layer (Colles' fascia). The fatty layer gives shape to the labia majora. The membranous layer of the superficial perineal fascia is attached to the ischiopubic ramus and the perineal membrane.

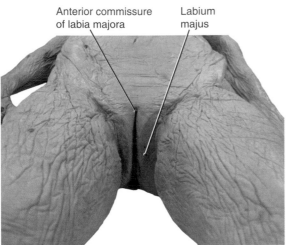

Fig. 15.19 Female cadaver in supine position.

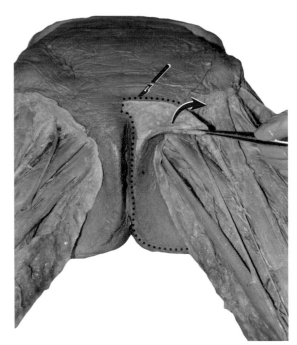

Fig. 15.21 *Dotted lines* demarcating the incision points and reflection of the skin laterally.

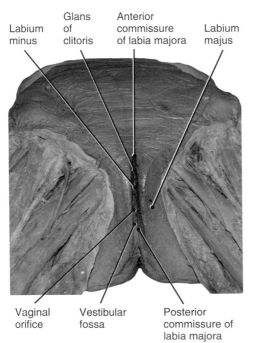

Labium minus   Glans of clitoris   Anterior commissure of labia majora   Labium majus

Vaginal orifice   Vestibular fossa   Posterior commissure of labia majora

Fig. 15.20 Female cadaver in supine position.

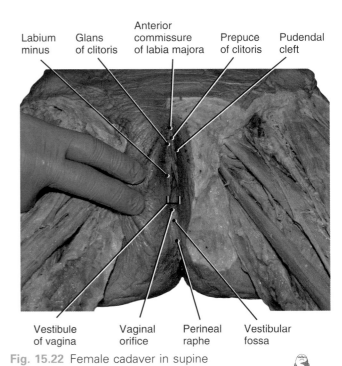

Labium minus   Glans of clitoris   Anterior commissure of labia majora   Prepuce of clitoris   Pudendal cleft

Vestibule of vagina   Vaginal orifice   Perineal raphe   Vestibular fossa

Fig. 15.22 Female cadaver in supine position, exposing the external genitalia.

DISSECTION **TIP**

Remnants of the round ligament of the uterus may be found as the removal of the superficial fascia is taking place, typically in younger cadavers.

○ Remove the superficial fatty layer of the superficial perineal fascia to expose the superficial perineal (Colles') fascia and the fat of the ischioanal fossa (Fig. 15.23).

○ Cut open the superficial perineal fascia to reveal the deep perineal (investing or Gallaudet's) fascia. This fascia covers the bulbospongiosus muscle located lateral to the labia minora (Fig. 15.24 and Plate 15.2).

○ Identify the bulbospongiosus muscle. Dissect lateral to the bulbospongiosus muscle to identify the ischiocavernosus muscle running along the ischiopubic ramus. Use blunt dissection to locate the deep and superficial branches of the perineal artery, vein, and nerve (Fig. 15.25).

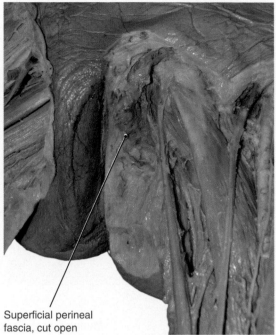

Superficial perineal fascia, cut open

Fig. 15.24 Superficial perineal (Colles') fascia cut open.

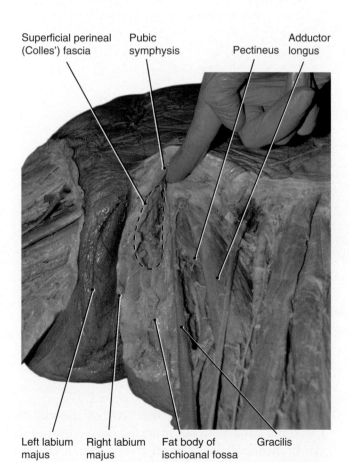

Superficial perineal (Colles') fascia   Pubic symphysis   Pectineus   Adductor longus

Left labium majus   Right labium majus   Fat body of ischioanal fossa   Gracilis

Fig. 15.23 Superficial perineal (Colles') fascia exposed, as well as the musculature of the left thigh.

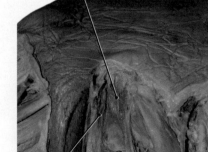

Ishiocavernosus, atrophied

Bulbospongiosus with deep perineal (investing or Gallaudet's) fascia   Deep and superficial perineal branches of perineal artery, vein, and nerve

Fig. 15.25 Bulbospongiosus and deep perineal fascia exposed, as well as superficial and deep branches of perineal artery, vein, and nerve.

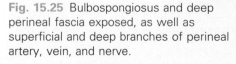

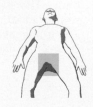

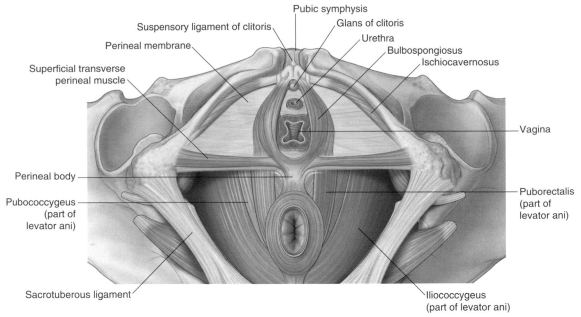

Muscles of the superficial perineal pouch in women

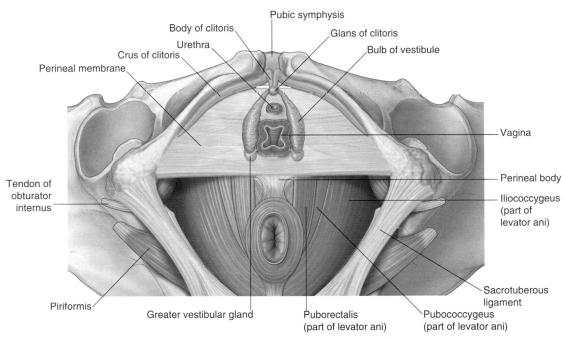

Erectile tissues of the superficial perineal pouch in women

Plate 15.2 Muscles and erectile tissues of the superficial perineal pouch in females.

ANATOMY **NOTE**

The bulbospongiosus muscle attaches anteriorly to the corpus cavernosus clitoris and posteriorly to the perineal body. The bulbospongiosus muscle in the female is separate and does not attach in the midline as in males. The ischiocavernosus muscle covers the surface of the crus of the clitoris.

○ Dissect further to reveal the crus of the clitoris. Clean the adipose tissue from the deep and superficial branches of the perineal artery, vein, and nerve (Fig. 15.26).
○ Reflect the bulbospongiosus muscle laterally to reveal the bulb of the vestibule (Fig. 15.27).
○ Cut the crus of the clitoris and reflect it laterally (Fig. 15.28).
○ Identify the perineal membrane (Fig. 15.29).

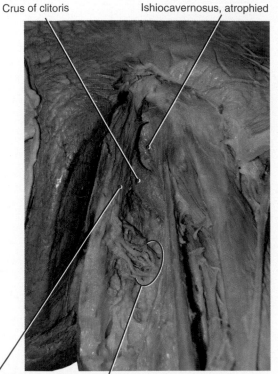

Crus of clitoris — Ishiocavernosus, atrophied

Bulbospongiosus with deep perineal (investing or Gallaudet's) fascia

Deep and superficial perineal branches of perineal artery, vein, and nerve

Fig. 15.26 Crus of clitoris exposed.

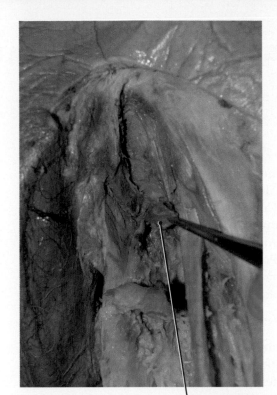

Crus of clitoris, cut and reflected

Fig. 15.28 Crus of clitoris cut and reflected.

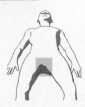

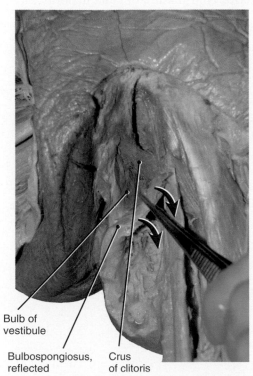

Bulb of vestibule

Bulbospongiosus, reflected

Crus of clitoris

Fig. 15.27 Bulbospongiosus reflected, exposing the bulb of vestibule.

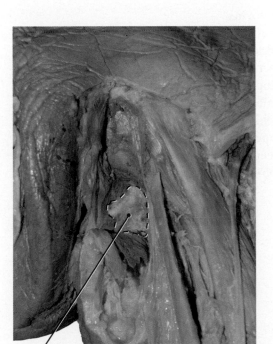

Perineal membrane

Fig. 15.29 Perineal membrane exposed.

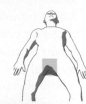

LABORATORY IDENTIFICATION CHECKLIST

NERVES
- [ ] Femoral
  - [ ] Motor branches
  - [ ] Cutaneous branches
- [ ] Obturator
  - [ ] Anterior branch
  - [ ] Posterior branch
- [ ] Ilioinguinal
- [ ] Pudendal

ARTERIES
- [ ] Femoral
- [ ] Obturator
- [ ] Deferential
- [ ] Perineal

VEINS
- [ ] Great saphenous
- [ ] Femoral
- [ ] Deep dorsal of penis

MUSCLES
- [ ] Sartorius
- [ ] Gracilis
- [ ] Adductor longus
- [ ] Pectineus
- [ ] Iliopsoas
- [ ] Bulbospongiosus
- [ ] Ischiocavernosus
- [ ] Superficial transverse perineus
- [ ] Deep transverse perineus
- [ ] Sphincter urethrae

CONNECTIVE TISSUE
- [ ] Superficial perineal fascia
- [ ] Corpora cavernosa
- [ ] Bulb of penis
- [ ] Bulb of vestibule
- [ ] Corpus spongiosum
- [ ] Crus of penis/clitoris
- [ ] Perineal membrane
- [ ] Perineal body
- [ ] Suspensory ligament of penis/clitoris
- [ ] Prepuce of penis/clitoris
- [ ] Glans of penis/clitoris
- [ ] Spermatic cord
- [ ] Scrotum
- [ ] Labia majora
- [ ] Labia minora
- [ ] Rectoprostatic fascia
- [ ] Pubic symphysis
- [ ] Anterior commissure of labia majora
- [ ] Glans of clitoris
- [ ] Vaginal orifice
- [ ] Vestibular fossa
- [ ] Posterior commissure of labia majora

BONES
- [ ] Right/left pubic bone
- [ ] Ischial spine

Clinical Application

Figs. VI.1 and VI.2 depict the pelvic cavity with viscera removed. Note the superior and inferior hypogastric plexuses.

Figs. VI.3 and VI.4 show large tumors in the uterus.

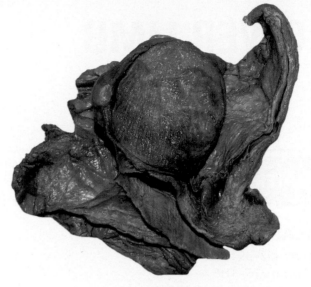

Fig. VI.3

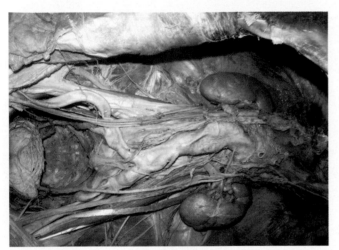

Fig. VI.1

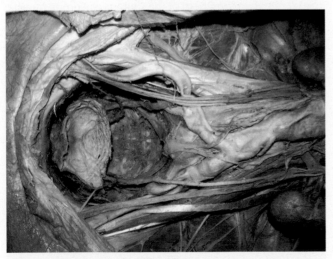

Fig. VI.2

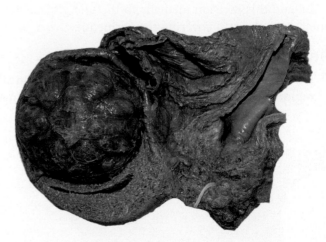

Fig. VI.4

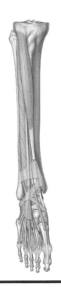

SECTION VII

LOWER LIMB

ATLAS REFERENCES

Netter: 492–494
McMinn: 316–319
Gray's Atlas: 301–303, 307, 314, 315

BEFORE YOU BEGIN

Typically, you will not need to make additional skin incisions if you continue the dissection on the same cadaver on which you performed the dissection of the back in Chapter 2 (Fig. 16.1).

If not, place the cadaver in the prone position, and incise the skin and subcutaneous tissues along the iliac crest to the posterior superior iliac spine (Figs. 16.2 and 16.3).

Extend this incision medially to the intergluteal cleft, anterior to the area covering the perineum.

SKIN AND SUPERFICIAL FASCIA

○ Reflect the skin and superficial fascia from the gluteal region and posterior thigh by making a longitudinal midline skin incision distally to the knee. Make a circumferential incision through the skin of the leg, just distal to the knee (see Figs. 16.2 and 16.3).

○ There is typically a large amount of adipose tissue over the gluteus maximus muscle. Remove the adipose tissue and deep fascia in the gluteal region, exposing the gluteus maximus muscle (Figs. 16.4 to 16.6).

DISSECTION **TIP**

In many atlases, you will find the gluteus maximus muscle shown with no fat. To create a clean specimen, remove the fat between the fibers of the gluteus maximus muscle (see Fig. 16.6).

Fig. 16.1 Surface anatomy of the gluteal region.

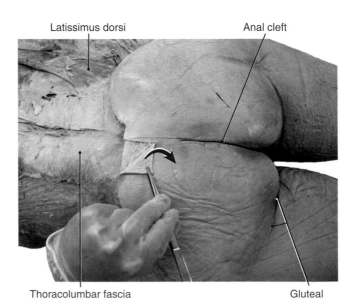

Fig. 16.2 Gluteal region with reflected skin, demonstrating dissection from the midline.

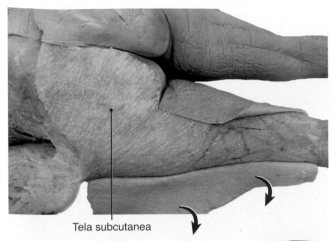

Tela subcutanea

Fig. 16.3 Gluteal and posterior thigh regions with dermis reflected, revealing membranous layer of subcutaneous tissue (tela subcutanea).

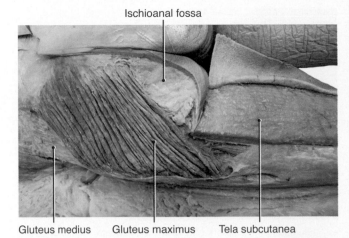

Ischioanal fossa

Gluteus medius   Gluteus maximus   Tela subcutanea

Fig. 16.5 Further gluteal region dissection, revealing the gluteus medius (covered with fascia) muscle superiorly, the gluteus maximus muscle inferiorly, and the ischioanal fossa and tela subcutanea medially.

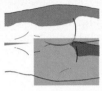

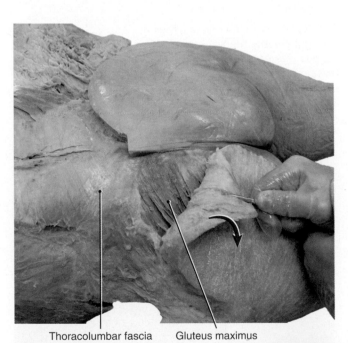

Thoracolumbar fascia   Gluteus maximus

Fig. 16.4 Gluteal region with thoracolumbar fascia superiorly and reflected subcutaneous tissue, revealing gluteus maximus muscle inferiorly.

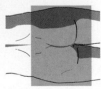

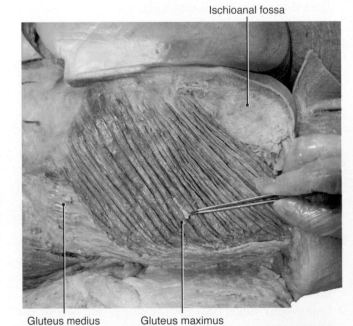

Ischioanal fossa

Gluteus medius   Gluteus maximus

Fig. 16.6 Closer view highlighting the gluteus medius (covered with fascia) muscle superiorly, the gluteus maximus muscle inferiorly, and the ischioanal fossa medially.

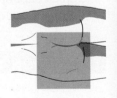

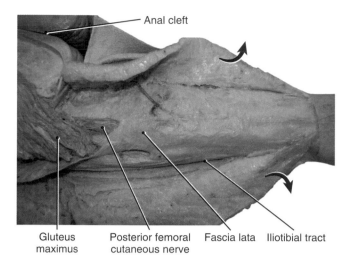

Anal cleft

Gluteus maximus | Posterior femoral cutaneous nerve | Fascia lata | Iliotibial tract

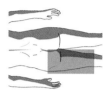

Fig. 16.7 Posterior thigh region with skin and subcutaneous tissue reflected, revealing the posterior cutaneous nerve, fascia lata, and iliotibial tract.

○ Reflect the skin over the posterior portion of the thigh. The adipose tissue and deep fascia will be removed later during the dissection (Fig. 16.7).

DISSECTION TIP

As you delineate the superior and inferior borders of the gluteus maximus muscle, protect the posterior femoral cutaneous nerve from damage by being cautious along the inferior border of the gluteus maximus muscle.

SUPERFICIAL MUSCLES

○ Palpate the sacrotuberous ligament at the medial border of the gluteus maximus muscle by placing your fingertips into the ischioanal fossa (Fig. 16.8).

○ Palpate the superior border of the gluteus maximus and insert your fingertips into the space between the gluteus maximus muscle and fascia over the gluteus medius muscle (Fig. 16.9).

○ Using your fingertips, lift the upper portion of the gluteus maximus muscle from the underlying gluteus medius muscle.

DISSECTION TIP

In most cadavers, the deep fascia and aponeurotic tissues along the superior border of the gluteus maximus muscle blend with those of the gluteus medius muscle. However, the muscular fibers of the gluteus medius muscle run almost perpendicular to the orientation of the gluteus maximus muscle, and the two muscles can be separated readily once you have clearly exposed their fibers.

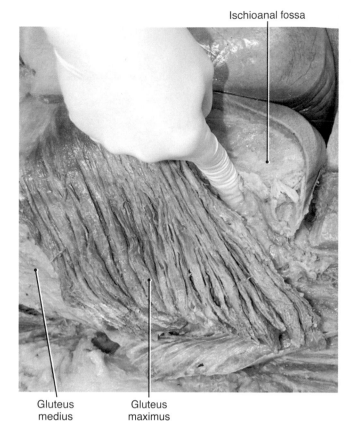

Ischioanal fossa

Gluteus medius | Gluteus maximus

Fig. 16.8 Fingertips in gluteal region highlight gluteus medius superiorly, gluteus maximus inferiorly, and ischioanal fossa medially (palpation of lateral wall of fossa–obturator internus).

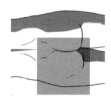

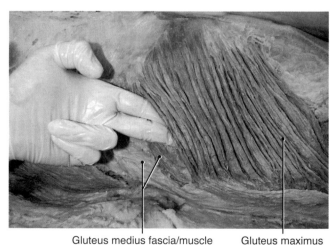

Gluteus medius fascia/muscle | Gluteus maximus

Fig. 16.9 Gluteal region after dissecting superior border of gluteus maximus muscle superficially, revealing deeper gluteus medius fascia and muscle.

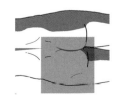

DEEP DISSECTION

○ Make an incision at the lateral border of the gluteus maximus muscle, separating it from its connection to the iliotibial tract (Fig. 16.10).

○ Lift the gluteus maximus medially toward the sacrum, and identify the greater trochanter and overlying trochanteric bursa (Figs. 16.11 and 16.12).

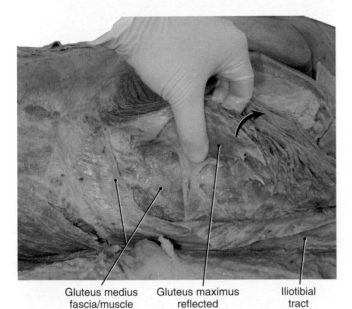

Gluteus medius   Gluteus maximus   Iliotibial
fascia/muscle   reflected   tract

Fig. 16.10 Reflecting the gluteus maximus muscle demonstrates the deeper lying muscle fibers of the gluteus medius muscle.

DISSECTION TIP

The trochanteric bursa appears as loose connective tissue over the greater trochanter, intermingled with adipose tissue. It often is cleaned away during routine dissection.

○ Reflect the gluteus maximus muscle medially from the gluteal tuberosity of the femur; remove the deep fascia and adipose tissue along its inferior border (Fig. 16.13).

○ Clean the sciatic and the posterior femoral cutaneous nerves from the adipose tissue, and trace them proximally from under the piriformis muscle (Fig. 16.14). Once you identify the posterior femoral cutaneous nerve, identify its perineal branch traveling medially.

DISSECTION TIP

To identify the posterior femoral cutaneous nerve, make a small opening through the fascia lata on the posterior aspect of the thigh, and identify the sciatic nerve. Medial to the sciatic nerve, you will be able to identify the posterior femoral cutaneous nerve. In some specimens, the sciatic nerve may split in the gluteal region, with one part traveling above or through and the other part below the piriformis muscle.

○ The gluteus maximus muscle is partially attached to the sacrotuberous ligament. Palpate the sacrotuberous

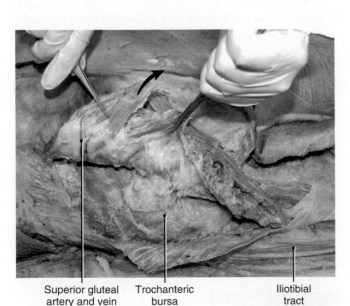

Superior gluteal   Trochanteric   Iliotibial
artery and vein   bursa   tract

Fig. 16.11 Reflection of superolateral border of gluteus maximus muscle, revealing superior gluteal artery and vein and trochanteric bursa.

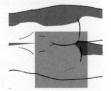

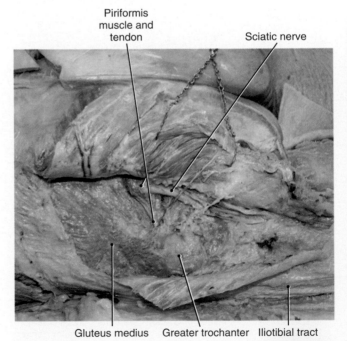

Piriformis
muscle and
tendon   Sciatic nerve

Gluteus medius   Greater trochanter   Iliotibial tract

Fig. 16.12 Gluteal region with reflected gluteus maximus muscle, revealing gluteus medius and piriformis muscles and sciatic nerve.

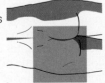

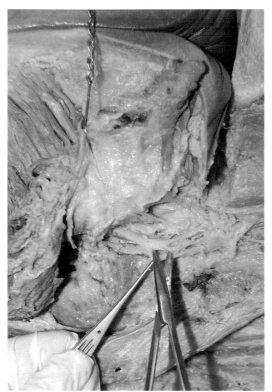

Fig. 16.13 Connective tissue cleaned around posterior femoral cutaneous and sciatic nerves.

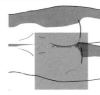

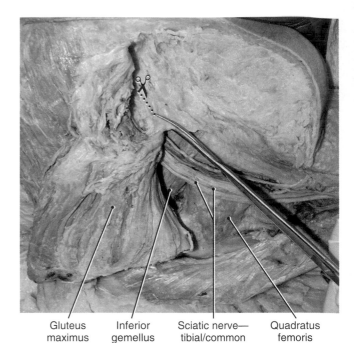

Gluteus maximus | Inferior gemellus | Sciatic nerve—tibial/common fibular nerves | Quadratus femoris

Fig. 16.15 Reflected gluteus maximus muscle revealing quadratus femoris muscle and tibial and common fibular nerves.

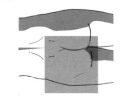

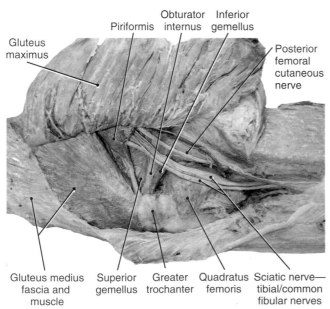

Gluteus maximus — Piriformis — Obturator internus — Inferior gemellus — Posterior femoral cutaneous nerve

Gluteus medius fascia and muscle — Superior gemellus — Greater trochanter — Quadratus femoris — Sciatic nerve—tibial/common fibular nerves

Fig. 16.14 Reflected gluteus maximus muscle, revealing gluteus medius, rotator muscles (piriformis, superior/inferior gemelli, obturator internus, quadratus femoris), sciatic nerve, and posterior femoral cutaneous nerve.

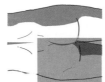

ligament as you did earlier (see Fig. 16.8); reflect the gluteus maximus muscle medially toward the sacrum, and expose the sacrotuberous ligament.

○ Use a scalpel to cut the attachment of the gluteus maximus muscle from the sacrotuberous ligament. With scissors, cut the lateral portion of the sacrotuberous ligament, and free the gluteus maximus muscle (Fig. 16.15).

○ Clean and expose the inferior gluteal vessels and nerve from the deep surface of the gluteus maximus muscle (Figs. 16.16 and 16.17).

○ Lift the posterior femoral cutaneous and sciatic nerves, and clean the adipose and connective tissues from the structures that lie deep to the gluteus maximus muscle, such as the piriformis, obturator internus, and superior and inferior gemellus muscles (Figs. 16.18 and 16.19).

○ Inferior to the obturator internus and gemelli muscles, identify the quadratus femoris muscle.

DISSECTION **TIP**

The obturator internus, superior gemellus, and inferior gemellus muscles often are seen as a combined tripartite tendon with indistinguishable borders. With scissors or a probe, separate these three muscles at the margin of the lesser sciatic foramen.

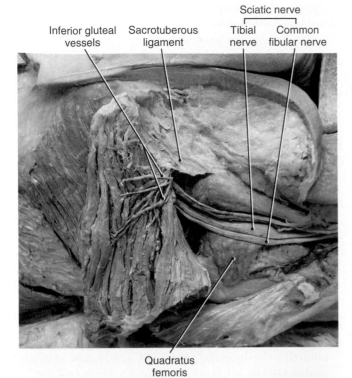

Inferior gluteal vessels | Sacrotuberous ligament | Sciatic nerve — Tibial nerve | Common fibular nerve

Quadratus femoris

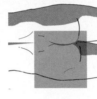

Fig. 16.16 Gluteus maximus muscle reflected superiorly, revealing inferior gluteal vessels, quadratus femoris muscle, and tibial and common fibular nerves.

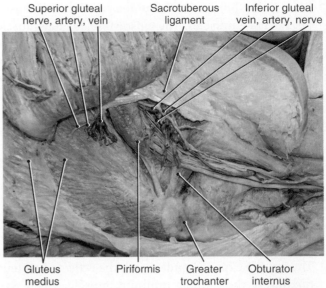

Superior gluteal nerve, artery, vein | Sacrotuberous ligament | Inferior gluteal vein, artery, nerve

Gluteus medius | Piriformis | Greater trochanter | Obturator internus

Fig. 16.18 Gluteal region with gluteus maximus reflected, revealing superior and inferior gluteal artery and vein oriented around piriformis muscle.

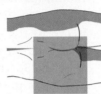

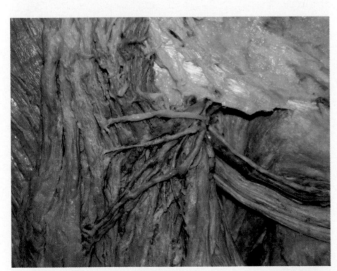

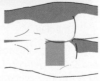

Fig. 16.17 Closer view of Fig. 16.16 showing gluteal region with gluteus maximus reflected, revealing inferior gluteal artery and vein and sacrotuberous ligament.

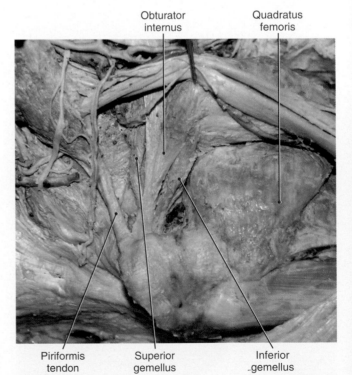

Obturator internus | Quadratus femoris

Piriformis tendon | Superior gemellus | Inferior gemellus

Fig. 16.19 Gluteal region close-up view highlighting lateral rotator muscles (piriformis, superior/inferior gemelli, obturator internus, quadratus femoris) with sciatic nerve reflected medially.

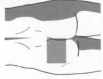

- Identify the borders of the gluteus medius and tensor fasciae latae muscles. The tensor fasciae latae muscle arises from the anterior portion of the iliac crest. Its tendon is covered by fascia lata and continues distally as the iliotibial tract. Place your fingertips at the inferior border of the gluteus medius muscle and lift it upward (Fig. 16.20).

- At the superior space between the gluteus maximus and gluteus medius muscles, identify the superficial branch of the superior gluteal artery (Figs. 16.21 and 16.22).

- Cut the attachment of the gluteus medius from the greater trochanter and reflect it superiorly. On its deep surface, identify the deep branch of the superior gluteal artery (see Fig. 16.22).

- The muscle exposed underneath the reflected gluteus medius is the gluteus minimus muscle. Deep and inferior to the sacrotuberous ligament, identify the nerve to the obturator internus, internal pudendal artery, its venae comitantes, and the pudendal nerve (Fig. 16.23). The venae comitantes are the pair of veins that accompany the internal pudendal artery.

DISSECTION TIP

The nerve to the quadratus femoris and inferior gemellus muscles is a small branch that may be found by retracting the sciatic nerve posteromedially; observe this small nerve traveling deep to the gemelli and obturator internus muscles.

PUDENDAL CANAL AND ISCHIOANAL FOSSA

Note: This part of the dissection involves opening the pudendal canal and dissecting the ischioanal fossa; it also may be performed separately with the dissection of the perineum.

- Dissect and clean away the adipose tissue of the structures inferior to the sacrotuberous ligament, and identify the internal pudendal artery, internal pudendal vein, and the pudendal nerve (Fig. 16.24).

- Identify the continuation of the obturator fascia at the ischioanal fossa, the *lunate fascia*. This fascia encircles the internal pudendal artery and vein and pudendal nerve branches (Figs. 16.25 and 16.26).

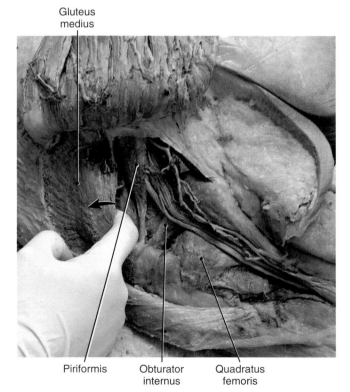

Gluteus medius

Piriformis   Obturator internus   Quadratus femoris

Fig. 16.20 Reflected gluteus maximus muscle reveals gluteus medius muscle, "lateral rotators" (piriformis, obturator internus, quadratus femoris muscles), and the sciatic nerve.

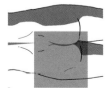

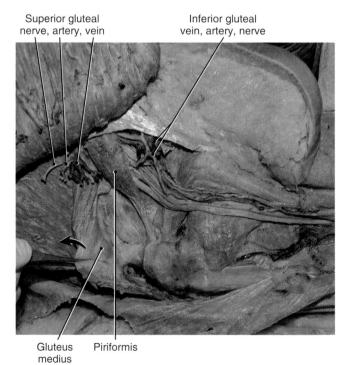

Superior gluteal nerve, artery, vein   Inferior gluteal vein, artery, nerve

Gluteus medius   Piriformis

Fig. 16.21 Gluteus maximus reflected, revealing piriformis muscle and superior and inferior gluteal neurovascular bundles.

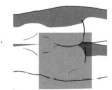

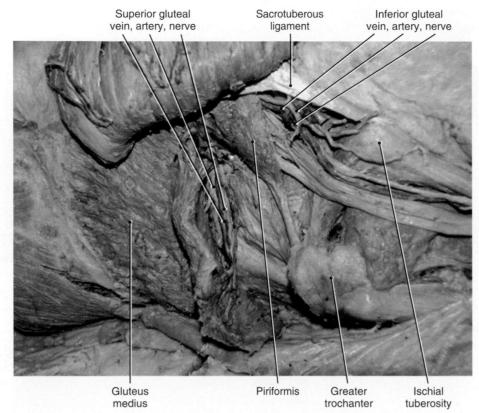

Superior gluteal vein, artery, nerve   Sacrotuberous ligament   Inferior gluteal vein, artery, nerve

Gluteus medius   Piriformis   Greater trochanter   Ischial tuberosity

Fig. 16.22 Gluteus maximus muscle reflected, highlighting piriformis muscle and superior and inferior gluteal neurovascular bundles.

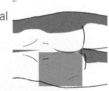

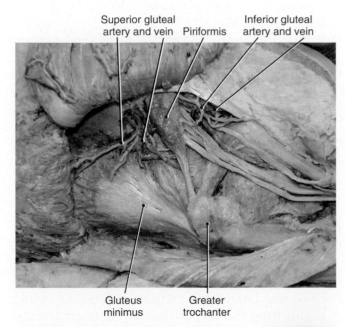

Superior gluteal artery and vein   Piriformis   Inferior gluteal artery and vein

Gluteus minimus   Greater trochanter

Fig. 16.23 Gluteal region with reflection of the gluteus maximus muscle medially and the gluteus medius muscle superiorly, revealing the gluteus minimus muscle and the superior gluteal neurovascular bundle lying superficial to the gluteus minimus muscle.

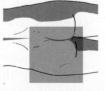

Gluteus maximus   Sacrotuberous ligament

Gluteus minimus   Quadratus femoris

Fig. 16.24 Gluteal region with reflection of the gluteus maximus muscle medially and gluteus medius muscle superiorly, revealing the gluteus minimus muscle and the superior gluteal neurovascular bundle lying superficial to the gluteus minimus muscle.

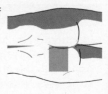

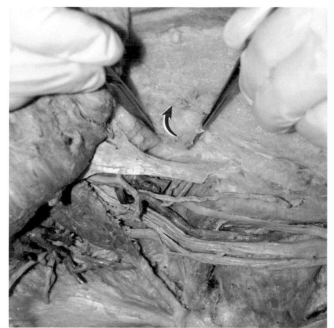

Fig. 16.25 Gluteal region with reflection of gluteus maximus, highlighting piriformis muscle, sacrotuberous ligament, and superior/inferior gluteal neurovascular bundles.

Gluteus maximus   Ischioanal fossa

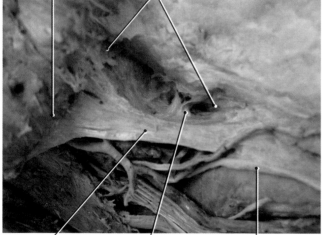

Sacrotuberous ligament   Neurovascular bundle of pudendal nerve, artery, and vein covered with lunate fascia   Posterior femoral cutaneous nerve

Fig. 16.26 Gluteus maximus reflected, revealing ischioanal fossa, sacrotuberous ligament, pudendal neurovascular bundle, and posterior femoral cutaneous nerve.

DISSECTION TIP

Identifying the lunate fascia and the point of entrance of the internal pudendal artery and vein and the pudendal nerve into the gluteal region is useful for exposing these structures when a large amount of adipose tissue is present.

Sacrotuberous ligament   Gluteus maximus fibers   Ischioanal fossa   Internal pudendal artery and vein

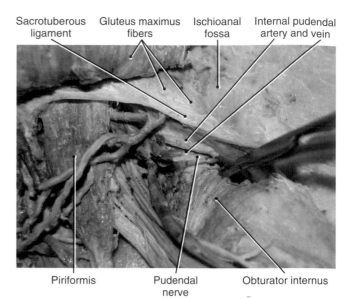

Piriformis   Pudendal nerve   Obturator internus

Fig. 16.27 Gluteus maximus muscle reflected, revealing sacrotuberous ligament, gluteus maximus fibers, ischioanal fossa border, obturator internus muscle, and pudendal neurovascular bundle.

○ Separate the inferior border of the sacrotuberous ligament with scissors, and cut its inferior attachment from the ischial tuberosity (Fig. 16.27).

○ Reflect the sacrotuberous ligament upward toward the reflected gluteus maximus muscle, and expose the contents of the pudendal canal (Alcock's canal) (Figs. 16.28 and 16.29).

○ Expose the pudendal, inferior rectal, and perineal nerves (Fig. 16.30).

○ Remove all the adipose tissue from the ischioanal fossa thoroughly so that the branches of the pudendal nerve and internal pudendal artery are fully identified (Figs. 16.31 and 16.32, Plate 16.1).

○ Expose the levator ani muscle and the fascia of the obturator internus muscle as well as the external anal sphincter (Figs. 16.33 and 16.34, Plate 16.2).

POSTERIOR THIGH

○ Palpate the iliotibial tract, the band into which the tensor fasciae latae and the gluteus maximus muscles (partially) insert.

○ Note the lateral intermuscular septum, which begins from the deep surface of the fascia lata and attaches to the *linea aspera* (rough line) of the femur.

○ Identify the space between the quadratus femoris and adductor magnus (adductor minimus) muscles, and find the medial femoral circumflex artery (Fig. 16.35).

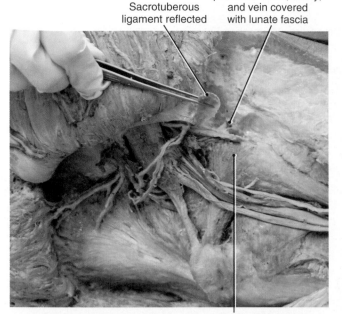

Sacrotuberous
ligament reflected

Neurovascular bundle of
pudendal nerve, artery,
and vein covered
with lunate fascia

Obturator internus

Fig. 16.28 Sacrotuberous ligament held between forceps with gluteus maximus muscle reflected, revealing ischioanal fossa border, obturator internus muscle, and pudendal neurovascular bundle within lunate fascia.

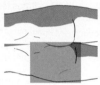

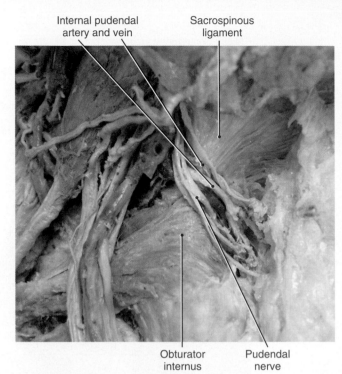

Internal pudendal
artery and vein

Sacrospinous
ligament

Obturator
internus

Pudendal
nerve

Fig. 16.30 Sacrotuberous ligament reflected, revealing obturator internus muscle, pudendal nerve, internal pudendal artery and vein, and sacrospinous ligament.

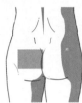

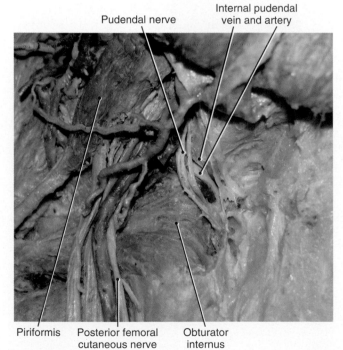

Pudendal nerve

Internal pudendal
vein and artery

Piriformis   Posterior femoral   Obturator
cutaneous nerve   internus

Fig. 16.29 Gluteus maximus muscle reflected, revealing piriformis muscle, posterior femoral cutaneous nerve, obturator internus muscle, ischioanal fossa, pudendal nerve, and internal pudendal artery and vein.

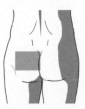

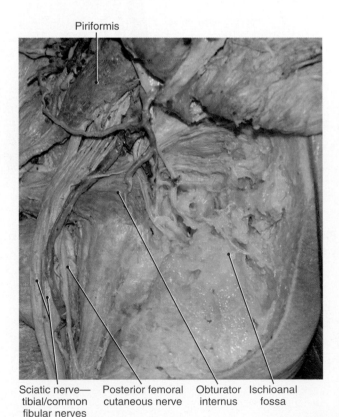

Piriformis

Sciatic nerve—
tibial/common
fibular nerves

Posterior femoral
cutaneous nerve

Obturator
internus

Ischioanal
fossa

Fig. 16.31 Reflected gluteus maximus muscle reveals piriformis and obturator internus muscles, tibial and common fibular nerves of sciatic nerve, posterior femoral cutaneous nerve, and ischioanal fossa.

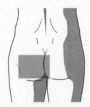

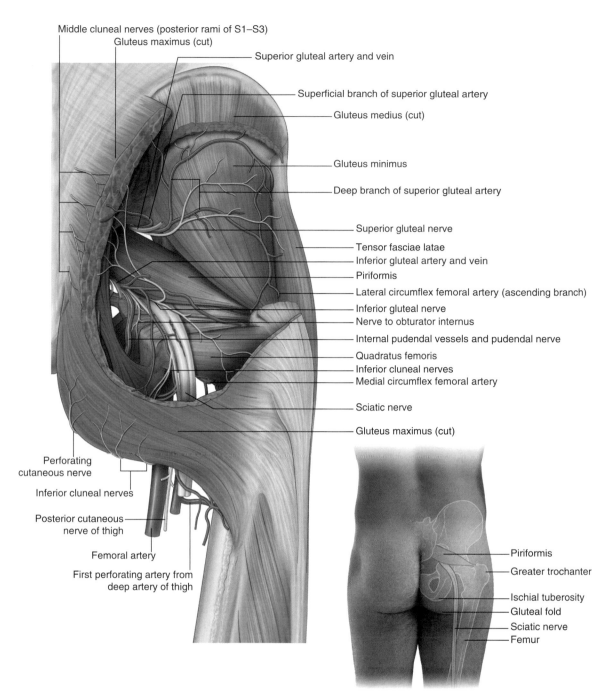

Middle cluneal nerves (posterior rami of S1–S3)
Gluteus maximus (cut)
Superior gluteal artery and vein
Superficial branch of superior gluteal artery
Gluteus medius (cut)
Gluteus minimus
Deep branch of superior gluteal artery
Superior gluteal nerve
Tensor fasciae latae
Inferior gluteal artery and vein
Piriformis
Lateral circumflex femoral artery (ascending branch)
Inferior gluteal nerve
Nerve to obturator internus
Internal pudendal vessels and pudendal nerve
Quadratus femoris
Inferior cluneal nerves
Medial circumflex femoral artery
Sciatic nerve
Gluteus maximus (cut)

Perforating cutaneous nerve
Inferior cluneal nerves
Posterior cutaneous nerve of thigh
Femoral artery
First perforating artery from deep artery of thigh

Piriformis
Greater trochanter
Ischial tuberosity
Gluteal fold
Sciatic nerve
Femur

Plate 16.1 Arteries and nerves of the gluteal region and sciatic nerve in the gluteal region as it relates to the surface (posterior view).

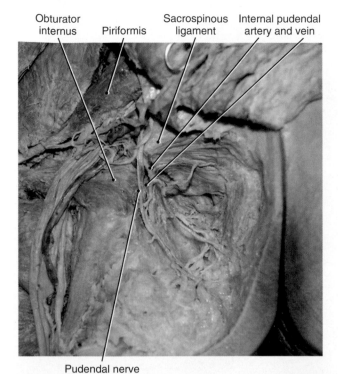

Obturator internus | Piriformis | Sacrospinous ligament | Internal pudendal artery and vein

Pudendal nerve

Fig. 16.32 Sacrotuberous ligament reflected, revealing obturator internus, pudendal nerve, internal pudendal artery and vein, and sacrospinous ligament.

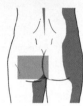

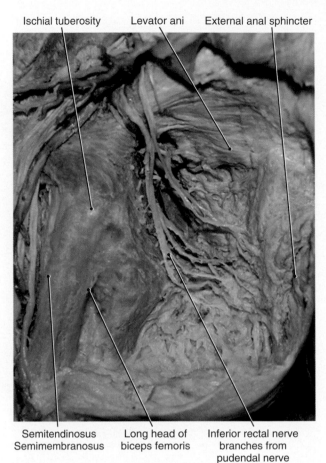

Ischial tuberosity | Levator ani | External anal sphincter

Semitendinosus Semimembranosus | Long head of biceps femoris | Inferior rectal nerve branches from pudendal nerve

Fig. 16.33 Superior aspect of posterior thigh and ischioanal fossa, highlighting ischial tuberosity, "hamstring" muscles (semitendinosus, semimembranosus, long head of biceps femoris), and inferior rectal nerve branches.

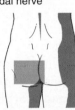

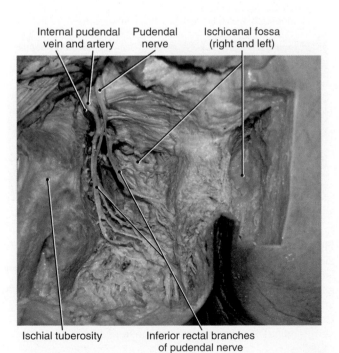

Internal pudendal vein and artery | Pudendal nerve | Ischioanal fossa (right and left)

Ischial tuberosity | Inferior rectal branches of pudendal nerve

Fig. 16.34 Bilateral ischioanal fossae highlighting subcutaneous fat, pudendal nerve, internal pudendal artery and vein, and inferior rectal nerve branches.

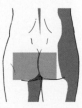

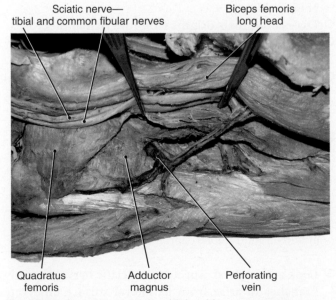

Sciatic nerve— tibial and common fibular nerves | Biceps femoris long head

Quadratus femoris | Adductor magnus | Perforating vein

Fig. 16.35 Superior posterior thigh with retracted tibial and common fibular nerves and long head of biceps femoris muscle, highlighting quadratus femoris and adductor longus muscles and perforating vein.

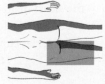

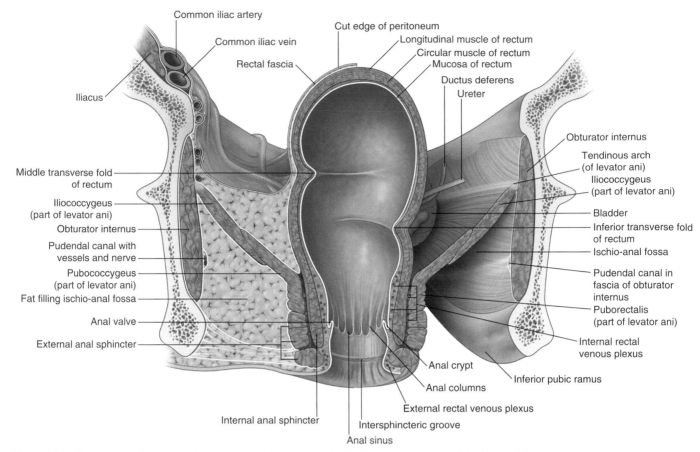

Plate 16.2 Coronal section through rectum and anal canal depicting the contents of ischioanal fossa.

○ With blunt dissection, separate the muscles of the posterior thigh ("hamstrings"), and identify the long and short heads of the biceps femoris muscle as well as the semitendinosus and semimembranous muscles (Fig. 16.36).

○ Dissect out their origins from the ischial tuberosity.

○ Retract the long head of the biceps femoris laterally to expose the sciatic nerve.

○ Note the division of the sciatic nerve into the tibial and common fibular (peroneal) nerves as it approaches the popliteal fossa (Fig. 16.37).

DISSECTION TIP

Typically, the division of the sciatic nerve into the tibial and common fibular nerves occurs near the popliteal fossa. However, some cadavers may have a high split of the sciatic nerve, or two nerves may exit from the inferior border of the piriformis muscle, with a lateral nerve (common fibular) and a medial nerve (tibial).

○ Look at the lateral aspect of the sciatic nerve. The only branches to arise from its lateral surface innervate the short head of the biceps femoris muscle (Fig. 16.38).

○ Clean the perforating arteries and veins, which provide the arterial supply and venous drainage of the posterior thigh (Figs. 16.39 to 16.41, Plate 16.3).

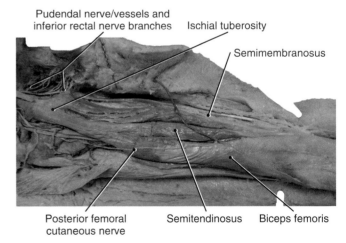

Fig. 16.36 Reflected skin and subcutaneous tissue of posterior thigh and ischioanal fossa, revealing pudendal nerve superiorly and inferior rectal nerve inferiorly, internal pudendal artery and vein, ischial tuberosity, and biceps femoris, semitendinosus, and semimembranosus muscles.

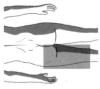

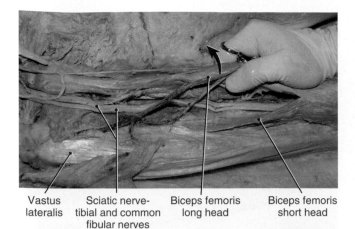

Vastus lateralis | Sciatic nerve-tibial and common fibular nerves | Biceps femoris long head | Biceps femoris short head

Fig. 16.37 Posterior thigh, highlighting sciatic nerve (tibial/common fibular nerves) and biceps femoris muscle (long and short heads).

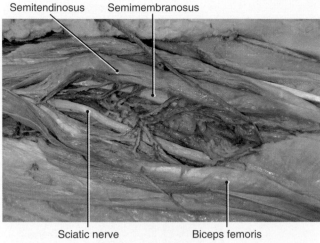

Semitendinosus | Semimembranosus

Sciatic nerve | Biceps femoris

Fig. 16.39 Posterior thigh, highlighting sciatic nerve between "hamstrings": biceps femoris lateral, semitendinosus medial and superficial, and semimembranosus muscle medial and deep.

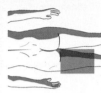

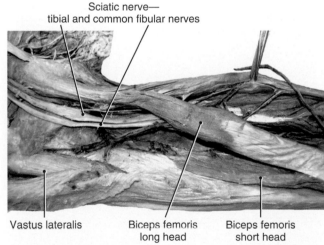

Sciatic nerve— tibial and common fibular nerves

Vastus lateralis | Biceps femoris long head | Biceps femoris short head

Fig. 16.38 Posterior thigh, showing tibial and common fibular nerves of sciatic nerve long and short heads of biceps femoris muscle.

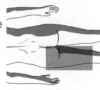

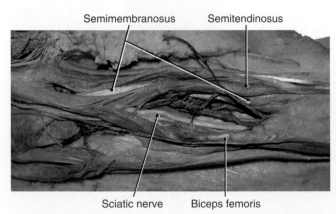

Semimembranosus | Semitendinosus

Sciatic nerve | Biceps femoris

Fig. 16.40 Posterior thigh, showing sciatic nerve between hamstring muscles (biceps femoris, semitendinosus, semimembranosus).

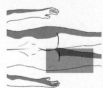

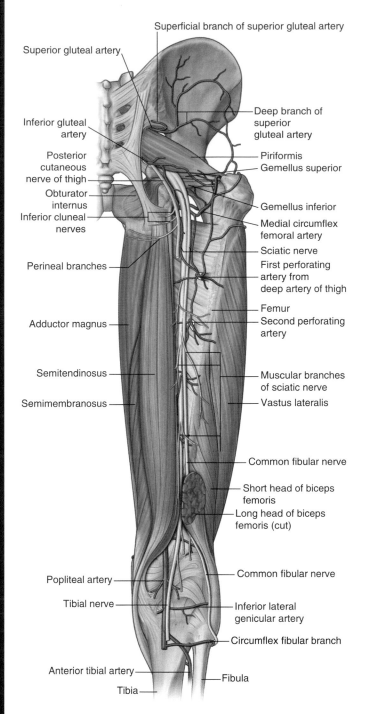

Arteries and nerves of the thigh (posterior view)

Plate 16.3 Arteries and nerves of the posterior thigh.

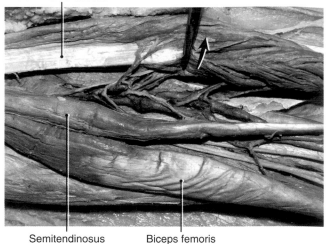

Fig. 16.41 Posterior thigh revealing musculature: biceps femoris laterally, semitendinosus reflected laterally, and semimembranosus medially.

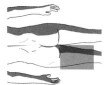

LABORATORY IDENTIFICATION CHECKLIST

NERVES
- ☐ Superior gluteal
- ☐ Inferior gluteal
- ☐ Pudendal
    - ☐ Inferior rectal
- ☐ Posterior femoral cutaneous
    - ☐ Sciatic
        - ☐ Tibial (medial)
        - ☐ Common fibular (lateral)

ARTERIES
- ☐ Superior gluteal
- ☐ Inferior gluteal
- ☐ Internal pudendal
    - ☐ Inferior rectal
- ☐ Medial femoral circumflex
- ☐ Perforating arteries

VEINS
- ☐ Superior gluteal
- ☐ Inferior gluteal
- ☐ Internal pudendal
- ☐ Perforating veins

MUSCLES
- ☐ Gluteus maximus
- ☐ Gluteus medius
- ☐ Gluteus minimus
- ☐ Piriformis
- ☐ Superior gemellus

- ☐ Obturator internus
- ☐ Inferior gemellus
- ☐ Quadratus femoris
- ☐ Semimembranosus
- ☐ Semitendinosus
- ☐ Biceps femoris
    - ☐ Long head
    - ☐ Short head
- ☐ Adductor minimus
- ☐ Tensor fasciae latae
- ☐ Levator ani
- ☐ External anal sphincter

LIGAMENTS
- ☐ Sacrotuberous
- ☐ Sacrospinous

FOSSA/CANAL
- ☐ Ischioanal fossa
- ☐ Alcock's canal

FASCIA
- ☐ Gluteal
- ☐ Obturator internus
- ☐ Lunate
- ☐ Fascia lata
- ☐ Iliotibial tract

BURSA
- ☐ Trochanteric bursa

ATLAS REFERENCES

Netter: 480–485, 490–491
McMinn: 320–327
Gray's Atlas: 299, 300, 306–317

BEFORE YOU BEGIN

Palpate the following bony landmarks on the cadaver or on yourself:

- Anterior superior iliac spine
- Pubic tubercle
- Pubic symphysis
- Greater trochanter of femur
- Medial and lateral femoral condyles
- Patella
- Tibial tuberosity
- Head and neck of fibula
- Medial and lateral malleoli of tibia and fibula, respectively

DISSECTION STEPS

- ○ Make a horizontal skin incision on the thigh 2 to 3 cm (~1 inch) inferior and parallel to the inguinal ligament.
- ○ Leave the skin intact over the external genitalia.
- ○ At the midpoint of this horizontal incision, make a vertical incision to the anterior portion of the patella.
- ○ Make an encircling incision around the knee (Fig. 17.1).
- ○ Reflect the skin medially over the thigh, and identify the superficial veins (Fig. 17.2).
- ○ Continue the dissection by making a vertical incision from the knee toward the ankle (Fig. 17.3).
- ○ Make a transverse incision between the malleoli.
- ○ Reflect the skin of the leg laterally (Fig. 17.4).
- ○ Start exposing the superficial veins of the leg and thigh (Fig. 17.5).
- ○ Identify the great saphenous vein and saphenous nerve (Fig. 17.6).
- ○ Clean the superficial fascia over the *great saphenous vein,* starting from the ankle toward the knee (Fig. 17.7).

ANATOMY **NOTE**

Around the knee, the saphenous nerve is located deep to the great saphenous vein. In the leg medial to the tibia, however, the great saphenous vein runs parallel with the saphenous nerve (Fig. 17.8). The great saphenous vein arises from the medial side of the dorsal venous arch of the foot and ascends anterior to the medial malleolus, along the medial side of the leg and thigh, finally draining into the femoral vein.

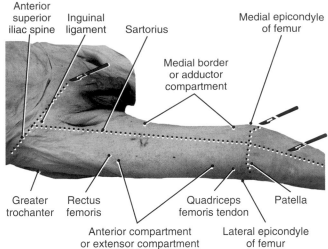

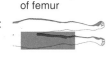

Fig. 17.1 Three thigh dissection incisions: horizontal cut inferior and parallel to inguinal ligament, vertical cut to anterior patella at midpoint of horizontal incision, and encircling cut around the knee.

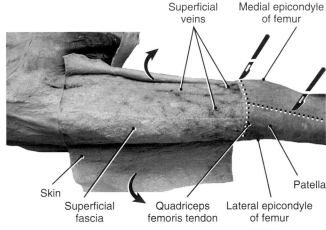

Fig. 17.2 Skin reflected medially over thigh, revealing superficial veins.

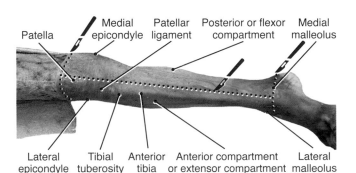

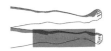

Fig. 17.3 Vertical incision from the knee toward the ankle and transverse incision between the malleoli.

- Identify the great saphenous nerve and note its relationship to the saphenous vein medial to the tibia.
- Remove the skin from the posterior aspect of the leg to the ankle (Fig. 17.9).
- Leave the superficial and deep fasciae (crural fascia) intact.
- Identify the *small* (lesser) *saphenous vein,* which begins from the lateral aspect of the dorsal venous arch of the foot.

ANATOMY **NOTE**

The small saphenous vein ascends just inferior to the lateral malleolus, accompanying the sural nerve, and finally drains into the popliteal vein (Fig. 17.10).

- Identify the sural nerve.
- Observe the sural nerve and the small saphenous vein as they penetrate the deep crural fascia to travel to the popliteal fossa (Fig. 17.11).
- On the anterior part of the leg, on its medial side over the patellar ligament, expose the infrapatellar branch of the saphenous nerve (Fig. 17.12).
- Follow the great saphenous vein toward the thigh, and clean the fat off the superficial fascia around the vein (Fig. 17.13).

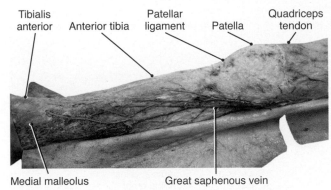

Fig. 17.6 Skin of leg reflected, showing great saphenous vein and tibialis anterior muscle.

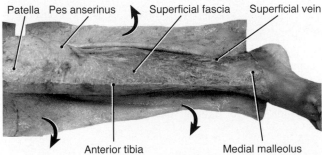

Fig. 17.4 Transverse cut between the malleoli, with skin of leg reflected laterally.

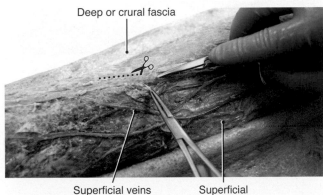

Fig. 17.7 Superficial fascia cleaned away over great saphenous vein.

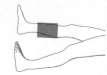

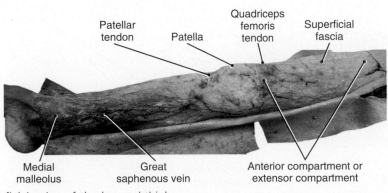

Fig. 17.5 Exposure of superficial veins of the leg and thigh.

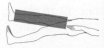

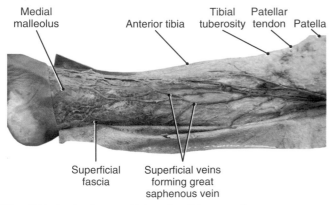

Medial malleolus | Anterior tibia | Tibial tuberosity | Patellar tendon | Patella

Superficial fascia | Superficial veins forming great saphenous vein

Fig. 17.8 In the leg medial to the tibia, note how the great saphenous vein runs parallel with the saphenous nerve.

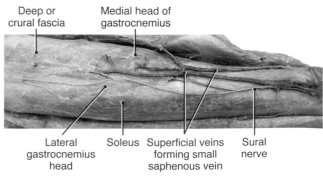
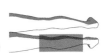

Deep or crural fascia | Medial head of gastrocnemius

Lateral gastrocnemius head | Soleus | Superficial veins forming small saphenous vein | Sural nerve

Fig. 17.11 Reflected view shows sural nerve and small saphenous vein penetrating deep (crural) fascia to travel to popliteal fossa.

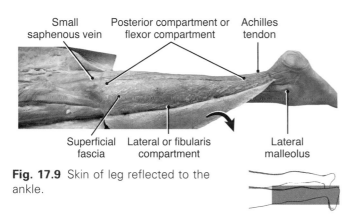

Small saphenous vein | Posterior compartment or flexor compartment | Achilles tendon

Superficial fascia | Lateral or fibularis compartment | Lateral malleolus

Fig. 17.9 Skin of leg reflected to the ankle.

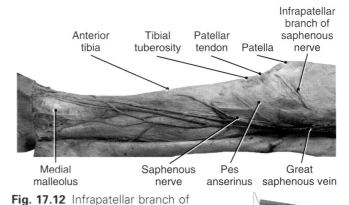

Anterior tibia | Tibial tuberosity | Patellar tendon | Patella | Infrapatellar branch of saphenous nerve

Medial malleolus | Saphenous nerve | Pes anserinus | Great saphenous vein

Fig. 17.12 Infrapatellar branch of saphenous nerve exposed on medial side of anterior leg over patellar ligament.

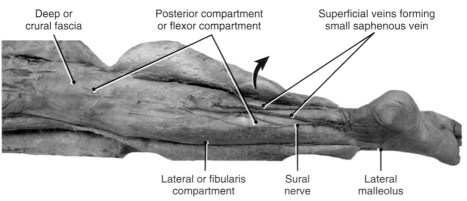

Deep or crural fascia | Posterior compartment or flexor compartment | Superficial veins forming small saphenous vein

Lateral or fibularis compartment | Sural nerve | Lateral malleolus

Fig. 17.10 Skin of leg reflected, revealing posterior and lateral compartments, deep fascia, and small saphenous vein.

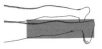

- Expose the great saphenous vein toward the *fossa ovalis* (saphenous hiatus), the opening in the deep fascia, where the vein travels through to drain into the femoral vein.
- Expose the superficial and deep perforating tributaries of the great saphenous vein (Fig. 17.14).
- Start cleaning fat from around the great saphenous vein, extending the dissection medially and laterally (Fig. 17.15).
- Do not cut through the deep fascia of the thigh, but identify the anterior cutaneous branches of the femoral nerve intermingled with the tributaries of the great saphenous vein.
- Lateral to the vein, identify the rectus femoris muscle.
- On top of and lateral to the muscle, identify the lateral femoral cutaneous nerves (Fig. 17.16).

DISSECTION TIP

Observe the lymphatics in the area of the fossa ovalis, but do not spend time exposing all of them. Realize that the inguinal lymph nodes are so named based on their position relative to the deep fascia. The deep inguinal lymph nodes are located deep to it, whereas the superficial nodes are superficial to the deep fascia.

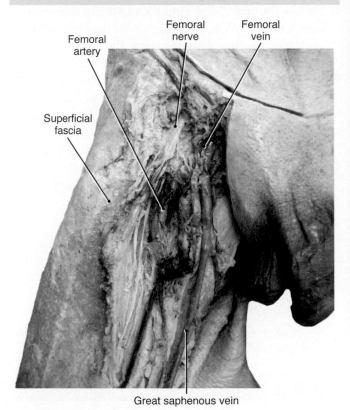

Fig. 17.15 Fat cleaned away around saphenous vein, with dissection extended medially and laterally.

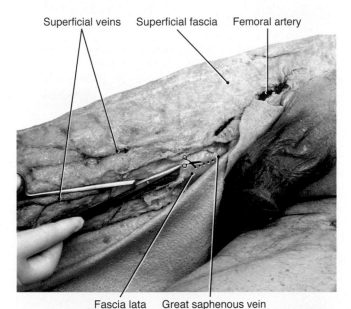

Fig. 17.13 Fat of superficial fascia cleaned away around great saphenous vein.

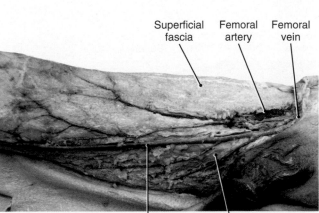
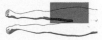

Fig. 17.14 View of great saphenous vein and its superficial and deep perforating tributaries.

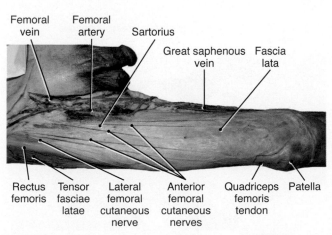

Fig. 17.16 Appreciate anterior cutaneous branches of femoral nerve intermingled with tributaries of great saphenous vein and rectus femoris muscle with lateral femoral cutaneous nerve.

- Cut the distal ends of the cutaneous nerves you previously dissected.
- Reflect the nerves medially and preserve them.
- Cut the deep fascia of the thigh, *fascia lata,* and expose the sartorius muscle (Fig. 17.17).
- Continue reflecting the fascia lata over the vastus medialis muscle (Fig. 17.18).
- Expose the quadriceps femoris muscles of the extensor compartment of the thigh; the vastus medialis, lateralis, and intermedius muscles; and the rectus femoris muscle and their tendons attaching to the patella.
- Continue the exposure by noting the fascia lata laterally and its thickened distal part, the *iliotibial tract,* attaching to the lateral condyle of the tibia (Fig. 17.19).
- Reflect the rectus femoris muscle medially, and expose the vastus intermedius muscle underneath (Fig. 17.20).
- Place the cutaneous nerves back in their original position over the dissected muscles, and appreciate their location (Fig. 17.21).

- Expose the femoral vein, and dissect out the *cribriform fascia,* which fills the saphenous hiatus (Fig. 17.22).
- Cut the femoral sheath around the femoral artery and vein.
- Note the relationship between the femoral artery and vein; the femoral artery is located lateral to the femoral vein. The femoral nerve lies lateral to the femoral artery (Fig. 17.23).

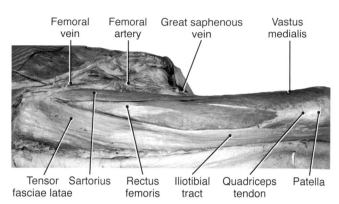

Femoral vein | Femoral artery | Great saphenous vein | Vastus medialis

Tensor fasciae latae | Sartorius | Rectus femoris | Iliotibial tract | Quadriceps tendon | Patella

Fig. 17.19 Exposed quadriceps femoris muscles of extensor compartment of thigh with tendon attaching to patella.

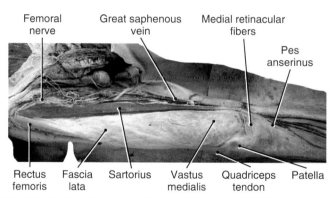

Femoral nerve | Great saphenous vein | Medial retinacular fibers | Pes anserinus

Rectus femoris | Fascia lata | Sartorius | Vastus medialis | Quadriceps tendon | Patella

Fig. 17.17 Distal ends of dissected cutaneous nerve reflected, with deep fascia (fascia lata) cut, exposing sartorius muscle.

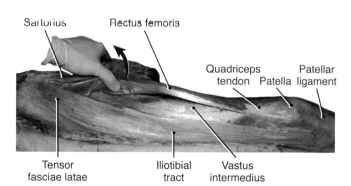

Sartorius | Rectus femoris | Quadriceps tendon | Patella | Patellar ligament

Tensor fasciae latae | Iliotibial tract | Vastus intermedius

Fig. 17.20 Rectus femoris muscle reflected medially, exposing vastus intermedius muscle.

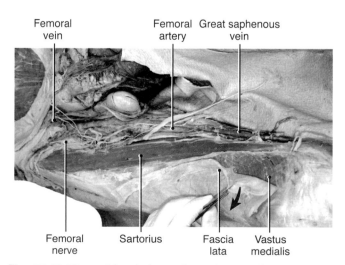

Femoral vein | Femoral artery | Great saphenous vein

Femoral nerve | Sartorius | Fascia lata | Vastus medialis

Fig. 17.18 View of fascia lata reflected over vastus medialis muscle.

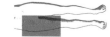

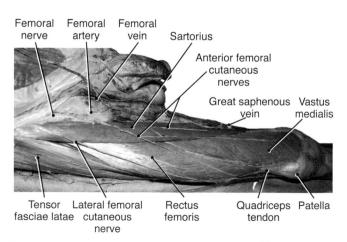

Femoral nerve | Femoral artery | Femoral vein | Sartorius

Anterior femoral cutaneous nerves

Great saphenous vein | Vastus medialis

Tensor fasciae latae | Lateral femoral cutaneous nerve | Rectus femoris | Quadriceps tendon | Patella

Fig. 17.21 Appreciate the position of the cutaneous nerves of the anterior thigh.

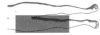

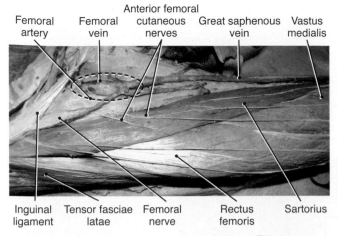

Femoral artery · Femoral vein · Anterior femoral cutaneous nerves · Great saphenous vein · Vastus medialis

Inguinal ligament · Tensor fasciae latae · Femoral nerve · Rectus femoris · Sartorius

Fig. 17.22 Femoral vein exposed, and the cribriform fascia that fills saphenous hiatus *(outlined oval)* is dissected.

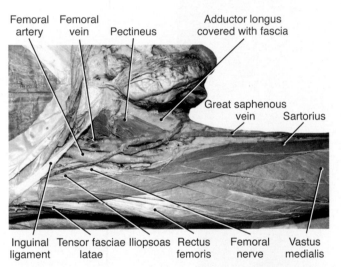

Femoral artery · Femoral vein · Pectineus · Adductor longus covered with fascia

Great saphenous vein · Sartorius

Inguinal ligament · Tensor fasciae latae · Iliopsoas · Rectus femoris · Femoral nerve · Vastus medialis

Fig. 17.23 Femoral sheath incised around femoral artery and vein to appreciate their relationship.

- ○ Clean the fascia covering the femoral artery and vein, and trace these vessels underneath the inguinal ligament to the femoral triangle.
- ○ Continue removing fat, and expose the adductor longus and gracilis muscles medially (Fig. 17.24).
- ○ Retract the femoral artery laterally from the femoral vein, and deep between these vessels note the iliopsoas muscle lying over the anterior aspect of the hip joint (Fig. 17.25).

ANATOMY **NOTE**

The area you just dissected is called the *femoral triangle,* formed by the inguinal ligament superiorly, the sartorius muscle laterally, and the adductor longus muscle medially. The pectineus and iliopsoas muscles form the floor of the triangle (Plate 17.1).

- ○ Cut the smaller venous tributaries draining to the femoral vein for better exposure of the femoral triangle.

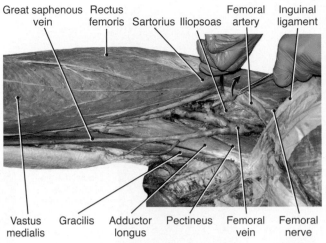

Great saphenous vein · Rectus femoris · Sartorius · Iliopsoas · Femoral artery · Inguinal ligament

Vastus medialis · Gracilis · Adductor longus · Pectineus · Femoral vein · Femoral nerve

Fig. 17.24 View of femoral artery and vein underneath inguinal ligament showing adductor longus and gracilis muscles.

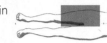

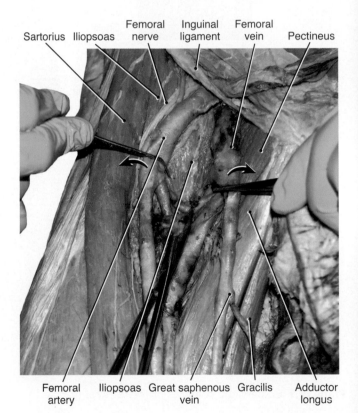

Sartorius · Iliopsoas · Femoral nerve · Inguinal ligament · Femoral vein · Pectineus

Femoral artery · Iliopsoas · Great saphenous vein · Gracilis · Adductor longus

Fig. 17.25 Femoral artery retracted laterally from femoral vein, highlighting deep-lying iliopsoas muscle over anterior aspect of capsule of hip joint.

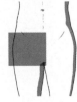

- ○ Medial to the iliopsoas muscle, note the pectineus muscle, and more medially, the adductor longus muscle.
- ○ Clean the femoral artery and vein proximal to the femoral canal, and trace the lateral femoral cutaneous nerve underneath the inguinal ligament, just medial to the anterior superior iliac spine (Fig. 17.26).

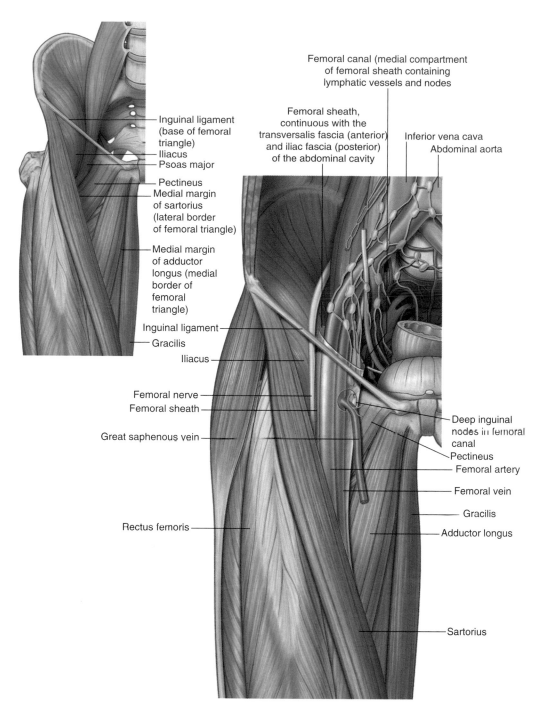

Inguinal ligament
(base of femoral
triangle)

Iliacus

Psoas major

Pectineus

Medial margin
of sartorius
(lateral border
of femoral triangle)

Medial margin
of adductor
longus (medial
border of
femoral
triangle)

Inguinal ligament

Gracilis

Iliacus

Femoral nerve

Femoral sheath

Great saphenous vein

Rectus femoris

Femoral canal (medial compartment
of femoral sheath containing
lymphatic vessels and nodes

Femoral sheath,
continuous with the
transversalis fascia (anterior)
and iliac fascia (posterior)
of the abdominal cavity

Inferior vena cava

Abdominal aorta

Deep inguinal
nodes in femoral
canal

Pectineus

Femoral artery

Femoral vein

Gracilis

Adductor longus

Sartorius

Plate 17.1 Borders and contents of the femoral triangle.

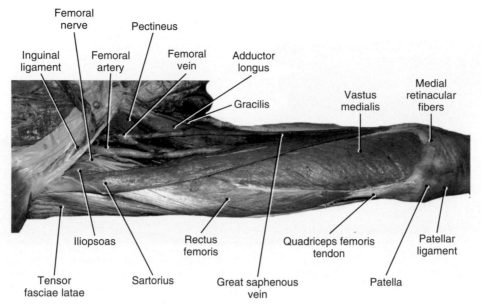

Fig. 17.26 Femoral artery and vein cleaned proximal to femoral canal, showing lateral femoral cutaneous nerve.

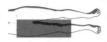

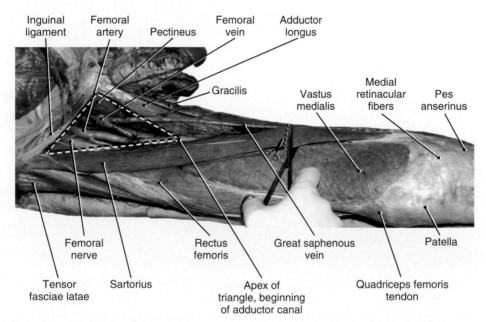

Fig. 17.27 Smaller tributaries draining the femoral vein cut to expose femoral triangle *(outline)* and appreciate the pectineus and adductor longus muscles.

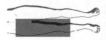

○ Cut the sartorius muscle at its distal quarter, and expose the adductor canal (Figs. 17.27 and 17.28).

ANATOMY **NOTE**

The adductor canal is formed by the adductor magnus, adductor longus, and vastus medialis muscles. The canal begins at the apex of the femoral triangle and ends at the adductor hiatus, which is the canal formed by the adductor magnus tendon at the posterior knee. After passing through the adductor hiatus and reaching the posterior part of the knee, the femoral artery and femoral vein are termed the *popliteal artery* and *popliteal vein* (Fig. 17.29).

○ Within the adductor canal, expose and identify the femoral artery, femoral vein, saphenous nerve, nerve to the vastus medialis muscle, and descending genicular artery (see Fig. 17.29).

○ Expose the aperture in the tendon of insertion of the adductor magnus, the adductor hiatus (Fig. 17.30).

○ Identify the nerve to the vastus medialis muscle, and trace the nerve to its termination on the muscle.

○ Distal to the level of the adductor hiatus, trace the saphenous nerve and expose it to the postero-medial aspect of the knee where it meets the great saphenous vein.

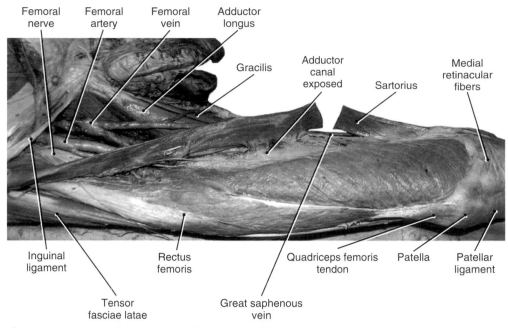

Fig. **17.28** View of cut sartorius muscle, exposing adductor canal.

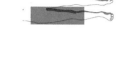

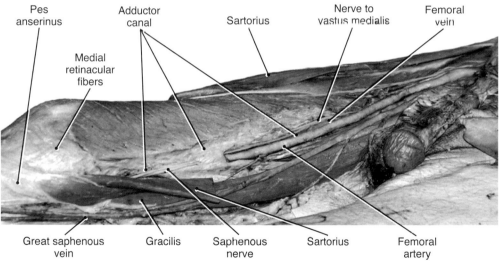

Fig. **17.29** View of femoral artery and vein, saphenous nerve, nerve to vastus medialis muscle, and descending genicular artery within adductor canal.

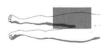

○ With scissors, cut the femoral vein a few centimeters inferior to the femoral canal and reflect it inferiorly (Figs. 17.31 and 17.32).

○ Fully expose the pectineus, adductor longus, and gracilis muscles.

○ Pull the femoral artery medially, and dissect out its branches (Figs. 17.33 and 17.34).

○ Identify the lateral circumflex femoral artery, and expose its descending branch supplying the vastus lateralis, which travels in the muscle between the vastus lateralis and vastus intermedius (this is a fairly constant dissection landmark).

ANATOMY **NOTE**

The lateral circumflex femoral artery also gives off several perforating branches to the vastus intermedius.

○ Continue the dissection by exposing the deep femoral artery (*profunda femoris*) deep to the adductor longus muscle (see Figs. 17.33 and 17.34, Plate 17.2).

○ Expose several of the perforating branches mainly supplying the posterior compartment of the thigh.

○ Identify the medial circumflex femoral artery, and expose it between the iliopsoas and pectineus muscles.

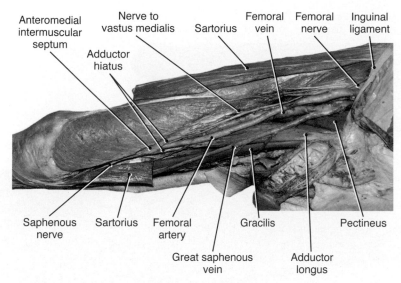

Fig. 17.30 View of adductor hiatus, the aperture in the tendon of insertion of the adductor magnus muscle.

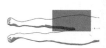

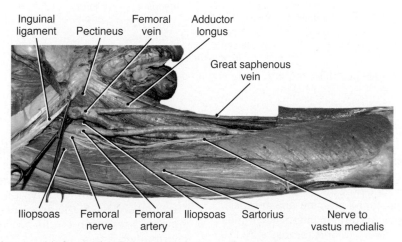

Fig. 17.31 View of musculature with femoral vein incised inferior to the femoral canal.

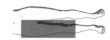

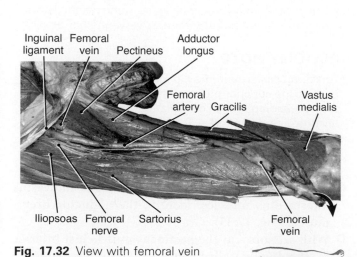

Fig. 17.32 View with femoral vein reflected inferiorly.

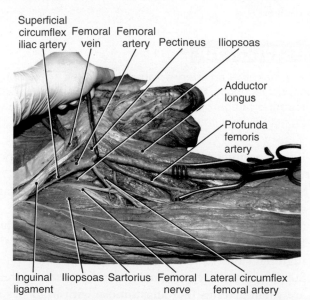

Fig. 17.33 Femoral artery pulled medially and its branches dissected.

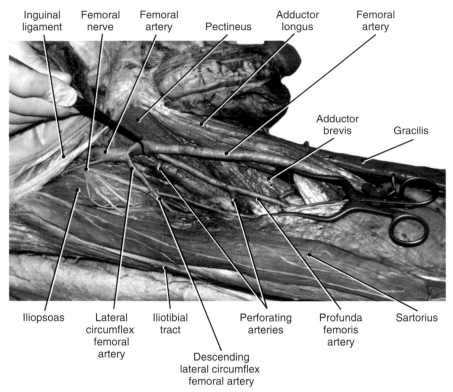

Inguinal ligament — Femoral nerve — Femoral artery — Pectineus — Adductor longus — Femoral artery — Adductor brevis — Gracilis

Iliopsoas — Lateral circumflex femoral artery — Iliotibial tract — Descending lateral circumflex femoral artery — Perforating arteries — Profunda femoris artery — Sartorius

Fig. 17.34 Appreciate the lateral circumflex femoral artery and its descending branch.

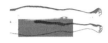

DISSECTION TIP

If it is large enough, dissect out the transverse branch of the lateral circumflex femoral artery running to the posterior surface of the femur below the greater trochanter and contributing to the so-called cruciate anastomosis. Look for an ascending branch from the lateral circumflex femoral artery that runs upward to anastomose with the deep circumflex iliac and superior gluteal arteries. In some specimens, a retractor is useful to retract the tissues between the adductor longus and vastus intermedius muscles.

DISSECTION TIP

Remember that an artery's name is based on its distribution, not its origin. The lateral circumflex femoral, medial circumflex femoral, and deep femoral arteries commonly originate from a common trunk.

If time permits, from the exposed femoral artery, look for the following arteries:

○ **Superficial circumflex iliac artery,** which travels toward the anterior superior iliac spine.
○ **Superficial epigastric artery,** which travels upward toward the anterior abdominal wall, crossing over the inguinal canal.
○ **Superficial and deep external pudendal vessels** typically are small arteries that anastomose with branches of the internal pudendal artery. Do not attempt to identify these two vessels.

ANATOMY NOTE

The so-called cruciate anastomosis classically involves the confluence of four arteries posterior to the upper part of the femur: (1) the transverse branch of the lateral circumflex femoral artery, (2) the medial circumflex femoral artery, (3) the descending branch of the inferior gluteal artery, and (4) the ascending branch of the first perforating artery.

DISSECTION TIP

From personal observations, the *transverse* branch of the lateral circumflex femoral artery is only rarely significant in this anastomosis, although the *ascending* branch does participate. Actually, the transverse branch of the lateral circumflex femoral artery may be very small or absent.

ANATOMY NOTE

Anastomoses around the hip also involve other vessels such as the superior gluteal, iliolumbar, deep circumflex iliac, ascending branch of the lateral circumflex femoral, and the obturator arteries. Therefore, with occlusion of the femoral artery, many possible routes can form collateral circulation from the iliac arteries to the lower extremity.

○ In the space between the adductor longus and vastus intermedius muscles, identify the adductor brevis muscle (Fig. 17.35).
○ With scissors, cut the pectineus muscle just inferior to the inguinal ligament, and reflect it laterally (Fig. 17.36).

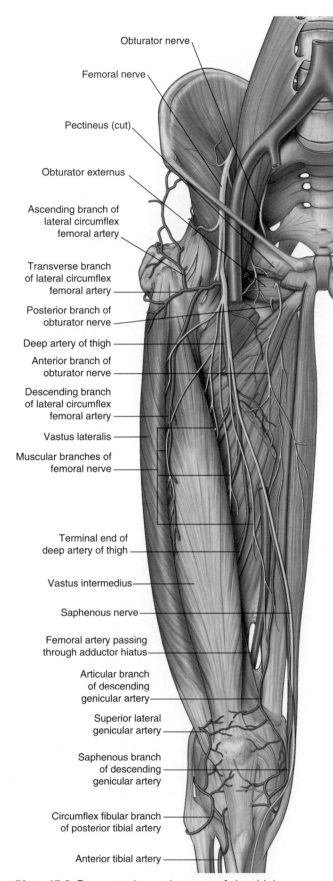

Obturator nerve

Femoral nerve

Pectineus (cut)

Obturator externus

Ascending branch of
lateral circumflex
femoral artery

Transverse branch
of lateral circumflex
femoral artery

Posterior branch of
obturator nerve

Deep artery of thigh

Anterior branch of
obturator nerve

Descending branch
of lateral circumflex
femoral artery

Vastus lateralis

Muscular branches of
femoral nerve

Terminal end of
deep artery of thigh

Vastus intermedius

Saphenous nerve

Femoral artery passing
through adductor hiatus

Articular branch
of descending
genicular artery

Superior lateral
genicular artery

Saphenous branch
of descending
genicular artery

Circumflex fibular branch
of posterior tibial artery

Anterior tibial artery

Plate 17.2 Deep arteries and nerves of the thigh.

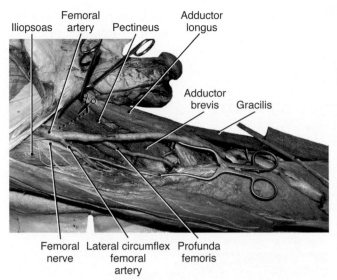

Iliopsoas · Femoral artery · Pectineus · Adductor longus · Adductor brevis · Gracilis

Femoral nerve · Lateral circumflex femoral artery · Profunda femoris

Fig. 17.35 Appreciate the adductor brevis muscle in space between adductor longus and vastus intermedius muscles.

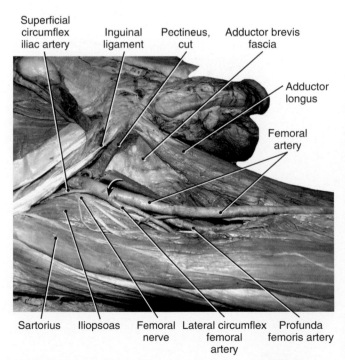

Superficial circumflex iliac artery · Inguinal ligament · Pectineus, cut · Adductor brevis fascia · Adductor longus · Femoral artery

Sartorius · Iliopsoas · Femoral nerve · Lateral circumflex femoral artery · Profunda femoris artery

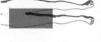

Fig. 17.36 View with pectineus muscle incised inferior to the inguinal ligament and reflected laterally.

○ Note the adductor brevis fascia over the proximal part of the adductor brevis muscle. Remove the fascia carefully, and expose the obturator artery and nerve (Figs. 17.37 and 17.38).

ANATOMY **NOTE**

The *obturator nerve* splits into two divisions: anterior and posterior. The *anterior division* courses anterior to the adductor brevis to innervate the adductor longus and brevis muscles.

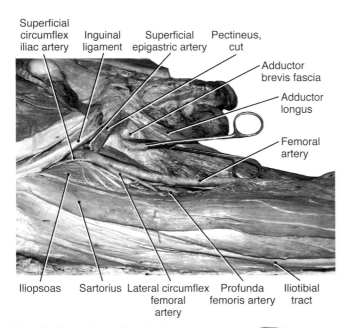

Superficial circumflex iliac artery · Inguinal ligament · Superficial epigastric artery · Pectineus, cut · Adductor brevis fascia · Adductor longus · Femoral artery

Iliopsoas · Sartorius · Lateral circumflex femoral artery · Profunda femoris artery · Iliotibial tract

Fig. 17.37 Adductor brevis fascia removed, exposing obturator artery and nerve.

○ Reflect the adductor brevis muscle laterally, and identify the *posterior division* of the obturator nerve innervating the adductor magnus.

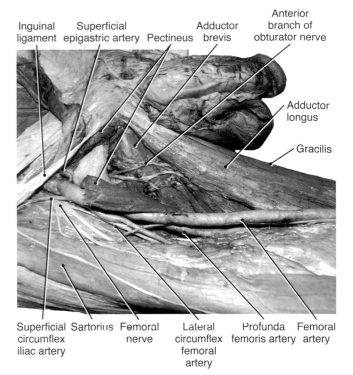

Inguinal ligament · Superficial epigastric artery · Pectineus · Adductor brevis · Anterior branch of obturator nerve · Adductor longus · Gracilis

Superficial circumflex iliac artery · Sartorius · Femoral nerve · Lateral circumflex femoral artery · Profunda femoris artery · Femoral artery

Fig. 17.38 Adductor brevis muscle reflected laterally, revealing posterior division of obturator nerve.

LABORATORY IDENTIFICATION CHECKLIST

NERVES
- [ ] Femoral
  - [ ] Branch to vastus medialis
  - [ ] Branch to rectus femoris
  - [ ] Branch to vastus lateralis
  - [ ] Branch to vastus intermedius
  - [ ] Saphenous
- [ ] Lateral femoral cutaneous
- [ ] Obturator
  - [ ] Anterior division
  - [ ] Posterior division
- [ ] Sciatic
  - [ ] Tibial
  - [ ] Common fibular
- [ ] Posterior cutaneous, of thigh

ARTERIES
- [ ] Femoral
- [ ] Superficial epigastric
- [ ] Superficial circumflex iliac
- [ ] Superficial external pudendal
- [ ] Deep external pudendal
- [ ] Profunda femoris
- [ ] Medial circumflex femoral
- [ ] Lateral circumflex femoral
- [ ] Perforating arteries
- [ ] Descending genicular
- [ ] Popliteal
- [ ] Superior genicular arteries
- [ ] Middle genicular
- [ ] Inferior genicular arteries
- [ ] Obturator
  - [ ] Acetabular branch

VEINS
- [ ] Great saphenous
- [ ] Small (lesser) saphenous
- [ ] Superficial epigastric
- [ ] Superficial circumflex iliac
- [ ] External pudendal
- [ ] Popliteal
- [ ] Profunda femoris
- [ ] Femoral

CONNECTIVE TISSUE
- [ ] Femoral fascia (fascia lata)
- [ ] Anteromedial intermuscular septum
- [ ] Medial intermuscular septum
- [ ] Lateral intermuscular septum
- [ ] Posterior intermuscular septum
- [ ] Vastoadductor membrane

LIGAMENTS
- [ ] *Hip*
  - [ ] Iliofemoral
  - [ ] Pubofemoral
  - [ ] Ischiofemoral
  - [ ] Ligamentum teres
  - [ ] Acetabular labrum/transverse acetabular
- [ ] *Knee*
  - [ ] Anterior cruciate
  - [ ] Posterior cruciate
  - [ ] Transverse
  - [ ] Tibial collateral
- [ ] Fibular (lateral) collateral
- [ ] Oblique popliteal

CARTILAGE
- [ ] Medial meniscus
- [ ] Lateral meniscus

MUSCLES
Anterior Compartment (Extensor Compartment)
- [ ] Sartorius
- [ ] Iliopsoas
- [ ] Iliacus
- [ ] Rectus femoris
- [ ] Vastus medialis
- [ ] Vastus lateralis
- [ ] Vastus intermedius
- [ ] Articularis genus
Femoral Triangle
- [ ] Borders
  - [ ] Inguinal ligament, superior border
  - [ ] Adductor longus, medial border
  - [ ] Sartorius, lateral border
- [ ] Floor
  - [ ] Iliacus
  - [ ] Psoas
  - [ ] Pectineus
- [ ] Contents (medial to lateral)
  - [ ] Femoral canal with lymphatics
  - [ ] Femoral vein
  - [ ] Femoral artery
  - [ ] Femoral nerve

Adductor Canal (Subsartorial, or Hunter's Canal)

Extends from femoral triangle apex to adductor hiatus

- ☐ Contents
    - ☐ Femoral artery
    - ☐ Femoral vein
    - ☐ Nerve to vastus medialis
    - ☐ Saphenous nerve
    - ☐ Descending genicular

Tendons/Retinacula

- ☐ Quadriceps femoris tendon
- ☐ Patellar ligament
- ☐ Medial retinaculum
- ☐ Lateral retinaculum

Medial Compartment (Adductor Compartment)

- ☐ Gracilis
- ☐ Pectineus
- ☐ Obturator externus
- ☐ Adductor longus
- ☐ Adductor brevis
- ☐ Adductor magnus
- ☐ Femoral head
- ☐ Ischial or hamstring head
- ☐ Adductor minimus

POSTERIOR COMPARTMENT (FLEXOR COMPARTMENT)

- ☐ Biceps femoris
    - ☐ Long head
    - ☐ Short head
- ☐ Semitendinosus muscle
- ☐ Semimembranosus muscle

Pes anserinus

- ☐ Sartorius
- ☐ Gracilis
- ☐ Semitendinosus

BURSAE

- ☐ Suprapatellar
- ☐ Prepatellar
- ☐ Infrapatellar

BONES

- ☐ Coxal (hip bone)
- ☐ Femur
- ☐ Patella
- ☐ Proximal tibia
- ☐ Proximal fibula

ATLAS REFERENCES

Netter: 495–514
McMinn: 328–343
Gray's Atlas: 318–329, 339–347

BEFORE YOU BEGIN

Identify the great and small (lesser) saphenous veins and the saphenous and sural nerves, from the previous dissection of the thigh and leg in Chapter 17.

POSTERIOR LEG

O Insert scissors or a probe between the **semitendinosus** and **biceps femoris** muscles into the popliteal fossa, and remove the superficial adipose tissue (Fig. 18.1).

O Insert scissors or a probe underneath the **crural fascia** (Fig. 18.2), and divide the fascia into two parts.

O Reflect the semitendinosus and biceps femoris muscles, and expose the contents of the popliteal fossa (Fig.

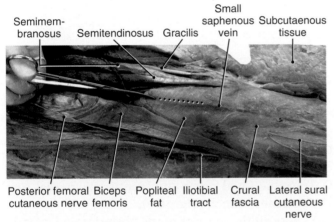

Semimem- Semitendinosus Gracilis Small saphenous vein Subcutaneous tissue
branosus

Posterior femoral Biceps Popliteal Iliotibial Crural Lateral sural
cutaneous nerve femoris fat tract fascia cutaneous nerve

Fig. 18.1 Scissors inserted between semitendinosus and biceps femoris muscles, into popliteal fossa, with superficial adipose tissue removed.

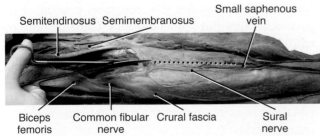

Semitendinosus Semimembranosus Small saphenous vein

Biceps Common fibular Crural fascia Sural
femoris nerve nerve

Fig. 18.2 *Dotted line* indicates crural fascia cut into two parts.

18.3). Note the sciatic nerve dividing into the tibial and common fibular nerves.

O Clean the fat and the lymphatics within the popliteal fossa and identify the following structures (Plate 18.1):

O Posterior femoral cutaneous nerve
O Small saphenous vein
O Tibial nerve
O Common fibular nerve
O Popliteal vein
O Popliteal artery

DISSECTION TIP

Identify the following landmarks (see also Chapter 17):

*   The **great saphenous vein** and the saphenous nerve accompany each other along the medial aspect of the leg and thigh.
*   The **small saphenous vein** and the sural nerve accompany each other along the posterior aspect of the leg. The small saphenous vein usually drains into the popliteal vein and often exhibits anastomoses with the great saphenous vein.
*   The **sural nerve** is formed by the union of the medial sural cutaneous nerve, a branch of the tibial nerve, and a communicating branch of the lateral sural cutaneous nerve arising from the common fibular nerve. The sural nerve terminates as the **lateral dorsal cutaneous nerve** on the lateral foot.
*   Clean the popliteal artery, and identify its division into **anterior and posterior tibial arteries**. Look for the popliteal artery's genicular branches, the superolateral, superomedial, inferolateral, inferomedial, and middle genicular arteries.
*   To find the **superolateral and superomedial genicular arteries**; remove the fat just superior to the lateral and medial condyles of the femur, at the origin of the medial and lateral heads of the gastrocnemius muscle, respectively.
*   The **middle genicular artery** is usually found arising from the anterior surface of the popliteal artery (deep from your view) just posterior to the knee joint.
*   The **inferolateral genicular artery** is usually found underneath the lateral head of the gastrocnemius muscle.
*   The **inferomedial genicular artery** is usually found underneath the medial head of the gastrocnemius muscle.

DISSECTION TIP

Do not try to identify every branch of the genicular arteries; some are too small. Similarly, exposing the anastomoses around the knee requires special preparation of the specimen (e.g., filling arteries with red latex).

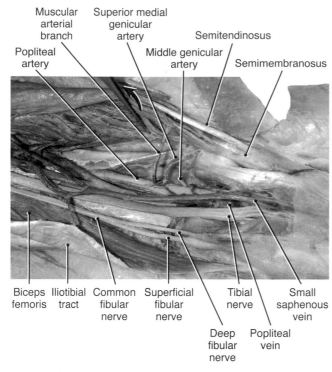

Muscular arterial branch — Popliteal artery — Superior medial genicular artery — Middle genicular artery — Semitendinosus — Semimembranosus

Biceps femoris — Iliotibial tract — Common fibular nerve — Superficial fibular nerve — Deep fibular nerve — Popliteal vein — Tibial nerve — Small saphenous vein

Fig. 18.3 Semitendinosus and biceps femoris muscles reflected laterally, exposing contents of the popliteal fossa.

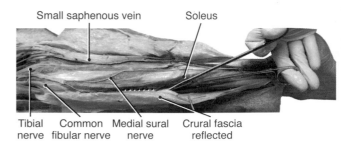

Small saphenous vein — Soleus

Tibial nerve — Common fibular nerve — Medial sural nerve — Crural fascia reflected

Fig. 18.4 Removing fascia, being careful not to disturb superficial veins and cutaneous nerves.

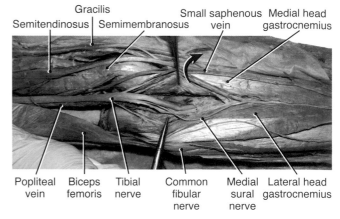

Gracilis — Semitendinosus — Semimembranosus — Small saphenous vein — Medial head gastrocnemius

Popliteal vein — Biceps femoris — Tibial nerve — Common fibular nerve — Medial sural nerve — Lateral head gastrocnemius

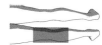

Fig. 18.5 Close-up view with medial and lateral heads of gastrocnemius muscle retracted laterally.

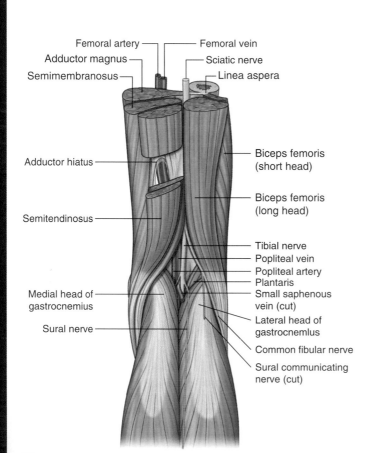

Femoral artery — Adductor magnus — Semimembranosus — Femoral vein — Sciatic nerve — Linea aspera

Adductor hiatus

Semitendinosus

Medial head of gastrocnemius

Sural nerve

Biceps femoris (short head) — Biceps femoris (long head) — Tibial nerve — Popliteal vein — Popliteal artery — Plantaris — Small saphenous vein (cut) — Lateral head of gastrocnemius — Common fibular nerve — Sural communicating nerve (cut)

Plate 18.1 Structures in the popliteal fossa.

- Completely remove the crural fascia from the underlying muscles of the posterior compartment of the leg, without disturbing the superficial veins and cutaneous nerves (Fig. 18.4).
- Identify the medial and lateral heads of the gastrocnemius muscle, and retract them laterally (Fig. 18.5).
- Trace the **tibial nerve** and identify its **medial sural cutaneous branch** (Fig. 18.6).
- Expose all the muscles of the posterior and lateral.
- Identify the **common fibular nerve** and trace its course from the thigh to the neck of the fibula compartments (Fig. 18.6).
- Separate the lateral head of the **gastrocnemius muscle** from the underlying soleus muscle (Fig. 18.7). Look for the *Achilles tendon,* the common tendon of the gastrocnemius and **soleus muscles** inserting onto the **calcaneus.**
- Preserve the **lateral sural cutaneous nerve** as you reflect the lateral head of the gastrocnemius. Similarly, preserve the **medial sural cutaneous nerve** and the **tibial nerve** as you reflect the medial head gastrocnemius muscle.
- Expose the underlying soleus muscle, and identify the tendon of the plantaris muscle on the posterior surface of the soleus.

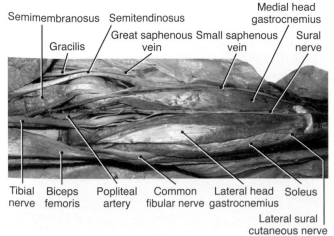
Semimembranosus   Semitendinosus
Gracilis
Great saphenous   Small saphenous   Medial head
vein   vein   gastrocnemius   Sural nerve

Tibial   Biceps   Popliteal   Common   Lateral head   Soleus
nerve   femoris   artery   fibular nerve   gastrocnemius

Lateral sural
cutaneous nerve

Fig. 18.6 Appreciate the tibial nerve and medial sural cutaneous branch as well as muscles of the posterior and lateral compartments of the leg.

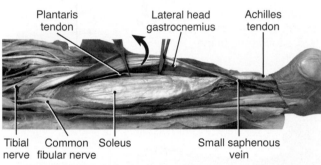

Plantaris   Lateral head   Achilles
tendon   gastrocnemius   tendon

Tibial   Common   Soleus
nerve   fibular nerve

Small saphenous
vein

Fig. 18.7 The gastrocnemius muscle reflected, preserving the lateral and medial sural cutaneous nerves and the tibial nerve, and exposing the underlying soleus muscle and the tendon of the plantaris muscle on the posterior surface of the soleus muscle.

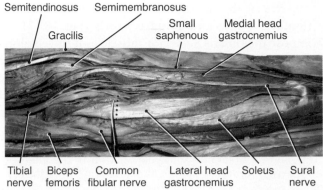

Semitendinosus   Semimembranosus
Gracilis
Small
saphenous   Medial head
gastrocnemius

Tibial   Biceps   Common   Lateral head   Soleus   Sural
nerve   femoris   fibular nerve   gastrocnemius   nerve

Fig. 18.8 Lateral head of gastrocnemius muscle cut at level of femoral condyle.

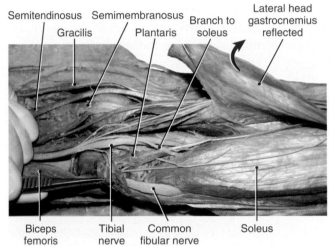

Semitendinosus   Semimembranosus   Branch to   Lateral head
Gracilis   Plantaris   soleus   gastrocnemius
reflected

Biceps   Tibial   Common   Soleus
femoris   nerve   fibular nerve

Fig. 18.9 Close-up view highlights muscle belly of plantaris muscle.

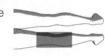

- Cut the lateral head of the gastrocnemius at the level of the femoral condyle (Fig. 18.8).
- Reflect the lateral head of the gastrocnemius muscle medially, and expose the tendon of the **plantaris** muscle. Identify the muscle belly of the plantaris muscle (Fig. 18.9).
- Identify the branch from the tibial nerve, the **nerve to the soleus** muscle.
- With forceps, lift the lateral border of the soleus muscle and separate it from the underlying fascia over the **flexor hallucis longus** and **flexor digitorum longus** muscles (Fig. 18.10).
- With scissors, cut the soleus muscle close to its attachment to the tibia and fibula, and reflect it medially (Fig. 18.11).
- Clean the fascia and expose the **flexor hallucis longus** and **flexor digitorum longus** muscles as well as the

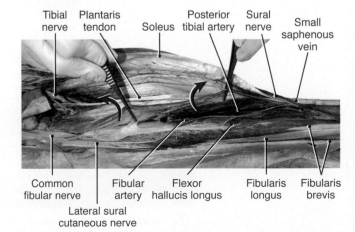

Tibial   Plantaris   Posterior   Sural   Small
nerve   tendon   Soleus   tibial artery   nerve   saphenous
vein

Common   Fibular   Flexor   Fibularis   Fibularis
fibular nerve   artery   hallucis longus   longus   brevis
Lateral sural
cutaneous nerve

Fig. 18.10 Lateral border of soleus muscle detached from underlying fascia over flexor hallucis longus and flexor digitorum longus muscles.

muscles of the lateral compartment of the leg, the **fibularis longus** and **fibularis brevis** (Fig. 18.12).

○ Expose the **tibialis posterior muscle** as it travels along the posterior surface of the interosseous membrane to reach the bones of the foot (Fig. 18.13). Trace the division of the **common fibular nerve** into **deep** and **superficial fibular nerves** (Plate 18.2).

ANATOMY **NOTE**

The anterior tibial artery travels anterior to the interosseous membrane, whereas the posterior tibial artery gives rise to a fibular branch that travels to the lateral compartment and deep to the flexor hallucis longus muscle. Soon after arriving from the common fibular nerve, the superficial fibular nerve enters the lateral compartment of the leg.

KNEE

○ Place the cadaver in the supine position, and observe the knee joint. Identify the tendon of the **quadriceps femoris muscle** attaching to the **patella**.

○ Identify the **patellar ligament** and the strong, thick fascia on the medial and lateral sides of the knee joint, the *medial and lateral retinacula* of the knee (Fig. 18.14).

○ Cut the medial and lateral retinacula, and expose the patellar ligament and the tendon of the quadriceps femoris muscle (Fig. 18.15).

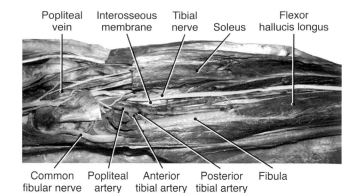
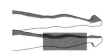

Fig. 18.13 Tibialis posterior muscle exposed along posterior surface of interosseous membrane.

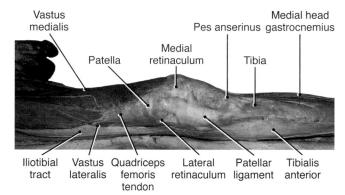
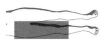

Fig. 18.14 Supine position, highlighting tendon of quadriceps femoris muscle, patellar ligament, and thick fascia on sides of knee joint (medial/lateral retinacula).

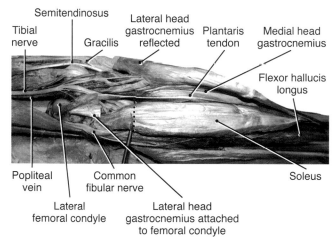

Fig. 18.11 Soleus muscle cut proximal to tibiofibular attachment and reflected medially.

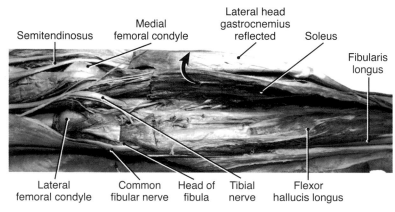
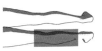

Fig. 18.12 Fascia cleaned, exposing flexor hallucis longus, flexor digitorum longus, and lateral compartment muscles.

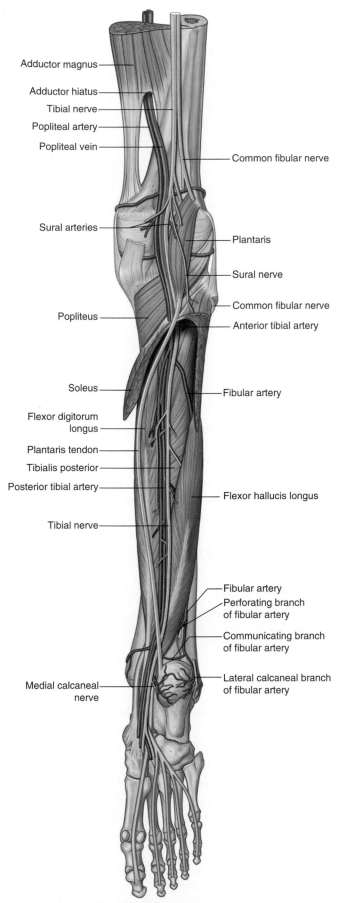

Adductor magnus

Adductor hiatus

Tibial nerve

Popliteal artery

Popliteal vein

Common fibular nerve

Sural arteries

Plantaris

Sural nerve

Common fibular nerve

Popliteus

Anterior tibial artery

Soleus

Fibular artery

Flexor digitorum longus

Plantaris tendon

Tibialis posterior

Posterior tibial artery

Flexor hallucis longus

Tibial nerve

Fibular artery

Perforating branch of fibular artery

Communicating branch of fibular artery

Medial calcaneal nerve

Lateral calcaneal branch of fibular artery

Plate 18.2 Arteries and nerves of the posterior leg.

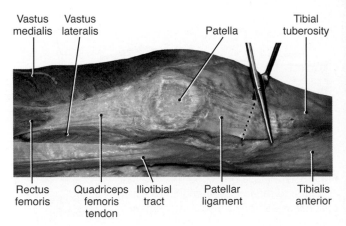

Vastus medialis

Vastus lateralis

Patella

Tibial tuberosity

Rectus femoris

Quadriceps femoris tendon

Iliotibial tract

Patellar ligament

Tibialis anterior

Fig. 18.15 Medial and lateral retinacula cut, exposing patellar ligament and quadriceps femoris tendon. Patellar ligament scissors-cut *(dotted line)* close to tibial tuberosity.

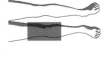

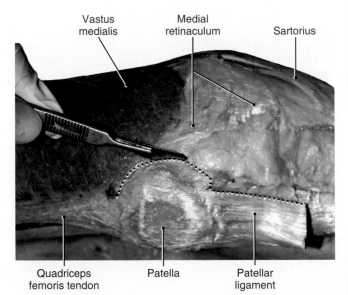

Vastus medialis

Medial retinaculum

Sartorius

Quadriceps femoris tendon

Patella

Patellar ligament

Fig. 18.16 Incision continued with scalpel lateral and medial to patella.

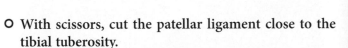

○ With scissors, cut the patellar ligament close to the tibial tuberosity.

○ Continue the incision with a scalpel lateral and medial to the patella to separate the patella from surrounding connective tissue (Fig. 18.16).

○ Detach the patella from its subcutaneous prepatellar and infrapatellar bursae and fat, and reflect it superiorly, preserving its attachment to the quadriceps femoris tendon (Fig. 18.17).

○ Cut the attachment of the vastus medialis muscle from the medial side of the knee, and expose this area (Fig. 18.18).

○ Similarly, cut the tendon of the biceps femoris muscle from the head of the fibula (Fig. 18.19).

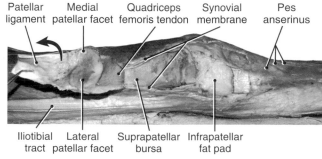

Patellar ligament | Medial patellar facet | Quadriceps femoris tendon | Synovial membrane | Pes anserinus

Iliotibial tract | Lateral patellar facet | Suprapatellar bursa | Infrapatellar fat pad

Fig. 18.17 Patella detached from bursae and fat and reflected superiorly, retaining quadriceps femoris muscle attachment.

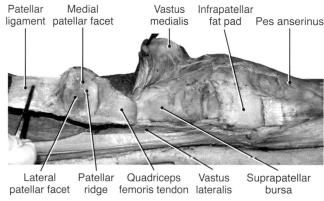

Patellar ligament | Medial patellar facet | Vastus medialis | Infrapatellar fat pad | Pes anserinus

Lateral patellar facet | Patellar ridge | Quadriceps femoris tendon | Vastus lateralis | Suprapatellar bursa

Fig. 18.18 Vastus medialis muscle reflected from medial side of knee.

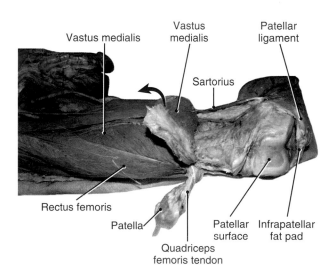

Vastus medialis | Vastus medialis | Patellar ligament

Sartorius

Rectus femoris

Patella | Patellar surface | Infrapatellar fat pad

Quadriceps femoris tendon

Fig. 18.19 Tendon of biceps femoris muscle incised from the head of fibula.

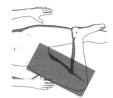

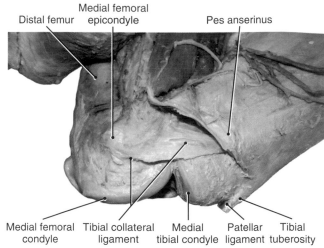

Medial femoral epicondyle
Distal femur | Pes anserinus

Medial femoral condyle | Tibial collateral ligament | Medial tibial condyle | Patellar ligament | Tibial tuberosity

Fig. 18.20 Knee flexed at joint to locate pes anserinus.

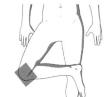

- After releasing these attachments, flex the knee joint (Fig. 18.20).
- On the medial side of the knee joint, inferior and medial to the tuberosity of the tibia, trace the common insertion of the tendons of the **sartorius, gracilis, and semitendinosus muscles,** the *pes anserinus.*
- Just superior to the pes anserinus, identify the *tibial (medial) collateral ligament.*

ANATOMY **NOTE**

The **tibial collateral ligament** is a thick band of connective tissue that extends from the medial femoral epicondyle to the medial tibial condyle; it also attaches to the medial meniscus.

- Using scissors, cut the **tibial collateral ligament** (Fig. 18.21). Similarly, cut the **biceps femoris tendon,** and identify a thick band of connective tissue extending between the lateral femoral condyle to the head of the fibula, the *fibular* collateral ligament.
- Remove the infrapatellar fat pad and **infrapatellar synovial fold** to expose the **anterior cruciate ligament** and the **medial and lateral menisci** between the femur and tibia (Fig. 18.22).
- Further expose the anterior cruciate ligament. With scissors, cut the anterior cruciate ligament (Fig. 18.23).
- Expose the **posterior cruciate ligament** by flexing the knee joint farther and observe the ligament as it is stretched (Fig. 18.24 and Plate 18.3).

Medial femoral condyle | Anterior cruciate ligament | Tibial collateral ligament | Medial meniscus

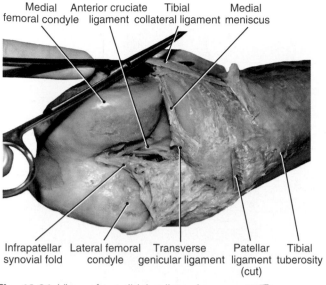

Infrapatellar synovial fold | Lateral femoral condyle | Transverse genicular ligament | Patellar ligament (cut) | Tibial tuberosity

Fig. 18.21 View of cut tibial collateral ligament.

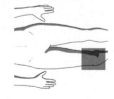

Anterior cruciate ligament | Medial femoral condyle | Medial meniscus | Great saphenous vein

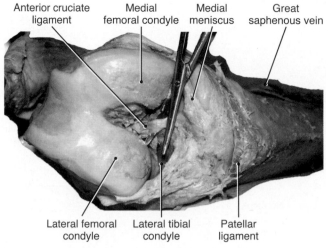

Lateral femoral condyle | Lateral tibial condyle | Patellar ligament

Fig. 18.23 View of cut anterior cruciate ligament.

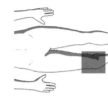

Infrapatellar synovial fold | Medial femoral condyle | Tibial collateral ligament | Medial meniscus | Tibial collateral ligament

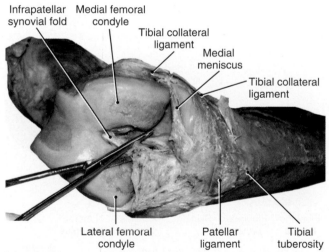

Lateral femoral condyle | Patellar ligament | Tibial tuberosity

Fig. 18.22 Removing infrapatellar fat pad and synovial fold, exposing anterior cruciate ligament and medial/lateral menisci.

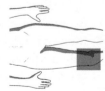

Medial femoral condyle | Medial tibial condyle | Medial meniscus | Patellar ligament

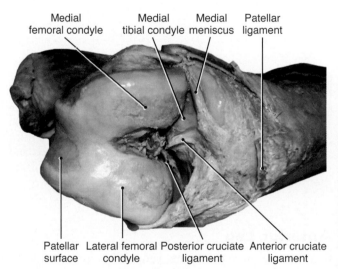

Patellar surface | Lateral femoral condyle | Posterior cruciate ligament | Anterior cruciate ligament

Fig. 18.24 In this view, appreciate the posterior cruciate ligament.

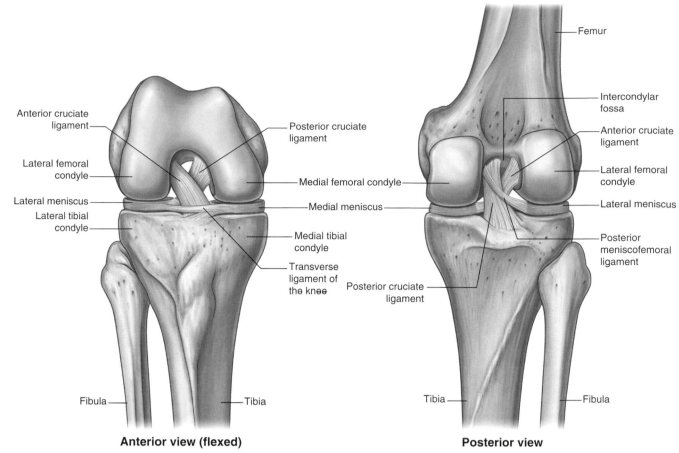

Anterior cruciate ligament

Lateral femoral condyle

Lateral meniscus

Lateral tibial condyle

Fibula — Tibia

Posterior cruciate ligament

Medial femoral condyle

Medial meniscus

Medial tibial condyle

Transverse ligament of the knee

Posterior cruciate ligament

Anterior view (flexed)

Femur

Intercondylar fossa

Anterior cruciate ligament

Lateral femoral condyle

Lateral meniscus

Posterior meniscofemoral ligament

Tibia — Fibula

Posterior view

Plate 18.3 Anterior and posterior views of the knee.

DISSECTION TIP

If time permits, cut the posterior part of the fibrous capsule of the knee joint. Again, identify the lateral and medial menisci and the posterior cruciate ligament. Find a thick connective tissue band between the lateral meniscus and the posterior cruciate ligament, the posterior menisco-femoral ligament.

Anterior Leg

○ With the cadaver supine, remove the remaining **skin** over the leg and expose the *crural fascia* (deep fascia) over the anterior compartment of the leg (Fig. 18.25).

○ Make a midline longitudinal incision along the lateral side of the anterior border of the tibia, reflecting the crural fascia laterally (Fig. 18.26).

○ Identify the *superior extensor retinaculum,* a flat, broad part of the deep fascia extending from the tibia to the fibula above the **lateral malleolus** (Fig. 18.27).

○ Identify the *tibialis anterior* muscle. Place your fingertip on its inferior border, and with blunt dissection, expose the **extensor digitorum longus muscle** (Fig. 18.28).

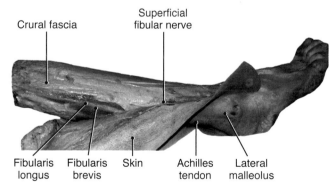

Crural fascia

Superficial fibular nerve

Fibularis longus   Fibularis brevis   Skin   Achilles tendon   Lateral malleolus

Fig. 18.25 Remaining skin over leg removed, exposing crural fascia over anterior compartment.

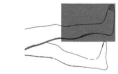

○ Trace its tendons towards the dorsum of the foot, where they run to the lateral four digits.

○ Find the **fibularis tertius muscle,** which is best seen distally lateral to the extensor digitorum longus muscle.

○ Appreciate the **extensor hallucis longus muscle** in the space between the tibialis anterior and extensor digitorum longus muscles (Fig. 18.29). Note that the tendon of the extensor hallucis longus inserts onto the base of the distal phalanx of the 1st digit.

DISSECTION TIP

To better visualize the deep part of the anterior compartment, place two retractors (one proximal and one distal) between the **tibialis anterior** and **fibularis longus** muscles (see Fig. 18.44).

○ Identify the *interosseous membrane* and the area between the extensor digitorum longus and tibialis anterior muscles (Fig. 18.30).

LATERAL LEG

○ Reflect the **fibularis longus** muscle inferiorly, and expose the **fibularis brevis** muscle as well as the **superficial fibular nerve** (Fig. 18.31).

ANATOMY **NOTE**

The fibularis longus is located superficially to the fibularis brevis muscle. Trace the insertion of the tendon of the fibularis brevis onto the tuberosity of the 5th metatarsal bone.

DISSECTION TIP

To highlight dissection landmarks, clean the fascia over the anteromedial surface of the tibia and expose the periosteum (Fig. 18.32).

ANKLE

○ Using a scalpel, make a shallow, circumferential incision on the dorsum of the foot (Fig. 18.33).

DISSECTION TIP

The skin of the dorsum of the foot is thin; therefore the incision must be shallow. Do not spend too much time exposing the entire dorsal venous arch.

○ Reflect the skin over the dorsum of the foot, and expose the tendons of the **extensor hallucis** and **extensor digitorum** muscles.

○ Identify and expose the **dorsal venous arch**, then trace the small saphenous vein at the lateral aspect of the

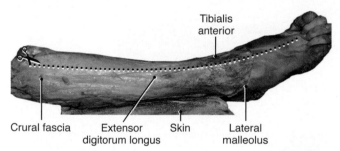

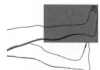

Fig. 18.26 *Dotted line* shows midline longitudinal incision along lateral side of anterior border of the tibia.

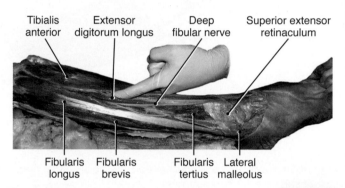

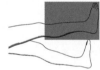

Fig. 18.28 Extensor digitorum longus tendons on dorsum of foot toward lateral four digits.

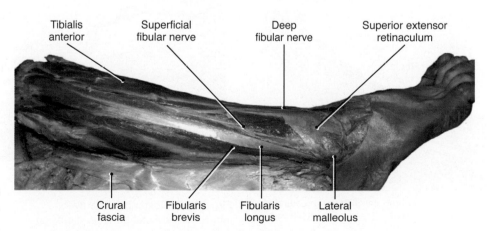

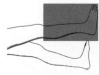

Fig. 18.27 In this view, appreciate the superior extensor retinaculum.

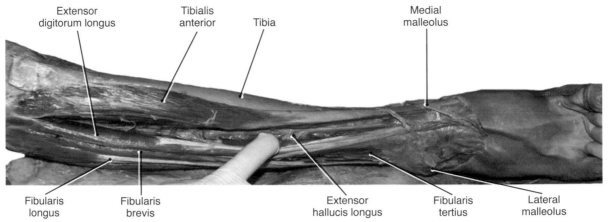

Fig. 18.29 View highlighting fibularis tertius, longus, and brevis muscles; anterior intermuscular septum; and extensor hallucis longus muscle.

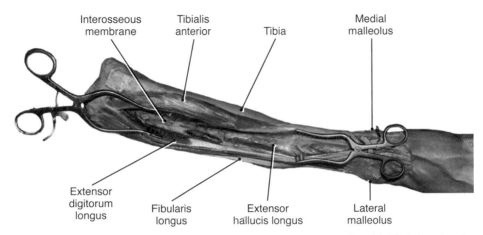
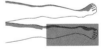

Fig. 18.30 Retractors placed between the tibialis anterior and fibularis longus muscles, highlighting the deep part of the anterior compartment.

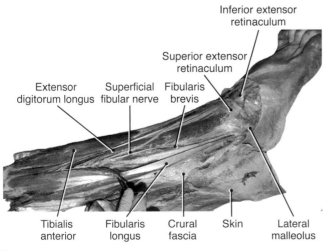

Fig. 18.31 Fibularis longus muscle reflected inferiorly, exposing fibularis brevis muscle as well as superficial fibular nerve.

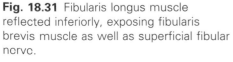

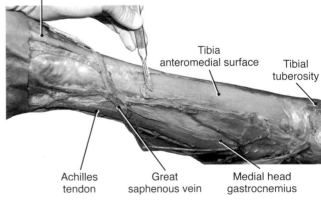

Fig. 18.32 Cleaning fascia over anteromedial tibial surface, exposing periosteum.

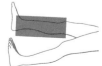

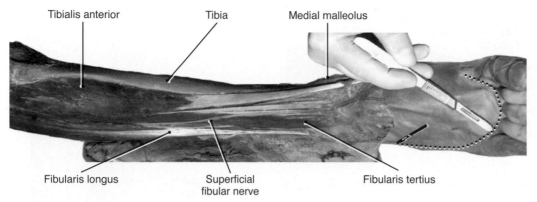

Fig. 18.33 Shallow circumferential incision *(dotted line)* on dorsum of foot.

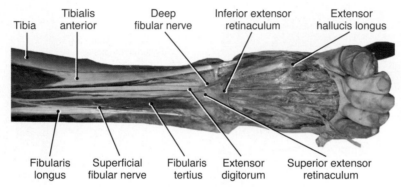

Fig. 18.34 Appreciate superior and inferior parts of extensor retinaculum.

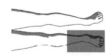

arch and the great saphenous vein at the medial portion of the dorsal venous arch traveling superiorly, anterior to the medial malleolus.

○ Identify the **extensor retinaculum**, divided into the superior and inferior parts.

ANATOMY **NOTE**

The superior extensor retinaculum extends from the tibia to the fibula above the lateral malleolus as a broad, flat part of the deep fascia (Fig. 18.34).

○ The inferior extensor retinaculum is a Y-shaped band of deep fascia forming a passage for the tendons of the extensor digitorum longus and fibularis tertius muscles. The inferior extensor retinaculum attaches to the *medial malleolus* (upper part) and to the *plantar aponeurosis* (lower band) (see Figs. 18.34 and 18.35).

○ Cut the superior and inferior portions of the extensor retinaculum over the tendons of the extensor digitorum muscle (Fig. 18.36).

○ Free the tendons of the extensor digitorum, extensor hallucis longus, tibialis anterior, and fibularis tertius

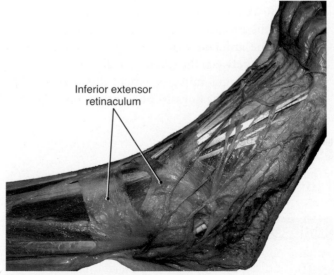

Fig. 18.35 Note the inferior extensor retinaculum as a Y-shaped band of deep fascia forming a passage for the tendons of the extensor digitorum longus and fibularis tertius muscles.

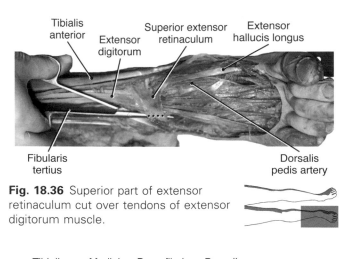

Fibularis
tertius

Dorsalis
pedis artery

Fig. 18.36 Superior part of extensor retinaculum cut over tendons of extensor digitorum muscle.

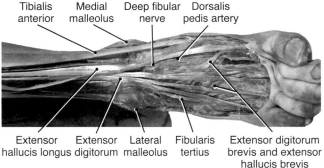

Fig. 18.37 Tendons of extensor digitorum, extensor hallucis longus, tibialis anterior, and fibularis tertius separated from underlying bursae and soft tissue.

muscles from the underlying bursae and soft tissues, toward their insertions (Fig. 18.37).

○ Identify the **extensor digitorum brevis** and its medial part, the **extensor hallucis brevis**, inserting onto the base of the proximal phalanx of the first digit.

○ Follow the **anterior tibial artery** to the level of the ankle joint between the extensor halluces and extensor digitorum longus muscles, where the anterior tibial artery becomes the **dorsalis pedis artery** (see Fig. 18.37 and Plate 18.4).

DISSECTION **TIP**

The dorsalis pedis artery is absent in approximately 20% of the population.

DISSECTION **TIP**

If time permits, continue the dissection as follows:
• Trace out the tendon of the extensor hallucis longus muscle to the distal phalanx of the 1st digit.
• Compare the extensor hallucis longus with the extensor digitorum longus muscle inserting onto the middle and distal phalanges.
• Follow the terminal branches of the dorsalis pedis artery: deep plantar branch and 1st metatarsal branch.

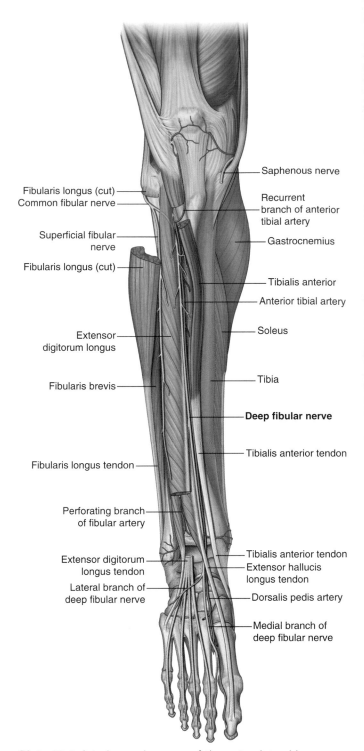

Plate 18.4 Arteries and nerves of the anterolateral leg.

○ Continue the dissection along the lateral aspect of ankle joint at the level of the *lateral malleolus* (see Fig. 18.38).

○ Expose the tendons of the fibularis brevis and fibularis longus muscles (Fig. 18.38).

○ Clean the fat around the lateral malleolus, and expose the structures of this region (see Fig. 18.38).

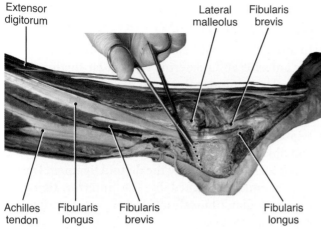

Extensor digitorum | Lateral malleolus | Fibularis brevis

Achilles tendon | Fibularis longus | Fibularis brevis | Fibularis longus

Fig. 18.38 View of exposed tendons of fibularis brevis and fibularis longus muscles.

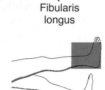

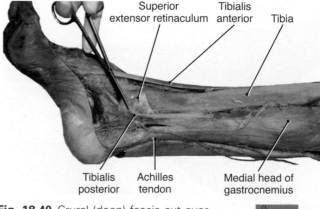

Superior extensor retinaculum | Tibialis anterior | Tibia

Tibialis posterior | Achilles tendon | Medial head of gastrocnemius

Fig. 18.40 Crural (deep) fascia cut over medial malleolus.

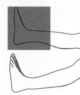

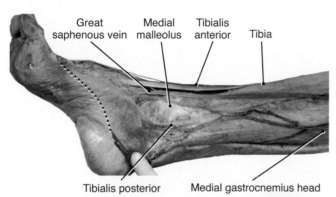

Great saphenous vein | Medial malleolus | Tibialis anterior | Tibia

Tibialis posterior | Medial gastrocnemius head

Fig. 18.39 View of skin incision over medial malleolus.

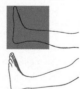

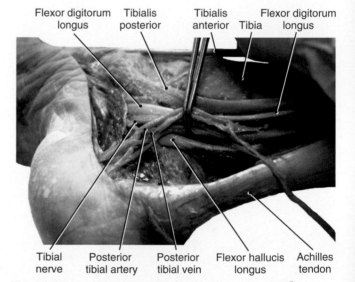

Flexor digitorum longus | Tibialis posterior | Tibialis anterior | Tibia | Flexor digitorum longus

Tibial nerve | Posterior tibial artery | Posterior tibial vein | Flexor hallucis longus | Achilles tendon

Fig. 18.41 Note the relationship of structures passing through the tarsal tunnel.

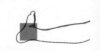

○ Cut the skin over the **medial malleolus** and expose the **crural fascia** (Fig. 18.39).

○ With scissors, cut the **crural fascia** over the medial malleolus (Fig. 18.40).

○ Identify the **flexor retinaculum** attaching between the medial malleolus and the medial surface of the calcaneus. This flexor retinaculum forms the **tarsal tunnel.**

○ Cut the **flexor retinaculum,** and expose the **tibial nerve, the posterior tibial artery, the tibialis posterior muscle, the flexor digitorum longus muscle,** and the **Achilles tendon.**

○ If time permits, expose the tendon of the **tibialis posterior muscle** to the **navicular bone,** one of its many insertion sites.

ANATOMY **NOTE**

The relationship of these structures to the medial malleolus is important for their recognition (Figs. 18.41 and 18.42). From anterior to posterior, the structures are arranged as follows (Plate 18.5):

• Tendon of tibialis posterior muscle
• Tendon of flexor digitorum longus muscle
• Posterior tibial artery and vein
• Tibial nerve
• Flexor hallucis longus muscle

To remember the relationship of these structures at the medial malleolus, use one of the following mnemonics:
Tom, Dick, And Harry
Tom Drives A Very Nervous Harry
Tom, Dick, and A Very Nervous Harry

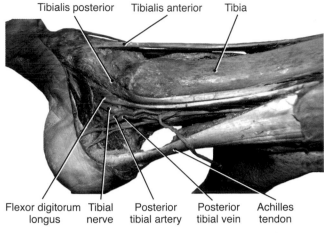

Tibialis posterior Tibialis anterior Tibia

Flexor digitorum Tibial Posterior Posterior Achilles
longus nerve tibial artery tibial vein tendon

Fig. 18.42 Appreciate the order of tendons, vessels, and nerves as they pass by the medial malleolus.

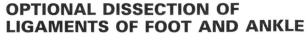

OPTIONAL DISSECTION OF LIGAMENTS OF FOOT AND ANKLE

○ Identify the lateral ligament of the ankle, formed by the **anterior** and **posterior talofibular ligaments** and the **calcaneofibular ligament**.

○ Identify the **interosseous talocalcaneal** ligament on the lateral side of the foot (Fig. 18.43).

○ Expose and cut the tendons of the tibialis anterior and tibialis posterior muscles at their insertion points.

○ Just underneath, identify the **deltoid ligament** (medial side of ankle), formed by **the anterior tibiotalar, tibionavicular, tibiocalcaneal, and posterior tibiotalar** parts (Fig. 18.44).

○ Look lateral and underneath the tendon of the tibialis posterior muscle for the **plantar calcaneonavicular** *(spring)* **ligament** connecting the calcaneus to the navicular bones.

○ Lateral to the calcaneonavicular ligament, expose the **long and short plantar ligaments** (Fig. 18.45).

See also Chapter 19.

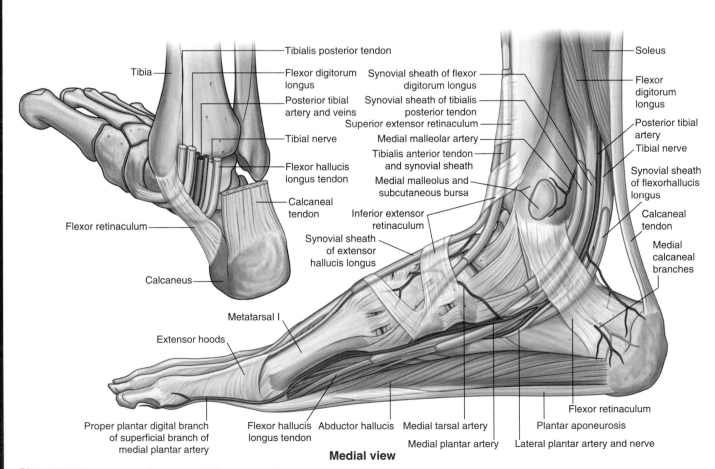

Medial view

Plate 18.5 Structures of the medial foot and ankle.

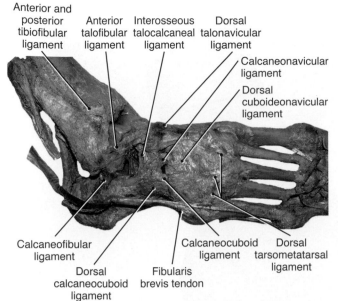

Anterior and posterior tibiofibular ligament
Anterior talofibular ligament
Interosseous talocalcaneal ligament
Dorsal talonavicular ligament
Calcaneonavicular ligament
Dorsal cuboideonavicular ligament
Calcaneofibular ligament
Dorsal calcaneocuboid ligament
Fibularis brevis tendon
Calcaneocuboid ligament
Dorsal tarsometatarsal ligament

Fig. 18.43 Optional dissection: lateral view of ankle, highlighting ligaments.

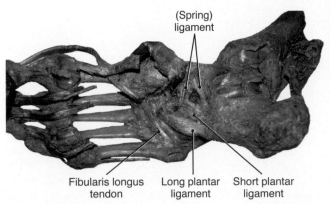

(Spring) ligament
Fibularis longus tendon
Long plantar ligament
Short plantar ligament

Fig. 18.45 Optional dissection: plantar view of foot, highlighting plantar calcaneonavicular (spring) ligament and long and short plantar ligaments.

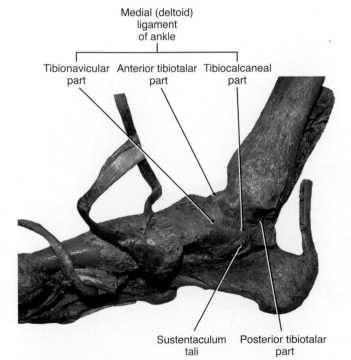

Medial (deltoid) ligament of ankle
Tibionavicular part
Anterior tibiotalar part
Tibiocalcaneal part
Sustentaculum tali
Posterior tibiotalar part

Fig. 18.44 Optional dissection: medial view of ankle, demonstrating deltoid (medial) ligament.

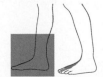

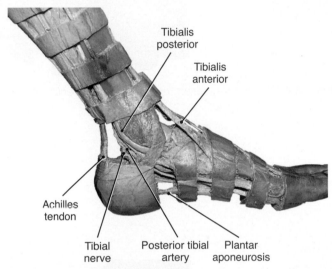

Tibialis posterior
Tibialis anterior
Achilles tendon
Tibial nerve
Posterior tibial artery
Plantar aponeurosis

Fig. 18.46 Special dissection: lateral view, demonstrating depth from skin to differing layers of foot, ankle, and leg, from superficial to deep.

DISSECTION TIP

The long plantar ligament crosses over the tendon of the fibularis longus muscle. The short plantar (plantar calcaneocuboid) ligament attaches to the cuboid bone. Sometimes, the long plantar ligament may be confused with the spring ligament attached to the navicular bone (see Fig. 18.45).

CREATIVE DISSECTION

○ In this dissection, we left strips of skin intact. We dissected the intervals in between to appreciate the depth from skin to the different layers of the foot, ankle, and leg from superficial to deep (Figs. 18.46 to 18.48).

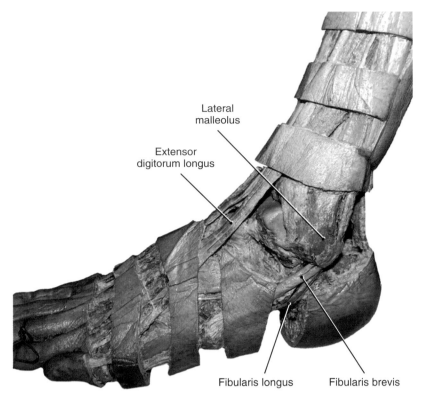

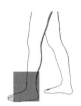

Fig. 18.47 Special dissection: medial view; appreciate depth from skin (superficial to deep) to different layers of the foot, ankle, and leg.

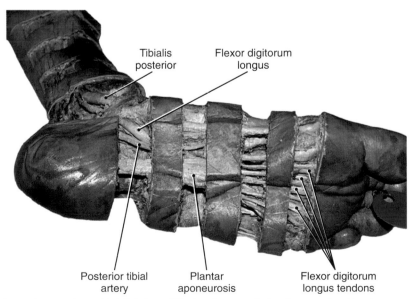

Fig. 18.48 Special dissection: plantar view, highlighting differing layers of the foot and ankle, from superficial to deep.

LABORATORY IDENTIFICATION CHECKLIST

NERVES

- ☐ Common fibular
  - ☐ Superficial fibular
  - ☐ Lateral sural cutaneous
- ☐ Sural communicating (normally formed from tibial and common fibular, but can form independently)
- ☐ Deep fibular
- ☐ Tibial nerve
  - ☐ Medial sural cutaneous
- ☐ Sural (normally formed from tibial and common fibular, but can form independently)

ARTERIES

- ☐ Popliteal
- ☐ Anterior tibial
- ☐ Posterior tibial
- ☐ Circumflex fibular
- ☐ Fibular

VEINS

- ☐ *Superficial*
  - ☐ Great (long) saphenous
  - ☐ Small (lesser) saphenous
- ☐ Deep
  - ☐ Popliteal
  - ☐ Posterior tibial
  - ☐ Fibular
  - ☐ Anterior tibial
  - ☐ Sural

MUSCLES

- ☐ *Anterior compartment*
- ☐ Tibialis anterior
- ☐ Extensor hallucis longus
- ☐ Extensor digitorum longus
- ☐ Fibularis tertius
- ☐ *Posterior compartment*

- ☐ Superficial
  - ☐ Gastrocnemius
  - ☐ Soleus
  - ☐ Plantaris
- ☐ Deep
  - ☐ Popliteus
  - ☐ Flexor hallucis longus
  - ☐ Flexor digitorum longus
  - ☐ Tibialis posterior
- ☐ *Lateral compartment*
- ☐ Fibularis longus
- ☐ Fibularis brevis

CONNECTIVE TISSUE

- ☐ Anterior intermuscular septum
- ☐ Transverse intermuscular septum
- ☐ Posterior intermuscular septum
- ☐ Interosseous membrane
- ☐ Superior extensor retinaculum

LIGAMENTS

- ☐ *Lateral ankle complex*
  - ☐ Anterior talofibular ligament
  - ☐ Calcaneofibular ligament
  - ☐ Posterior talofibular ligament
- ☐ *Medial ankle complex*
  - ☐ Deltoid
    - ☐ Anterior tibiotalar part
    - ☐ Tibionavicular part
    - ☐ Tibiocalcaneal part
    - ☐ Posterior tibiotalar part
    - ☐ Long
    - ☐ Short
    - ☐ Spring

BONES

- ☐ Fibula
- ☐ Tibia

ATLAS REFERENCES
Netter: 516–528
McMinn: 344–354
Gray's Atlas: 350–363

BEFORE YOU BEGIN
Identify and palpate the **calcaneus**, the **lateral longitudinal arch**, and the five **metatarsal heads** (Fig. 19.1).

SKIN AND SUBCUTANEOUS TISSUE
○ Make a longitudinal incision starting from the lateral side of the calcaneus and following the lateral side of the lateral longitudinal arch, terminating at the 1st metatarsal head (Fig. 19.2).

DISSECTION **TIP**

You also could begin the incision from the plantar surface of the 1st metatarsal head and then end at the calcaneus.

DISSECTION **TIP**

An alternate incision involves making a longitudinal cut from the calcaneus to the first digit and a second, transverse incision from the first digit to the lateral longitudinal arch, then removing the skin laterally from the foot.

○ Reflect the skin medially while maintaining its attachment to the calcaneus (Fig. 19.3). Observe the fatty,

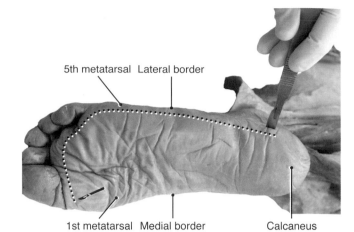

5th metatarsal   Lateral border

1st metatarsal   Medial border   Calcaneus

Fig. 19.2 Longitudinal incision starts from lateral side of calcaneus and follows lateral longitudinal arch.

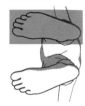

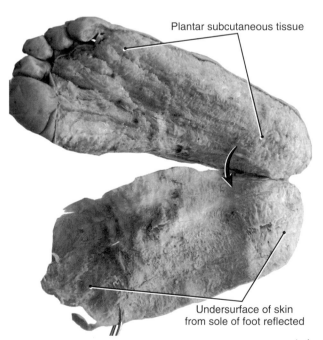

Plantar subcutaneous tissue

Undersurface of skin from sole of foot reflected

Fig. 19.3 Skin completely reflected over plantar portion of foot, maintaining attachment to calcaneus.

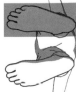

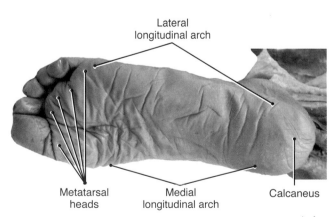

Lateral longitudinal arch

Metatarsal heads   Medial longitudinal arch   Calcaneus

Fig. 19.1 View of the plantar surface of the foot for identifying calcaneus, lateral longitudinal arch, and five metatarsal heads.

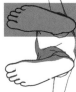

plantar subcutaneous tissue, and the thick layer of connective tissue, the **plantar aponeurosis**.

○ With a scalpel, make an incision from the lateral side of the calcaneus, reflecting the **plantar subcutaneous tissue** over the plantar aponeurosis medially (Fig. 19.4).

○ Remove the fat and expose the plantar aponeurosis with its fibrous slips to the digits.

(SUPERFICIAL) 1ST LAYER OF PLANTAR FOOT MUSCLES

ANATOMY **NOTE**

The three muscles that make up the 1st and most superficial layer of muscles of the plantar surface of the foot are abductor hallucis, flexor digitorum brevis, and abductor digiti minimi.

○ On the lateral side of the foot, identify the **abductor digiti minimi** muscle and the underlying **flexor digiti minimi** muscle (Fig. 19.5).

○ With a scalpel, cut the plantar aponeurosis at its junction with the flexor digiti minimi muscle, and reflect it toward the calcaneus (see Figs. 19.5 and 19.6).

○ Just underneath the plantar aponeurosis, separate the **flexor digitorum brevis** muscle, which arises from the deep surface of the aponeurosis (see Fig. 19.6).

○ Carefully dissect out the fibrous attachments between the plantar aponeurosis and the digits (Fig. 19.7).

○ Identify and clean the **abductor hallucis** muscle located on the medial side of the foot (see Fig. 19.7).

○ Lateral to the abductor hallucis muscle, clean and expose the tendons of the **flexor digitorum brevis** muscle (see Fig. 19.7).

○ Lateral **to the flexor digitorum brevis**, identify and clean the abductor digiti minimi muscle (see Fig. 19.7).

○ Between the abductor hallucis and flexor digitorum brevis muscles, identify and expose the **medial plantar nerve** (see Fig. 19.7).

○ Identify the digital branches of the medial plantar nerve (see Fig. 19.7).

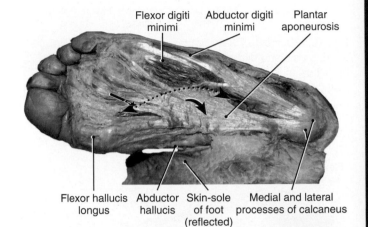

Flexor digiti minimi   Abductor digiti minimi   Plantar aponeurosis

Flexor hallucis longus   Abductor hallucis   Skin-sole of foot (reflected)   Medial and lateral processes of calcaneus

Fig. 19.5 Fat removal exposes the plantar aponeurosis and fibrous slips to the digits.

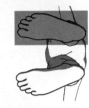

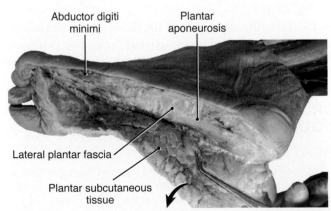

Abductor digiti minimi   Plantar aponeurosis

Lateral plantar fascia

Plantar subcutaneous tissue

Fig. 19.4 Lateral side of calcaneus incised, reflecting fat over plantar aponeurosis medially.

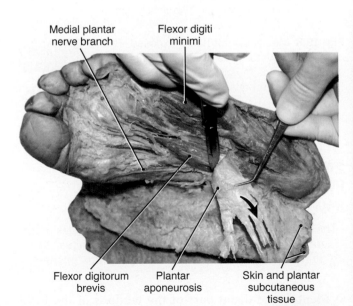

Medial plantar nerve branch   Flexor digiti minimi

Flexor digitorum brevis   Plantar aponeurosis   Skin and plantar subcutaneous tissue

Fig. 19.6 Abductor digiti minimi muscle and underlying flexor digiti minimi on lateral side of foot, with plantar aponeurosis reflected toward calcaneus, and flexor digitorum brevis muscle separated.

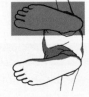

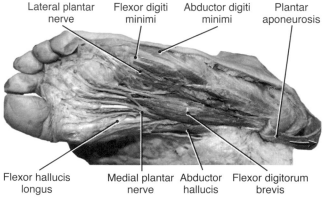

Lateral plantar nerve — Flexor digiti minimi — Abductor digiti minimi — Plantar aponeurosis

Flexor hallucis longus — Medial plantar nerve — Abductor hallucis — Flexor digitorum brevis

Fig. 19.7 Dissected view between plantar aponeurosis and digits reveals digital branches of medial plantar nerve, abductor hallucis muscle, and tendons of flexor digitorum brevis and abductor digiti minimi muscles.

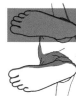

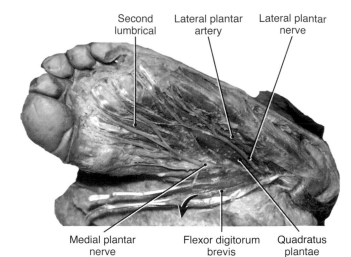

Second lumbrical — Lateral plantar artery — Lateral plantar nerve

Medial plantar nerve — Flexor digitorum brevis — Quadratus plantae

Fig. 19.9 View of lateral plantar nerve and artery underneath flexor digitorum brevis muscle.

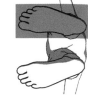

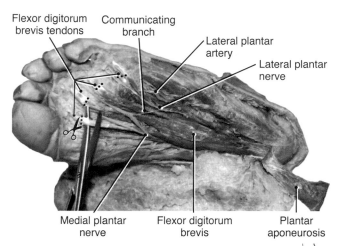

Flexor digitorum brevis tendons — Communicating branch — Lateral plantar artery — Lateral plantar nerve

Medial plantar nerve — Flexor digitorum brevis — Plantar aponeurosis

Fig. 19.8 Medial plantar nerve exposed between abductor hallucis and flexor digitorum brevis muscles, with distal parts of flexor digitorum brevis tendons incised.

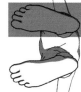

2ND LAYER OF PLANTAR FOOT MUSCLES

ANATOMY **NOTE**

The muscles that make up the 2nd layer of muscles of the plantar region of the foot are flexor hallucis longus, flexor digitorum longus, lumbricals, and quadratus plantae.

○ Identify the distal part of the tendons of the flexor digitorum brevis muscle, and cut them using scissors (Fig. 19.8).

DISSECTION **TIP**

Be careful not to cut the medial plantar nerve.

○ Reflect the tendons (with the belly of the flexor digitorum brevis) posteriorly (Fig. 19.9).
○ Just underneath the flexor digitorum brevis, clean and expose the **lateral plantar nerve** and **lateral plantar artery** as they travel to the lateral side of the foot (see Fig. 19.9 and Plate 19.1).
○ Identify and clean the tendon of the **flexor hallucis longus** muscle located on the medial side of the foot and inserting onto the base of the distal phalanx of the 1st digit (Fig. 19.10).
○ Lateral to the flexor hallucis longus muscle, identify the tendons of the **flexor digitorum longus** muscle inserting onto the distal phalanges of the remaining four digits (see Fig. 19.10).
○ Arising from the tendons of the flexor digitorum longus, identify the four **lumbrical muscles** (see Fig. 19.10).
○ Lateral to the main belly of the flexor digitorum longus, identify a small muscle arising from the calcaneus and inserting onto the flexor digitorum, the **quadratus plantae muscle** (see Fig. 19.10).

3RD LAYER OF PLANTAR FOOT MUSCLES

ANATOMY **NOTE**

The muscles that occupy the 3rd layer of muscles of the plantar aspect of the foot are adductor hallucis, flexor hallucis brevis, abductor digiti minimi, and flexor digiti minimi brevis.

○ With scissors, cut the tendon of the flexor digitorum longus at the posterior aspect of the foot near the calcaneus (Fig. 19.11).

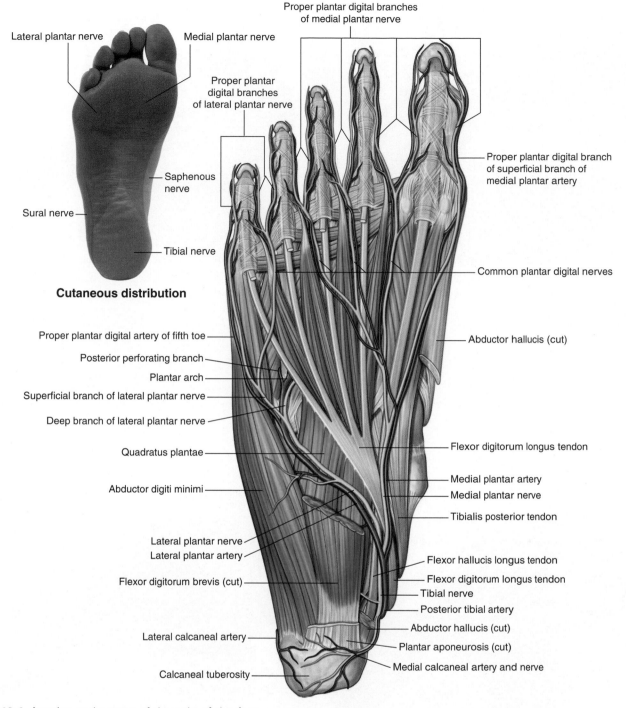

Lateral plantar nerve

Medial plantar nerve

Proper plantar digital branches
of medial plantar nerve

Proper plantar
digital branches
of lateral plantar nerve

Proper plantar digital branch
of superficial branch of
medial plantar artery

Saphenous
nerve

Sural nerve

Tibial nerve

Common plantar digital nerves

Cutaneous distribution

Proper plantar digital artery of fifth toe

Abductor hallucis (cut)

Posterior perforating branch

Plantar arch

Superficial branch of lateral plantar nerve

Deep branch of lateral plantar nerve

Flexor digitorum longus tendon

Quadratus plantae

Medial plantar artery

Abductor digiti minimi

Medial plantar nerve

Tibialis posterior tendon

Lateral plantar nerve

Flexor hallucis longus tendon

Lateral plantar artery

Flexor digitorum longus tendon

Flexor digitorum brevis (cut)

Tibial nerve

Posterior tibial artery

Abductor hallucis (cut)

Lateral calcaneal artery

Plantar aponeurosis (cut)

Medial calcaneal artery and nerve

Calcaneal tuberosity

Plate 19.1 Arteries and nerves of the sole of the foot.

- Continue the dissection by transecting the quadratus plantae muscle close to its calcaneal origin (Fig. 19.12).
- Reflect the transected muscle toward the toes (Fig. 19.13).
- Clean the small amounts of fascia and fat (Fig. 19.14).
- Identify the two heads of the **adductor hallucis** muscle, the oblique head and transverse head (see Fig. 19.14).

- Posterior to the two heads of the adductor hallucis muscle, identify the fibularis longus tendon and its attachments (see Fig. 19.14).
- Cut the tendon of the flexor hallucis longus muscle, and reflect it toward the great toe, exposing the **flexor hallucis brevis** muscle underneath.
- On the lateral side of the foot, retract the tendon of the abductor digiti minimi muscle, and medially and deep to it, identify the **flexor digiti minimi brevis** muscle.

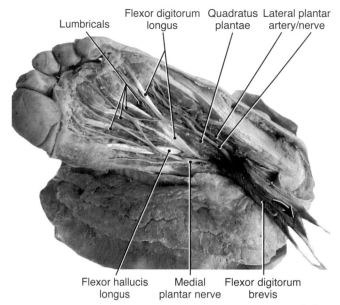

Lumbricals · Flexor digitorum longus · Quadratus plantae · Lateral plantar artery/nerve

Flexor hallucis longus · Medial plantar nerve · Flexor digitorum brevis

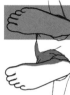

Fig. 19.10 View highlighting tendon of flexor hallucis longus muscle on medial side of foot.

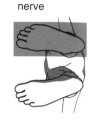

Communicating branch between medial and lateral plantar nerves · Flexor digitorum longus · Quadratus plantae

Flexor hallucis longus · Medial plantar nerve · Lateral plantar nerve

Fig. 19.12 Quadratus plantae muscle transected.

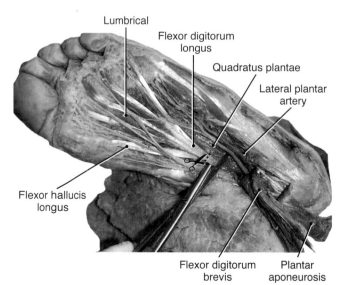

Lumbrical · Flexor digitorum longus · Quadratus plantae · Lateral plantar artery

Flexor hallucis longus

Flexor digitorum brevis · Plantar aponeurosis

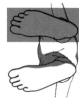

Fig. 19.11 Tendon of flexor digitorum longus incised at posterior aspect of foot near calcaneus.

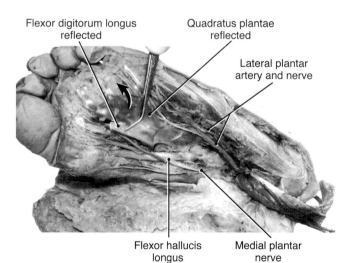

Flexor digitorum longus reflected · Quadratus plantae reflected · Lateral plantar artery and nerve

Flexor hallucis longus · Medial plantar nerve

Fig. 19.13 Quadratus plantae muscle reflected toward the toes.

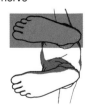

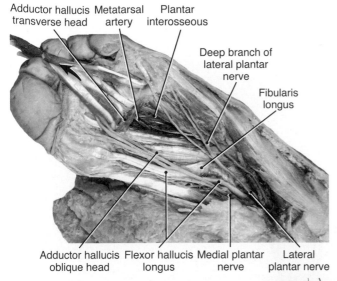

Adductor hallucis Metatarsal Plantar
transverse head artery interosseous

Deep branch of
lateral plantar
nerve

Fibularis
longus

Adductor hallucis Flexor hallucis Medial plantar Lateral
oblique head longus nerve plantar nerve

Fig. 19.14 Tendon of flexor hallucis longus reflected toward the great toe, exposing the flexor hallucis brevis muscle; tendon of abductor digiti minimi reflected to locate the flexor digiti minimi brevis muscle.

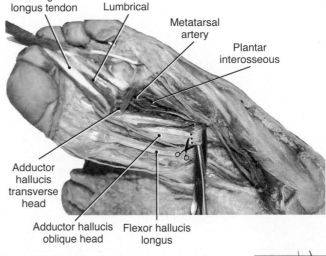

Flexor digitorum
longus tendon Lumbrical

Metatarsal
artery

Plantar
interosseous

Adductor
hallucis
transverse
head

Adductor hallucis Flexor hallucis
oblique head longus

Fig. 19.15 Plantar interosseous muscles exposed in space between the two heads of the adductor hallucis muscle, with the oblique head cut.

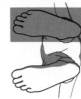

(DEEP) 4TH LAYER OF PLANTAR FOOT MUSCLES

○ Trace the **lateral plantar nerve** from its origin to its final distribution, and identify its superficial and **deep branches** (see Fig. 19.1 and Plate 19.2).

○ In the space between the two heads of the adductor hallucis muscle, expose the **interosseous muscles** (see Fig. 19.14).

○ With scissors, cut the oblique head of the adductor hallucis muscle (Fig. 19.15).

○ Fully expose and trace the fibularis longus tendon to its insertion onto the 1st cuneiform and 1st metatarsal bones (Fig. 19.16).

OPTIONAL DISSECTION

○ Follow the lateral plantar artery along the lateral plantar nerve and identify the deep branch of the lateral plantar nerve at the lateral side of the oblique head of the adductor hallucis muscle (see Plate 19.1).

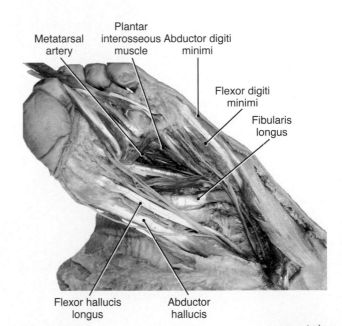

Plantar
Metatarsal interosseous Abductor digiti
artery muscle minimi

Flexor digiti
minimi

Fibularis
longus

Flexor hallucis Abductor
longus hallucis

Fig. 19.16 Identify the fibularis longus tendon and insertion onto the 1st cuneiform and 1st metatarsal bones.

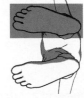

ANATOMY **NOTE**

At this point, the lateral plantar artery gives off a branch to form the plantar arch, just underneath the oblique head of the adductor hallucis muscle.

ANATOMY **NOTE**

In the space between the 1st and 2nd metatarsals, the deep plantar arch joins the plantar branch of the dorsalis pedis artery.

○ Identify the **plantar arch** and trace its branches, the **metatarsal branches**, which provide **plantar digital vessels** to the digits (see Plate 19.1).

○ Follow the plantar arch to the base of the 1st metatarsal and identify the **plantar branch to the dorsalis pedis artery** (see Plate 19.1).

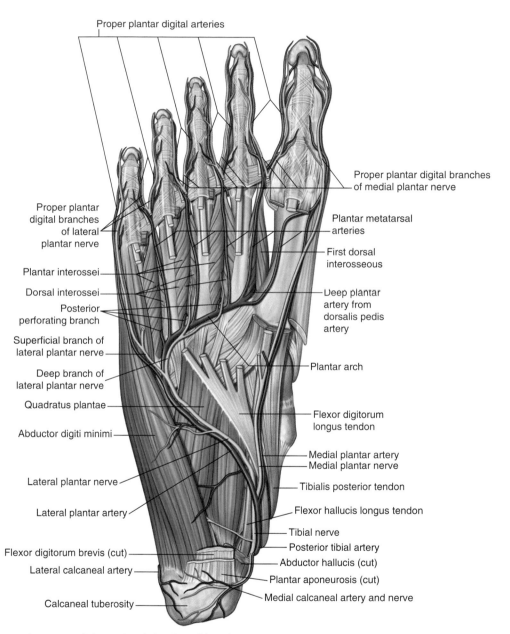

Proper plantar digital arteries

Proper plantar
digital branches
of lateral
plantar nerve

Plantar interossei

Dorsal interossei

Posterior
perforating branch

Superficial branch of
lateral plantar nerve

Deep branch of
lateral plantar nerve

Quadratus plantae

Abductor digiti minimi

Lateral plantar nerve

Lateral plantar artery

Flexor digitorum brevis (cut)

Lateral calcaneal artery

Calcaneal tuberosity

Proper plantar digital branches
of medial plantar nerve

Plantar metatarsal
arteries

First dorsal
interosseous

Deep plantar
artery from
dorsalis pedis
artery

Plantar arch

Flexor digitorum
longus tendon

Medial plantar artery
Medial plantar nerve

Tibialis posterior tendon

Flexor hallucis longus tendon

Tibial nerve
Posterior tibial artery

Abductor hallucis (cut)

Plantar aponeurosis (cut)

Medial calcaneal artery and nerve

Plate 19.2 Arteries and nerves of the sole of the foot (deep).

LABORATORY IDENTIFICATION CHECKLIST

NERVES
- ☐ Medial plantar
  - ☐ Common plantar digital
    - ☐ Plantar digital
- ☐ Lateral plantar
  - ☐ Common plantar digital
    - ☐ Plantar digital
- ☐ Superficial fibular
  - ☐ Dorsal digital branches
- ☐ Deep fibular
  - ☐ Dorsal digital branches
- ☐ Medial calcaneal
- ☐ Lateral calcaneal

ARTERIES
- ☐ Dorsalis pedis
  - ☐ Lateral tarsal
  - ☐ Arcuate
  - ☐ Deep plantar
- ☐ Dorsal metatarsal
  - ☐ Dorsal digital
- ☐ Medial plantar
- ☐ Plantar metatarsal
  - ☐ Common plantar digital
    - ☐ Plantar digital
- ☐ Lateral plantar
- ☐ *Plantar arch*
  - ☐ Plantar metatarsal
    - ☐ Common plantar digital
      - ☐ Plantar digital

VEINS
- ☐ Dorsal venous arch

MUSCLES
- ☐ *Dorsal muscles and tendons*
  - ☐ Extensor hallucis brevis
  - ☐ Extensor digitorum brevis
  - ☐ Extensor hallucis longus tendon
  - ☐ Extensor digitorum longus tendons
  - ☐ Tibialis anterior tendon
- ☐ *Plantar muscles and leg muscle tendons*
- ☐ Abductor hallucis

- ☐ Flexor hallucis brevis
  - ☐ Medial head
  - ☐ Lateral head
- ☐ Flexor hallucis longus tendon
- ☐ Flexor digitorum brevis
- ☐ Flexor digiti minimi brevis
- ☐ Abductor digiti minimi
- ☐ Flexor digitorum longus tendons
- ☐ Quadratus plantae
- ☐ Lumbricals
- ☐ Fibularis longus tendon
- ☐ Tibialis posterior tendon
- ☐ Fibularis brevis tendon
- ☐ Adductor hallucis
  - ☐ Transverse head
  - ☐ Oblique head
- ☐ Plantar interossei
- ☐ Dorsal interossei

LIGAMENTS
- ☐ Plantar calcaneonavicular (spring) ligament
- ☐ Long plantar ligament
- ☐ Plantar calcaneocuboid (short plantar) ligament

CONNECTIVE TISSUE
- ☐ Plantar aponeurosis
- ☐ Inferior extensor retinaculum

BONES
- ☐ *Tarsal bones*
  - ☐ Calcaneus
  - ☐ Talus
  - ☐ Cuboid
  - ☐ Navicular
  - ☐ Medial cuneiform
  - ☐ Middle cuneiform
  - ☐ Lateral cuneiform
  - ☐ Metatarsals
  - ☐ Phalanges
    - ☐ Proximal
    - ☐ Middle
    - ☐ Distal

CLINICAL APPLICATIONS

TROCHANTERIC BURSITIS INJECTION

Gray's Anatomy for Students: 296-299
Netter: 481, 482, 494

Clinical Application

Introduce local anesthetic using an intrabursal injection to relieve pain of inflamed trochanteric bursa.

Anatomic Landmarks (Figs. VII.1 and VII.2)

- Skin
- Subcutaneous tissue
- Iliotibial fascia
- Tensor fasciae latae
- Trochanteric bursa
- Greater trochanter

PREPATELLAR BURSITIS ASPIRATION/INJECTION

Gray's Anatomy for Students: 325–326
Netter: 498–502

Clinical Application

Introduce local anesthesia into prepatellar bursa to withdraw fluid and relieve pain from prepatellar bursa.

Anatomic Landmarks (Figs. VII.3)

- Skin
- Patella
- Subcutaneous tissue
- Prepatellar bursa

SUPRAPATELLAR BURSITIS ASPIRATION/INJECTION

Gray's Anatomy for Students: 325, 326
Netter: 498, 502

Clinical Application

Introduce local anesthesia into suprapatellar bursa to relieve pain from prepatellar bursa.

Anatomic Landmarks (Fig. VII.4)

- Skin
- Subcutaneous tissue
- Suprapatellar bursa

PLANTAR FASCITIS INJECTION

Gray's Anatomy for Students: 356
Netter: 523

Clinical Application

Injection of local anesthetic at the point of maximal tenderness within the plantar fascia or plantar aponeurosis, often near its attachment to the medial process of the calcaneal tuberosity, to relieve pain caused by inflamed fascia.

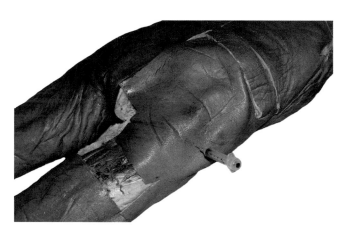

Fig. VII.1

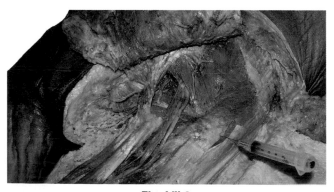

Fig. VII.2

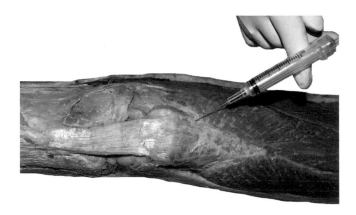

Fig. VII.3

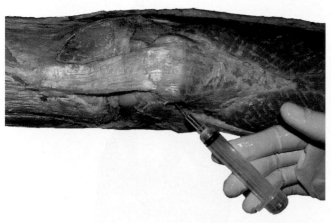

Fig. VII.4

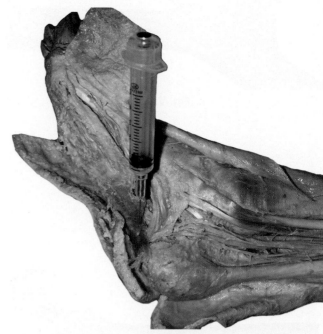

Fig. VII.6

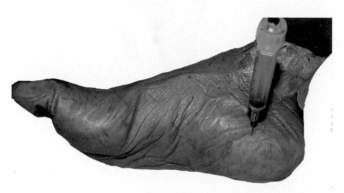

Fig. VII.5

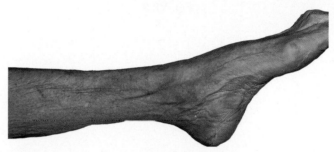

Fig. VII.7

Anatomic Landmarks (Figs. VII.5 and VII.6)

- Skin
- Subcutaneous tissue/fat pad
- Plantar fascia/aponeurosis
- Calcaneal tuberosity

ARTHROCENTESIS: KNEE

Gray's Anatomy for Students: 325, 326
Netter: 498–501

Clinical Application

Introduce needle into the knee joint to withdraw fluid and to inject medication.

Anatomic Landmarks

- Skin
- Subcutaneous tissue
- Patella
- Intercondylar notch
- Joint cavity

GREAT SAPHENOUS VEIN CUTDOWN OR CANNULATION

Gray's Anatomy for Students: 364
Netter: 473, 475

Clinical Application

Procedure to cannulate great saphenous vein for infusion of fluids.

Anatomic Landmarks (Figs. VII.7 and VII.8)

- Medial malleolus
- Skin
- Subcutaneous tissue
- Great saphenous vein
- Saphenous nerve

FEMUR AND KNEE REPLACEMENT

Fig. VII.9 depicts a head of the femur replacement.
Fig. VII.10 depicts a knee replacement.

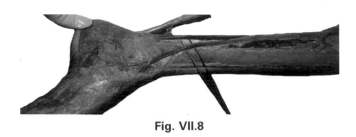

Fig. VII.8

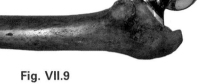

Fig. VII.9

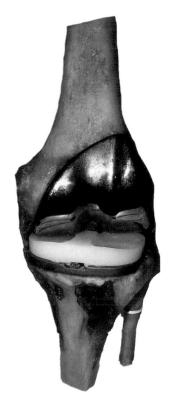

Fig. VII.10

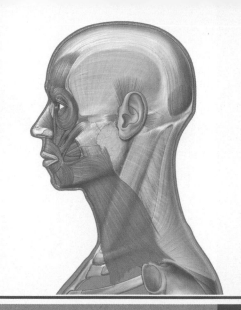

CHAPTER 20 | NECK

ATLAS REFERENCES

Netter: 8, 9, 31, 32, 35, 38–41, 141–142
McMinn: 28–37
Gray's Atlas: 536, 539–551

BEFORE YOU BEGIN

Palpate the following landmarks on your neck or the cadaver:

- Mental protuberance
- Hyoid bone
- Laryngeal prominence ("Adam's apple")
- Cricoid cartilage
- Jugular notch
- Thyroid gland

ANATOMIC TRIANGLES

ANATOMY NOTE

The neck may be divided into smaller topographic areas, the *triangles* of the neck. Specifically, the "carotid triangle" and the "root of the neck" are involved in many surgical procedures on the neck. There are two major triangles of the neck, the anterior and posterior cervical triangles (Fig. 20.1). The *anterior cervical triangle* is demarcated anteriorly by the midline of the neck; its base is the lower border of the mandible, and the posterior border is the anterior boundary of the sternocleidomastoid muscle. The *posterior cervical triangle* is bounded by the posterior border of the sternocleidomastoid muscle, the middle third of the clavicle, and the anterior border of the trapezius muscle. The cervical triangles may be subdivided as follows:

Anterior cervical triangle
1. Digastric triangle
2. Submental triangle
3. Carotid triangle
4. Muscular triangle

Posterior cervical triangle
5. Occipital triangle
6. Supraclavicular triangle

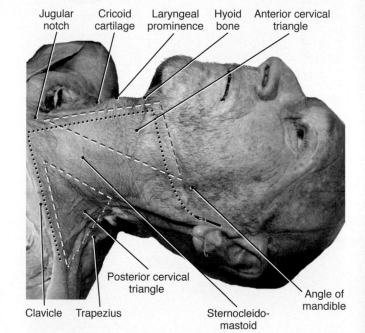

Fig. 20.1 Anterolateral view of surface anatomy of the neck, highlighting hyoid bone, laryngeal prominence, sternal notch, angle of mandible, sternoclcidomastoid muscle and anterior and posterior triangles of the neck.

NECK DISSECTION

- ○ Make a midline incision through the skin from the jugular notch to the mental protuberance.
- ○ A second incision should be made from the jugular notch laterally, along the clavicles bilaterally, to the acromion processes.
- ○ Make a final incision from the mental protuberance along the inferior border of the mandible, toward the earlobe (Fig. 20.2). Carefully reflect the skin over the neck.

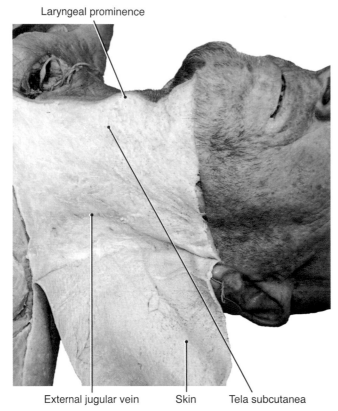

Laryngeal prominence

External jugular vein   Skin   Tela subcutanea

Fig. 20.2 Skin of neck reflected laterally, revealing tela subcutanea (subcutaneous tissue), laryngeal prominence, superficial lobe of submandibular gland, external jugular vein, and midline of the neck.

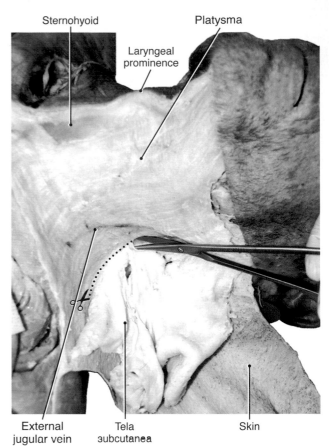

Sternohyoid   Platysma
Laryngeal
prominence

External   Tela   Skin
jugular vein   subcutanea

Fig. 20.4 Separation of lateral border of platysma muscle from tela subcutanea.

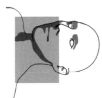

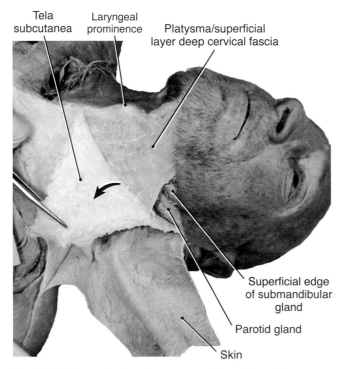

Tela   Laryngeal
subcutanea prominence   Platysma/superficial
                          layer deep cervical fascia

Superficial edge
of submandibular
gland

Parotid gland

Skin

Fig. 20.3 Skin and tela subcutanea reflected laterally, revealing platysma muscle, superficial layer of deep cervical fascia, superficial lobe of submandibular gland and sternocleidomastoid muscle.

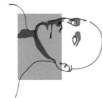

DISSECTION **TIP**

The skin over the neck is thin. Pay special attention during its reflection for the subcutaneous tissue so that you do not reflect the platysma muscle with the skin.

○ Start the dissection by reflecting the subcutaneous tissue from the mental protuberance inferiorly and laterally toward the clavicles to expose the platysma muscle (Fig. 20.3).
○ The platysma is pierced by the transverse cervical and supraclavicular nerves of the cervical plexus. Reflect the subcutaneous tissue over the platysma muscle (Fig. 20.4).
○ Separate the lateral border of the platysma from the subcutaneous tissue. Identify the sternocleidomastoid muscle posterior to the platysma muscle.
○ At the level of the clavicle, cut and reflect the platysma upward, toward the mandible (Figs. 20.5 and 20.6).
○ Similarly, at the angle of the mandible, cut and reflect the platysma anteriorly (Fig. 20.7).

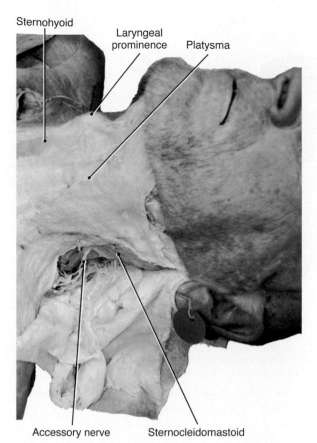

Fig. 20.5 Identification of accessory nerve at interval junction between platysma, sternocleidomastoid, and trapezius muscles.

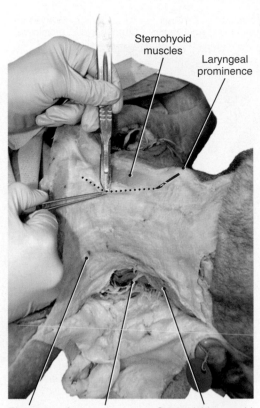

Fig. 20.6 Dissection of medial border of platysma muscle from underlying tissues.

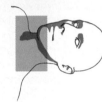

○ Preserve the attachment of the platysma muscle along the mandible (Fig. 20.8).

DISSECTION TIP

At this stage, it is possible to identify the cervical branch of the facial nerve, which innervates the platysma muscle, coursing from the inferior border of the parotid gland toward the platysma.

○ About 1 cm inferior to the angle of the mandible, expose the marginal mandibular branch of the facial nerve.

ANATOMY NOTE

The cervical branch of the facial nerve passes superficial to the facial vein and artery. The facial vein usually drains into the internal jugular vein through the retromandibular vein.

○ Notice the investing *cervical fascia* covering the sternocleidomastoid muscle (see Fig. 20.8). Observe the external jugular vein running lateral to the sternocleidomastoid muscle.

ANATOMY NOTE

The investing cervical fascia encircles the trapezius and sternocleidomastoid muscles before reaching the midline of the neck. In the gap between these muscles, this fascia forms the "roof" of the posterior cervical triangle. The "floor" of the posterior cervical triangle is provided by another fascia, the *prevertebral fascia,* which covers the musculature of the lateral and anterior aspects of the vertebral column. Between these two fascial layers there is a potential space.

○ Clean the superficial investing fascia over the sternocleidomastoid muscle (Fig. 20.9 and Plate 20.1).

DISSECTION TIP

Use care when you reflect the fascia not to sever any of the cutaneous nerves arising deep to the posterior edge of the sternocleidomastoid muscle.

○ Identify the external jugular vein running superficial to the sternocleidomastoid muscle, as well as the

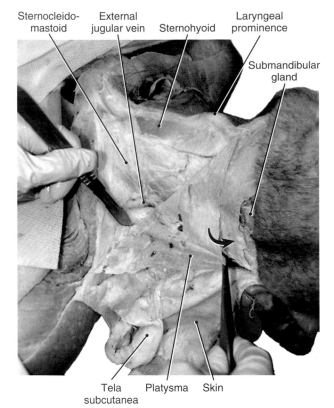

Fig. 20.7 Anterolateral view of neck with skin, tela subcutanea, and platysma reflected laterally, revealing sternocleidomastoid muscle, external jugular vein, sternohyoid muscle, thyroid cartilage, and submandibular gland.

Sternocleido-mastoid · External jugular vein · Sternohyoid · Laryngeal prominence · Submandibular gland · Tela subcutanea · Platysma · Skin

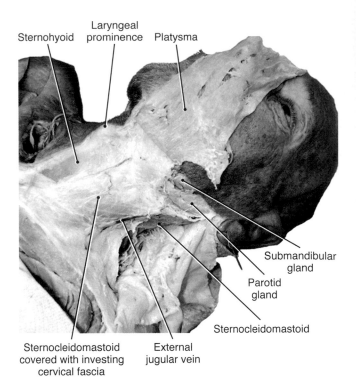

Fig. 20.8 Complete reflection of platysma muscle and exposure of underlying structures.

Sternohyoid · Laryngeal prominence · Platysma · Submandibular gland · Parotid gland · Sternocleidomastoid · Sternocleidomastoid covered with investing cervical fascia · External jugular vein

following cutaneous nerve branches of the cervical plexus:

- ○ Lesser occipital nerve (C2-C3)
- ○ Great auricular nerve (C2-C3)
- ○ Transverse cervical nerve (C2-C3)
- ○ Supraclavicular nerves (C3-C4)

○ These nerves emerge, from top to bottom, along the posterior border of the sternocleidomastoid muscle in the following order: the lesser occipital, great auricular, and transverse cervical nerves.

○ Once you expose these nerves, look for the accessory nerve; it appears posterior to the sternocleidomastoid, about two-thirds the distance up its posterior edge, and then crosses the posterior triangle to reach the trapezius muscle.

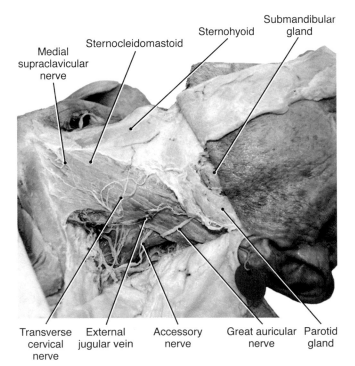

Fig. 20.9 Anterolateral view of neck with skin and tela subcutanea reflected laterally and platysma reflected superiorly.

Medial supraclavicular nerve · Sternocleidomastoid · Sternohyoid · Submandibular gland · Transverse cervical nerve · External jugular vein · Accessory nerve · Great auricular nerve · Parotid gland

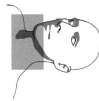

DISSECTION TIP

In many specimens the transverse cervical nerve, which is a cutaneous nerve, communicates with the cervical branch of the facial nerve, which is a motor nerve.

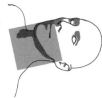

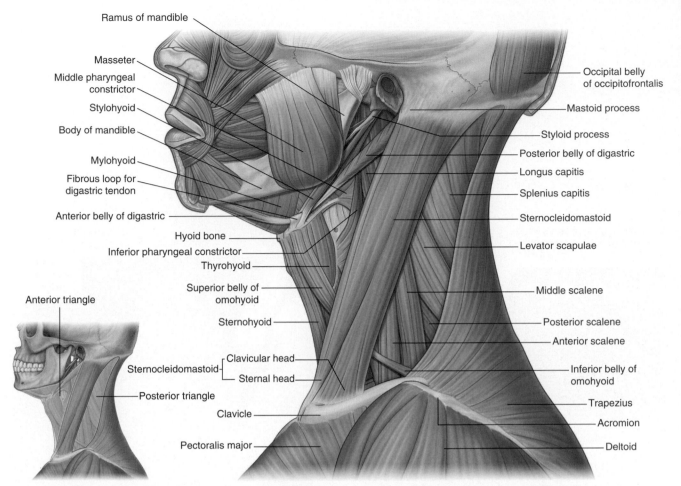

Plate 20.1 Lateral view of the muscles and triangle of the neck.

○ Identify the external jugular vein, which arises at the junction of the posterior auricular vein and the posterior division of the retromandibular vein. This vein terminates in the subclavian vein.

DISSECTION TIP

The external jugular vein may be absent in the presence of a large anterior jugular vein.

○ With scissors, detach the medial border of the sternocleidomastoid muscle from its fascial investment (Fig. 20.10).
○ Cut the origin of the sternocleidomastoid muscle from the clavicle and the manubrium of the sternum (Fig. 20.11).
○ Reflect the sternocleidomastoid muscle upward, away from its fascia. Leave the posterior layer of the superficial cervical fascia intact.
○ Trace the accessory nerve from the posterior aspect of the sternocleidomastoid muscle, and preserve this nerve for later dissection.

○ Dissect out the fascia, and separate the parotid gland from the sternocleidomastoid muscle without damaging the great auricular and lesser occipital nerves.

ANATOMY NOTE

In some specimens the accessory nerve will exhibit communications with C3 and C4 ventral rami. The accessory nerve in the posterior triangle is found between the superficial investing fascia and the prevertebral fascia.

DISSECTION TIP

In some cadavers the parotid gland may cover the most proximal portion of the sternocleidomastoid muscle (Fig. 20.12). It is important to separate the parotid gland from the sternocleidomastoid to reflect the muscle as laterally as possible. The more the sternocleidomastoid is reflected, the more space that will be available for later dissection.

○ Reflect the superficial layer of the investing fascia, and note its contribution to the formation of the carotid sheath (Fig. 20.13).

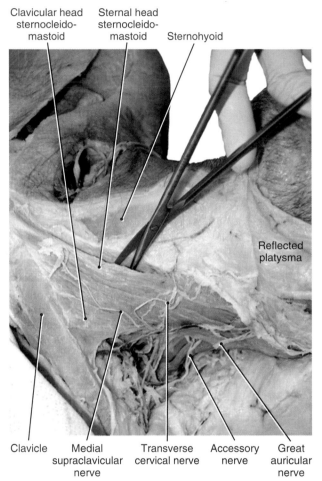

Clavicular head sternocleido-mastoid   Sternal head sternocleido-mastoid   Sternohyoid

Reflected platysma

Clavicle   Medial supraclavicular nerve   Transverse cervical nerve   Accessory nerve   Great auricular nerve

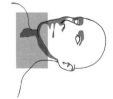

Fig. 20.10 Medial border of underlying tissues detached.

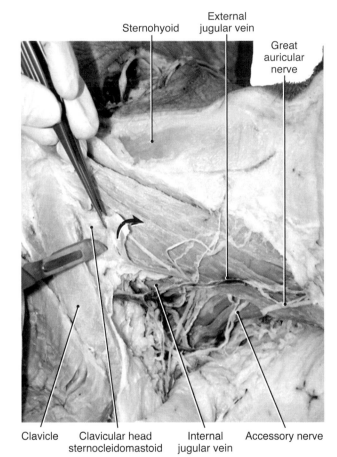

Sternohyoid   External jugular vein   Great auricular nerve

Clavicle   Clavicular head sternocleidomastoid   Internal jugular vein   Accessory nerve

Fig. 20.11 Sternocleidomastoid muscle detached from clavicle.

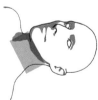

Investing layer superficial cervical fascia | Laryngeal prominence | Sternohyoid | Submandibular gland

Reflected platysma

Lateral supraclavicular nerve | Reflected sternocleidomastoid | Accessory nerve

Parotid gland

Fig. 20.12 Anterolateral view of neck with skin, tela subcutanea, and sternocleidomastoid muscle reflected laterally and platysma reflected superiorly.

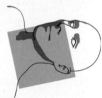

Carotid sheath | Sternohyoid | Submandibular gland

Laryngeal prominence

Investing layer superficial cervical fascia | Internal jugular vein | Sternocleidomastoid | Parotid gland

Fig. 20.13 Carotid sheath cleaned over internal jugular vein.

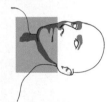

○ Identify the carotid sheath, omohyoid muscle, and internal jugular vein.
○ Clean the carotid sheath over the internal jugular vein.

DISSECTION TIP

As you expose the internal jugular vein from the carotid sheath and superficial layer of the investing cervical fascia, look for the deep cervical lymph nodes. These lymph nodes are often prominent where the omohyoid crosses the internal jugular vein (jugulo-omohyoid node) and where the digastric muscle crosses the internal jugular vein (jugulodigastric node).

○ Identify the *ansa cervicalis.* The ansa cervicalis usually lies superficial to the internal jugular vein, outside the carotid sheath (Fig. 20.14). There are two techniques for the identification of the ansa cervicalis:
  1. Look superficial and lateral to the internal jugular vein in the lower part of the neck, and identify the ansa cervicalis.
  2. Identify and clean the strap muscles. Follow their nerve supply backward, and trace it to the ansa cervicalis.

Specifically, identify the sternohyoid muscle, and follow its small nerve branches proximally.
○ Pull the internal jugular vein laterally, and expose the other contents of the carotid sheath, the *vagus nerve* and *common carotid artery* (Fig. 20.15).
○ Clean the connective tissue, and identify the "strap muscles": the omohyoid (superior and inferior bellies), sternohyoid, sternothyroid, and thyrohyoid muscles (Fig. 20.16).
○ Clear away the carotid sheath, and fully expose the internal jugular vein, common carotid artery, and vagus nerve (Fig. 20.17).

DISSECTION TIP

With scissors, pull the common carotid artery from the carotid sheath (see Fig. 20.17), to avoid severing important arteries and nerves.

○ Clean the connective tissue, fat, and carotid sheath, and expose the cervical plexus (Fig. 20.18).

Ansa cervicalis   Sternohyoid   Internal jugular   Submandibular
                                  vein   lymph node

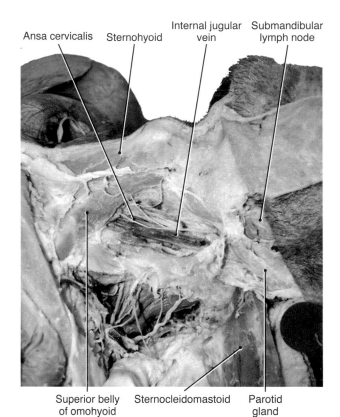

Superior belly   Sternocleidomastoid   Parotid
of omohyoid   gland

Fig. 20.14 Superior belly of omohyoid muscle exposed, revealing ansa cervicalis superficial to internal jugular vein.

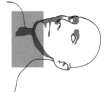

Sternohyoid   Superior belly   Laryngeal   Submandibular
               of omohyoid   prominence   gland

                                 Common
                                 carotid
                                 artery

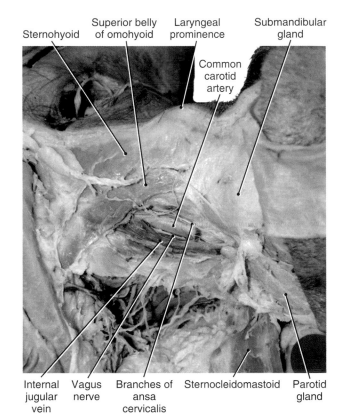

Internal   Vagus   Branches of   Sternocleidomastoid   Parotid
jugular   nerve   ansa   gland
vein   cervicalis

Fig. 20.15 Anterolateral view of neck with skin, tela subcutanea, and sternocleidomastoid muscle reflected laterally and platysma muscle reflected superiorly. Internal jugular vein pulled laterally to expose the other contents of the carotid sheath: vagus nerve and common carotid artery.

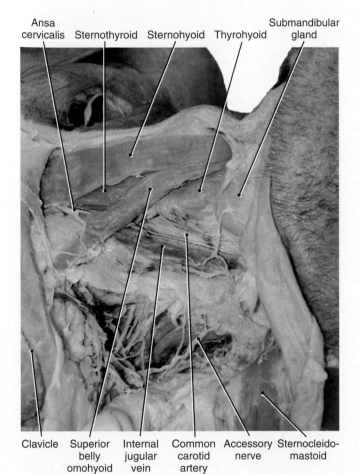

Ansa cervicalis   Sternothyroid   Sternohyoid   Thyrohyoid   Submandibular gland

Clavicle   Superior belly omohyoid   Internal jugular vein   Common carotid artery   Accessory nerve   Sternocleido-mastoid

Fig. 20.16 Connective tissue cleaned, highlighting strap muscles (omohyoid superior/inferior bellies, sternohyoid, sternothyroid, thyrohyoid).

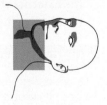

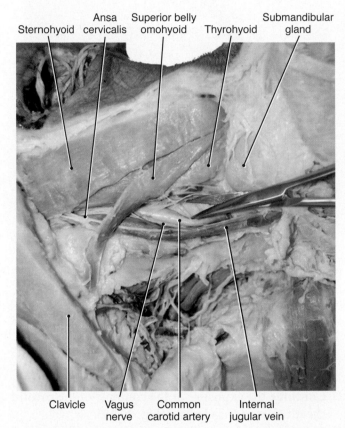

Sternohyoid   Ansa cervicalis   Superior belly omohyoid   Thyrohyoid   Submandibular gland

Clavicle   Vagus nerve   Common carotid artery   Internal jugular vein

Fig. 20.17 Remaining carotid sheath cleaned, fully exposing vagus nerve and carotid artery.

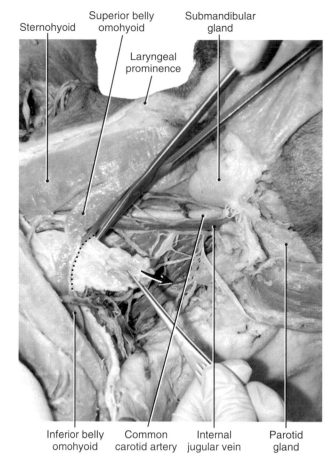

Sternohyoid | Superior belly omohyoid | Submandibular gland
Laryngeal prominence

Inferior belly omohyoid | Common carotid artery | Internal jugular vein | Parotid gland

Fig. 20.18 Adipose tissue removed from posterior cervical triangle, leaving intact nerves and arteries.

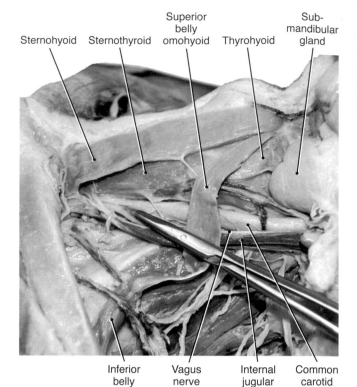

Sternohyoid | Sternothyroid | Superior belly omohyoid | Thyrohyoid | Sub-mandibular gland

Inferior belly omohyoid | Vagus nerve | Internal jugular vein | Common carotid artery

Fig. 20.19 Carotid sheath cleaned inferiorly, revealing vagus nerve and carotid artery toward root of neck.

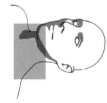

- Continue the exposure of the contents of the carotid sheath toward the clavicle (Fig. 20.19).
- Identify the submandibular gland, and pull it toward the midline.
- Clean the carotid sheath toward the angle of the mandible, and identify (if prominent) the *jugulodigastric lymph nodes* (Fig. 20.20).
- Clean away fat and connective tissue around the common carotid artery and medial to the carotid sheath and identify the superior thyroid artery (Fig. 20.21). This artery runs between the thyrohyoid muscle and the carotid sheath. Do not try to identify the origin of this artery yet.
- Remove the jugulodigastric lymph nodes, and by pulling the parotid gland laterally, expose the posterior belly of the digastric muscle (Fig. 20.22).
- Expose the digastric muscle, with its posterior and anterior bellies, and the stylohyoid muscle.
- Observe the tendon insertion of the stylohyoid muscle onto the hyoid and its relationship with the posterior belly of the digastric muscle.

- Identify the hyoid bone, and expose the mylohyoid muscle, which is partially hidden by the anterior belly of the digastric muscle (see Fig. 20.22).
- Expose the distal portion of the common carotid artery at its division into the internal and external carotid arteries (Fig. 20.23).
- Identify the origin of the *superior thyroid artery* from the external carotid artery, and trace it to its termination in the thyroid gland.

DISSECTION **TIP**

To create more space for exposing the branches of the external carotid artery, detach the submandibular gland from its base (Fig. 20.24) and mobilize it medially.

- Dissect out the facial artery, which passes deep to the submandibular gland before emerging at the angle of the mandible (Fig. 20.25).
- Mobilize the submandibular gland medially, and expose the stylohyoid muscle and the posterior belly of the digastric muscle. Identify the hypoglossal nerve running parallel to the digastric posterior belly (Fig. 20.26).

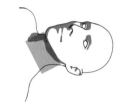

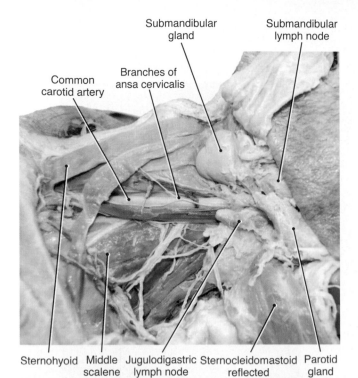

Common carotid artery

Submandibular gland

Branches of ansa cervicalis

Submandibular lymph node

Sternohyoid   Middle scalene   Jugulodigastric lymph node   Sternocleidomastoid reflected   Parotid gland

Fig. 20.20 Appreciate jugulodigastric lymph nodes and parotid and submandibular glands.

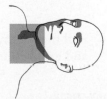

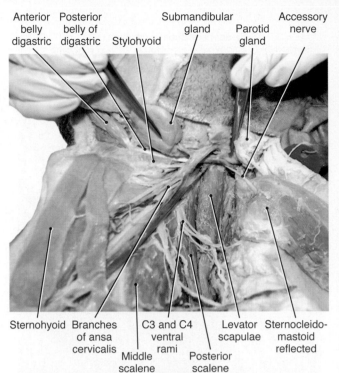

Anterior belly digastric   Posterior belly of digastric   Stylohyoid   Submandibular gland   Parotid gland   Accessory nerve

Sternohyoid   Branches of ansa cervicalis   Middle scalene   C3 and C4 ventral rami   Posterior scalene   Levator scapulae   Sternocleido-mastoid reflected

Fig. 20.22 Submandibular and parotid glands lifted to expose external and internal carotid arteries.

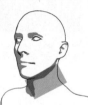

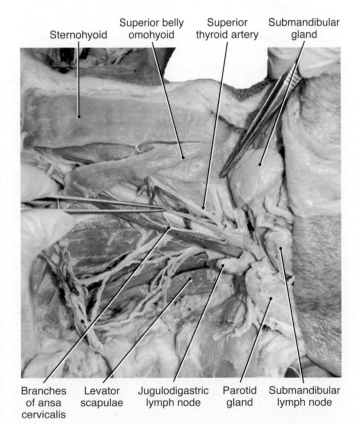

Sternohyoid   Superior belly omohyoid   Superior thyroid artery   Submandibular gland

Branches of ansa cervicalis   Levator scapulae   Jugulodigastric lymph node   Parotid gland   Submandibular lymph node

Fig. 20.21 Fat and connective tissue removed around common carotid artery and medial to carotid sheath to highlight superior thyroid artery.

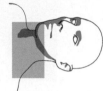

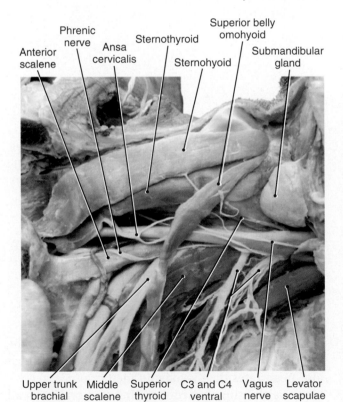

Phrenic nerve   Ansa cervicalis   Sternothyroid   Superior belly omohyoid   Submandibular gland

Anterior scalene   Sternohyoid

Upper trunk brachial plexus   Middle scalene   Superior thyroid artery   C3 and C4 ventral rami   Vagus nerve   Levator scapulae

Fig. 20.23 Anterolateral view of neck revealing neurovascular structures of anterior and posterior cervical triangles.

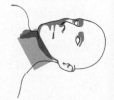

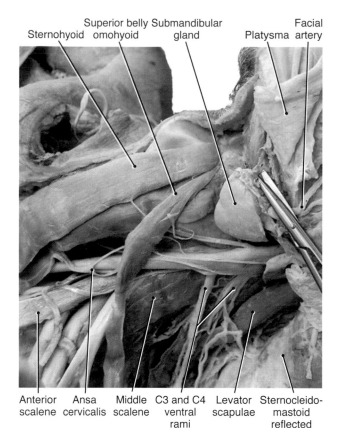

Superior belly Submandibular Facial
Sternohyoid omohyoid gland Platysma artery

Anterior | Ansa | Middle | C3 and C4 | Levator | Sternocleido-
scalene | cervicalis | scalene | ventral rami | scapulae | mastoid reflected

Fig. 20.24 Submandibular gland detached from base to create more space for exposing branches of the external carotid artery.

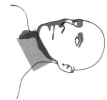

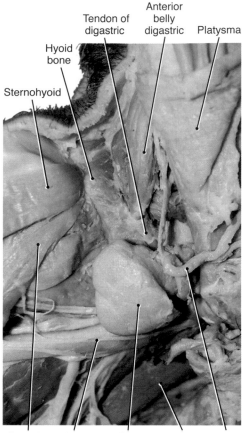

Anterior
Tendon of | belly
Hyoid | digastric | digastric | Platysma
bone
Sternohyoid

Superior | Ansa | Sub- | Levator | Facial
belly | cervicalis | mandibular | scapulae | artery
omohyoid | | gland

Fig. 20.25 Dissection of facial artery, which passes deep to submandibular gland before emerging at the angle of mandible.

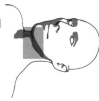

○ Note the small branch of the superior thyroid artery, the *superior laryngeal artery,* which travels medially and penetrates the thyrohyoid membrane (Fig. 20.27).

ANATOMY **NOTE**

The superior laryngeal artery has a variable origin. If it does not arise from the superior thyroid artery, the superior laryngeal may arise directly from the external carotid artery.

○ Parallel to the superior laryngeal artery, expose the internal branch of the superior laryngeal nerve, which also penetrates the thyrohyoid membrane.
○ Observe the superior root of the ansa cervicalis all the way to the hypoglossal nerve. Note that the ansa cervicalis travels within the connective tissue sheath of the hypoglossal nerve.
○ At the origin of the internal carotid artery, look for a dilation of its wall, the *carotid sinus* (Fig. 20.28).

ANATOMY **NOTE**

The carotid sinus contains nerve fibers responsible for detecting blood pressure changes at this location.

○ Using scissors, expose the division of the common carotid artery, and identify the *carotid body* (Fig. 20.29), a small mass of specialized cells that act as chemoreceptors (Plate 20.2).

ANATOMY **NOTE**

A branch of the glossopharyngeal nerve (carotid sinus nerve, or Hering's nerve) is responsible for the nerve supply to the carotid body and sinus.

○ Pull the common carotid artery laterally (Fig. 20.30), and expose the *lingual artery.*

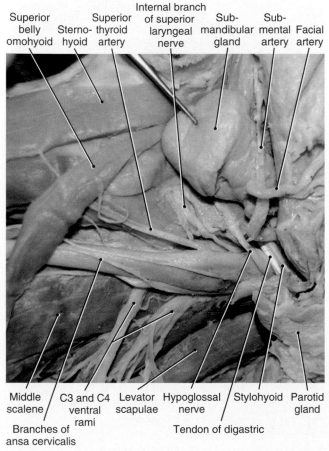

Superior belly omohyoid | Sterno-hyoid | Superior thyroid artery | Internal branch of superior laryngeal nerve | Sub-mandibular gland | Sub-mental artery | Facial artery

Middle scalene | C3 and C4 ventral rami | Levator scapulae | Hypoglossal nerve | Stylohyoid | Parotid gland

Branches of ansa cervicalis | Tendon of digastric

Fig. 20.26 Submandibular gland lifted to expose internal laryngeal and hypoglossal nerves, posterior belly of digastric muscle, and facial artery.

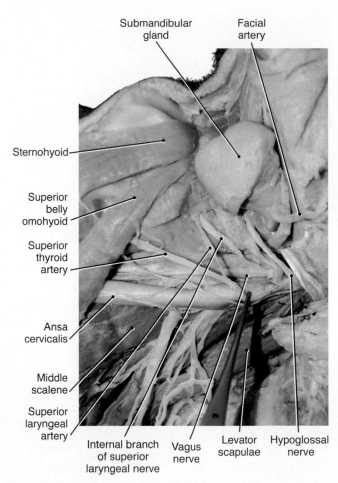

Submandibular gland | Facial artery

Sternohyoid

Superior belly omohyoid

Superior thyroid artery

Ansa cervicalis

Middle scalene

Superior laryngeal artery

Internal branch of superior laryngeal nerve | Vagus nerve | Levator scapulae | Hypoglossal nerve

Fig. 20.27 Anterolateral view of neck.

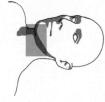

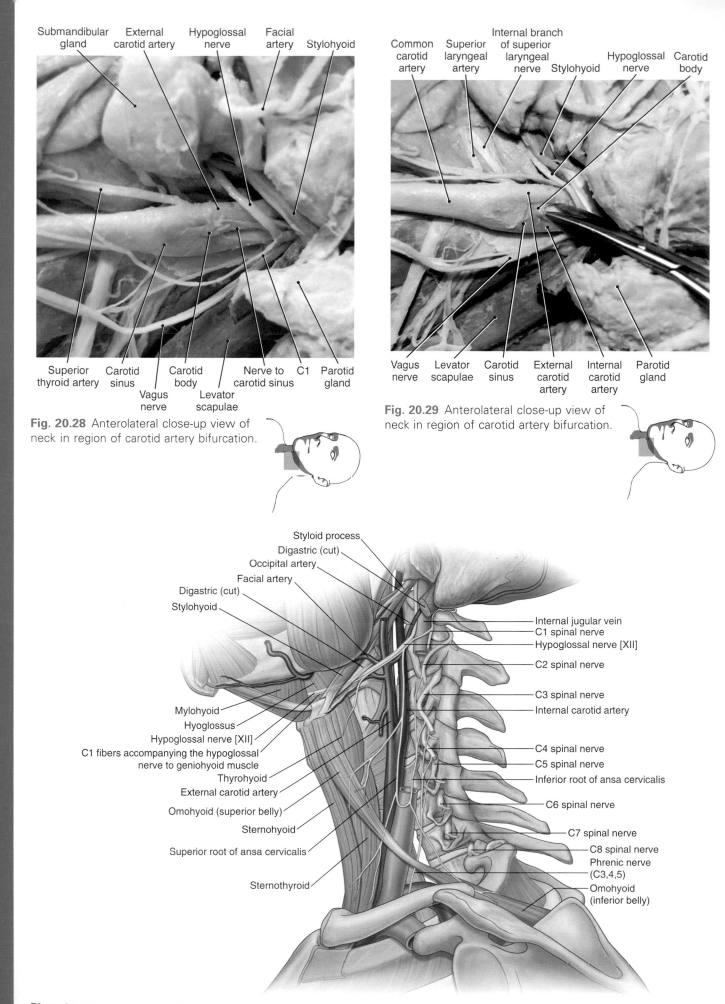

Submandibular gland | External carotid artery | Hypoglossal nerve | Facial artery | Stylohyoid

Superior thyroid artery | Carotid sinus | Vagus nerve | Carotid body | Levator scapulae | Nerve to carotid sinus | C1 | Parotid gland

Fig. 20.28 Anterolateral close-up view of neck in region of carotid artery bifurcation.

Internal branch of superior laryngeal nerve

Common carotid artery | Superior laryngeal artery | Stylohyoid | Hypoglossal nerve | Carotid body

Vagus nerve | Levator scapulae | Carotid sinus | External carotid artery | Internal carotid artery | Parotid gland

Fig. 20.29 Anterolateral close-up view of neck in region of carotid artery bifurcation.

Styloid process
Digastric (cut)
Occipital artery
Facial artery
Digastric (cut)
Stylohyoid

Mylohyoid
Hyoglossus
Hypoglossal nerve [XII]
C1 fibers accompanying the hypoglossal nerve to geniohyoid muscle
Thyrohyoid
External carotid artery
Omohyoid (superior belly)
Sternohyoid
Superior root of ansa cervicalis

Sternothyroid

Internal jugular vein
C1 spinal nerve
Hypoglossal nerve [XII]
C2 spinal nerve
C3 spinal nerve
Internal carotid artery
C4 spinal nerve
C5 spinal nerve
Inferior root of ansa cervicalis
C6 spinal nerve
C7 spinal nerve
C8 spinal nerve
Phrenic nerve (C3,4,5)
Omohyoid (inferior belly)

Plate 20.2 Lateral view of the neck exposing cervical spinal nerves, ansa cervicalis, and hypoglossal nerve.

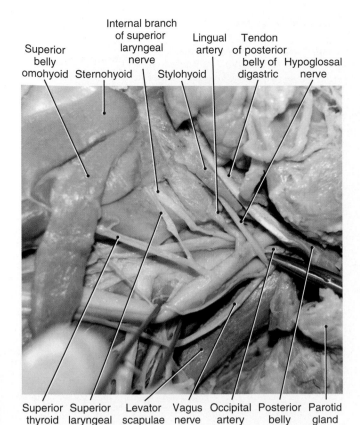

Superior belly omohyoid | Sternohyoid | Internal branch of superior laryngeal nerve | Stylohyoid | Lingual artery | Tendon of posterior belly of digastric | Hypoglossal nerve

Superior thyroid artery | Superior laryngeal artery | Levator scapulae | Vagus nerve | Occipital artery | Posterior belly digastric | Parotid gland

Fig. 20.30 Anterolateral view of neck with skin, tela subcutanea, sternocleidomastoid reflected laterally and platysma reflected superiorly. Common carotid artery pulled laterally to reveal nerves and arteries.

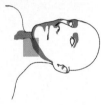

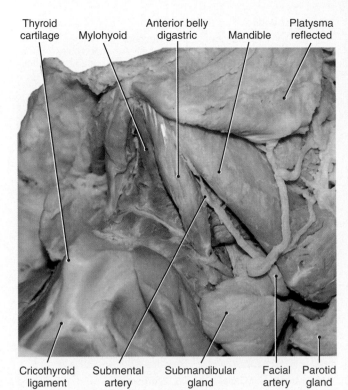

Thyroid cartilage | Mylohyoid | Anterior belly digastric | Mandible | Platysma reflected

Cricothyroid ligament | Submental artery | Submandibular gland | Facial artery | Parotid gland

Fig. 20.31 Anteroinferior view of midline of neck with skin, tela subcutanea, and platysma reflected.

ANATOMY NOTE

The lingual artery is commonly the second branch of the external carotid artery in the majority of cases.

○ If time permits, trace the lingual artery to the point where it passes deep to the hyoglossus muscle.

○ At the lateral border of the external carotid artery, expose the *occipital artery*, which passes posteriorly, crossing over the hypoglossal nerve (see Fig. 20.30 and Plate 20.2).

ANATOMY NOTE

In the majority of cases, the occipital artery gives rise to the artery of the sternocleidomastoid muscle.

○ Opposite the occipital artery, at the medial border of the external carotid artery and superior to the lingual artery, identify the *facial artery*, and trace it to the submandibular gland at the angle of the mandible (Fig. 20.31).

ANATOMY NOTE

In some cadavers the facial and lingual arteries may have a common origin, the *faciolingual trunk*. Similarly, the lingual and the superior thyroid arteries may originate as a common trunk.

○ Posterior to the origin of the external carotid artery, identify the ascending pharyngeal artery, which travels between the internal carotid and the lateral aspect of the pharynx.

○ Clean any muscle attachments and connective tissue from the clavicle to expose the *brachial plexus* in the supraclavicular area (Fig. 20.32).

○ Cover the neck and thorax with paper towels to protect the dissected structures from bone dust (Fig. 20.33).

○ With an electric saw, cut the clavicle at the jugular notch and at its distal one third (Fig. 20.34).

○ With scissors, detach the clavicle from the underlying connective tissue and subclavius muscle (Figs. 20.35 and 20.36).

○ Reflect the subclavius muscle laterally, and expose the root of the neck and the brachial plexus (Fig. 20.37).

○ Identify the anterior scalene muscle (Fig. 20.38), and on its surface identify the phrenic nerve (Fig. 20.39).

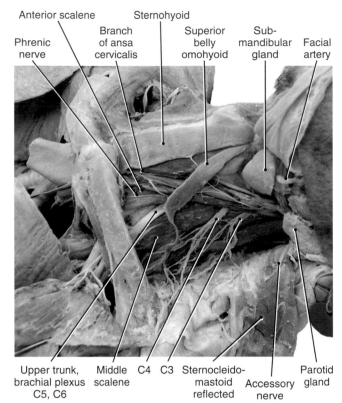

Anterior scalene   Sternohyoid
Phrenic nerve   Branch of ansa cervicalis   Superior belly omohyoid   Sub-mandibular gland   Facial artery

Upper trunk, brachial plexus C5, C6   Middle scalene   C4   C3   Sternocleido-mastoid reflected   Accessory nerve   Parotid gland

Fig. 20.32 Cleaned clavicle and adipose tissue removed, further revealing key neurovascular structures.

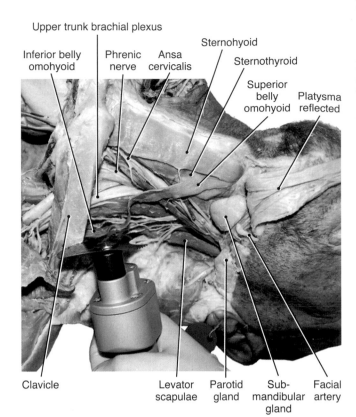

Upper trunk brachial plexus
Inferior belly omohyoid   Phrenic nerve   Ansa cervicalis   Sternohyoid   Sternothyroid   Superior belly omohyoid   Platysma reflected

Clavicle   Levator scapulae   Parotid gland   Sub-mandibular gland   Facial artery

Fig. 20.34 Clavicle cut at jugular notch and its distal one third.

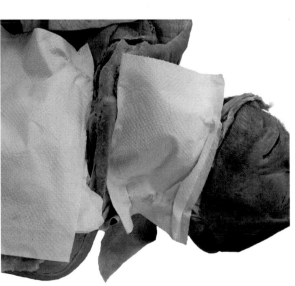

Fig. 20.33 Neck and thorax covered with paper towels to protect the dissected structures from bone dust when using a bone saw.

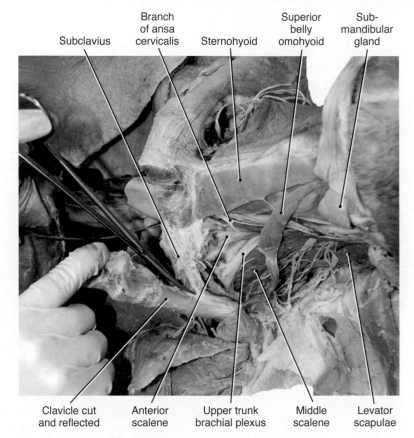

Subclavius — Branch of ansa cervicalis — Sternohyoid — Superior belly omohyoid — Sub-mandibular gland

Clavicle cut and reflected — Anterior scalene — Upper trunk brachial plexus — Middle scalene — Levator scapulae

Fig. 20.35 Clavicle detached from underlying connective tissue and subclavius muscle.

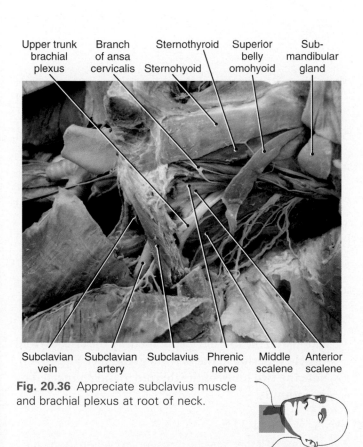

Upper trunk brachial plexus — Branch of ansa cervicalis — Sternohyoid — Sternothyroid — Superior belly omohyoid — Sub-mandibular gland

Subclavian vein — Subclavian artery — Subclavius — Phrenic nerve — Middle scalene — Anterior scalene

Fig. 20.36 Appreciate subclavius muscle and brachial plexus at root of neck.

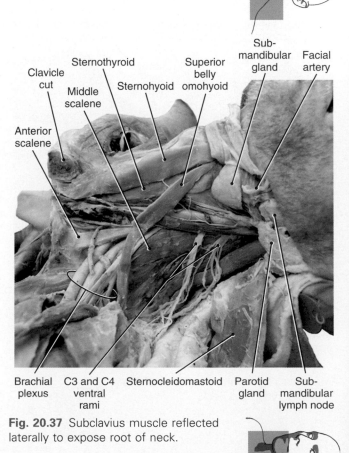

Clavicle cut — Anterior scalene — Middle scalene — Sternothyroid — Sternohyoid — Superior belly omohyoid — Sub-mandibular gland — Facial artery

Brachial plexus — C3 and C4 ventral rami — Sternocleidomastoid — Parotid gland — Sub-mandibular lymph node

Fig. 20.37 Subclavius muscle reflected laterally to expose root of neck.

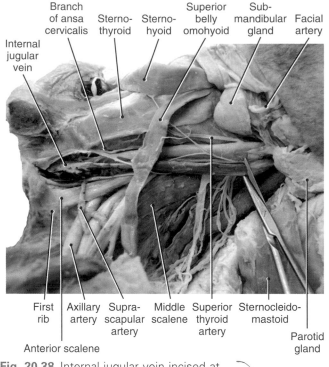

Fig. 20.38 Internal jugular vein incised at level of bifurcation of common carotid artery and removed from the neck.

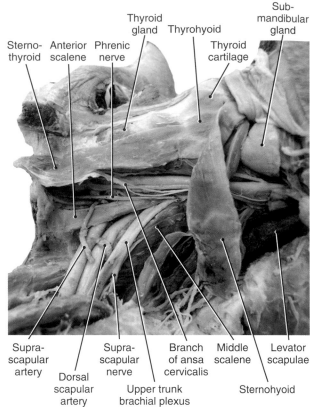

Fig. 20.40 Appreciate supraclavicular nerves and phrenic nerve crossed by branches of thyrocervical trunk.

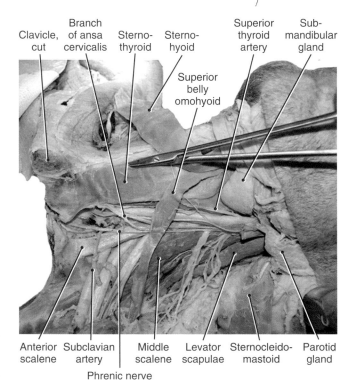

Fig. 20.39 Appreciate the course of the phrenic nerve in the neck.

○ With scissors, cut the internal jugular vein at the level of the bifurcation of the common carotid artery, and remove it from the neck.

○ Trace the supraclavicular nerves, noting their origin from cervical nerves 3 and 4 (C3, C4) (see Fig. 20.39).

○ On the anterior surface of the anterior scalene muscle, note the phrenic nerve is crossed by branches of the thyrocervical trunk, the transverse cervical and suprascapular arteries (Fig. 20.40).

○ Cut the inferior attachments of the sternohyoid and sternothyroid muscles, and reflect them upward to expose the *thyroid gland* (Figs. 20.41 and 20.42).

○ Notice the branches from the ansa cervicalis innervating the strap muscles.

○ Follow the superior thyroid artery medial to its termination into the thyroid gland. Identify the cricothyroid muscle superior to the thyroid gland (see Fig. 20.40).

○ Note the two lobes of the thyroid gland connected by the isthmus.

ANATOMY **NOTE**

A pyramidal lobe may be present, traveling from the thyroid gland toward the hyoid bone.

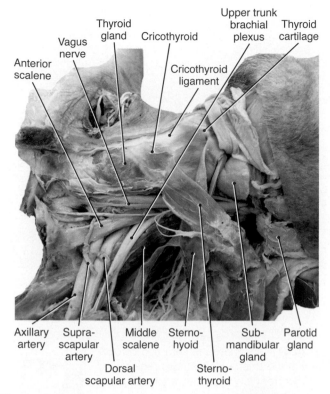

Fig. 20.41 Inferior attachments of sternohyoid and sternothyroid muscles reflected upward to expose thyroid gland.

Labels (Fig. 20.41):
Anterior scalene · Vagus nerve · Thyroid gland · Cricothyroid · Upper trunk brachial plexus · Thyroid cartilage · Cricothyroid ligament · Axillary artery · Suprascapular artery · Dorsal scapular artery · Middle scalene · Sternohyoid · Sternothyroid · Submandibular gland · Parotid gland

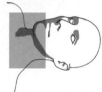

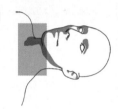

Fig. 20.42 Thyroid gland and cricothyroid muscle exposed.

Labels (Fig. 20.42):
Aortic arch · Common carotid artery · Anterior scalene · Thyroid gland · Cricothyroid ligament · Thyroid cartilage · Cricothyroid · First rib · Suprascapular artery · Transverse cervical artery · Dorsal scapular artery · Sternothyoid · Sternohyoid · Submandibular gland · Facial artery

○ If time permits, cut the isthmus of the thyroid gland, and reflect the gland laterally from the trachea.

○ Look on the posterior surface of the thyroid gland for the *parathyroid glands,* typically found close to the posterior branches of the superior and inferior thyroid arteries.

○ If time permits, identify the superior and middle thyroid veins, and trace them back to the internal jugular vein.

○ Pull the common carotid artery laterally, and trace the superior thyroid artery (Fig. 20.43).

○ Locate the internal laryngeal branch of the superior laryngeal nerve, and trace its origin back to the superior laryngeal nerve.

○ Pull the internal laryngeal nerve away from its origin, and identify the external laryngeal branch. Follow this nerve as it descends into the neck medial to the common carotid artery, running along the superior thyroid artery.

○ Clean the superior thyroid artery, and find the external laryngeal nerve piercing the cricothyroid muscle.

○ Pull the common carotid artery laterally to expose the space between the anterior scalene muscle and trachea (Fig. 20.44).

○ Clean the connective tissue in this space, and identify the inferior thyroid artery, thyrocervical trunk, and recurrent laryngeal nerve (Fig. 20.45).

ANATOMY **NOTE**

The *inferior thyroid artery* is a branch of the thyrocervical trunk that supplies the inferior pole of the thyroid gland.

○ Dissect the fat and connective tissue medial to the trachea (tracheoesophageal groove), and identify the *recurrent laryngeal nerve* (Fig. 20.46).

ANATOMY **NOTE**

The left recurrent laryngeal nerve arises from the left vagus nerve in the thorax as the vagus nerve crosses the arch of the aorta. The right recurrent laryngeal nerve arises from the right vagus nerve as it crosses the right subclavian artery.

ANATOMY **NOTE**

The *inferior thyroid artery* crosses the recurrent laryngeal nerve at the inferior pole of the thyroid artery (Fig. 20.47). This is an important surgical landmark.

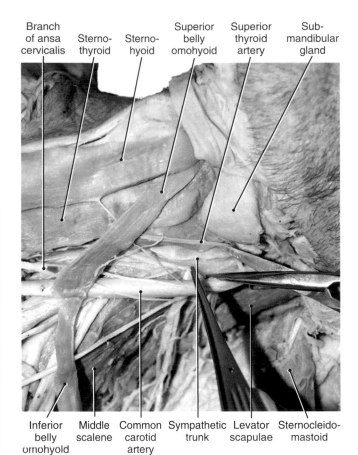

Branch of ansa cervicalis — Sterno-thyroid — Sterno-hyoid — Superior belly omohyoid — Superior thyroid artery — Sub-mandibular gland

Inferior belly omohyoid — Middle scalene — Common carotid artery — Sympathetic trunk — Levator scapulae — Sternocleido-mastoid

Fig. 20.43 Common carotid artery pulled laterally to trace superior thyroid artery, internal laryngeal nerve, superior laryngeal artery, and external laryngeal nerve.

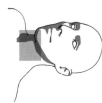

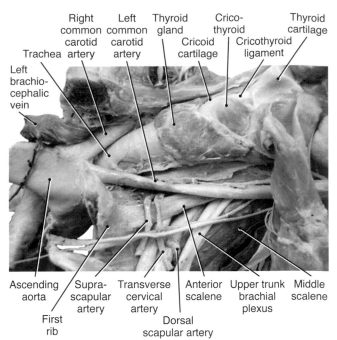

Right common carotid artery — Left common carotid artery — Thyroid gland — Crico-thyroid — Thyroid cartilage

Trachea — Cricoid cartilage — Cricothyroid ligament

Left brachio-cephalic vein

Ascending aorta — Supra-scapular artery — Transverse cervical artery — Anterior scalene — Upper trunk brachial plexus — Middle scalene

First rib — Dorsal scapular artery

Fig. 20.44 Appreciate the common carotid artery in the tracheoesophageal region, with recurrent laryngeal nerve along the tracheoesophageal groove.

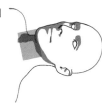

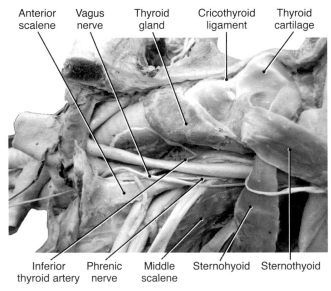

Anterior scalene — Vagus nerve — Thyroid gland — Cricothyroid ligament — Thyroid cartilage

Inferior thyroid artery — Phrenic nerve — Middle scalene — Sternohyoid — Sternothyroid

Fig. 20.45 Appreciate the inferior thyroid artery, a key surgical landmark.

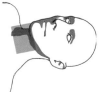

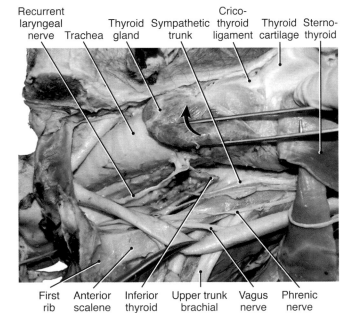

Recurrent laryngeal nerve — Trachea — Thyroid gland — Sympathetic trunk — Crico-thyroid ligament — Thyroid cartilage — Sterno-thyroid

First rib — Anterior scalene — Inferior thyroid artery — Upper trunk brachial plexus — Vagus nerve — Phrenic nerve

Fig. 20.46 Common carotid artery pulled laterally, revealing branches of thyrocervical trunk. Note the relationship between the recurrent laryngeal nerve and inferior thyroid artery.

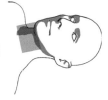

ANATOMY NOTE

When the inferior thyroid artery arises from the aortic arch, brachiocephalic trunk, or common carotid or vertebral artery, it is called the *thyroidea ima* (lowest thyroid) artery. This variation is present in approximately 5% of the population.

ANATOMY NOTE

In some specimens a nonrecurrent laryngeal nerve is present. This variation is caused by a delay in the development of the aortic arches, resulting in the right vagus nerve giving off a transversely oriented, nonrecurrent laryngeal nerve, which passes directly toward the larynx without reaching the thorax. This anatomic situation is usually associated with a retroesophageal right subclavian artery.

○ Trace the previously identified transverse cervical and suprascapular arteries deep to their origin from the thyrocervical trunk (see Fig. 20.47).

ANATOMY NOTE

The transverse cervical or suprascapular arteries may be absent. In such cases the dorsal scapular artery may be large and may arise from the subclavian artery, crossing over the first rib.

○ Lift the contents of the carotid sheath (internal jugular vein, common carotid artery, vagus nerve), and look posterior for the cervical part of the sympathetic trunk,

or sympathetic trunk (see Fig. 20.50). Note that the sympathetic trunk and the roots of the cervical plexus lie behind the carotid sheath.

○ The sympathetic trunk lies within a dense fascial layer, the prevertebral fascia. Clean the prevertebral fascia (and remnants of carotid sheath) posterior to the common carotid artery.

○ Trace the sympathetic trunk inferiorly, and identify the superior, middle, and inferior cervical ganglia (see Fig. 20.53).

DISSECTION TIP

The middle cervical ganglion is variable in origin and is often not present. The superior cervical ganglion can be identified at the level of the angle of the mandible. However, during the retropharyngeal dissection, it will be fully exposed.

○ Once the thyrocervical trunk is identified and its branches exposed, pull it laterally and look for the *vertebral artery*, which ascends medial and deep to it (see Figs. 20.47 and 20.48).

○ Near the origin of the vertebral artery, identify the inferior cervical ganglion and/or the stellate ganglion (Figs. 20.49 and 20.50).

○ The inferior cervical ganglion is large and often fused with the first thoracic trunk ganglion, forming the stellate (cervicothoracic) ganglion (Fig. 20.51).

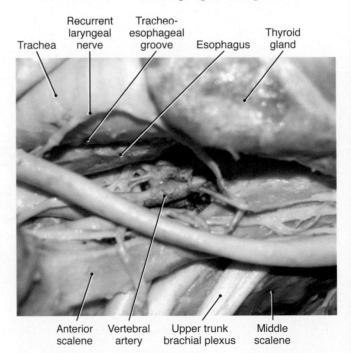

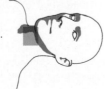

Fig. 20.47 Medial to the thyrocervical trunk, identify the vertebral artery arising as the first branch of the subclavian artery.

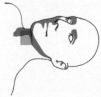

Fig. 20.48 Common carotid artery and thyrocervical trunk pulled laterally to identify the vertebral artery and sympathetic trunk.

○ After identifying the stellate ganglion or inferior cervical ganglion, cut 2 to 3 cm of the inferior portion of the common carotid artery (Fig. 20.52). Immediately beneath this artery, identify the *thoracic duct.*

ANATOMY **NOTE**

On the left side, the thoracic duct will empty into the junction between the internal jugular and subclavian veins. On the right side, the smaller right lymphatic duct will terminate at the junction of the right internal jugular and right subclavian veins.

Vertebral artery | Stellate ganglion | Trachea | Inferior thyroid artery | Thyroid gland | Cervical sympathetic trunk

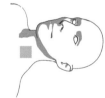

Thyrocervical trunk | Ascending cervical artery | Common carotid artery | Internal jugular vein

Fig. 20.49 Retractors used (as necessary) to keep common carotid artery and thyrocervical trunk reflected laterally, highlighting the sympathetic trunk with its stellate ganglion and vertebral artery.

Stellate ganglion | Inferior thyroid artery | Cervical sympathetic trunk

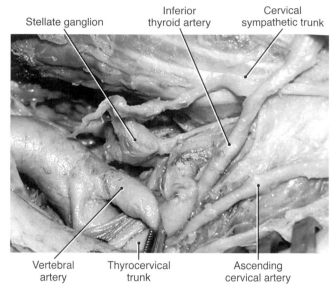

Vertebral artery | Thyrocervical trunk | Ascending cervical artery

Fig. 20.51 Stellate ganglion, vertebral artery, and sympathetic trunk fully dissected and exposed.

Stellate ganglion | Trachea | Inferior thyroid artery | Thyroid gland | Cervical sympathetic trunk

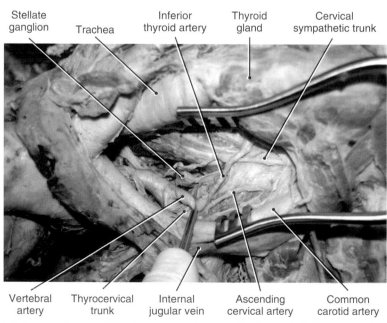

Vertebral artery | Thyrocervical trunk | Internal jugular vein | Ascending cervical artery | Common carotid artery

Fig. 20.50 Appreciate the stellate ganglion, vertebral artery, and sympathetic trunk fully exposed.

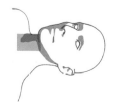

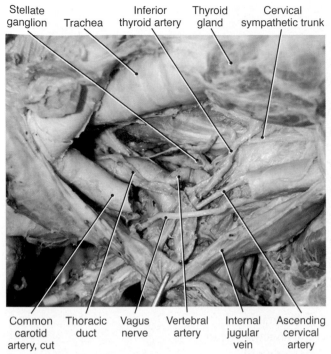

Stellate ganglion | Trachea | Inferior thyroid artery | Thyroid gland | Cervical sympathetic trunk

Common carotid artery, cut | Thoracic duct | Vagus nerve | Vertebral artery | Internal jugular vein | Ascending cervical artery

Fig. 20.52 Left common carotid artery cut, revealing the throracic duct.

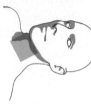

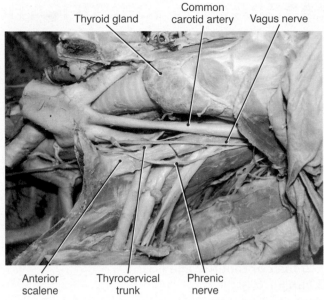

Thyroid gland | Common carotid artery | Vagus nerve

Anterior scalene | Thyrocervical trunk | Phrenic nerve

Fig. 20.53 Anterior scalene muscle cut midway from its attachment onto first rib.

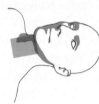

DISSECTION TIP

The thoracic duct is located close to the stellate or inferior cervical ganglion and is often severed during this dissection.

OPTIONAL DISSECTION

ANATOMY NOTE

The subclavian artery gives rise to the following branches:
1. Thyrocervical trunk
2. Vertebral artery
3. Internal thoracic artery
4. Costocervical trunk

- The *costocervical trunk* is located on the deep surface of the subclavian artery posterior to the anterior scalene muscle. It usually gives off the highest intercostal artery, which supplies the uppermost intercostal spaces.
- Cut the anterior scalene muscle midway from its attachment to the first rib (Fig. 20.53).
- Look at the posterior surface of subclavian artery, and trace the costocervical trunk (Fig. 20.54).

DISSECTION TIP

This dissection can also take place from the internal surface of the already-dissected thorax.

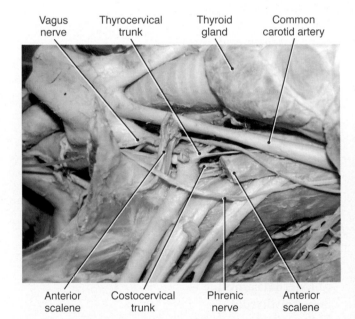

Vagus nerve | Thyrocervical trunk | Thyroid gland | Common carotid artery

Anterior scalene | Costocervical trunk | Phrenic nerve | Anterior scalene

Fig. 20.54 Anterior scalene muscle and posterior surface of subclavian artery lifted, revealing origin of costocervical trunk.

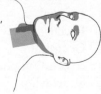

ANATOMY NOTE

The other branch of the costocervical trunk is the deep cervical artery, which ascends in the neck posterior to the transverse processes of the cervical vertebrae.

LABORATORY IDENTIFICATION CHECKLIST

NERVES

Cervical Plexus
- ☐ Great auricular
- ☐ Transverse cervical
- ☐ Supraclavicular nerves
- ☐ Lesser occipital
- ☐ C1 fibers to thyrohyoid muscle
- ☐ Ansa cervicalis (C1-C3)
    - ☐ Superior root (C1)
    - ☐ Inferior root (C2 and C3)
- ☐ Phrenic (C3-C5)

Cranial Nerves (CN)
- ☐ Accessory (CN XI)
- ☐ Hypoglossal nerve (CN XII)
- ☐ Vagus nerve (CN X)
- ☐ Nerve to mylohyoid/anterior digastric muscle (CN V; from inferior alveolar nerve)
- ☐ Cervical branch from facial (CN VII)

Autonomic Nerves
- ☐ Vagus
- ☐ Superior laryngeal
    - ☐ External laryngeal
    - ☐ Internal laryngeal
    - ☐ Recurrent laryngeal
    - ☐ Inferior laryngeal
- ☐ Cervical sympathetic trunk

Ganglia
- ☐ Superior cervical
- ☐ Middle cervical
- ☐ Stellate

ARTERIES
- ☐ Common carotid
    - ☐ Internal carotid
    - ☐ External carotid
- ☐ Superior thyroid
    - ☐ Superior laryngeal
- ☐ Lingual
- ☐ Facial
- ☐ Occipital
- ☐ Ascending pharyngeal
- ☐ Subclavian
- ☐ Vertebral
- ☐ Thyrocervical trunk
    - ☐ Inferior thyroid
    - ☐ Transverse scapular
    - ☐ Suprascapular
- ☐ Dorsal scapular

VEINS
- ☐ External jugular
- ☐ Anterior jugular
- ☐ Internal jugular
    - ☐ Superior thyroid
    - ☐ Middle thyroid
- ☐ Subclavian
- ☐ Inferior thyroid veins

MUSCLES
- ☐ Platysma
- ☐ Sternocleidomastoid
    - ☐ Sternal head
    - ☐ Clavicular head
- ☐ Sternohyoid
- ☐ Omohyoid
- ☐ Sternothyroid
- ☐ Thyrohyoid
- ☐ Anterior belly of digastric
- ☐ Mylohyoid
- ☐ Posterior belly of digastric
- ☐ Stylohyoid
- ☐ Splenius capitis
- ☐ Levator scapulae
- ☐ Posterior scalene
- ☐ Middle scalene
- ☐ Anterior scalene
- ☐ Trapezius

FASCIA
- ☐ Superficial fascia
- ☐ Tela subcutanea
- ☐ Deep fascia
    - ☐ Investing layer
    - ☐ Pretracheal layer
    - ☐ Prevertebral layer

BONES
- ☐ Mandible
- ☐ Hyoid
- ☐ Manubrium
- ☐ Clavicle
- ☐ Cervical vertebrae (C1-C7)
    - ☐ Atlas (C1)
    - ☐ Axis (C2)
- ☐ Occipital
- ☐ Temporal
    - ☐ Mastoid process
    - ☐ Styloid process

CONNECTIVE TISSUE

- ☐ Thyroid cartilage
- ☐ Cricoid cartilage
- ☐ Cricothyroid ligament
- ☐ Stylohyoid ligament
- ☐ Stylomandibular ligament
- ☐ Thyrohyoid membrane

GLANDS

- ☐ Submandibular gland
- ☐ Thyroid gland
  - ☐ Right lobe
  - ☐ Left lobe
  - ☐ Pyramidal lobe
- ☐ Parathyroid glands

ATLAS REFERENCES
Netter: 42, 53–54, 83–85
McMinn: 38–41
Gray's Atlas: 503–506

BEFORE YOU BEGIN
Review the superficial anatomy of the face:
- Glabella
- Root of nose, dorsum of nose
- Tip of nose
- Ala
- Columella nasi
- Philtrum
- Mental protuberance
- Modiolus
- Vermillion border

Palpate the following facial landmarks on the cadaver:
- Jugular notch
- Mental protuberance
- Nasion
- Glabella
- Vertex
- External occipital protuberance (inion)
- Mastoid process
- Ramus, angle, and body of mandible
- Zygomatic arch
- Infraorbital margin
- Supraorbital margin
- Superciliary arch

SKIN AND SUPERFICIAL FASCIA
○ **With a marker, outline the dissection for the cadaver as follows (Fig. 21.1):**
1. Make a line from the mental protuberance to the vertex. The line should encircle the lips, nostrils, and eyelids.
2. Make a second line from the mental protuberance to the lobule of the ear.
3. Make a third line from the vertex to the upper part of the helix of the ear.

○ Identify the six major surface regions (temporal, frontal, zygomatic, maxillary, mandibular, mental).

○ Based on the lines drawn, make an incision between the angle of the mandible and the mental protuberance (Fig. 21.2).

○ Carefully reflect the flaps of skin (from medial to lateral) created by the incisions (Figs. 21.3 and 21.4).

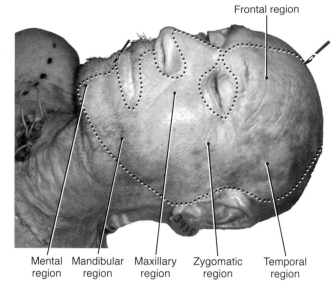

Fig. 21.1 Anterolateral facial view with stippled lines for incisions, showing the six major surface regions.

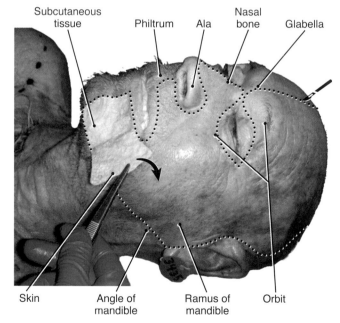

Fig. 21.2 Anterolateral facial view with skin reflected from the mental region and facial landmarks.

ANATOMY **NOTE**

Beneath the skin, notice the surface of the face covered almost entirely by fat. This fibrofatty tissue is also known as the **superficial musculoaponeurotic space** or system (SMAS) (Fig. 21.5).

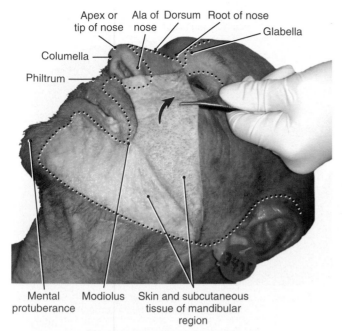

Apex or Ala of Dorsum Root of nose
tip of nose nose
Glabella
Columella
Philtrum

Mental   Modiolus   Skin and subcutaneous
protuberance   tissue of mandibular
                          region

Fig. 21.3 Anterolateral facial view with skin reflected from the mandibular region.

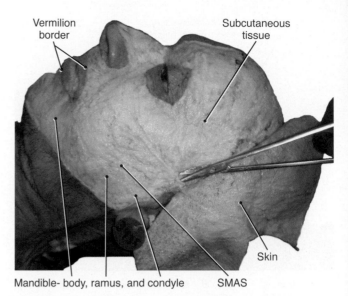

Vermilion   Subcutaneous
border   tissue

                                                  Skin

Mandible- body, ramus, and condyle   SMAS

Fig. 21.5 Lateral facial view with skin reflected from mandibular, maxillary, zygomatic, frontal, and temporal regions.

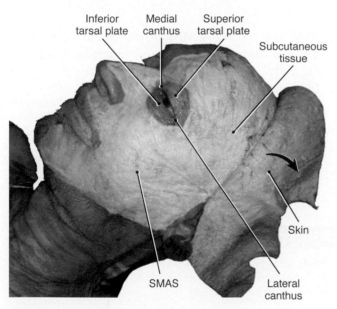

Inferior   Medial   Superior
tarsal plate canthus   tarsal plate
                         Subcutaneous
                         tissue

                                      Skin

SMAS   Lateral
                             canthus

Fig. 21.4 Lateral facial view with skin reflected from mandibular, maxillary, zygomatic, frontal, and temporal regions.

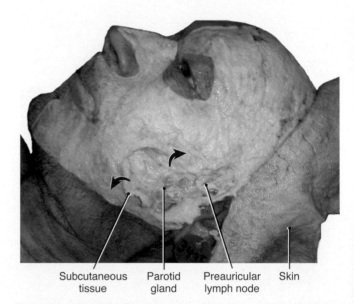

Subcutaneous   Parotid   Preauricular   Skin
tissue   gland   lymph node

Fig. 21.6 Lateral facial view with skin reflected and SMAS removed from the mandibular region.

separating technique with your scissors, reflect as much fat as possible.

○ Identify the substance of the parotid gland, which typically extends into the space between the zygomatic arch and the angle of the mandible (Fig. 21.6).

ANATOMY **NOTE**

The parotid gland is covered by a dense fibrous capsule, which sends septae into the gland, dividing it into lobules.

○ Begin to reflect the SMAS medially over the mandibular region to reveal the parotid gland (see Fig. 21.5).
○ Continue to remove the SMAS from the mandibular region (Fig. 21.7).

DISSECTION **TIP**

The muscles of facial expression vary in thickness. Pay special attention when removing the skin and SMAS to avoid cutting any muscles, because many attach directly into the skin.

PAROTID GLAND

○ Situated in front of the ear (auricle), the parotid gland is covered with variable amounts of fat. Using the

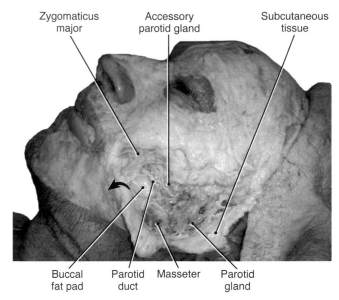

Fig. 21.7 Lateral facial view with skin reflected and SMAS removed from the mandibular region.

Zygomaticus major — Accessory parotid gland — Subcutaneous tissue

Buccal fat pad — Parotid duct — Masseter — Parotid gland

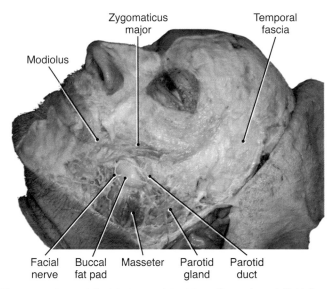

Modiolus — Zygomaticus major — Temporal fascia

Facial nerve — Buccal fat pad — Masseter — Parotid gland — Parotid duct

Fig. 21.8 Lateral facial view with skin reflected and SMAS removed from mandibular, maxillary, and temporal regions.

○ Identify the **parotid duct**, usually found emerging from the anterior edge of the parotid gland, about 1 inch (2.5 cm) inferior to the zygomatic arch (Figs. 21.7 and 21.8).

ANATOMY **NOTE**

From this point, the parotid duct passes horizontally across the masseter muscle, then turns around the anterior edge of the masseter and pierces the buccinator muscle (Fig. 21.9).

○ Remove the SMAS from the maxillary and temporal regions (see Fig. 21.8).

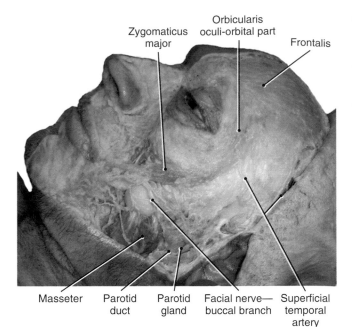

Zygomaticus major — Orbicularis oculi-orbital part — Frontalis

Masseter — Parotid duct — Parotid gland — Facial nerve—buccal branch — Superficial temporal artery

Fig. 21.9 Lateral facial view with skin reflected and subcutaneous tissue removed from the mandibular, maxillary, and orbital regions.

○ Note the following structures: zygomaticus major muscle, masseter muscle, and temporal fascia (see Figs. 21.7 and 21.8).
○ Identify the buccal fat pad.

ANATOMY **NOTE**

The buccal fat pad is an encapsulated mass of adipose tissue, which lies between the masseter and buccinator muscles.

DISSECTION **TIP**

An accessory parotid gland can often be identified along the parotid duct in its course across the masseter muscle (see Figs. 21.7 and 21.8).

MIMETIC MUSCLES

○ Clean the mimetic muscles, taking care to preserve the branches of the facial nerve, which innervate them.
○ Remove the SMAS from the orbital region and identify the frontalis and orbicularis oculi muscles (see Fig. 21.9 and Plate 21.1).
○ Identify the parts of the orbicularis oculi muscles:
  ○ Orbital
  ○ Palpebral
  ○ Lacrimal
○ Identify the superficial temporal artery just superior to the zygomatic arch in front of the external acoustic meatus (see Fig. 21.9).

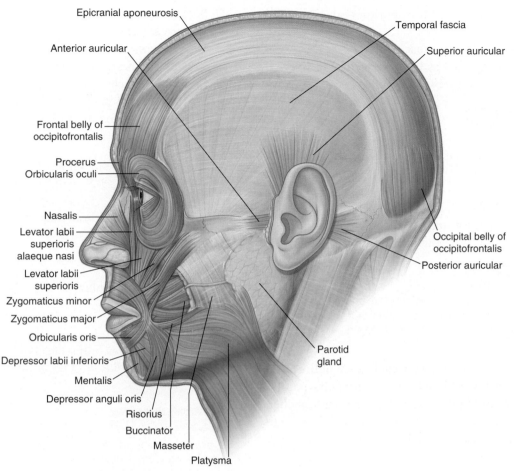

Plate 21.1 Lateral view of the muscles of facial expression.

ANATOMY **NOTE**

The auriculotemporal nerve can be found just posterior to this artery.

DISSECTION **TIP**

The transverse facial artery runs superior to the parotid duct, but because of its small size, identifying this artery is often difficult.

○ Identify several of the mimetic muscles (Fig. 21.10):
○ The muscle surrounding the lips is the *orbicularis oris.*

DISSECTION **TIP**

Often you will need to remove additional skin from the margins of the lips to expose the orbicularis oris fully. Fibers from several other facial muscles merge with the orbicularis oris, including the buccinator and the elevators and depressors of the angles of the mouth.

○ Identify the zygomaticus major muscles.
○ Identify the zygomaticus minor muscles.
○ Identify the depressor anguli oris muscles.
○ Identify the depressor labii inferioris muscles.

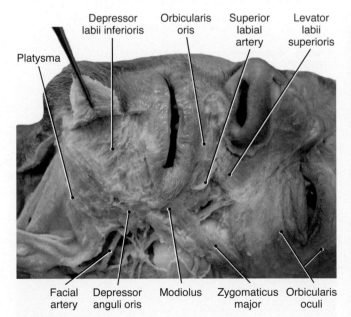

Fig. 21.10 Anterior view of mandible and neck with skin removed, revealing muscles.

○ Identify the levator labii superioris alaeque nasi muscles.
○ Identify the buccinator muscle.
○ The platysma muscle has been identified in the dissection of the neck (see Chapter 20).

DISSECTION TIP

Some platysma fibers pass up over the lower border of the mandible and mingle with the depressor muscles of the lips and with the risorius muscle more laterally.

FACIAL NERVE

○ Identify the *buccal branch* of the facial nerve, which usually runs alongside the parotid duct (Fig. 21.11).

DISSECTION TIP

Tracing the branches of the facial nerve can be challenging. In some specimens, some of the parotid lymph nodes may be encountered as the gland is dissected.

○ After you have exposed the buccal branch of the facial nerve, carefully trace it into the substance of the parotid gland until you find its junction(s) with other branches.
○ Dissect out the other branches of the facial nerve to their target muscles (Fig. 21.12). Landmarks for other branches of the facial nerve follow:
  ○ *Temporal* branch: Dissect near the posterior part of the zygomatic arch.
  ○ *Zygomatic* branch: Dissect around the zygomaticus major muscle at the base of the zygomatic bone.
  ○ *Buccal* branch: Runs parallel to the parotid duct and crosses the masseter muscle.
  ○ *Marginal mandibular* branch: Dissect at the posteroinferior margin of the mandible.
  ○ *Cervical* branch: Dissect deep to the platysma muscle, approximately one fingerbreadth posterior to the angle of the mandible.

ANATOMY NOTE

The facial nerve typically bifurcates into temporofacial and cervicofacial divisions (see Fig. 21.12).

○ Identify the terminal branches of the facial nerve:
  ○ Temporal
  ○ Zygomatic
  ○ Buccal
  ○ Marginal mandibular
  ○ Cervical

ANATOMY NOTE

The terminal branches of the facial nerve often connect to one another or with infraorbital branches of the trigeminal nerve.

DISSECTION TIP

Several branches of the facial nerve are not identified with the cadaver in the supine position, including the posterior auricular nerve, which innervates musculature of the external ear and the occipitalis muscle, and the digastric branch, which supplies the posterior belly of the digastric muscle and the stylohyoid muscle.

Parotid duct   Superior labial artery   Accessory parotid gland

Orbicularis oculi

Parotid gland   Buccal, zygomatic, temporal branches of CN VII

Fig. 21.11 Anterolateral view of face with skin and subcutaneous tissue removed.

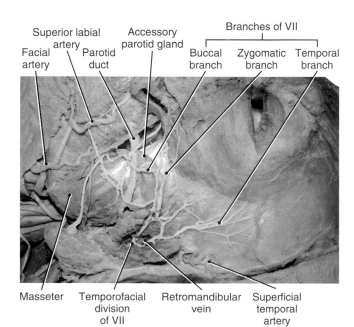

Superior labial artery   Accessory parotid gland   Branches of VII
Facial artery   Parotid duct   Buccal branch   Zygomatic branch   Temporal branch

Masseter   Temporofacial division of VII   Retromandibular vein   Superficial temporal artery

Fig. 21.12 Anterolateral view of face with skin and subcutaneous tissue removed.

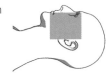

BUCCAL FAT PAD

- After you expose all terminal branches of the facial nerve, identify and remove the *buccal fat pad*, an encapsulated mass of adipose tissue, which lies between the masseter and buccinator muscles (Figs. 21.13 and 21.14).
- Trace the parotid duct to its point of penetration into the buccinator muscle.
- Lift the buccal fat bad with forceps, and use scissors to cut its attachments to nearby structures (Figs. 21.14 and 21.15).
- Pay special attention to preserve the neurovascular structures in the area as you remove the fat pad.

DISSECTION **TIP**

As you remove the buccal fat pad, you will probably notice branches of the buccal artery and nerve. The buccal nerve usually is located between the masseter and buccinator muscles and follows the anterior border of the temporalis muscle to its insertion onto the coronoid process of the mandible. Do not spend time completely exposing the temporalis now; this occurs during the infratemporal area dissection (Chapter 22).

ARTERIES OF THE FACE

- Identify the superior labial artery within the substance of the orbicularis oris muscle.

- Expose the *superior labial artery*, and trace it backward toward the angle of the mandible (see Fig. 21.11).
- The *facial artery* is hidden along part of its course by the submandibular gland and by several mimetic muscles. Identify the facial artery as it becomes superficial at the inferior border of the mandible near its angle. It then crosses the cheek, passes near the

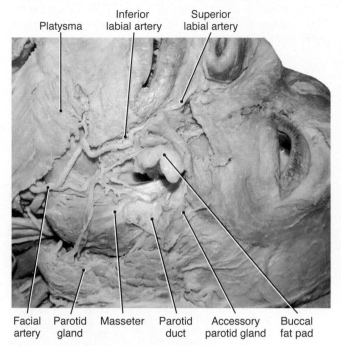

Fig. 21.14 Anterolateral view of face with skin and subcutaneous tissue removed.

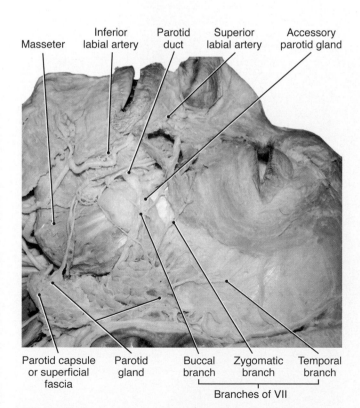

Fig. 21.13 Anterolateral view of face with skin and subcutaneous tissue removed, revealing temporofacial division of the facial nerve and its branches.

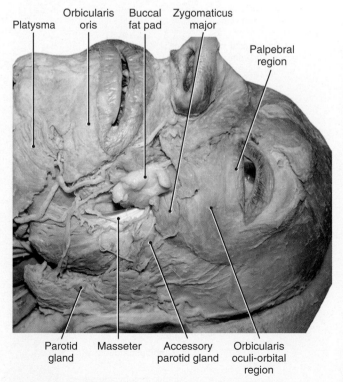

Fig. 21.15 Anterolateral view of face with skin and subcutaneous tissue removed.

angle of the mouth, and ends near the medial angle of the eye as the *angular artery* (Plate 21.2).

○ Medially reflect any of the mimetic muscles covering the facial artery. Once the facial artery is exposed, continue exposing the terminal part, the angular artery.

DISSECTION TIP

The facial artery will terminate in approximately 50% of the specimens as the angular artery. The course of the facial artery is tortuous and in contact with the facial vein, which lies just posterior to it.

○ With scissors, remove the platysma, depressor labii inferioris, and depressor anguli oris muscles medially over the periosteum of the mandible (see Fig. 21.17).

TRIGEMINAL NERVE

○ Expose the fibers of the platysma muscle (Fig. 21.16).

○ With scissors, remove the platysma, depressor labii inferioris, and depressor anguli oris muscles medially over the periosteum of the mandible (Fig. 21.17).

○ Identify the mental foramen and the mental nerve (Fig. 21.18).

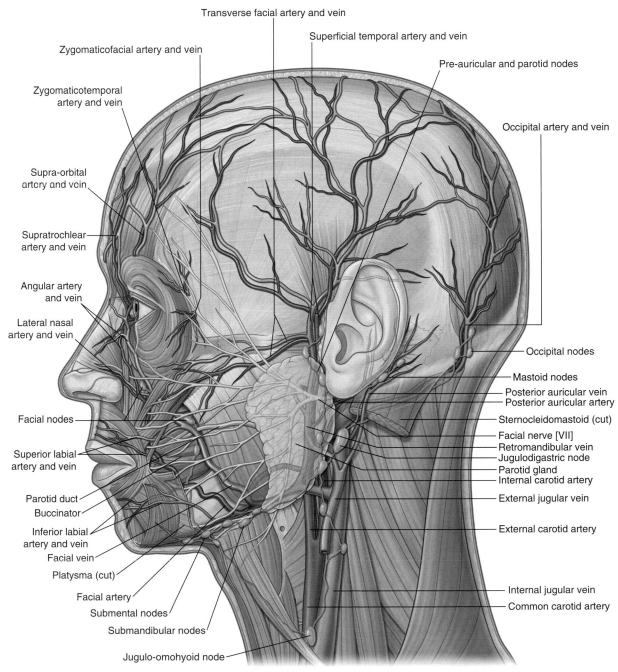

Transverse facial artery and vein
Superficial temporal artery and vein
Zygomaticofacial artery and vein
Pre-auricular and parotid nodes
Zygomaticotemporal artery and vein
Occipital artery and vein
Supra-orbital artery and vein
Supratrochlear artery and vein
Angular artery and vein
Lateral nasal artery and vein
Occipital nodes
Mastoid nodes
Posterior auricular vein
Posterior auricular artery
Facial nodes
Sternocleidomastoid (cut)
Facial nerve [VII]
Retromandibular vein
Superior labial artery and vein
Jugulodigastric node
Parotid gland
Internal carotid artery
Parotid duct
External jugular vein
Buccinator
Inferior labial artery and vein
External carotid artery
Facial vein
Platysma (cut)
Facial artery
Internal jugular vein
Common carotid artery
Submental nodes
Submandibular nodes
Jugulo-omohyoid node

Plate 21.2 Lateral view of muscles of the facial expression with accompanying nerves and arteries.

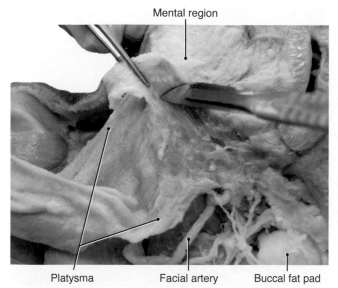

Fig. 21.16 Anterolateral view of the face and neck with skin and subcutaneous tissue removed.

Mental region

Platysma Facial artery Buccal fat pad

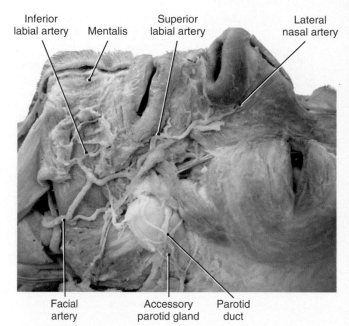

Fig. 21.18 Anterolateral view of face and neck with skin and subcutaneous tissue removed.

Inferior labial artery Mentalis Superior labial artery Lateral nasal artery

Facial artery Accessory parotid gland Parotid duct

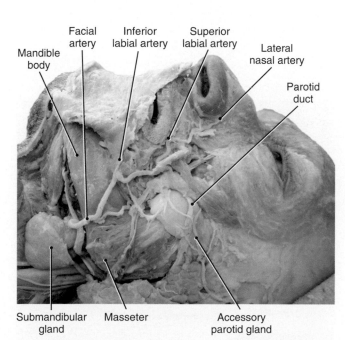

Fig. 21.17 Anterolateral view of face and neck with skin and subcutaneous tissue removed.

Facial artery Inferior labial artery Superior labial artery Lateral nasal artery

Mandible body Parotid duct

Submandibular gland Masseter Accessory parotid gland

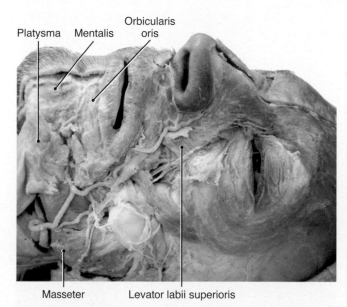

Fig. 21.19 Anterolateral view of face and neck with skin and subcutaneous tissue removed.

Platysma Mentalis Orbicularis oris

Masseter Levator labii superioris

DISSECTION TIP

One way to identify the infraorbital and mental nerves is to draw an imaginary line from the supraorbital notch vertically to the mandible, which will pass over, or near, the infraorbital and mental foramina.

○ Detach the inferior part of the orbicularis oris superiorly from the inferior orbital rim (medial to zygomaticus major muscle) (Fig. 21.19).

○ Detach the levator labii superioris alaeque nasi medially, and identify the infraorbital nerve (Figs. 21.20 to 21.22).

○ Reflect the superior part of the orbicularis oculi muscle, and identify the superior tarsal plate (Figs. 21.23 and 21.24).

○ Reflect the superior tarsal plate, and notice the fascia of the levator palpebrae superioris muscle (Fig. 21.25).

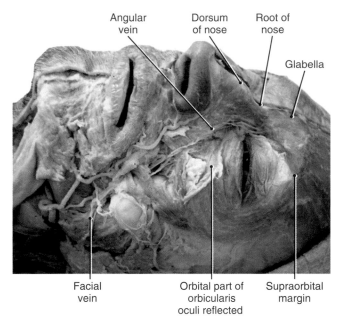

Fig. 21.20 Anterolateral view of face and neck with skin and subcutaneous tissue removed and orbital part of orbicularis oculi reflected.

Labels: Angular vein, Dorsum of nose, Root of nose, Glabella, Facial vein, Orbital part of orbicularis oculi reflected, Supraorbital margin

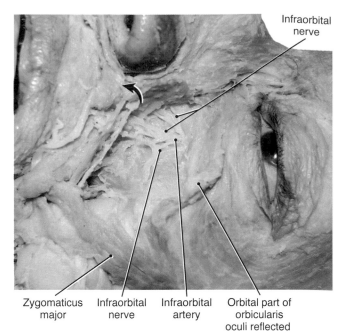

Fig. 21.22 Anteroinferior view of orbital region with skin and subcutaneous tissue removed and orbital part of orbicularis oculi reflected.

Labels: Infraorbital nerve, Zygomaticus major, Infraorbital nerve, Infraorbital artery, Orbital part of orbicularis oculi reflected

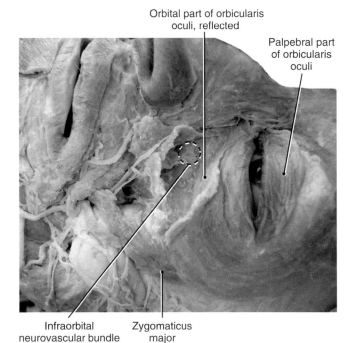

Fig. 21.21 Anteromedial view of nasal, orbital, and maxillary region with skin and subcutaneous tissue removed.

Labels: Orbital part of orbicularis oculi, reflected, Palpebral part of orbicularis oculi, Infraorbital neurovascular bundle, Zygomaticus major

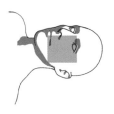

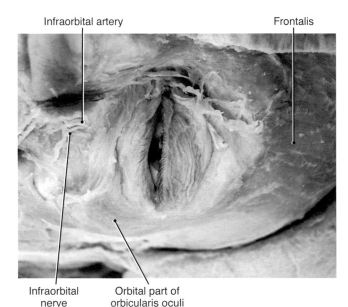

Fig. 21.23 Anteroinferior view of orbital region with skin and subcutaneous tissue removed.

Labels: Infraorbital artery, Frontalis, Infraorbital nerve, Orbital part of orbicularis oculi

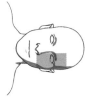

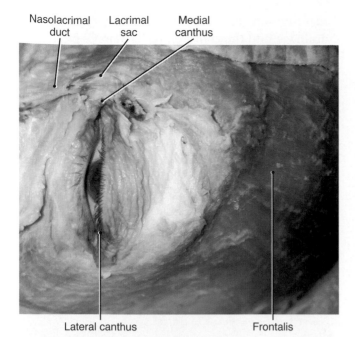

Nasolacrimal duct • Lacrimal sac • Medial canthus

Lateral canthus • Frontalis

Fig. 21.24 Anterior view of orbital region with skin and subcutaneous tissue removed.

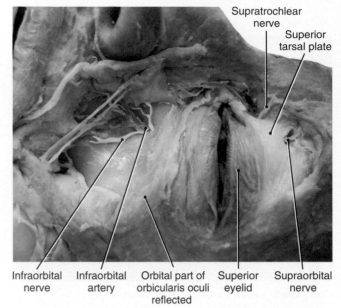

Supratrochlear nerve • Superior tarsal plate

Infraorbital nerve • Infraorbital artery • Orbital part of orbicularis oculi reflected • Superior eyelid • Supraorbital nerve

Fig. 21.26 Anterior superior view of orbital region with skin removed.

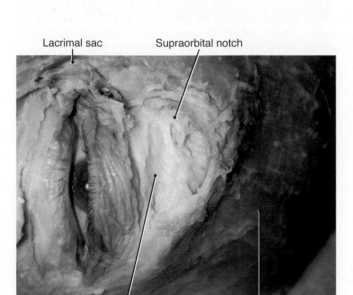

Lacrimal sac • Supraorbital notch

Fascia over levator palpebrae superioris • Frontalis

Fig. 21.25 Anterior view of orbital region with skin and subcutaneous tissue removed.

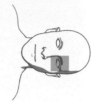

○ Palpate the supraorbital notch, and with scissors, separate the muscle fibers and the connective tissue superficial (inferior and superior) to the notch to expose the *supraorbital nerve* (Fig. 21.26).

○ Identify the superficial temporal vein. This vein joins the maxillary vein to form the retromandibular vein.

DISSECTION **TIP**

In most specimens the supraorbital nerve, artery, and vein emerge through the orbital septum and superior tarsal plate (see Fig. 21.26), whereas the supratrochlear nerve emerges medially (Fig. 21.27).

○ You may remove the parotid gland now (Fig. 21.28), or during the dissection of the infratemporal fossa (Chapter 22).

VEINS OF THE FACE

○ Identify the *retromandibular vein* deep to the facial nerve.

ANATOMY **NOTE**

The retromandibular vein splits into anterior and posterior divisions; the posterior division joins the posterior auricular vein to form the external jugular vein, and the anterior division joins the facial vein to form the common facial vein.

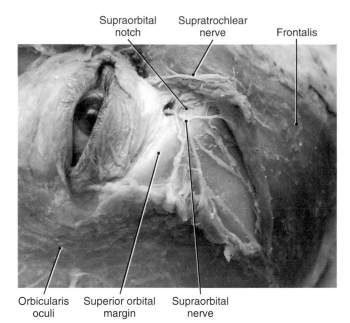

Fig. 21.27 Anterosuperior view of orbital region with skin and subcutaneous tissue removed.

Supraorbital notch · Supratrochlear nerve · Frontalis

Orbicularis oculi · Superior orbital margin · Supraorbital nerve

- ○ Identify and trace the *facial vein,* and look for its drainage into the common facial vein (Fig. 21.29).
- ○ The facial vein begins at the medial orbit as the angular vein, then courses with the facial artery toward the angle of the mandible (see Fig. 21.20).
- ○ Identify the junction of the posterior division of the retromandibular vein with the posterior auricular vein, forming the external jugular vein.
- ○ Trace the facial vein's drainage into the anterior division of the retromandibular vein, creating the common facial vein, which drains into the internal jugular vein.

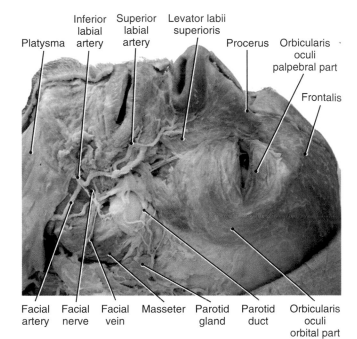

Platysma · Inferior labial artery · Superior labial artery · Levator labii superioris · Procerus · Orbicularis oculi palpebral part · Frontalis

Facial artery · Facial nerve · Facial vein · Masseter · Parotid gland · Parotid duct · Orbicularis oculi orbital part

Fig. 21.29 Anterolateral view of face and neck with skin and subcutaneous tissue removed.

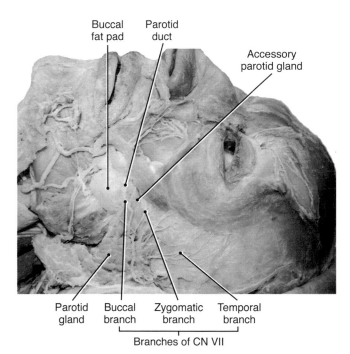

Buccal fat pad · Parotid duct · Accessory parotid gland

Parotid gland · Buccal branch · Zygomatic branch · Temporal branch

Branches of CN VII

Fig. 21.28 Anterolateral view of face with skin and subcutaneous tissue removed.

LABORATORY IDENTIFICATION CHECKLIST

NERVES

Trigeminal nerve branches (cutaneous)
- ☐ Supratrochlear nerve
- ☐ Supraorbital nerve
- ☐ Zygomaticotemporal nerve
- ☐ Zygomaticofacial nerve
- ☐ Auriculotemporal nerve
- ☐ Infratrochlear nerve
- ☐ Infraorbital nerve
- ☐ Mental nerve

Facial nerve branches (motor)
- ☐ Facial nerve trunk (deep within parotid gland)
- ☐ Temporal branches
- ☐ Zygomatic branches
- ☐ Buccal branches
- ☐ Marginal mandibular branches
- ☐ Cervical branches

ARTERIES

- ☐ External carotid (within parotid gland)
- ☐ Superficial temporal
- ☐ Maxillary
- ☐ Transverse facial
- ☐ Facial
  - ☐ Superior labial
  - ☐ Inferior labial
  - ☐ Angular

VEINS

- ☐ Facial
- ☐ Angular
- ☐ Retromandibular (within parotid gland)

MUSCLES

- ☐ Occipitofrontalis
  - ☐ Frontalis belly
  - ☐ Galea aponeurotica
  - ☐ Occipitalis belly
- ☐ Procerus
- ☐ Orbicularis oculi
  - ☐ Orbital part
  - ☐ Palpebral part
  - ☐ Lacrimal part
- ☐ Levator labii superioris alaeque nasi
- ☐ Levator labii superioris
- ☐ Levator anguli oris
- ☐ Risorius
- ☐ Zygomaticus major/minor
- ☐ Buccinator
- ☐ Orbicularis oris
- ☐ Depressor anguli oris
- ☐ Depressor labii inferioris
- ☐ Mentalis
- ☐ Platysma

BONES

- ☐ Frontal
- ☐ Zygomatic
- ☐ Temporal
- ☐ Maxillary
- ☐ Mandible

GLAND

- ☐ Parotid
  - ☐ Parotid duct (Stensen's duct)

ATLAS REFERENCES
Netter: 9, 10, 55–62, 64, 81–84
McMinn: 42, 44, 76
Gray's Atlas: 507, 527–533

BEFORE YOU BEGIN

- The infratemporal fossa dissection requires the use of an electric saw or a hammer and chisel. Make sure that you wear eye protection when you use these tools.
- Cut the terminal branches of the facial nerve, and reflect the nerves posteriorly toward the parotid gland (Fig. 22.1).
- Similarly, cut the parotid duct as it penetrates the buccinator muscle (Fig. 22.2), and reflect it posteriorly toward the parotid gland (see Fig. 22.1).
- Palpate the zygomatic arch, and expose it from the surrounding adipose tissue and temporal fascia (Fig. 22.3).

DISSECTION STEPS

○ Identify the temporalis muscle, and trace its course medial to the zygomatic arch (Fig. 22.4).

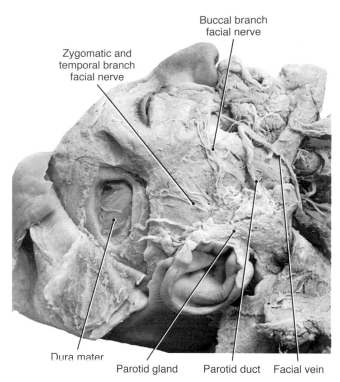

Fig. 22.2 Lateral view of face with skin reflected, revealing superficial structures.

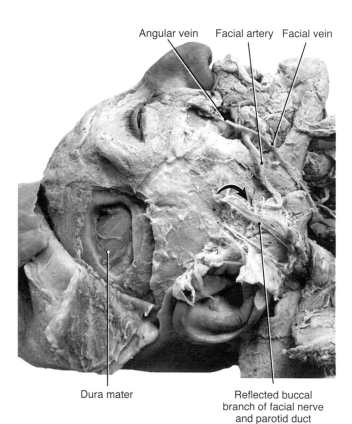

Fig. 22.1 Lateral view of face, with parotid duct and branches of facial nerve reflected.

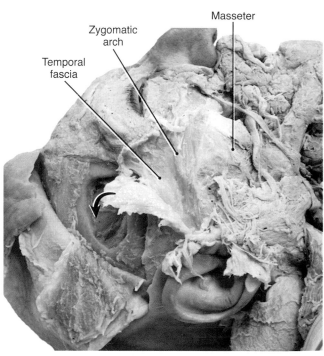

Fig. 22.3 Lateral view of face, with skin and subcutaneous tissue removed and temporal fascia reflected.

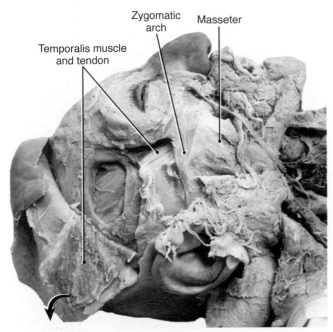

Fig. 22.4 Lateral view of face, with skin, subcutaneous tissue, and temporal fascia removed.

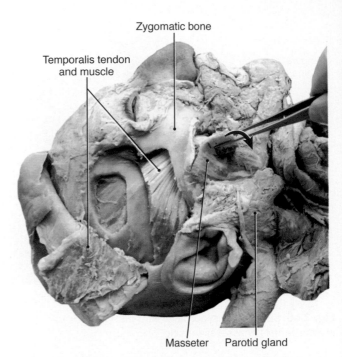

Fig. 22.6 Reflection of masseter muscle from inferior border of zygomatic arch.

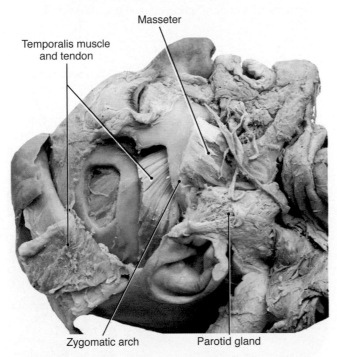

Fig. 22.5 Lateral view with skin and subcutaneous tissue removed.

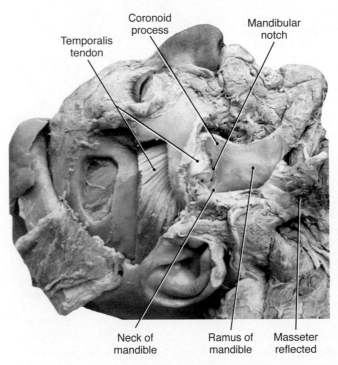

Fig. 22.7 Lateral view of face with superficial skin and subcutaneous skin removed and masseter muscle reflected.

○ Clean the lateral surface of the masseter muscle, and expose its borders (Fig. 22.5).

○ Detach the masseter muscle from the inferior border of the zygomatic arch (Fig. 22.6), and reflect it inferiorly toward the angle of the mandible.

○ Clean the remaining soft tissues over the mandible, and expose its surface (Fig. 22.7).

○ Identify the temporal, zygomatic, and mandibular bony regions.

○ Just deep to the anterior border of the ramus of the mandible, in the fat and connective tissue of the anterior edge of the temporalis muscle, identify and clean the *buccal nerve,* a branch of the mandibular division (V3) of the trigeminal nerve.

○ Place scissors or a probe underneath the zygomatic arch.

○ Using a saw, cut the zygomatic arch just anterior to the attachment of the masseter muscle (Fig. 22.8).

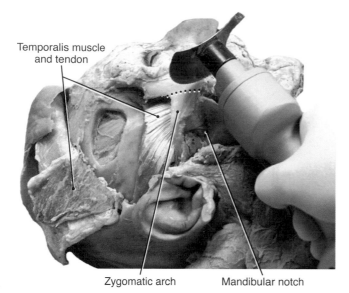

Fig. 22.8 Saw cut of zygomatic arch just anterior to attachment of masseter muscle.

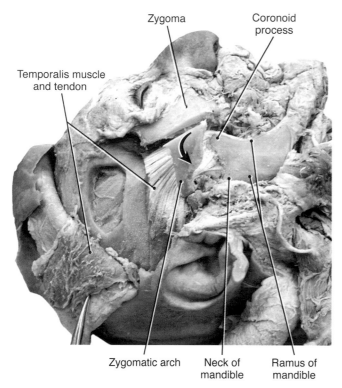

Fig. 22.9 Lateral view of face, revealing zygomatic arch osteotomy anterior to masseter attachment, with a second cut anterior to temporomandibular joint.

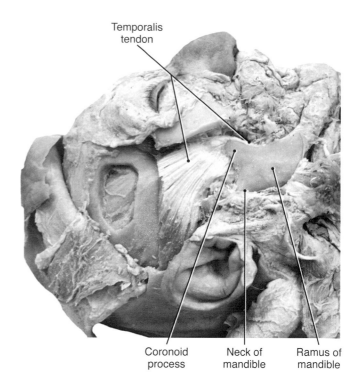

Fig. 22.10 Removal of zygomatic arch, exposing attachments of temporalis muscle and bony landmarks of mandible.

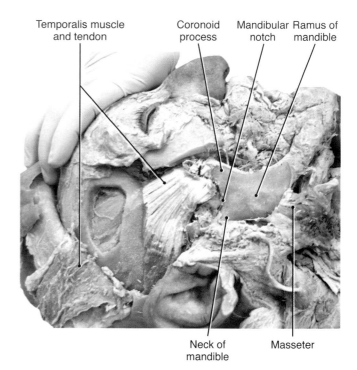

Fig. 22.11 Detachment of temporalis muscle from coronoid process and mandibular notch.

- Make a second cut through the arch just posterior to the masseter and anterior to the temporomandibular joint (Fig. 22.9).
- Detach the cut piece of zygomatic bone (Fig. 22.10).
- With scissors, cut the *temporalis muscle* from the coronoid process and ramus of the mandible (Fig. 22.11).
- Reflect the temporalis upward, and clean the soft tissues and fat over the mandibular notch (Fig. 22.12).

- Place your scissors or a probe or scalpel handle immediately beneath the ramus of the mandible (Fig. 22.13).
- Push the soft tissues, musculature, and vessels inferiorly.

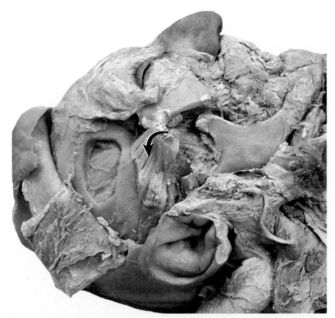

Fig. 22.12 Reflection of temporalis muscle upward *(arrow)*.

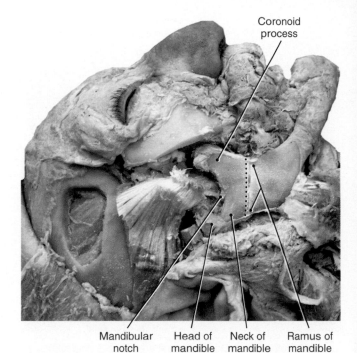

Coronoid
process

Mandibular | Head of | Neck of | Ramus of
notch | mandible | mandible | mandible

Fig. 22.14 Saw cut horizontally through ramus of mandible below coronoid process.

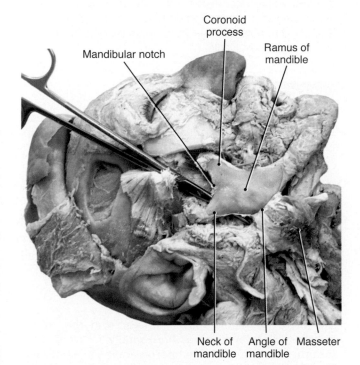

Coronoid
process

Mandibular notch | Ramus of
mandible

Neck of | Angle of | Masseter
mandible | mandible

Fig. 22.13 Placing scissors underneath the ramus of mandible and pushing soft tissues, muscles, and vessels inferiorly preserves underlying structure when the mandible is cut with electric saw.

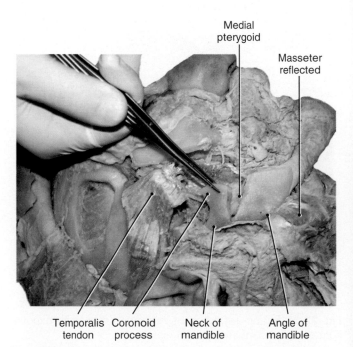

Medial
pterygoid

Masseter
reflected

Temporalis | Coronoid | Neck of | Angle of
tendon | process | mandible | mandible

Fig. 22.15 Severed coronoid process and the temporalis muscle reflected superiorly to open up dissection area.

DISSECTION TIP

This maneuver (see Fig. 22.13) is important for preserving underlying structures when the mandible is cut. You may leave the probe or scissors in place to protect the inferior alveolar neurovascular bundle and lingual nerve when you perform the cut (see next step).

○ With an electric saw, cut horizontally through the ramus of the mandible 2 to 3 inches (5–7.5 cm) below the coronoid process, leaving the articular process in place (Fig. 22.14).

○ Reflect the severed coronoid process and the temporalis muscle superiorly (Figs. 22.15 to 22.17).

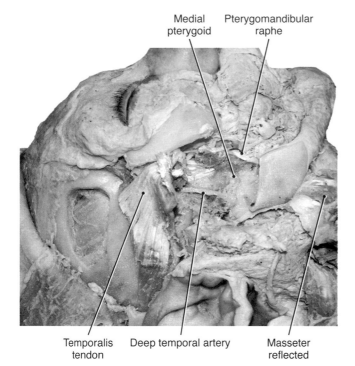

Medial pterygoid   Pterygomandibular raphe

Temporalis tendon   Deep temporal artery   Masseter reflected

Fig. 22.16 Appreciate medial pterygoid muscle with all soft tissues removed.

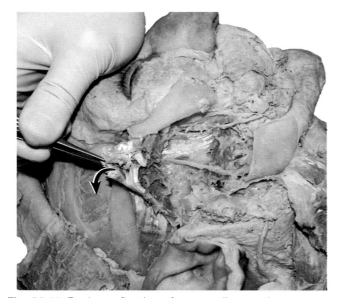

Fig. 22.17 Further reflection of temporalis muscle to expose contents of the infratemporal fossa.

DISSECTION **TIP**

Take special care when you reflect the coronoid process and the temporalis muscle so as not to injure the buccal nerve.

○ As the temporalis is reflected superiorly, observe the deep temporal arteries supplying this muscle.

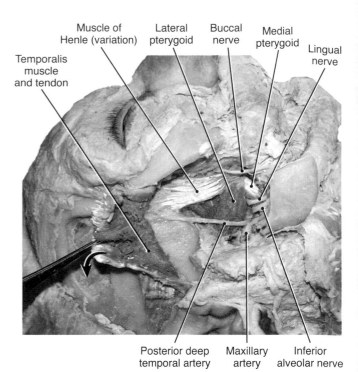

Temporalis muscle and tendon   Muscle of Henle (variation)   Lateral pterygoid   Buccal nerve   Medial pterygoid   Lingual nerve

Posterior deep temporal artery   Maxillary artery   Inferior alveolar nerve

Fig. 22.18 Appreciate medial and lateral pterygoid muscles. The maxillary artery is located deep to lateral pterygoid in this specimen; note also the uncommon pterygoideus proprius (muscle of Henle).

DISSECTION **TIP**

You can choose either to sever the arteries or to keep them. In this dissection, we choose to keep the deep temporal vessels (see Figs. 22.16 and 22.17).

○ Once temporalis has been reflected, identify the medial pterygoid muscle (see Figs. 22.15 to 22.17).

○ Once the temporalis muscle is reflected and the soft tissues are cleaned, identify and expose the *lateral pterygoid muscle,* which lies just beneath the temporalis (Fig. 22.18).

ANATOMY **NOTE**

The lateral pterygoid muscle arises from the lateral pterygoid plate and passes horizontally to insert onto the articular disc of the temporomandibular joint (see Fig. 22.18).

ANATOMY **NOTE**

In some cadavers, a variant muscle may be seen in the infratemporal fossa. In this specimen, a pterygoideus proprius was identified (muscle of Henle). This muscle originates from the anterior infratemporal crest, runs vertically downward to insert onto the lateral pterygoid plate, and crosses superficially to the lateral pterygoid muscle (see Fig. 22.18). Typically, the muscle of Henle has no functional significance, but it may compress the mandibular nerve, resulting in possible trigeminal neuralgia.

- Clean the soft tissues and fat at the inferior border of the lateral pterygoid muscle (Fig. 22.19 and Plate 22.1).
- Identify the *inferior alveolar nerve* and inferior alveolar artery superficial to the medial pterygoid muscle (see Figs. 22.18 and 22.19).
- Clean the inferior alveolar nerve and trace it to the mandibular foramen.

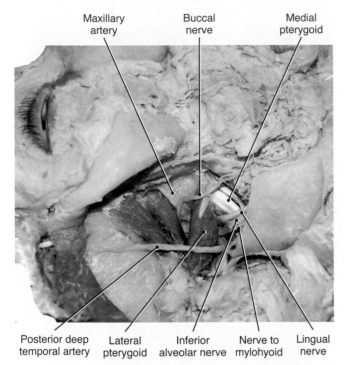

Fig. 22.19 Soft tissue in space between medial and lateral pterygoid muscles cleaned, exposing key structures.

Plate 22.1 Nerves and vessels of the infratemporal fossa.

- Look at the lateral surface of the inferior alveolar nerve, and note the small branch that runs parallel with it, the nerve to the mylohyoid muscle (see Fig. 22.19).

ANATOMY **NOTE**

The nerve to the mylohyoid arises just before the inferior alveolar nerve enters the mandibular foramen. The nerve to the mylohyoid travels inferiorly, beneath the ramus and body of the mandible, to innervate the mylohyoid muscle and the anterior belly of the digastric muscle.

- Lateral to the inferior alveolar nerve, identify the *lingual nerve* (Figs. 22.20 and 22.21).
- Medial to the inferior alveolar nerve, identify the *buccal nerve*.
- Immediately underneath these nerves, observe the medial pterygoid muscle passing from the pterygoid plate to its insertion onto the inferior and posterior parts of the medial surface of the mandibular ramus.
- Identify and expose the maxillary artery (see Fig. 22.19 to 22.21 and see Fig. 22.29).

ANATOMY **NOTE**

In the majority of cadavers, the lateral pterygoid muscle is crossed superficially by branches of the maxillary artery; in the remaining specimens, the artery travels deep to the muscle (see Fig. 22.21).

- Proceed by carefully detaching the lateral pterygoid muscle from its origin on the pterygoid plate with scissors and forceps (Figs. 22.22 to 22.24).

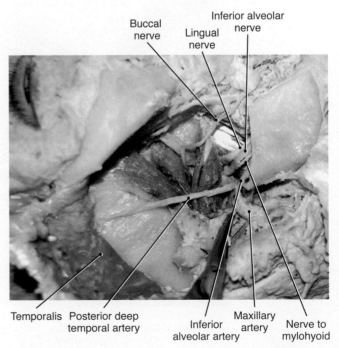

Fig. 22.20 The maxillary artery is exposed.

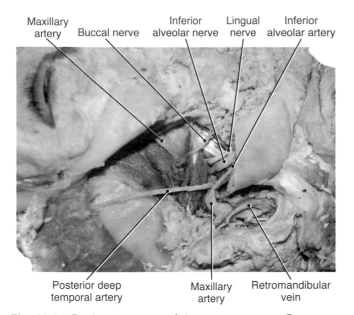

Maxillary artery · Buccal nerve · Inferior alveolar nerve · Lingual nerve · Inferior alveolar artery

Posterior deep temporal artery · Maxillary artery · Retromandibular vein

Fig. 22.21 Further exposure of the maxillary artery and accompanying maxillary and retromandibular veins.

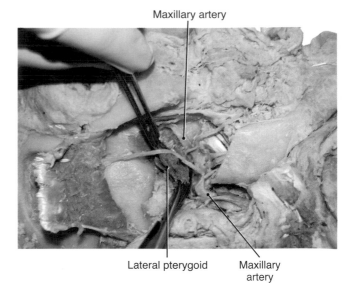

Maxillary artery

Lateral pterygoid · Maxillary artery

Fig. 22.22 Lateral pterygoid muscle removed with scissors and forceps.

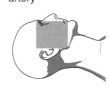

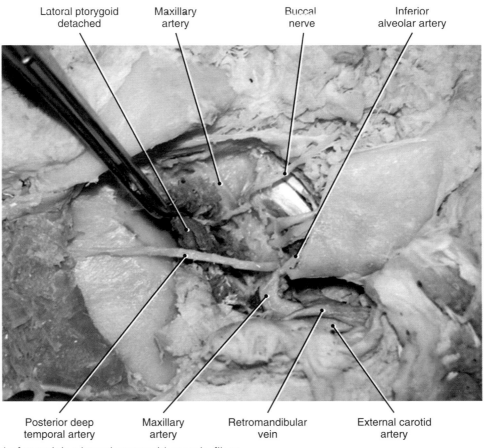

Lateral ptorygoid detached · Maxillary artery · Buccal nerve · Inferior alveolar artery

Posterior deep temporal artery · Maxillary artery · Retromandibular vein · External carotid artery

Fig. 22.23 Removal of remaining lateral pterygoid muscle fibers.

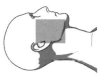

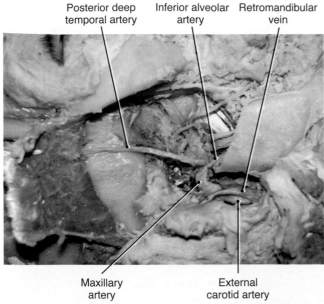

Posterior deep temporal artery · Inferior alveolar artery · Retromandibular vein

Maxillary artery · External carotid artery

Fig. 22.24 Complete removal of lateral pterygoid muscle. Note soft tissues around maxillary artery; carefully remove all soft tissues.

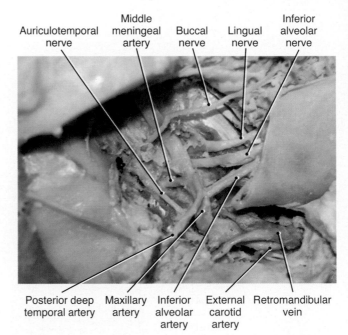

Auriculotemporal nerve · Middle meningeal artery · Buccal nerve · Lingual nerve · Inferior alveolar nerve

Posterior deep temporal artery · Maxillary artery · Inferior alveolar artery · External carotid artery · Retromandibular vein

Fig. 22.25 Complete removal of soft tissues, revealing neurovascular structures.

DISSECTION **TIP**

Removing the lateral pterygoid muscle can be a challenge. Be patient, and detach its muscle fibers carefully, paying special attention to the branches of the maxillary artery underneath it (see Figs. 22.22 through 22.24).

- Carefully remove all soft tissues around the maxillary artery.
- Posterior to the inferior alveolar artery and nerve and anterior to the medial pterygoid muscle, identify the sphenomandibular ligament.

DISSECTION **TIP**

This ligament is thin and may resemble a nerve, and it is often confused with the inferior alveolar nerve.

- Once the lateral pterygoid muscle is removed, expose the maxillary artery and its branches (Fig. 22.25).
- Note the retromandibular vein formed by the junction of the superficial temporal and maxillary veins (see Fig. 22.25).
- Identify the middle meningeal artery, which typically runs vertically toward the sphenoid bone, to enter the foramen spinosum (see Figs. 22.25 and 22.27).
- Identify the two roots of the auriculotemporal nerve, which, in the majority of cases, you will find encircling

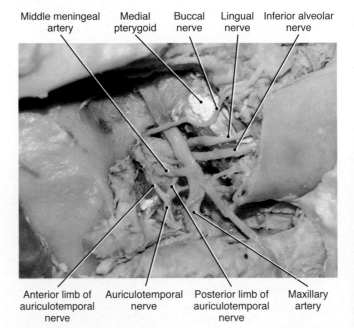

Middle meningeal artery · Medial pterygoid · Buccal nerve · Lingual nerve · Inferior alveolar nerve

Anterior limb of auriculotemporal nerve · Auriculotemporal nerve · Posterior limb of auriculotemporal nerve · Maxillary artery

Fig. 22.26 Lateral view of infratemporal fossa, revealing medial pterygoid muscle and neurovascular structures.

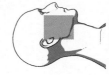

the middle meningeal artery (Figs. 22.26 and 22.27 and Plates 22.2 and 22.3).

- Lift the lingual nerve, and trace it superiorly until you see it joined on its posterior surface by a small nerve, the *chorda tympani,* which is a branch of the

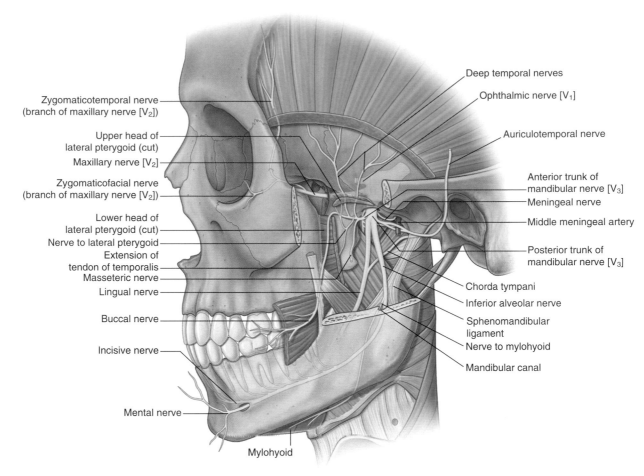

Zygomaticotemporal nerve (branch of maxillary nerve [V₂])

Upper head of lateral pterygoid (cut)

Maxillary nerve [V₂]

Zygomaticofacial nerve (branch of maxillary nerve [V₂])

Lower head of lateral pterygoid (cut)

Nerve to lateral pterygoid

Extension of tendon of temporalis

Masseteric nerve

Lingual nerve

Buccal nerve

Incisive nerve

Mental nerve

Mylohyoid

Deep temporal nerves

Ophthalmic nerve [V₁]

Auriculotemporal nerve

Anterior trunk of mandibular nerve [V₃]

Meningeal nerve

Middle meningeal artery

Posterior trunk of mandibular nerve [V₃]

Chorda tympani

Inferior alveolar nerve

Sphenomandibular ligament

Nerve to mylohyoid

Mandibular canal

Plate 22.2 Nerves of the infratemporal fossa.

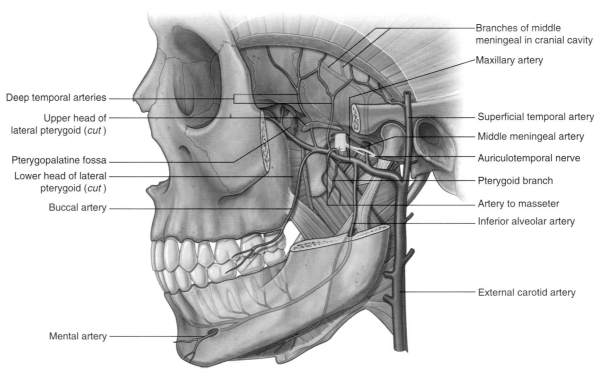

Deep temporal arteries

Upper head of lateral pterygoid (cut)

Pterygopalatine fossa

Lower head of lateral pterygoid (cut)

Buccal artery

Mental artery

Branches of middle meningeal in cranial cavity

Maxillary artery

Superficial temporal artery

Middle meningeal artery

Auriculotemporal nerve

Pterygoid branch

Artery to masseter

Inferior alveolar artery

External carotid artery

Plate 22.3 Arteries of the temporal and infratemporal fossae.

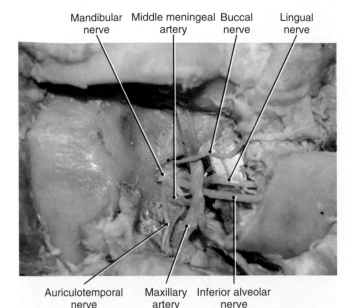

Fig. 22.27 Lateral view of infratemporal fossa, revealing the medial pterygoid muscle and neurovascular structures.

Labels (Fig. 22.27): Mandibular nerve; Middle meningeal artery; Buccal nerve; Lingual nerve; Auriculotemporal nerve; Maxillary artery; Inferior alveolar nerve

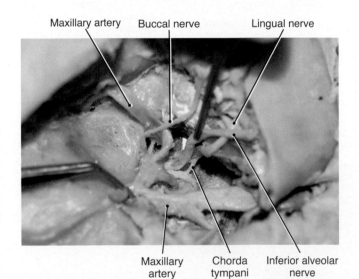

Fig. 22.28 Lingual nerve lifted and followed posteriorly to its connection with chorda tympani nerve.

Labels (Fig. 22.28): Maxillary artery; Buccal nerve; Lingual nerve; Maxillary artery; Chorda tympani; Inferior alveolar nerve

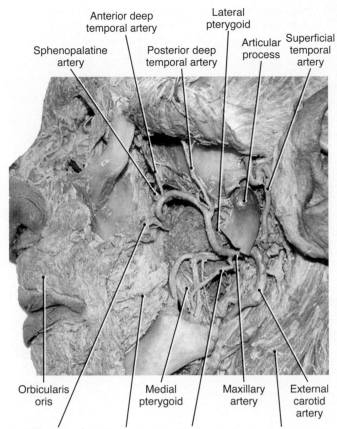

Fig. 22.29 A different specimen, with branches of maxillary artery exposed superficial to lateral pterygoid muscle.

Labels (Fig. 22.29): Sphenopalatine artery; Anterior deep temporal artery; Posterior deep temporal artery; Lateral pterygoid; Articular process; Superficial temporal artery; Orbicularis oris; Medial pterygoid; Maxillary artery; External carotid artery; Posterior superior alveolar artery; Buccinator; Inferior alveolar artery; Sternocleidomastoid

facial nerve (Fig. 22.28). If this nerve is not evident, clean the soft tissue around the lingual nerve more posteriorly.

○ Clean the lingual and inferior alveolar nerves, and trace their passage deep to the medial pterygoid muscle.

○ Deep to the infratemporal fossa, trace and follow the termination of the maxillary artery, the *sphenopalatine artery*, toward the sphenopalatine foramen (Figs. 22.29 and 22.30).

○ Typically, two additional branches are easily identifiable. Identify the *infraorbital artery* as it ascends to enter the infraorbital canal, and the *posterior superior alveolar artery* as it descends to enter the infratemporal surface of the maxilla (see Fig. 22.30).

○ Identify the mandibular canal and the inferior alveolar nerve (Figs. 22.31 to 22.33).

○ With an electric drill, cut the mandible in a direction demarcating a line between the mandibular canal and mental foramen (see Fig. 22.32).

○ With fine forceps, lift the small branches of the inferior alveolar nerve terminating on the teeth (Fig. 22.34).

○ Using a bone saw, make a shallow parasagittal cut through the temporomandibular joint. Identify the articular disc, the two synovial cavities, and the articular capsule of that joint.

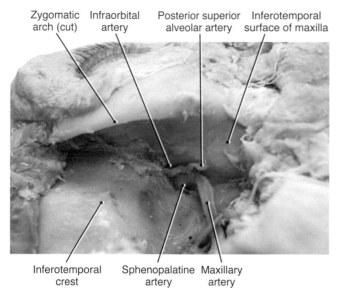

Zygomatic arch (cut) Infraorbital artery Posterior superior alveolar artery Inferotemporal surface of maxilla

Inferotemporal crest Sphenopalatine artery Maxillary artery

Fig. 22.30 Deep view of infratemporal fossa, revealing termination of maxillary artery.

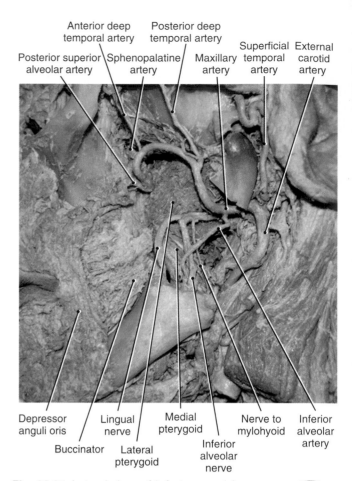

Anterior deep temporal artery Posterior deep temporal artery Superficial temporal artery External carotid artery

Posterior superior alveolar artery Sphenopalatine artery Maxillary artery

Depressor anguli oris Lingual nerve Medial pterygoid Nerve to mylohyoid Inferior alveolar artery

Buccinator Lateral pterygoid Inferior alveolar nerve

Fig. 22.31 Lateral view of infratemporal fossa.

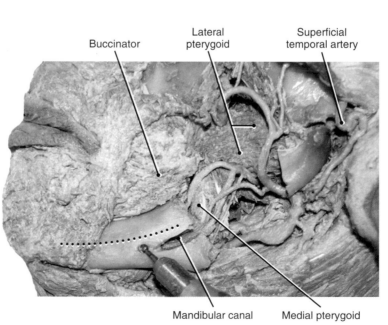

Buccinator Lateral pterygoid Superficial temporal artery

Mandibular canal Medial pterygoid

Fig. 22.32 Mandible drilled in direction demarcated *(broken line)* between mandibular canal and mental foramen.

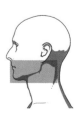

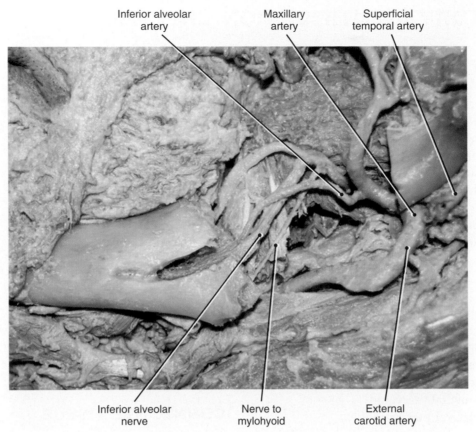

Fig. 22.33 Exposure of contents of mandibular canal.

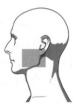

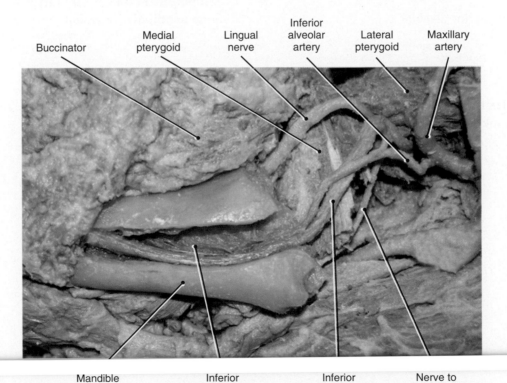

Fig. 22.34 Further exposure of inferior alveolar nerve within mandibular canal. Note small branches to the teeth.

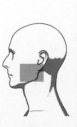

LABORATORY IDENTIFICATION CHECKLIST

NERVES
☐ Trigeminal, mandibular division (V3)
☐ Auriculotemporal
☐ Inferior alveolar
☐ Nerve to mylohyoid
☐ Lingual
☐ Chorda tympani
☐ Buccal (long buccal of trigeminal)

ARTERIES
☐ Maxillary
  ☐ Middle meningeal
  ☐ Inferior alveolar
  ☐ Deep temporal arteries
  ☐ Muscular branches
    ☐ Masseteric artery
    ☐ Artery to medial pterygoid
    ☐ Artery to lateral pterygoid
  ☐ Sphenopalatine (terminal branch of maxillary artery)
  ☐ Posterior superior alveolar
  ☐ Infraorbital
  ☐ Buccal

VEINS
☐ Pterygoid plexus (often difficult to isolate in cadaveric tissue)

MUSCLES
☐ Masseter
☐ Temporalis
☐ Lateral pterygoid
☐ Medial pterygoid

BONES
☐ Temporal
☐ Sphenoid
☐ Mandible
  ☐ Head
  ☐ Coronoid process
  ☐ Notch
  ☐ Ramus
  ☐ Angle
  ☐ Neck

CONNECTIVE TISSUE
☐ Temporomandibular joint capsule
☐ Temporomandibular joint (articular) disc
☐ Stylomandibular ligament

ATLAS REFERENCES

Netter: 111–126, 149–158
McMinn: 51–53, 62–72
Gray's Atlas: 490–502

BEFORE YOU BEGIN

The skin of the face has been previously removed (see Chapter 21).

DISSECTION STEPS

○ Continue the removal of the facial skin toward the occipital region, and separate the skin from the subcutaneous tissue (Fig. 23.1).

○ Identify and expose the superficial temporal artery and its branches (Fig. 23.2).

○ Once the superficial temporal artery has been fully exposed, separate the subcutaneous tissue and fat from the underlying galea aponeurotica, or *epicranial aponeurosis* (see Fig. 23.2).

○ This aponeurosis is a flattened tendon that connects the occipitalis and frontalis muscles, forming the occipitofrontalis muscle.

○ Cut and detach the frontalis muscle from the frontal bone.

○ With forceps, grasp the frontalis muscle and reflect it posteriorly (Fig. 23.3).

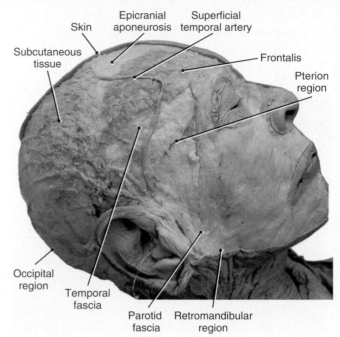

Fig. 23.2 Lateral view of exposed superficial temporal artery and branches.

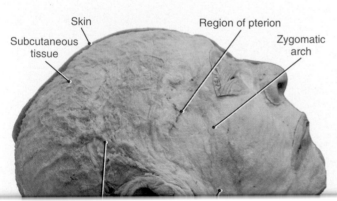

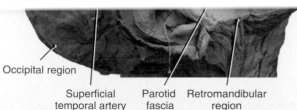

Fig. 23.1 Lateral view of external cranium and face.

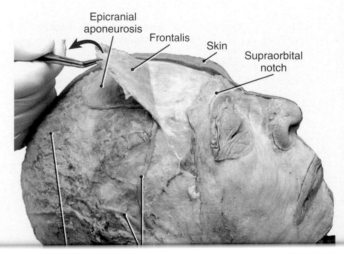

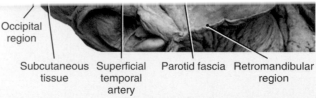

Fig. 23.3 Frontalis muscle detached from frontal bone and reflected posteriorly.

- On the internal surface of the frontalis muscle, note the loose areolar tissue, and on the surface of the cranium, note the *pericranium* (Fig. 23.4).
- At this part of the dissection, identify all the previously dissected layers of the *scalp* (Plate 23.1):
  - *Skin*
  - Connective tissue (subcutaneous tissue)
- *Aponeurotic layer*
- *Loose areolar tissue*
- *Pericranium*
- To expose the brain, the *calvaria,* or "skullcap," must be removed. The calvaria consists primarily of the parietal, frontal, and occipital bones. Dissect away the occipitofrontalis muscle and expose the pericranium, leaving the temporalis fascia intact (Fig. 23.5).
- With a scalpel, reflect the temporal fascia and expose the temporalis muscle (Fig. 23.6).

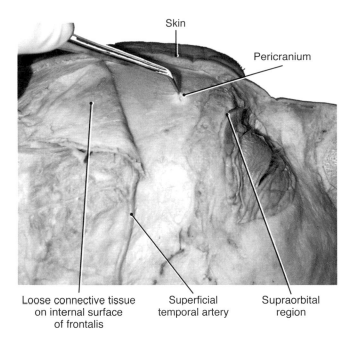

Fig. 23.4 Appreciate the loose areolar tissue at the internal surface of frontalis muscle and the pericranium on cranial surface.

Skin

Pericranium

Loose connective tissue on internal surface of frontalis

Superficial temporal artery

Supraorbital region

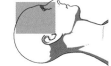

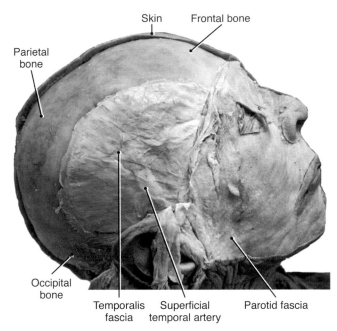

Skin   Frontal bone

Parietal bone

Occipital bone

Temporalis fascia   Superficial temporal artery   Parotid fascia

Fig. 23.5 Occipitofrontalis muscle removed, exposing pericranium and leaving temporalis fascia intact.

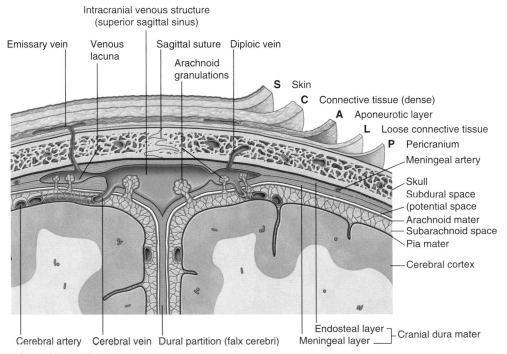

Intracranial venous structure (superior sagittal sinus)

Emissary vein   Venous lacuna   Sagittal suture   Diploic vein

Arachnoid granulations

S Skin

C Connective tissue (dense)

A Aponeurotic layer

L Loose connective tissue

P Pericranium

Meningeal artery

Skull

Subdural space (potential space)

Arachnoid mater

Subarachnoid space

Pia mater

Cerebral cortex

Cerebral artery   Cerebral vein   Dural partition (falx cerebri)

Endosteal layer ⎤ Cranial dura mater
Meningeal layer ⎦

Plate 23.1 Scalp and cranial meninges.

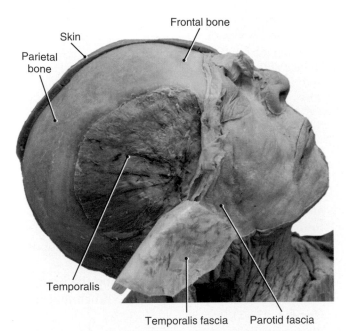

Fig. 23.6 Temporalis fascia reflected, exposing temporalis muscle.

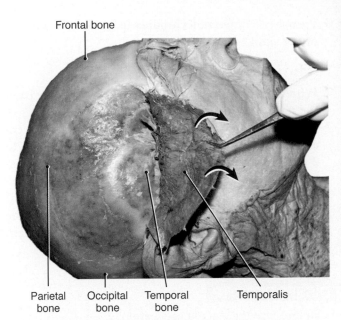

Fig. 23.8 Temporalis muscle reflected toward zygomatic bone, exposing pterion.

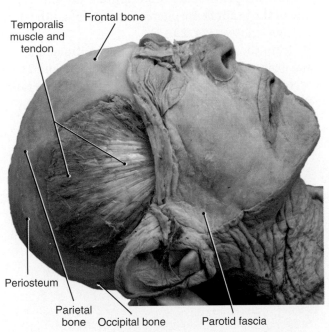

Fig. 23.7 Appreciate the temporalis muscle and tendinous fibers.

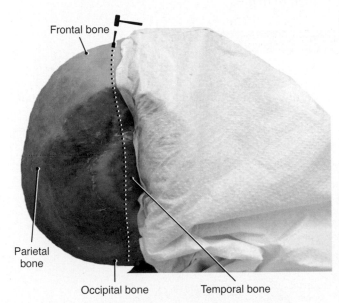

Fig. 23.9 Lateral view of external cranium and face (covered).

DISSECTION OF THE SKULL

fibers (Fig. 23.7).
O Reflect the temporalis toward the zygomatic bone, and expose the *pterion* (Fig. 23.8).
O Once the temporalis muscle is completely reflected and the calvaria fully exposed, identify the frontal, parietal, temporal, and occipital bones, as well as the sagittal, coronal, and lambdoid sutures.

O Place a plastic or wooden block under the head or shoulders to elevate the body from the dissection table.

DISSECTION TIP

Place paper towels around the face and temporalis muscles to protect them from bone dust (Fig. 23.9).

- We use two different techniques to expose the contents of the skull.

Technique 1

- With a marker, draw a stippled midsagittal line from the nasion to the external occipital protuberance.
- Draw a second, circumferential line passing 1 to 2 cm above the superciliary arches and ears to reach 1 to 2 cm above the external occipital protuberance posteriorly (see Fig. 23.9).
- With an electric saw, make a cut 2 to 3 cm (~1 inch) lateral to the midline, on both sides. In this way, the superior sagittal sinus and the falx cerebri will remain intact (Fig. 23.10).

DISSECTION TIP

Caution! Use the electric saw carefully.

- Make a shallow, circumferential cut of approximately 1 cm in depth.

DISSECTION TIP

Do not place the saw too deeply, because you will cut the dura and the brain. To complete the cut toward the external occipital protuberance, it is necessary to rotate the cadaver.

Once the first cut is complete, use the chisel and mallet to break through the bone and detach the two bone flaps (Fig. 23.11).

DISSECTION TIP

Detaching the bone flap from the underlying dura mater can be challenging. Place the forceps or a chisel into the gap (created by the saw cut) between the two adjacent bones, and use it to lift it up from the dura. If the dura is attached to the calvaria, use a probe to reflect the endosteal layer away from the calvaria, leaving the dura mater intact.

- After removal of the calvaria, examine the dura mater and identify the middle meningeal artery and its branches (see Figs. 23.11 and 23.13).
- Cut and reflect the dura, and expose the subdural space (Fig. 23.12).
- Observe the arachnoid layer covering the brain and the cerebral veins penetrating the arachnoid mater (see Fig. 23.12).
- Place your hands on one of the cerebral hemispheres and retract it laterally (Fig. 23.14).
- Notice the midline connection between the two hemispheres, the corpus callosum (see Fig. 23.14).
- With a scalpel, make a midsagittal cut, and reflect one of the brain hemispheres, leaving intact the dural venous sinuses (Fig. 23.15).
- Perform the same technique to the contralateral side, and expose the sinuses bilaterally (Figs. 23.16 and 23.17).
- Identify the *falx cerebri*, a dural partition separating the right from the left cerebral hemispheres.

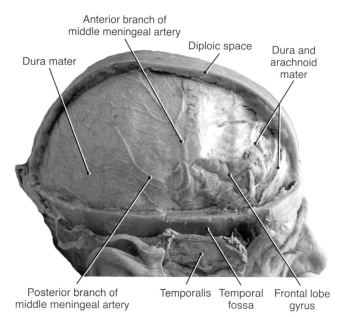

Fig. 23.11 Lateral view of right hemisphere after craniotomy.

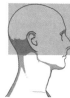

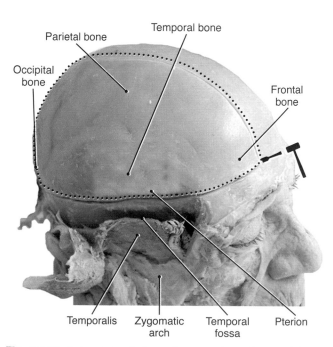

Fig. 23.10 Anterolateral view of external cranium and face.

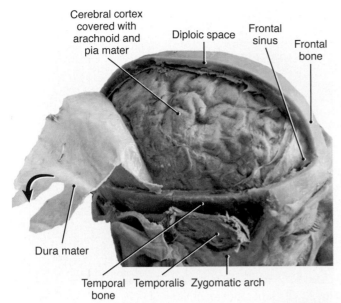

Fig. 23.12 Dura mater reflected, exposing subdural space. Observe the arachnoid layer covering the brain and cerebral veins penetrating it.

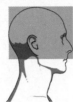

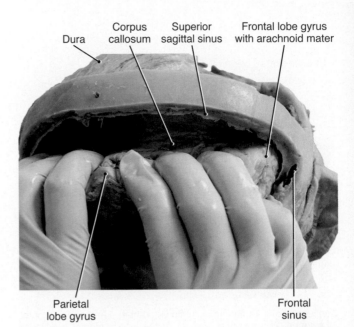

Fig. 23.14 Cerebral hemisphere retracted laterally; note the frontal and superior sagittal sinuses and corpus callosum. Appreciate the connection between the two hemispheres, the corpus callosum.

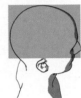

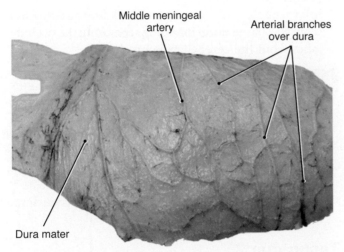

Fig. 23.13 External surface of removed dura mater, revealing the middle meningeal artery and arterial branches to dura mater.

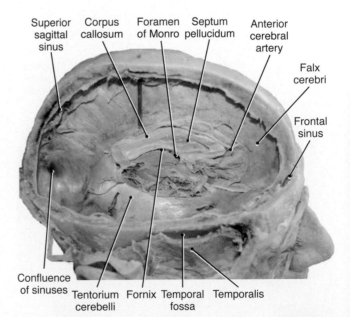

Fig. 23.15 With a midsagittal cut, the brain hemisphere is reflected, leaving the dural venous sinuses in place.

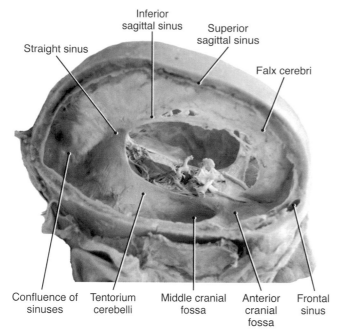

Figure labels: Straight sinus, Inferior sagittal sinus, Superior sagittal sinus, Falx cerebri, Confluence of sinuses, Tentorium cerebelli, Middle cranial fossa, Anterior cranial fossa, Frontal sinus

Fig. 23.16 Postcraniotomy lateral view of right hemisphere.

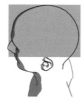

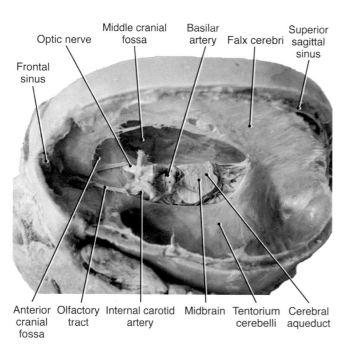

Figure labels: Optic nerve, Middle cranial fossa, Basilar artery, Falx cerebri, Superior sagittal sinus, Frontal sinus, Anterior cranial fossa, Olfactory tract, Internal carotid artery, Midbrain, Tentorium cerebelli, Cerebral aqueduct

Fig. 23.17 Lateral view of left hemisphere after craniotomy.

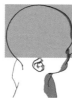

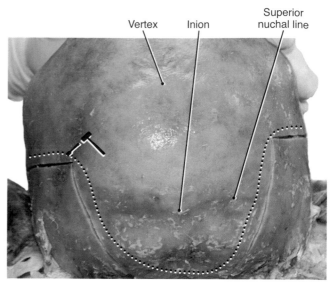

Figure labels: Vertex, Inion, Superior nuchal line

Fig. 23.18 Superoposterior view of external cranium revealing the superior nuchal line, inion, posterior craniotomy *(dashed line),* and vertex.

○ Superior to the falx cerebri, identify the *superior sagittal sinus,* which joins the two transverse sinuses at the confluence of sinuses ("torcular herophili," or wine-press of Herophilus).

○ Inferolateral to the falx cerebri, look for the *tentorium cerebelli,* a large dural infolding separating the occipital lobes from the cerebellar hemispheres.

DISSECTION **TIP**

If time permits, remove the midportion of the calvaria, and expose the superior sagittal sinus. Incise the dura forming the sinus, and notice its internal structure. In the majority of specimens the superior sagittal sinus will drain into the right transverse sinus.

○ At this point, the dissection can continue as outlined later.

Technique 2

○ With a pen, draw a circumferential line passing 1 to 2 cm above the superciliary ridges and ears to reach 1 to 2 cm above the external occipital protuberance posteriorly (Figs. 23.18 and 23.19).

○ With an electric saw, make a shallow, circumferential cut of about 1 cm along this line (Fig. 23.20).

DISSECTION **TIP**

Use the electric saw carefully. To complete the cut at the external occipital protuberance, the cadaver must be rotated. Do not insert the saw too deeply, or you may sever the dura mater and the brain (Fig. 23.21).

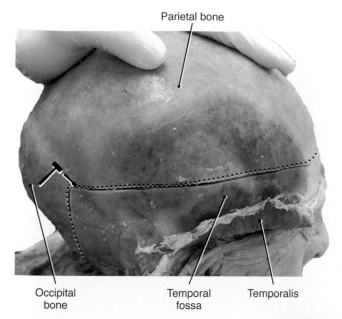

Parietal bone

Occipital bone   Temporal fossa   Temporalis

Fig. 23.19 Postcraniotomy lateral view of external cranium, revealing frontal bone, parietal bone, temporal bone/fossa, and temporalis muscle reflected inferiorly over zygomatic arch.

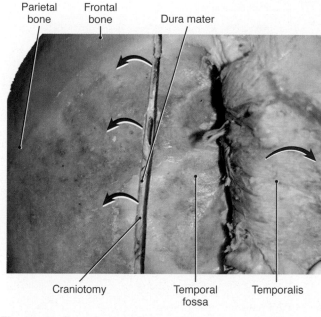

Parietal bone   Frontal bone   Dura mater

Craniotomy   Temporal fossa   Temporalis

Fig. 23.21 Once first cut is complete, use chisel and mallet to break through the bone and detach it from the dura.

DISSECTION **TIP**

The bone cut can extend below the external occipital protuberance, to the posterolateral aspects of the foramen magnum, including the posterior portions of the atlas and axis. With this extension, removal of the brain and spinal cord is easier. However, this extension will sever the muscles of the suboccipital triangle. If you want to preserve the suboccipital muscles, make the cut pass through the external occipital protuberance instead (Fig. 23.22).

○ Second, complete the bone removal with a chisel and mallet to break through the bone, and detach it from the underlying dura mater (Fig. 23.23).

DISSECTION **TIP**

Detaching the bone from the underlying dura can be challenging. Place the chisel in the gap (created by saw cut) between the adjacent bones, slightly rotating it to lift the bone from the dura. If the dura is still connected to the calvaria, use a probe to reflect the endosteal layer from the calvaria, leaving the dura intact.

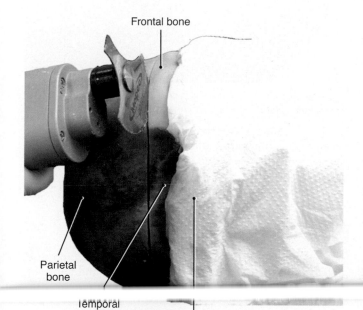

Frontal bone

Parietal bone

Temporal fossa

Reflected temporalis over zygomatic arch

Fig. 23.20 Posterolateral view of external cranium, revealing wedge resection cut.

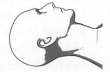

○ Inspect the internal surface of the calvaria and identify the small openings for emissary veins.
○ Note the small pits (granular *fovea*) produced by the *arachnoid granulations* (large arachnoid *villi* that protrude into dural venous sinuses) (Fig. 23.24).
○ Look for the frontal sinus extending into the calvaria.

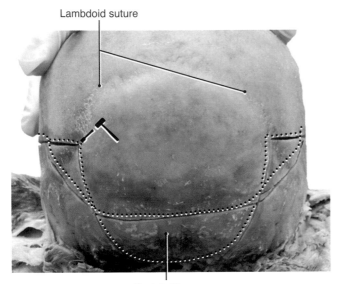

Lambdoid suture

Occipital bone

Fig. 23.22 Posterior view of external cranium shows of the cranium *(dashed line)*, lambdoid suture, and occipital bone, preserving the muscles of the suboccipital triangle.

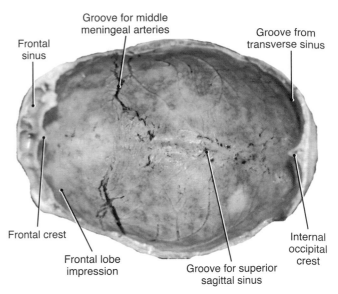

Groove for middle meningeal arteries

Frontal sinus

Groove from transverse sinus

Frontal crest

Frontal lobe impression

Groove for superior sagittal sinus

Internal occipital crest

Fig. 23.24 Craniotomy with calvaria removed, revealing internal surface.

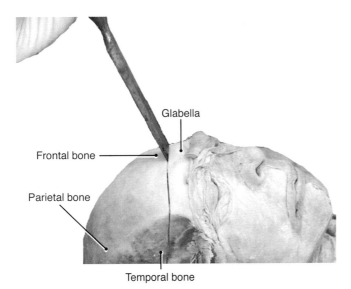

Glabella

Frontal bone

Parietal bone

Temporal bone

Fig. 23.23 Anterolateral view of external cranium and face revealing sagittal suture line for craniotomy, with chisel inserted into scoring line and glabella.

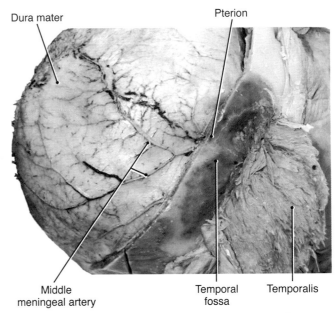

Dura mater

Pterion

Middle meningeal artery

Temporal fossa

Temporalis

Fig. 23.25 Lateral view showing dura mater, middle meningeal artery branches, pterion, temporal fossa, and temporalis muscle.

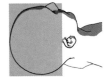

○ Note the spongy bone occupying the space between the outer and inner compact bony layers (tables), the *diploic space.*
○ Identify the impressions made by the superior sagittal sinus and the middle meningeal arteries.
○ Inspect the dura mater and identify the middle meningeal artery and its branches (Fig. 23.25).
○ Identify the superior sagittal sinus and look for the *lateral lacunae* (Fig. 23.26). The lateral lacunae are lateral venous extensions of the superior sagittal sinus.

DISSECTION **TIP**

If time permits, with a scalpel make an incision into the lateral lacunae, and note their opening to the superior sagittal sinus.

○ Cut the dura 2 to 3 cm (~1 inch) lateral to the midline, and reflect it inferiorly (Figs. 23.27 and 23.28).
○ Inspect the subdural space and the arachnoid layer pierced with cerebral veins.
○ Identify the arachnoid mater, and make a small incision to expose the pia mater.

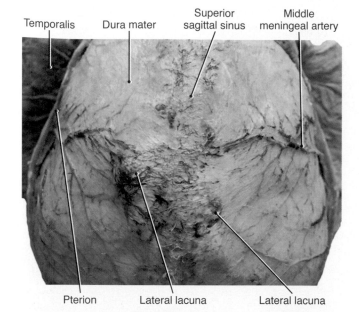

Fig. 23.26 Superior view of craniotomy, revealing superior sagittal sinus, middle meningeal artery, lateral lacuna, dura mater, temporalis muscle, and pterion.

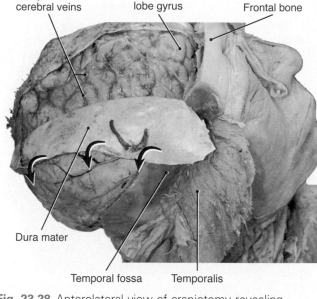

Fig. 23.28 Anterolateral view of craniotomy revealing reflected dura mater, temporal bone region, temporalis muscle, frontal bone region, frontal lobe gyri covered with arachnoid and pia mater, and superior cerebral veins of parietal lobe.

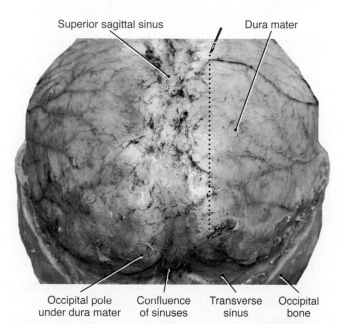

Fig. 23.27 Dura mater cut laterally from midline (dashed line) and reflected inferiorly.

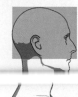

Fig. 23.29 Lateral view of craniotomy with dura mater reflected laterally, revealing key gyri, central sulcus, and frontal sinus.

- Notice how the cerebral arteries and veins are covered with pia mater.
- On the brain, identify the central sulcus, precentral gyrus, postcentral gyrus, and the frontal and occipital lobes (Fig. 23.29).

- On the other side of the brain, remove the pia mater (Fig. 23.30).
- With forceps, pull the superior sagittal sinus and the falx cerebri laterally, and observe the corpus callosum (Fig. 23.31).

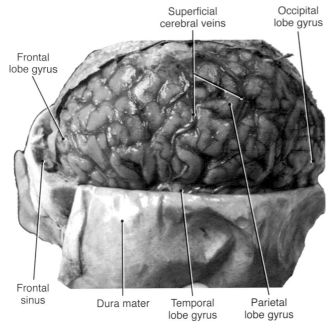

Superficial cerebral veins
Occipital lobe gyrus
Frontal lobe gyrus
Frontal sinus
Dura mater
Temporal lobe gyrus
Parietal lobe gyrus

Fig. 23.30 Pia mater removed from the brain.

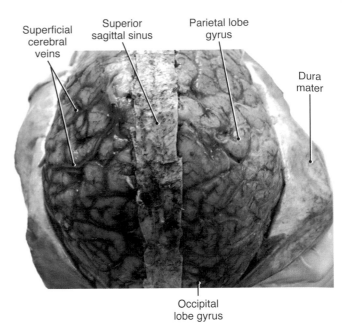

Superficial cerebral veins
Superior sagittal sinus
Parietal lobe gyrus
Dura mater
Occipital lobe gyrus

Fig. 23.32 Appreciate the superior sagittal sinus, lacunae, and tuft-like arachnoid granulations.

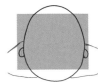

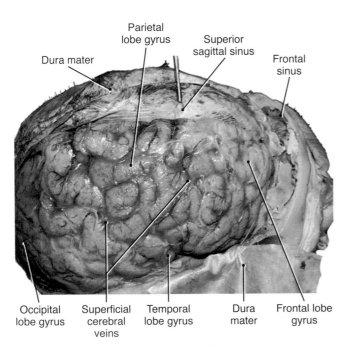

Parietal lobe gyrus
Superior sagittal sinus
Frontal sinus
Dura mater
Occipital lobe gyrus
Superficial cerebral veins
Temporal lobe gyrus
Dura mater
Frontal lobe gyrus

Fig. 23.31 Superior sagittal sinus and falx cerebri pulled laterally, revealing corpus callosum.

○ Observe the superior sagittal sinus, and identify the lacunae joining it.
○ Look for the tuft-like projections, the arachnoid granulations (Fig. 23.32).

ANATOMY **NOTE**

Appreciate the relationships of the following:
- The *falx cerebri* separates the two cerebral hemispheres.
- The *falx cerebelli* separates the two cerebellar hemispheres.
- The *tentorium cerebelli* separates the cerebellum from the occipital lobes.

○ Gently lift the cerebral hemispheres.
○ Inferior to the frontal lobes identify the attachment of the falx cerebri at the *crista galli*.
○ Cut this attachment from the crista galli and from the cerebral veins draining into the superior sagittal sinus.
○ Pull the detached falx cerebri and superior sagittal sinus posteriorly (Fig. 23.33).
○ Gently lift the cerebral hemispheres by placing your fingertips underneath the frontal lobes of the brain (Fig. 23.34).
○ Look at the space between the cribriform plate of the ethmoid bone and the frontal lobes for the internal carotid artery, olfactory tracts, olfactory bulbs, optic nerve, optic chiasm, and anterior cerebral artery (Fig. 23.35).

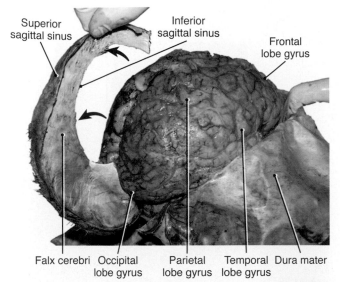

Fig. 23.33 Anterolateral view with dura mater reflected laterally.

Superior sagittal sinus
Inferior sagittal sinus
Frontal lobe gyrus
Falx cerebri
Occipital lobe gyrus
Parietal lobe gyrus
Temporal lobe gyrus
Dura mater

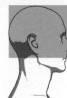

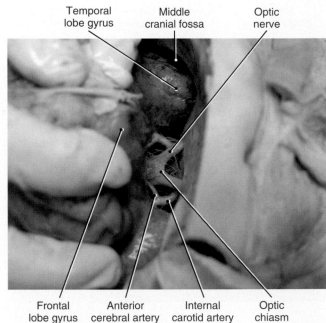

Temporal lobe gyrus
Middle cranial fossa
Optic nerve
Frontal lobe gyrus
Anterior cerebral artery
Internal carotid artery
Optic chiasm

Fig. 23.35 In space between cribriform plate of ethmoid bone and frontal lobes, appreciate the internal carotid artery, olfactory tracts/ bulbs, optic nerve/chiasm, and anterior cerebral artery.

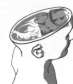

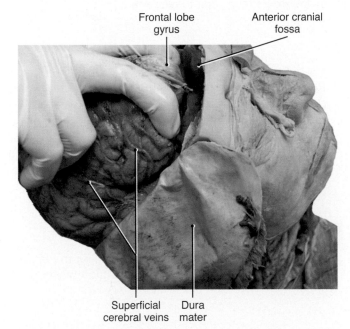

Frontal lobe gyrus
Anterior cranial fossa
Superficial cerebral veins
Dura mater

Fig. 23.34 Gently lift cerebral hemispheres by placing fingertips underneath frontal lobes.

○ With scissors, cut the aforementioned structures (Fig. 23.36).

the brainstem and the basilar artery (Figs. 23.37 and 23.38).

○ At this point, lift the occipital lobes of the cerebral hemisphere, and appreciate the tentorium cerebelli and the straight sinus (Fig. 23.39).

○ With a scalpel, carefully make a circumferential cut along the lateral attachment of the tentorium cerebelli.

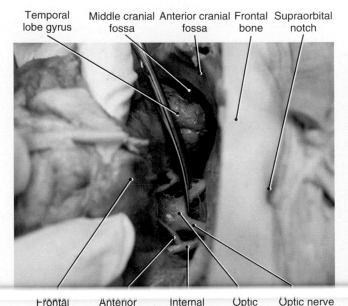

Temporal lobe gyrus
Middle cranial fossa
Anterior cranial fossa
Frontal bone
Supraorbital notch

Frontal lobe gyrus
Anterior cerebral artery
Internal carotid artery
Optic chiasm
Optic nerve

Fig. 23.36 Insert a pair of scissors and cut the optic nerve and internal carotid artery.

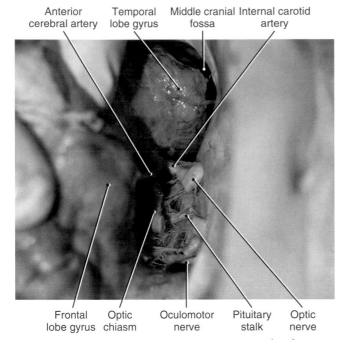

Fig. 23.37 View with frontal lobes reflected superoposteriorly revealing temporal lobe, middle cranial fossa, cut optic nerves, internal carotid artery, anterior cerebral artery, optic chiasm cut, oculomotor nerve, and pituitary stalk.

Anterior cerebral artery · Temporal lobe gyrus · Middle cranial fossa · Internal carotid artery

Frontal lobe gyrus · Optic chiasm · Oculomotor nerve · Pituitary stalk · Optic nerve

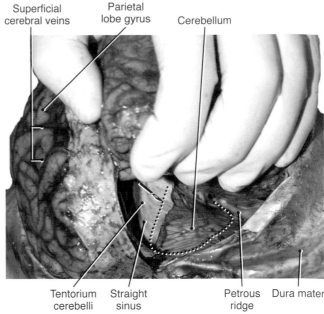

Superficial cerebral veins · Parietal lobe gyrus · Cerebellum

Tentorium cerebelli · Straight sinus · Petrous ridge · Dura mater

Fig. 23.39 Occipital lobes lifted to visualize tentorium cerebelli and straight sinus; circumferential cut from lateral attachment of tentorium cerebelli alongside transverse sinus toward petrous ridge to tentorial notch.

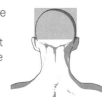

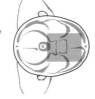

Basilar artery · Temporal lobe gyrus · Middle cranial fossa · Anterior cranial fossa

Optic chiasm · Internal carotid artery · Oculomotor nerve · Internal carotid artery · Optic nerve

Fig. 23.38 Anterosuperior view of craniotomy with frontal lobes reflected superiorly and posteriorly, revealing anterior/middle cranial fossae, temporal lobe, optic nerve cut, internal carotid artery cut, basilar artery, optic chiasm cut, and oculomotor nerve.

- Return to the frontal lobes and pull them upward (Fig. 23.40).
- Cut the facial, vestibulocochlear, trigeminal, abducens, and trochlear nerves.
- Because the tentorium cerebelli has been cut, pull the brain farther back and note the vertebral arteries forming the basilar artery (Fig. 23.41).

DISSECTION TIP

The point at which you need to stop pulling the brain backward is when you visualize the junction where the vertebral arteries form the basilar artery.

- Once you observe the vertebral arteries, cut the hypoglossal, accessory, glossopharyngeal, and vagus nerves.
- At this point, place a scalpel as deeply as possible within the foramen magnum, and cut the spinal cord (Fig. 23.42).
- Retract the brain from the base of the skull, leaving intact the dural venous sinuses (Fig. 23.43).
- Once the brain is removed, identify the different dural venous sinuses, the superior sagittal sinus, inferior sagittal sinus, confluence of the sinuses, straight sinus, transverse sinus, sigmoid sinus, and the great vein of Galen (see Fig. 23.18).

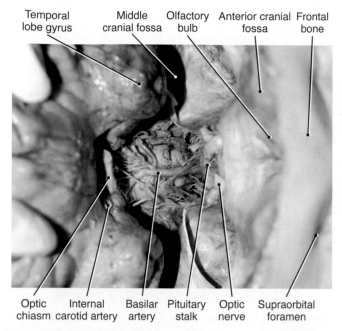

Temporal lobe gyrus | Middle cranial fossa | Olfactory bulb | Anterior cranial fossa | Frontal bone

Optic chiasm | Internal carotid artery | Basilar artery | Pituitary stalk | Optic nerve | Supraorbital foramen

Fig. 23.40 Anterosuperior view of craniotomy with frontal lobes reflected superiorly and posteriorly revealing frontal bone, supraorbital foramen, anterior cranial fossa, olfactory tract cut, optic nerve cut, middle cranial fossa, temporal lobe, internal carotid artery cut, optic nerves cut, pituitary stalk cut, and basilar artery.

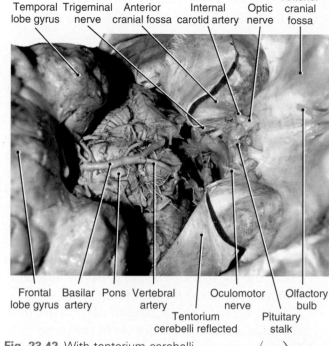

Temporal lobe gyrus | Trigeminal nerve | Anterior cranial fossa | Internal carotid artery | Optic nerve | Anterior cranial fossa

Frontal lobe gyrus | Basilar artery | Pons | Vertebral artery | Oculomotor nerve | Olfactory bulb | Tentorium cerebelli reflected | Pituitary stalk

Fig. 23.42 With tentorium cerebelli reflected, appreciate hypoglossal, accessory, glossopharyngeal, and vagus nerves.

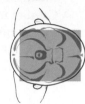

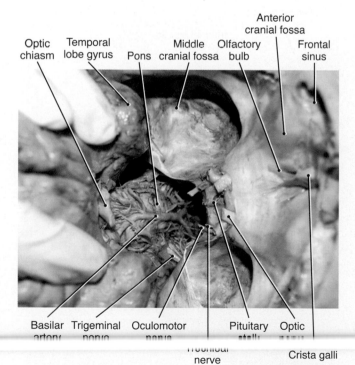

Optic chiasm | Temporal lobe gyrus | Pons | Middle cranial fossa | Olfactory bulb | Anterior cranial fossa | Frontal sinus

Basilar artery | Trigeminal nerve | Oculomotor nerve | Trochlear nerve | Pituitary stalk | Optic | Crista galli

Fig. 23.41 Appreciate the facial, vestibulocochlear, trigeminal, abducens, and trochlear nerves; brain pulled farther back to visualize vertebral arteries forming basilar artery.

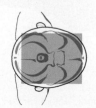

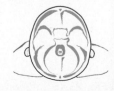

Olfactory tract | Foramen cecum | Oculomotor nerve | Anterior cranial fossa | Olfactory bulb | Crista galli | Optic nerve | Middle cranial fossa | Tentorium cerebelli reflected

Trigeminal | Abducens | Accessory | Vagus | Glossopharyngeal | Brainstem

Fig. 23.43 Brain retracted from base of skull, leaving dural venous sinuses intact.

EXAMINATION OF THE BRAIN

○ Once the brain is removed, dissect away the arachnoid and pia mater from its ventral surface.

○ Identify the cranial nerves on the brain (Figs. 23.44 and 23.45, Plate 23.2), as follows:

○ **Cranial nerve I:** The *olfactory bulbs and tracts* usually are found in contact with the frontal lobes of the brain.

○ **Cranial nerve II:** The *optic nerves* and the *optic chiasm* are usually well preserved in most cadavers. Posterior to the optic chiasm, identify the pituitary stalk.

○ **Cranial nerve III:** The *oculomotor nerve* passes between the posterior cerebral and superior cerebellar arteries, near the termination of the basilar artery.

○ **Cranial nerve IV:** The *trochlear nerve* is the smallest cranial nerve (less the olfactory nerves) and often is cut during brain removal. It passes anteriorly around the sides of the midbrain.

○ **Cranial nerve V:** The *trigeminal nerve* arises from the middle of the lateral aspect of the pons.

○ **Cranial nerve VI:** The *abducens nerve* arises from the inferior border of the pons, immediately superior to the medullary pyramids.

○ **Cranial nerve VII:** The *facial nerve* arises on the lateral aspect of the junction of the pons and the medulla oblongata, medial to the origin of cranial nerve VIII.

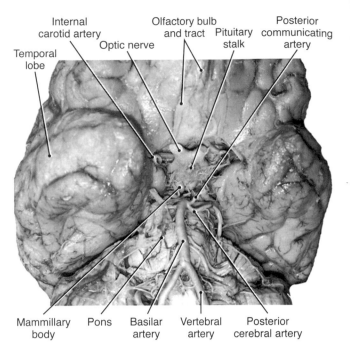

Fig. 23.44 Inferior aspect of brain, revealing olfactory bulb and tract, optic nerve, pituitary stalk, temporal lobe, mammillary bodies, and arteries (internal carotid, posterior communicating, basilar, vertebral, posterior cerebral).

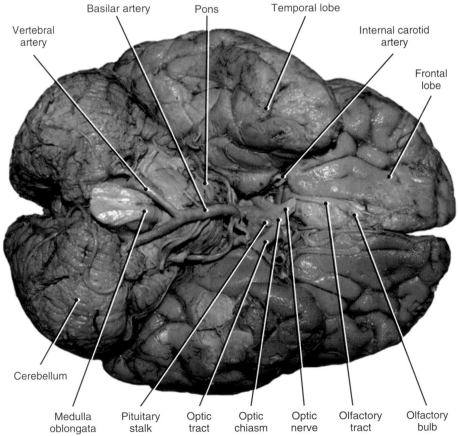

Fig. 23.45 Inferior aspect of brain, revealing olfactory bulb and tract, frontal lobe, optic chiasm, optic nerve, optic tract, internal carotid artery, pituitary stalk, temporal lobe, pons, medulla oblongata, basilar artery, vertebral artery, and cerebellum.

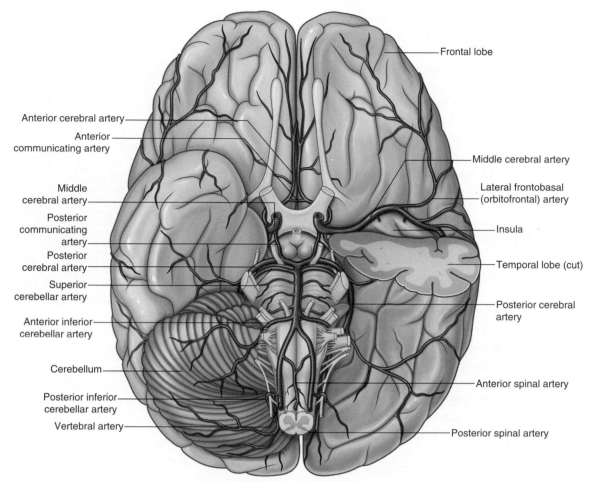

Anterior cerebral artery

Anterior communicating artery

Middle cerebral artery

Posterior communicating artery

Posterior cerebral artery

Superior cerebellar artery

Anterior inferior cerebellar artery

Cerebellum

Posterior inferior cerebellar artery

Vertebral artery

Frontal lobe

Middle cerebral artery

Lateral frontobasal (orbitofrontal) artery

Insula

Temporal lobe (cut)

Posterior cerebral artery

Anterior spinal artery

Posterior spinal artery

Plate 23.2 Arterial supply of the brain and cranial nerves.

○ **Cranial nerve VIII:** The *vestibulocochlear nerve* arises lateral to the facial nerve.

○ **Cranial nerve IX:** The *glossopharyngeal nerve* arises at the groove posterior to the olive on the medulla oblongata.

○ **Cranial nerve X:** The *vagus nerve* arises from the medulla oblongata by 8 to 10 rootlets between the olive and the inferior cerebellar peduncle.

○ **Cranial nerve XI:** The *accessory nerve* arises from cranial rootlets from the medulla oblongata and from rootlets of the upper five cervical levels of the spinal cord.

○ **Cranial nerve XII:** The *hypoglossal nerve* arises by a series of rootlets from the medulla oblongata on the ventrolateral sulcus between the pyramid and the olive.

○ Identify the following arteries contributing to the formation of the arterial circle of Willis (see Figs. 23.43 and 23.44, Plate 23.2):

○ The *anterior cerebral* arteries, connected by the anterior communicating artery

○ The *internal carotid* arteries, connected by posterior communicating arteries to the posterior cerebral arteries

ANATOMY **NOTE**

Common variations encountered in the formation of the circle of Willis include the following:
- Absent anterior communicating artery
- Absent posterior communicating artery
- Large posterior communicating artery
- Posterior cerebral artery arises from the internal carotid (fetal posterior cerebral artery).

POINT OF **DEBATE**

Some anatomists do not consider the accessory nerve a "cranial nerve" because (1) it does not arise from the brain, and (2) it enters the skull through the foramen magnum. The definition of a cranial nerve states that it should arise from the brain and exit through one of the skull foramina.

DISSECTION **TIP**

- The *anterior choroidal artery* arises near the origin of the posterior communicating artery and passes posterolaterally along the optic tract.
- The *trochlear nerve* and *oculomotor nerve* pass between the superior cerebellar and posterior cerebral arteries.

- Make a midsagittal incision through the brain, separating the right from the left hemisphere.
- Identify the thalamus, hypothalamus, and the three parts of the brainstem—midbrain, pons, and medulla oblongata (see Fig. 23.45).
- Identify the corpus callosum and fornix.
- Note the lateral ventricles, which open into the third ventricle through the foramen of Monro.
- Identify the foramen of Monro (Fig. 23.46).
- Note that the third ventricle is continuous inferiorly with the cerebral aqueduct, connecting the third with the fourth ventricles.

EXAMINATION OF THE CRANIAL BASE

- Identify the tentorium cerebelli and the anterior clinoid process.
- Visualize the dura covering the trigeminal nerve as it passes into the middle cranial fossa.
- With scissors, make a small cut in the dura covering the trigeminal nerve, and pull it upward (Fig. 23.47 and Plate 23.3).
- Pull the dura covering the trigeminal nerve away from the middle cranial fossa, and expose *Meckel's cave*, the area where the trigeminal (semilunar) ganglion resides (Fig. 23.48).
- Gently dissect out the soft tissues around Meckel's (trigeminal) cave and expose the trigeminal ganglion (Fig. 23.49).
- Continue the dissection distally to the trigeminal ganglion.
- Identify the ophthalmic (V1), maxillary (V2), and mandibular (V3) divisions of the trigeminal nerve entering into the superior orbital fissure, foramen

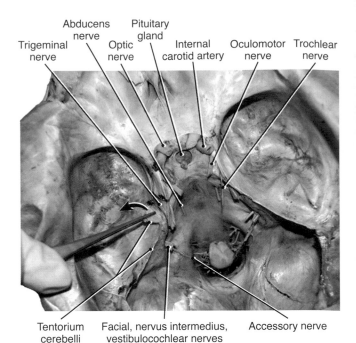

Abducens nerve · Pituitary gland · Trigeminal nerve · Optic nerve · Internal carotid artery · Oculomotor nerve · Trochlear nerve

Tentorium cerebelli · Facial, nervus intermedius, vestibulocochlear nerves · Accessory nerve

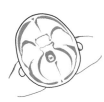

Fig. 23.47 Appreciate the tentorium cerebelli, anterior clinoid process, and dura mater covering the trigeminal nerve pulled upward.

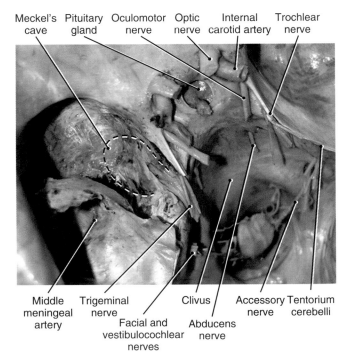

Meckel's cave · Pituitary gland · Oculomotor nerve · Optic nerve · Internal carotid artery · Trochlear nerve

Middle meningeal artery · Trigeminal nerve · Facial and vestibulocochlear nerves · Abducens nerve · Clivus · Accessory nerve · Tentorium cerebelli

Fig. 23.48 Trigeminal nerve dura pulled from middle cranial fossa, exposing pituitary gland, Meckel's cave *(dashed arch)*, and clivus (bony surface of posterior cranial fossa).

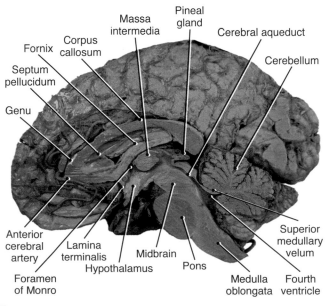

Massa intermedia · Pineal gland · Cerebral aqueduct · Cerebellum · Fornix · Corpus callosum · Septum pellucidum · Genu · Superior medullary velum · Anterior cerebral artery · Lamina terminalis · Midbrain · Pons · Medulla oblongata · Fourth ventricle · Foramen of Monro · Hypothalamus

Fig. 23.46 Sagittal section of cerebellum and brainstem.

rotundum, and foramen ovale, respectively (see Figs. 23.49 and 23.50).

- Continue laterally by identifying the internal carotid arteries passing underneath the optic nerves.
- Posterior to the optic chiasm and optic nerves, identify the infundibulum of the pituitary gland *(hypophysis)* and the diaphragma sella (Fig. 23.51 and Plate 23.3).
- Identify the cavernous sinus, appreciating that the walls of the cavernous sinuses are formed by dura mater.
- Identify the oculomotor nerve as it passes underneath the free edge of the tentorium toward the posterior clinoid process.
- At the posterior clinoid process, identify the trochlear nerve.
- Inferior to the sella turcica, note the *abducens nerve* penetrating the dural wall of the cavernous sinus (Fig. 23.52).
- Remove the dura from the middle cranial fossa as well as from the medial side of the cavernous sinus (Fig. 23.53).
- Separate the soft tissue around the oculomotor nerve and internal carotid artery.

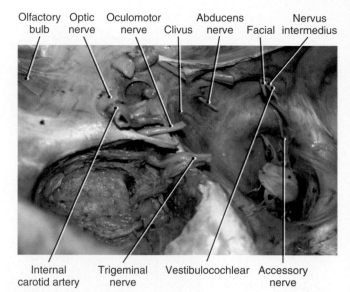

Fig. 23.50 Anterolateral view of anterior, middle, and posterior cranial fossae.

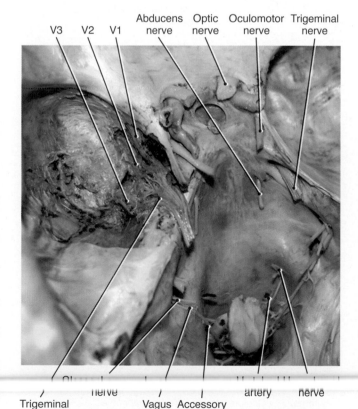

Fig. 23.49 Dissection continued distally to trigeminal ganglion revealing ophthalmic *(V1)*, maxillary *(V2)*, and mandibular *(V3)* divisions of trigeminal nerve and key neurovascular structures.

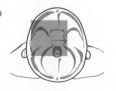

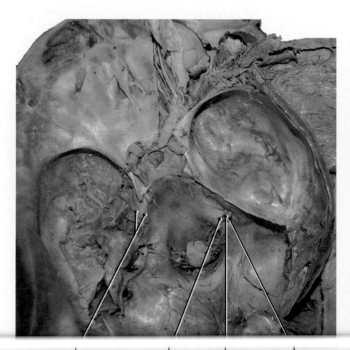

Fig. 23.51 Appreciate foramina for trigeminal nerve branches and facial, intermediate, and vestibulocochlear nerves.

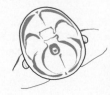

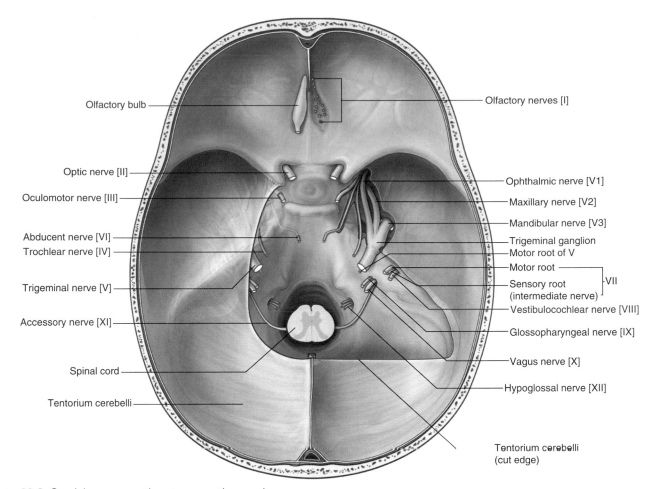

Olfactory bulb

Olfactory nerves [I]

Optic nerve [II]

Ophthalmic nerve [V1]

Oculomotor nerve [III]

Maxillary nerve [V2]

Mandibular nerve [V3]

Abducent nerve [VI]

Trigeminal ganglion

Trochlear nerve [IV]

Motor root of V

Motor root

Trigeminal nerve [V]

Sensory root
(intermediate nerve)

VII

Vestibulocochlear nerve [VIII]

Accessory nerve [XI]

Glossopharyngeal nerve [IX]

Vagus nerve [X]

Spinal cord

Hypoglossal nerve [XII]

Tentorium cerebelli

Tentorium cerebelli
(cut edge)

Plate 23.3 Cranial nerves as they traverse the cranium.

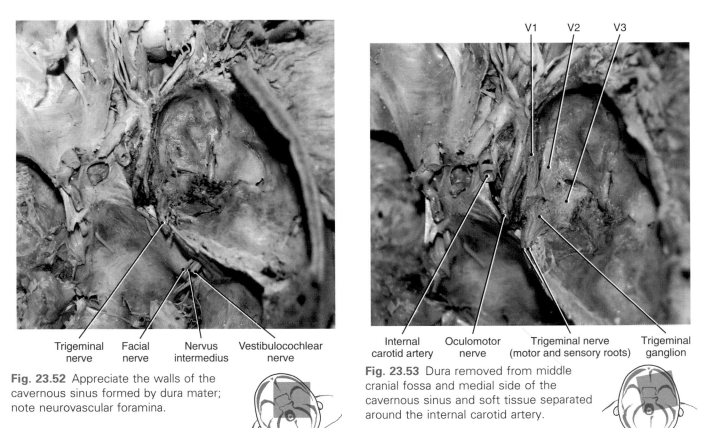

V1   V2   V3

Trigeminal   Facial   Nervus   Vestibulocochlear
nerve   nerve   intermedius   nerve

Internal   Oculomotor   Trigeminal nerve   Trigeminal
carotid artery   nerve   (motor and sensory roots)   ganglion

Fig. 23.52 Appreciate the walls of the cavernous sinus formed by dura mater; note neurovascular foramina.

Fig. 23.53 Dura removed from middle cranial fossa and medial side of the cavernous sinus and soft tissue separated around the internal carotid artery.

- Notice the S-shaped course of the internal carotid artery (carotid siphon) within the cavernous sinus.
- Identify the abducens nerve running lateral to the internal carotid artery within the cavernous sinus.
- Incise the dura at the entrance of the abducens nerve, and follow it into the cavernous sinus.

ANATOMY **NOTE**

The internal carotid artery and the abducens nerve are covered by a layer that separates them from adjacent venous blood (Fig. 23.54).

- Identify the sigmoid sinus, and cut open the dura that covers it.
- Pull the dura covering off the superior and inferior petrosal sinuses.
- Identify the internal acoustic meatus, and trace the facial and vestibulocochlear nerves as they enter the foramen.
- Look inferior to the internal acoustic meatus for the jugular foramen, and trace the glossopharyngeal, vagus, and accessory nerves (see Figs. 23.47 and 23.51).
- Note the upper cervical spinal fibers of the accessory nerve entering through the foramen magnum. Inferior to the jugular foramen and superior to the foramen magnum, identify the hypoglossal canal with the hypoglossal nerve (see Figs. 23.47 and 23.51).

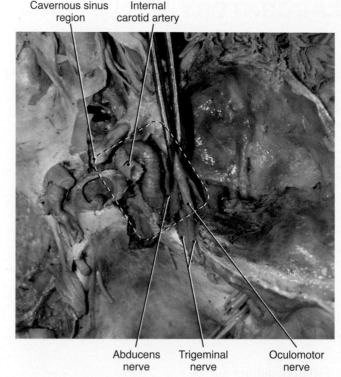

Cavernous sinus region   Internal carotid artery

Abducens nerve   Trigeminal nerve   Oculomotor nerve

Fig. 23.54 Dashed lines indicate cavernous sinus region with abducens nerve running lateral to internal carotid artery.

LABORATORY IDENTIFICATION CHECKLIST

BRAIN/BRAINSTEM
- ☐ Frontal lobe
  - ☐ Precentral gyrus
- ☐ Central sulcus
- ☐ Parietal lobe
  - ☐ Postcentral gyrus
- ☐ Occipital lobe
  - ☐ Occipital lobe gyri
- ☐ Temporal lobe
  - ☐ Temporal lobe gyri
- ☐ Corpus callosum
  - ☐ Genu
- ☐ Septum pellucidum
- ☐ Fornix
- ☐ Midbrain
- ☐ Hypothalamus
- ☐ Lamina terminalis
- ☐ Pineal gland
- ☐ Medulla oblongata
- ☐ Fourth ventricle
- ☐ Pons
- ☐ Mammillary body
- ☐ Foramen of Monro
- ☐ Cerebral aqueduct
- ☐ Pituitary stalk/gland
- ☐ Cerebellum

NERVES
- ☐ Olfactory bulb
- ☐ Olfactory tract
- ☐ Optic nerve
- ☐ Optic chiasm
- ☐ Oculomotor nerve
- ☐ Trochlear nerve
- ☐ Trigeminal nerve
  - ☐ V1 (ophthalmic) division
  - ☐ V2 (maxillary) division
  - ☐ V3 (mandibular) division
- ☐ Abducens nerve
- ☐ Facial nerve
- ☐ Nervus intermedius
- ☐ Vestibulocochlear nerve
- ☐ Glossopharyngeal nerve
- ☐ Vagus nerve
- ☐ Accessory nerve
- ☐ Hypoglossal nerve

ARTERIES
- ☐ Internal carotid
- ☐ Basilar
- ☐ Middle meningeal
  - ☐ Anterior branch
  - ☐ Posterior branch
- ☐ Superficial temporal
- ☐ Anterior cerebral
- ☐ Middle cerebral
- ☐ Posterior cerebral
- ☐ Posterior communicating
- ☐ Vertebral

VEINS/SINUSES
- ☐ Confluence of sinuses
- ☐ Superior sagittal sinus
- ☐ Inferior sagittal sinus
- ☐ Transverse sinus
- ☐ Straight sinus
- ☐ Emissary veins
- ☐ Superficial cerebral veins
- ☐ Cavernous sinus

MUSCLE
- ☐ Temporalis

CONNECTIVE TISSUE
- ☐ Skin
- ☐ Subcutaneous tissue
- ☐ Epicranial aponeurosis
- ☐ Dura mater
- ☐ Lateral lacunae
- ☐ Falx cerebri
- ☐ Tentorium cerebelli
- ☐ Arachnoid mater
- ☐ Pia mater
- ☐ Temporalis fascia
- ☐ Parotid fascia

BONES/FOSSAE/SINUSES
- ☐ Frontal bone
  - ☐ Frontal sinus
  - ☐ Supraorbital notch/foramen
  - ☐ Glabella

- ☐ Ethmoid bone
  - ☐ Crista galli
- ☐ Temporal bone
- ☐ Parietal bone
- ☐ Occipital bone
  - ☐ Internal occipital crest
  - ☐ Inion
  - ☐ Superior nuchal line
- ☐ Zygomatic arch
- ☐ Diploic space

- ☐ Pterion
- ☐ Sagittal suture
- ☐ Lambdoid suture
- ☐ Parietal foramen
- ☐ Temporal fossa
- ☐ Anterior cranial fossa
- ☐ Middle cranial fossa
- ☐ Posterior cranial fossa
- ☐ Retromandibular region

ATLAS REFERENCES
Netter: 94–104
McMinn: 54–57
Gray's Atlas: 508–519

BEFORE YOU BEGIN
Remove all soft tissues with a scalpel and expose the frontal and temporal bones. Reflect the temporalis muscle as laterally as possible.

OSTEOTOMY OF ORBITAL ROOF
- With an electric saw or a mallet and chisel, make a second vertical cut through the frontal bone, lateral to the supraorbital notch (Fig. 24.1).
- Extend this cut posteriorly through the roof of the orbit between the optic nerve and ethmoidal sinuses (Fig. 24.2).
- With an electric saw or a mallet and chisel, make a second vertical cut through the squamous part of the temporal bone.
- Continue the cut horizontally toward the orbital process of the zygomatic bone at the infraorbital margin (see Fig. 24.2).

> **DISSECTION TIP**
>
> Once all bones are cut, the orbital roof and the orbital process of the zygomatic bone can be reflected en bloc, while the periorbita (periosteal covering of orbital bones) is left intact (Fig. 24.3). This is referred to as an *orbito-zygomatic approach.*

- Complete the reflection of the orbital roof anteriorly but do not detach it from the orbit (Fig. 24.4).

ORBIT
- With sharp scissors, make a small cut in the periorbital fascia (Fig. 24.5).
- Identify the frontal nerve and its two branches, the supraorbital and supratrochlear nerves (Fig. 24.6).
- Clean and expose the frontal nerve and note the levator palpebrae superioris muscle lying underneath it (Fig. 24.7).
- Lateral and inferior to the levator palpebrae superioris, expose the superior rectus muscle (Fig. 24.8).
- Medial to the levator palpebrae superioris muscle, remove a small portion of the periorbital fat and identify the *nasociliary nerve* (Fig. 24.9 and Plate 24.1).

Squamous part of
temporal bone

Greater wing of
sphenoid bone

Temporalis
muscle

Frontal process of
zygomatic bone

Fig. 24.1 Anterolateral view of external orbit after craniotomy, with reflected temporalis muscle revealing bony landmarks; *dotted lines* indicate cuts through the frontal bone and orbital roof.

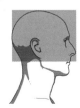

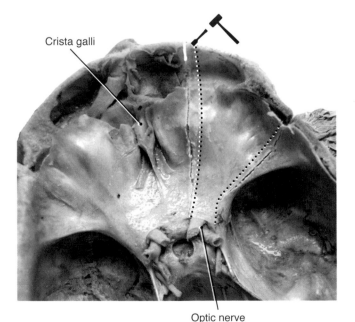

Crista galli

Optic nerve

Fig. 24.2 Craniotomy view of anterior cranial fossa, or superior roof of the orbit; *dotted lines* over dura represent osteotomy cuts.

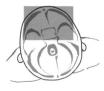

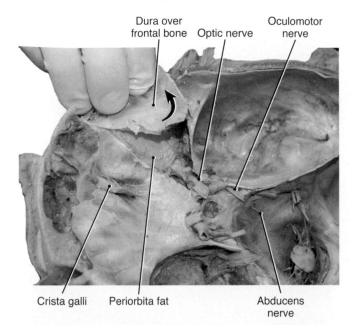

Fig. 24.3 Craniotomy view highlighting anterior cranial fossa and dura mater, periorbital fat, crista galli, frontal bone, and nerves (optic, oculomotor, abducens).

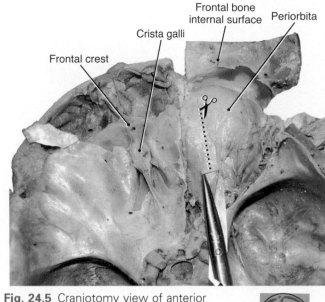

Fig. 24.5 Craniotomy view of anterior cranial fossa with osteotomy to roof of right orbit, revealing scissors cutting periorbita.

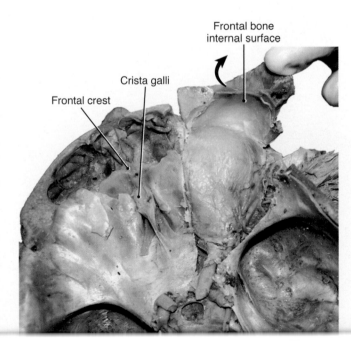

Fig. 24.4 Craniotomy view of anterior cranial fossa with osteotomy performed to the roof of right orbit.

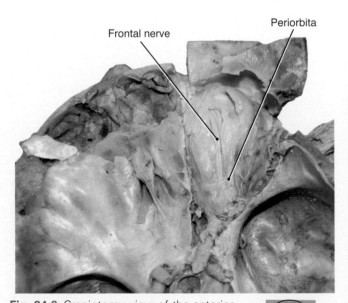

Fig. 24.6 Craniotomy view of the anterior cranial fossa with osteotomy to orbital

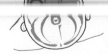

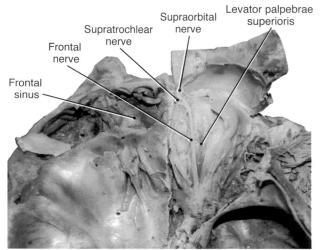

Fig. 24.7 Craniotomy view of anterior cranial fossa with osteotomy to roof of orbit.

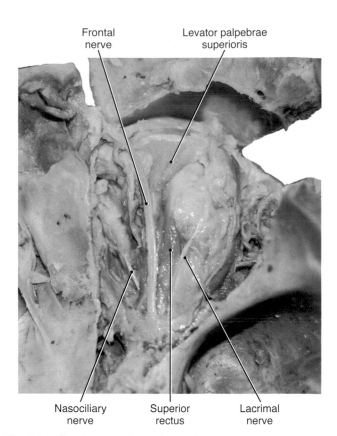

Fig. 24.8 Craniotomy view of anterior cranial fossa with orbital roof osteotomy, revealing neurovascular landmarks.

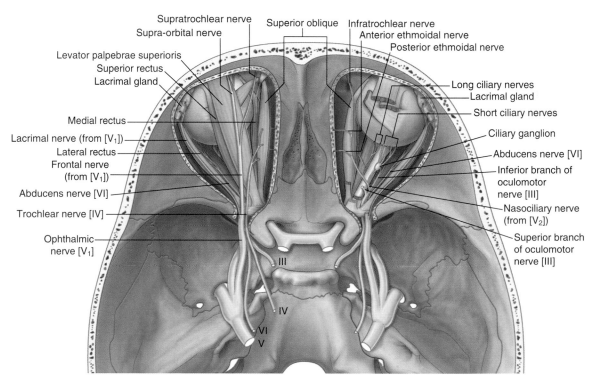

Plate 24.1 Superior view of the nerves and musculature of the orbit.

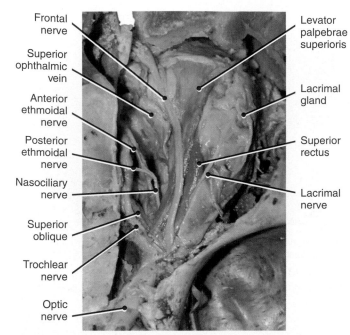

Frontal nerve
Superior ophthalmic vein
Anterior ethmoidal nerve
Posterior ethmoidal nerve
Nasociliary nerve
Superior oblique
Trochlear nerve
Optic nerve

Levator palpebrae superioris
Lacrimal gland
Superior rectus
Lacrimal nerve

Fig. 24.9 Craniotomy view of anterior cranial fossa with osteotomy to roof of orbit highlighting neurovascular musculature.

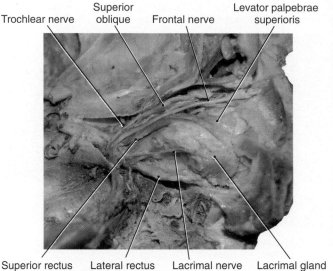

Trochlear nerve
Superior oblique
Frontal nerve
Levator palpebrae superioris

Superior rectus
Lateral rectus
Lacrimal nerve
Lacrimal gland

Fig. 24.10 Craniotomy view of anterior cranial fossa with osteotomy to roof of orbit highlighting neurovascular musculature.

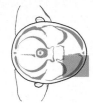

ANATOMY **NOTE**

The nasociliary nerve is located in the interval between the levator palpebrae superioris and the superior oblique muscles and crosses the optic nerve from lateral to medial (see Fig. 24.9).

○ Trace the terminal branches of the nasociliary nerve— the posterior ethmoidal, anterior ethmoidal, and infratrochlear nerves.

DISSECTION **TIP**

The branches of the nasociliary nerve are small and delicate. The infratrochlear nerve is especially delicate and easily severed during dissection. The posterior ethmoidal nerve is often absent.

○ The superior oblique muscle is usually hidden medially under the orbital roof. Break away portions of the orbital roof to identify and clean the superior oblique muscle.
○ Clean the periorbital fat around the superior

ing the superior surface of the muscle proximally (see Fig. 24.9).
○ Distal to the interval between the superior oblique and levator palpebrae superioris muscles, look for a flat vessel, the superior ophthalmic vein.
○ Remove all small tributaries of the ophthalmic veins (see Fig. 24.9).

○ On the lateral surface of the superior rectus muscle, trace and expose the lacrimal nerve and lacrimal gland (see Fig. 24.9).

DISSECTION **TIP**

The lacrimal gland is located distally and is often confused with periorbital fat. Lift and pull up on the lacrimal nerve to trace it to the lacrimal gland.

○ Deep to the lacrimal nerve, expose the lateral rectus muscle (Fig. 24.10).
○ Pull the lateral rectus muscle laterally, and expose the *abducens nerve* on its medial side (Fig. 24.11).
○ Look for the *superior ophthalmic vein* in the space between the superior rectus and lateral rectus muscles (Fig. 24.12).
○ After identifying the superior ophthalmic vein, remove the periorbital fat between the superior and lateral rectus muscles (Fig. 24.13).
○ Observe the optic nerve, surrounded by short and long ciliary nerves (Fig. 24.14).
○ Identify the *ciliary ganglion* on the lateral surface of the optic nerve and medial to the lateral rectus muscle (see Fig. 24.14).

DISSECTION TIP

Another important landmark is the ciliary ganglion. It is connected by a small branch (motor root of ciliary ganglion) with the inferior division of the oculomotor nerve. The ganglion may be confused with periorbital fat.

○ At the interval between the optic nerve and the lateral rectus muscle, identify the *ophthalmic artery* (Fig. 24.15).

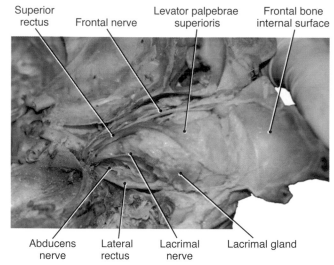

Superior rectus — Frontal nerve — Levator palpebrae superioris — Frontal bone internal surface

Abducens nerve — Lateral rectus — Lacrimal nerve — Lacrimal gland

Fig. 24.11 Craniotomy view of anterior cranial fossa with orbital osteotomy.

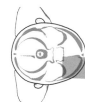

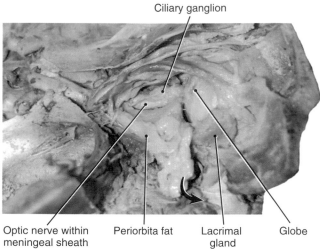

Ciliary ganglion

Optic nerve within meningeal sheath — Periorbita fat — Lacrimal gland — Globe

Fig. 24.13 Craniotomy view of anterior cranial fossa with osteotomy to roof of orbit.

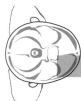

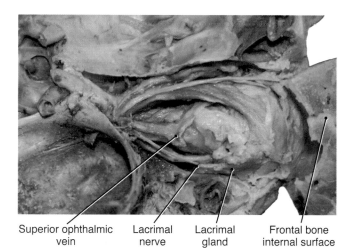

Superior ophthalmic vein — Lacrimal nerve — Lacrimal gland — Frontal bone internal surface

Fig. 24.12 Craniotomy view of anterior cranial fossa with osteotomy to orbital roof, highlighting superior ophthalmic vein.

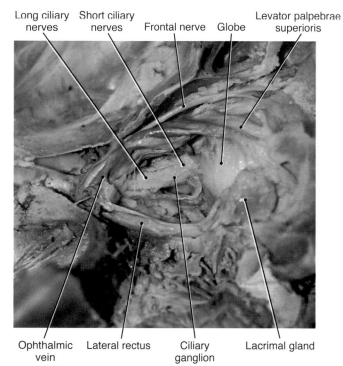

Long ciliary nerves — Short ciliary nerves — Frontal nerve — Globe — Levator palpebrae superioris

Ophthalmic vein — Lateral rectus — Ciliary ganglion — Lacrimal gland

Fig. 24.14 Craniotomy view of anterior cranial fossa with osteotomy to orbital roof, revealing frontal nerve, reflected levator palpebrae superioris muscle, and highlighting long and short ciliary nerves and ciliary ganglion.

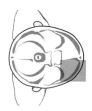

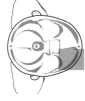

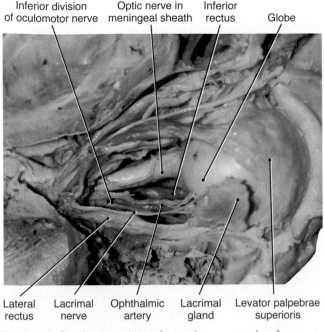

Inferior division of oculomotor nerve | Optic nerve in meningeal sheath | Inferior rectus | Globe

Lateral rectus | Lacrimal nerve | Ophthalmic artery | Lacrimal gland | Levator palpebrae superioris

Fig. 24.15 Craniotomy view of anterior cranial fossa with osteotomy.

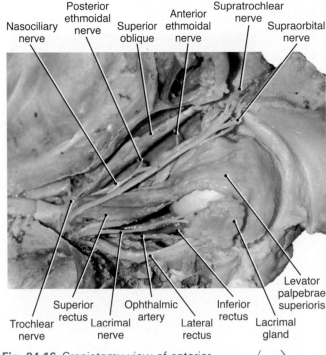

Nasociliary nerve | Posterior ethmoidal nerve | Superior oblique | Anterior ethmoidal nerve | Supratrochlear nerve | Supraorbital nerve

Trochlear nerve | Superior rectus | Lacrimal nerve | Ophthalmic artery | Lateral rectus | Inferior rectus | Lacrimal gland | Levator palpebrae superioris

Fig. 24.16 Craniotomy view of anterior cranial fossa with osteotomy to orbital roof.

ANATOMY **NOTE**

After entering the orbit, the ophthalmic artery gives off a central retinal branch to the optic nerve and usually crosses over the nerve and passes toward the medial wall of the orbit.

○ Inferior to the optic nerve, remove the periorbital fat and identify the inferior division of the oculomotor nerve, which runs parallel to the inferior rectus muscle (see Fig. 24.15).

○ Clean the periorbital fat inferior to the superior oblique muscle.

○ Trace the anterior and posterior ethmoidal nerves to their entrance into the anterior and posterior ethmoidal foramina, respectively (Fig. 24.16 and Plate 24.2).

ANATOMY **NOTE**

The four recti muscles arise from a fibrous ring that

orbital fissure. The superior oblique and levator palpebrae muscles arise from points superior and medial to this anulus (anulus of Zinn) (Fig. 24.17).

○ Reflect the nasociliary nerve and ophthalmic artery posteriorly and expose the medial rectus muscle (Fig. 24.18).

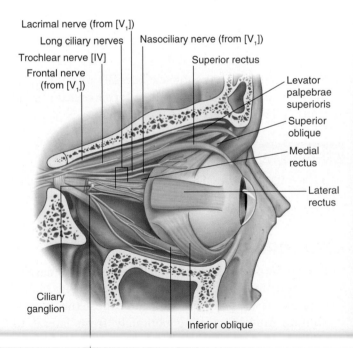

Lacrimal nerve (from [V₁])
Long ciliary nerves | Nasociliary nerve (from [V₁])
Trochlear nerve [IV]
Frontal nerve (from [V₁]) | Superior rectus

Levator palpebrae superioris
Superior oblique
Medial rectus
Lateral rectus

Ciliary ganglion

Inferior oblique

Inferior branch of oculomotor nerve [III]

Plate 24.2 Lateral view of the nerves and musculature of the orbit.

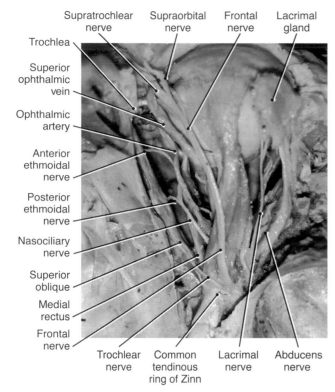

Supratrochlear nerve — Supraorbital nerve — Frontal nerve — Lacrimal gland
Trochlea
Superior ophthalmic vein
Ophthalmic artery
Anterior ethmoidal nerve
Posterior ethmoidal nerve
Nasociliary nerve
Superior oblique
Medial rectus
Frontal nerve

Trochlear nerve — Common tendinous ring of Zinn — Lacrimal nerve — Abducens nerve

Fig. 24.17 Craniotomy view of anterior cranial fossa with osteotomy to roof of orbit.

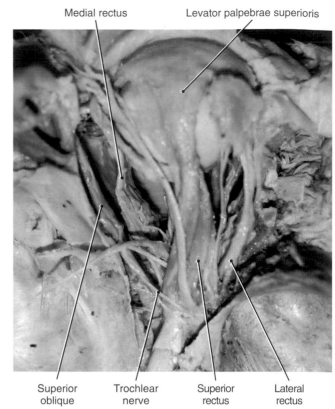

Medial rectus — Levator palpebrae superioris

Superior oblique — Trochlear nerve — Superior rectus — Lateral rectus

Fig. 24.18 Craniotomy view revealing trochlear nerve and key muscles.

○ Pull the lateral rectus muscle laterally and the optic nerve medially, and expose the inferior rectus muscle (Fig. 24.19 and Plate 24.3).

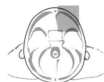

DISSECTION **TIP**

To trace the inferior oblique muscle, the inferior rectus muscle, and the nerve to the inferior oblique muscle, you need to dissect inferior to the globe.

INFRAORBITAL APPROACH

○ Detach the orbital septum from the infraorbital margin.
○ Lift the orbit and periorbital fat superiorly (Fig. 24.20).
○ Clean away the periorbital fat, and expose the inferior oblique muscle running obliquely from lateral to medial (Fig. 24.21).
○ Remove all periorbital fat, and identify the inferior rectus muscle and the nerve to the inferior oblique muscle (Fig. 24.22).
○ Lift the orbicularis oculi muscle and identify the medial palpebral ligament (Fig. 24.23).
○ Reflect all musculature from the frontal process of the maxilla (Fig. 24.24).

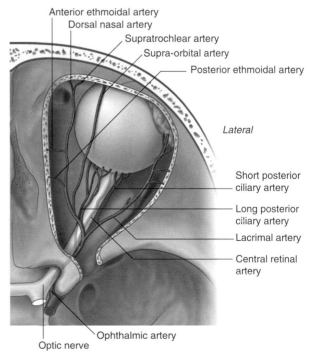

Anterior ethmoidal artery
Dorsal nasal artery
Supratrochlear artery
Supra-orbital artery
Posterior ethmoidal artery

Lateral

Short posterior ciliary artery
Long posterior ciliary artery
Lacrimal artery
Central retinal artery

Ophthalmic artery
Optic nerve

Plate 24.3 Superior view of the arteries of the orbit.

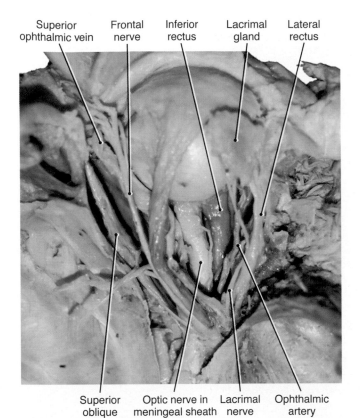

Superior ophthalmic vein Frontal nerve Inferior rectus Lacrimal gland Lateral rectus

Superior oblique Optic nerve in meningeal sheath Lacrimal nerve Ophthalmic artery

Fig. 24.19 Craniotomy view of anterior cranial fossa with osteotomy to roof of orbit revealing frontal nerve, ophthalmic vein, optic nerve, lacrimal nerve, and lacrimal gland.

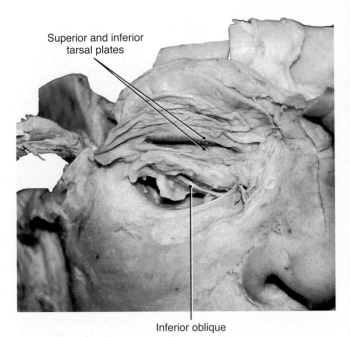

Superior and inferior tarsal plates

Inferior oblique

Fig. 24.21 Anterior view of external orbit with craniotomy showing infraorbital approach, highlighting tarsal plates.

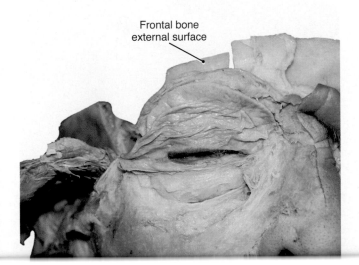

Frontal bone external surface

Fig. 24.20 Anterior view of external orbit with craniotomy and vertical frontal bone osteotomy.

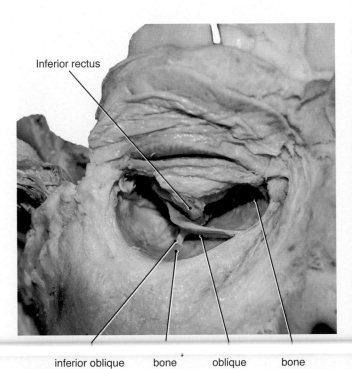

Inferior rectus

inferior oblique   bone   oblique   bone

Fig. 24.22 Anterior view of orbit with eyeball removed.

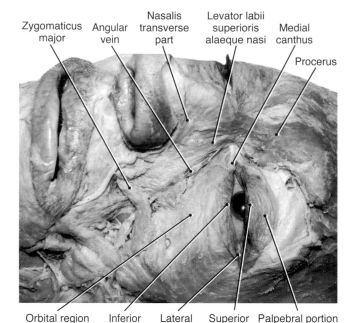

Fig. 24.23 Anterior view of external orbit with skin reflected superiorly, revealing canthi, tarsal plates, angular vein, and key muscles.

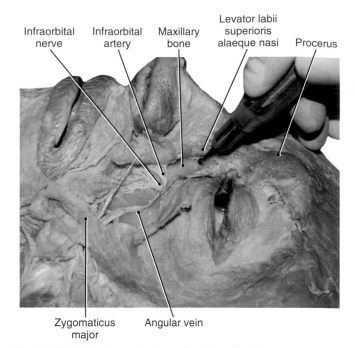

Fig. 24.25 Anterolateral view of orbit with skin and subcutaneous tissue removed and orbital part of orbicularis oculi muscle reflected.

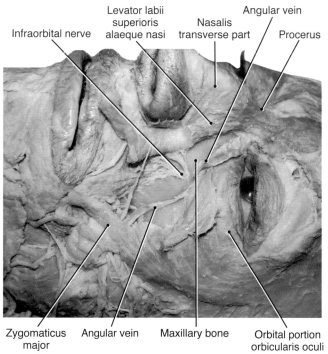

Fig. 24.24 Anterior view of external orbit, nose, and maxilla.

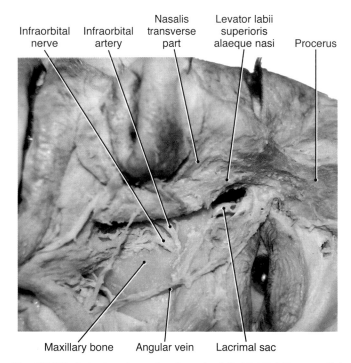

Fig. 24.26 Anterior view of external orbit, highlighting medial region with skin and subcutaneous tissue removed.

○ With an electric saw, cut the area inferior to the medial canthus and the inferomedial portion of the infraorbital margin (Fig. 24.25).

○ Identify the nasolacrimal duct within the lacrimal canal (Fig. 24.26 and Plate 24.4).

ANATOMY **NOTE**

Excess lacrimal fluid is drained by the *puncta* into *canaliculi,* which drain the fluid to the lacrimal sac. From this sac, the nasolacrimal duct passes into the nasal cavity.

○ If time permits, remove the eyeball en bloc with the surrounding extraocular muscles (Fig. 24.27).

DISSECTION **TIP**

The sclera is usually compressed and distorted. To restore its original shape, inject water into the eyeball with a hypodermic needle attached to a syringe (Fig. 24.28). Once the shape of the *sclera* has been restored, observe its extraocular muscle attachments (Fig. 24.29).

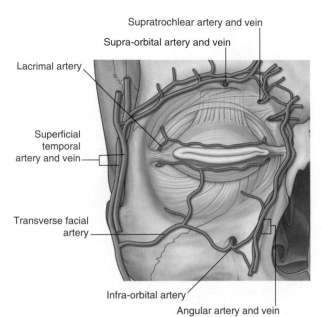

Supratrochlear artery and vein
Supra-orbital artery and vein
Lacrimal artery
Superficial temporal artery and vein
Transverse facial artery
Infra-orbital artery
Angular artery and vein

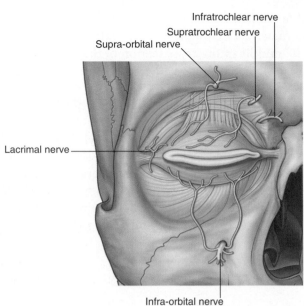

Infratrochlear nerve
Supratrochlear nerve
Supra-orbital nerve
Lacrimal nerve
Infra-orbital nerve

Plate 24.4 Anterior view of the lacrimal apparatus.

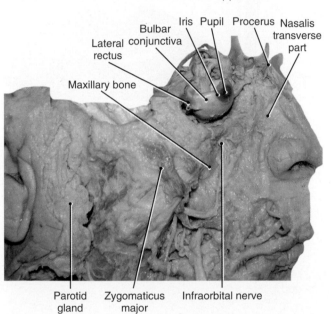

Iris Pupil Procerus Nasalis transverse part
Bulbar conjunctiva
Lateral rectus
Maxillary bone
Parotid gland
Zygomaticus major
Infraorbital nerve

Fig. 24.27 Lateral craniotomy view of orbit with skin and subcutaneous tissue removed and osteotomy to zygomatic bone, revealing globe, musculature, and parotid gland.

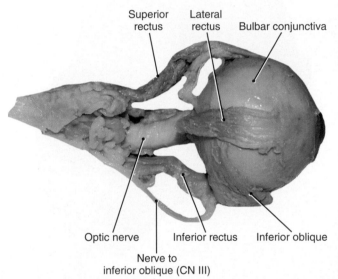

Superior rectus
Lateral rectus
Bulbar conjunctiva
Optic nerve
Inferior rectus
Inferior oblique
Nerve to inferior oblique (CN III)

Fig. 24.29 Superior view of globe with extraocular muscles removed from orbit.

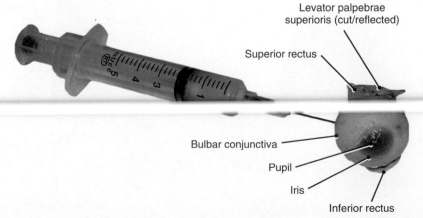

Levator palpebrae superioris (cut/reflected)
Superior rectus
Bulbar conjunctiva
Pupil
Iris
Inferior rectus

Fig. 24.28 Anterosuperior view of globe removed from orbit, with fluid injected to maintain morphologic shape.

- With a scalpel, cut the *optic nerve* and note the thick dura mater encircling it.
- At the middle of the cross section of the optic nerve, observe the small lumen that represents the central retinal artery (Fig. 24.30).
- Have a classmate hold the sclera firmly with their fingers (Fig. 24.31).
- Carefully incise the sclera with a scalpel (Fig. 24.32).
- On the hemisected orbit, identify the *limbus,* which is the junction of the cornea and the sclera (Fig. 24.33).
- The space between the iris and cornea is the anterior chamber. This is usually filled with the aqueous humor, but in the cadaver it will be empty (Fig. 24.34).

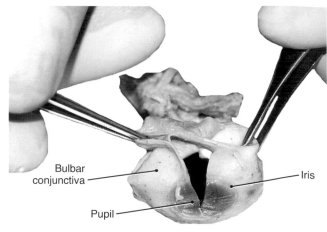

Fig. 24.32 Anterosuperior view of globe removed from orbit.

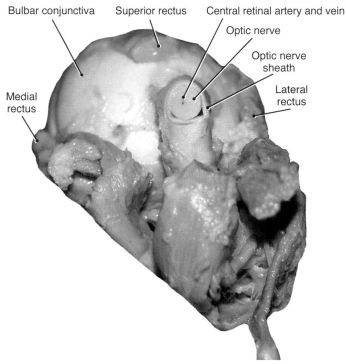

Fig. 24.30 Posterior view of globe with extraocular muscles removed from orbit.

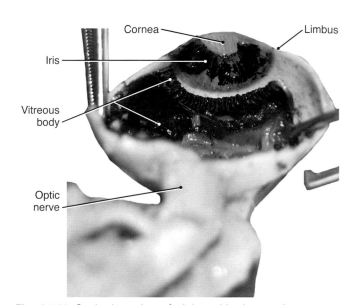

Fig. 24.33 Sagittal section of globe with vitreous humor removed.

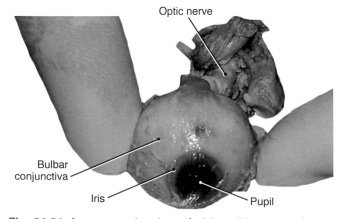

Fig. 24.31 Anterosuperior view of globe with extraocular muscles cut and reflected.

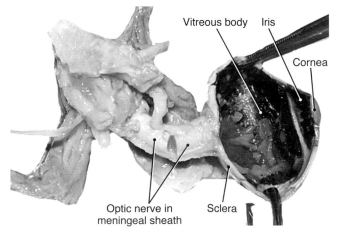

Fig. 24.34 Sagittal section of globe removed from orbit.

LABORATORY IDENTIFICATION CHECKLIST

NERVES
- ☐ Trochlear
- ☐ Frontal
  - ☐ Supratrochlear
  - ☐ Supraorbital
- ☐ Lacrimal
- ☐ Nasociliary
  - ☐ Posterior ethmoidal (inconstant)
  - ☐ Anterior ethmoidal
  - ☐ Infratrochlear
  - ☐ Long ciliary
- ☐ Oculomotor
  - ☐ Superior division
  - ☐ Inferior division
- ☐ Abducens
- ☐ Optic
- ☐ Short ciliary nerves (8–10)
- ☐ Infraorbital nerve

GANGLION/FASCIA/FAT
- ☐ Ciliary ganglion
- ☐ Periorbita
- ☐ Periorbital fat
- ☐ Trochlea
- ☐ Anulus of Zinn

ARTERIES
- ☐ Ophthalmic
  - ☐ Anterior ethmoidal
  - ☐ Posterior ethmoidal
  - ☐ Central retinal
  - ☐ Lacrimal

VEINS
- ☐ Superior ophthalmic
- ☐ Inferior ophthalmic

MUSCLES
- ☐ Procerus
  - *Recti*
- ☐ Superior rectus
- ☐ Inferior rectus
- ☐ Medial rectus
- ☐ Lateral rectus
  - *Obliques*
- ☐ Superior oblique
- ☐ Inferior oblique
- ☐ Levator palpebrae superioris

BONES
- ☐ Frontal
- ☐ Lacrimal
- ☐ Maxilla
- ☐ Ethmoid
- ☐ Zygomatic

GLAND
- ☐ Lacrimal

SINUSES
- ☐ Frontal
- ☐ Ethmoidal
  - ☐ Anterior cells
  - ☐ Middle cells
  - ☐ Posterior cells

ATLAS REFERENCES

Netter: 105–110
McMinn: 60–61
Gray's Atlas: 520–525

BEFORE YOU BEGIN

Identify the following bones in your atlas, text, and on a skull:

- Petrous part of temporal bone
- Squamous part of temporal bone
- Petrosquamous fissure (at junction of petrous and squamous parts)
- Arcuate eminence (overlies anterior semicircular canal)
- Internal acoustic meatus
- Hiatus of facial canal (greater petrosal nerve exits temporal bone from here)
- Groove for superior petrosal sinus
- Tegmen tympani (roof of middle ear between petrosquamous fissure and hiatus of facial canal)
- Jugular foramen
- Tympanic part of temporal bone (provides much of bony wall of external auditory meatus)
- Mandibular fossa
- Petrotympanic fissure (for passage of chorda tympani)
- Styloid process and stylomastoid foramen

External Ear

The ear is subdivided into the external, the middle, and the internal ear.

On the external ear of a classmate, identify the following structures (Fig. 25.1):

- Helix
- Antihelix and crura of antihelix
- Triangular fossa
- Concha
- Lobule
- Tragus
- Antitragus
- Intertragic notch
- External acoustic meatus

OPTIONAL DISSECTION (MIDDLE EAR)

- Students in most anatomy courses do not dissect the ear because it is a time-consuming dissection. This chapter presents a new, time-efficient method for exposing the structures of the middle ear.
- If time permits, create a skin flap from the helix to expose part of the elastic fibrocartilage.

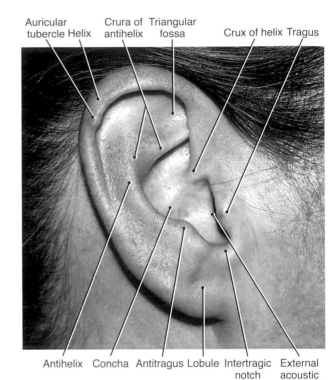

Fig. 25.1 External view of external ear with several surface features.

- Create a second skin flap at the lobule and note the dense, fibrous connective tissue.
- With your scalpel, make an incision posterior to the auricle toward the neck.
- Dissect away most of the soft tissue and the external acoustic meatus (Fig. 25.2).
- Remove any debris present in the remaining part of the external meatus.

DISSECTION TIP

With the aid of an otoscope, attempt to inspect the tympanic membrane. Remove any wax (cerumen) that may obstruct your view.

- Draw a line along the bony roof of the middle ear, the *tegmen tympani,* demarcating the length of the canal from the external acoustic meatus to the tympanic membrane.
- Draw two dashed lines at the outer borders of the meatus (Fig. 25.3).

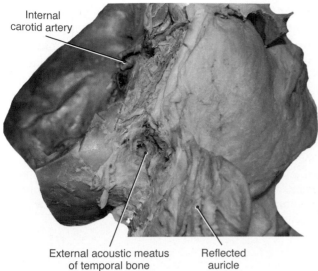

Fig. 25.2 Postcraniotomy horizontal section reveals lateral view of middle cranial fossa with external ear reflected, highlighting the external acoustic meatus of temporal bone.

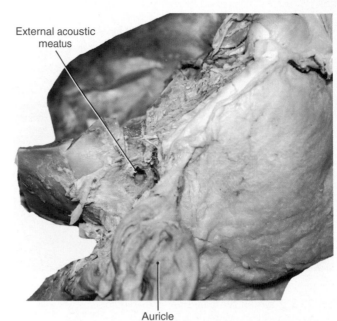

Fig. 25.4 Postcraniotomy horizontal section reveals lateral view of middle cranial fossa with external ear reflected.

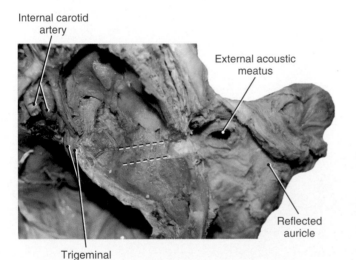

Fig. 25.3 Horizontal section after craniotomy shows middle cranial fossa with external ear reflected, highlighting the external acoustic meatus, trigeminal nerve, and internal carotid artery. *Dashed lines* demarcate lateral borders of the external acoustic meatus on tegmen tympani (roof of middle ear).

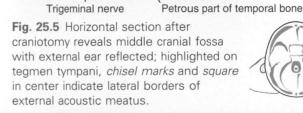

Fig. 25.5 Horizontal section after craniotomy reveals middle cranial fossa with external ear reflected; highlighted on tegmen tympani, *chisel marks* and *square* in center indicate lateral borders of external acoustic meatus.

○ With a chisel and a mallet, remove a small piece of bone, and expose the outer portion of the canal for inspection (Fig. 25.4).

○ With a cotton swab or forceps, clean the acoustic meatus of debris and cerumen (Fig. 25.5).

DISSECTION TIP

Do not place the swab or forceps too deeply into the canal, to prevent damage to the tympanic membrane.

○ Continue the removal of bone with the chisel and the mallet on the surface of the tegmen tympani (see Fig. 25.5). The external acoustic meatus is about 3 to 4 cm

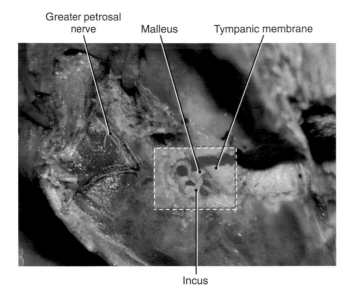

Greater petrosal nerve   Malleus   Tympanic membrane

Incus

Fig. 25.6 Tegmen tympani over the middle ear is removed, exposing tympanic membrane and two ear ossicles.

long. Once the tegmen tympani is removed to the epitympanic recess (area superior to tympanic membrane) and using bone rongeurs, remove small pieces of bone and expose the tympanic membrane and the three auditory ossicles – malleus, incus, and stapes (Fig. 25.6 and Plate 25.1).

DISSECTION **TIP**

When exposing the tegmen tympani to reveal malleus, incus, and stapes, grasp the outer part of the tympanic membrane and pull it gently upward to maintain the position of the ossicles.

○ At the final stage of dissection, cut the connective tissue layer covering the meatus, and appreciate the orientation of the tympanic membrane (see Fig. 25.6).
○ The membrane is positioned obliquely in spaces in the external acoustic meatus at an angle of about 55 degrees (Fig. 25.7).

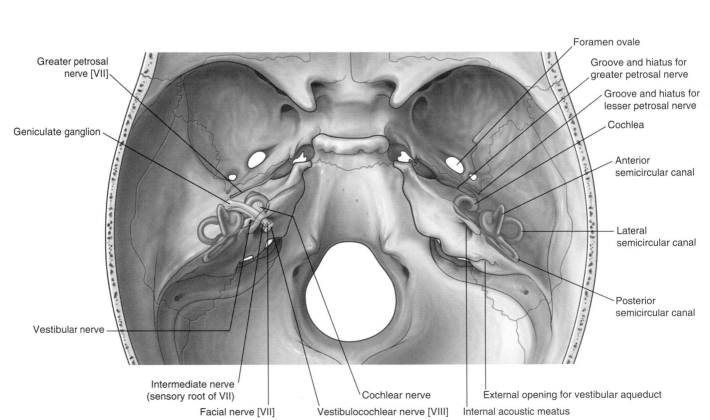

Greater petrosal nerve [VII]

Geniculate ganglion

Vestibular nerve

Intermediate nerve (sensory root of VII)

Facial nerve [VII]

Cochlear nerve

Vestibulocochlear nerve [VIII]

Internal acoustic meatus

External opening for vestibular aqueduct

Foramen ovale

Groove and hiatus for greater petrosal nerve

Groove and hiatus for lesser petrosal nerve

Cochlea

Anterior semicircular canal

Lateral semicircular canal

Posterior semicircular canal

Plate 25.1 Superior projection of internal ear in the temporal bone.

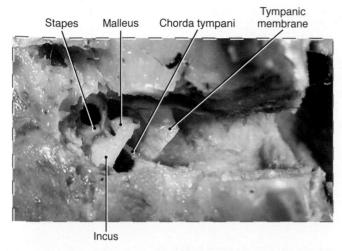

Stapes   Malleus   Chorda tympani   Tympanic membrane

Incus

Fig. 25.7 Magnified view of middle cranial fossa with acoustic meatus and middle ear exposed, revealing tympanic membrane, ossicles (malleus, incus, stapes), and chorda tympani.

○ Note the following relationships:
   ○ Stapedius muscle inserting onto the stapes.
   ○ Tendon of the tensor tympani muscle inserting onto the malleus.
   ○ Malleus attached to the tympanic membrane.

DISSECTION **TIP**

Dissecting the internal ear cavity is time-consuming; more importantly, however, inspection requires a dissecting microscope to identify auricular structures clearly.

LABORATORY IDENTIFICATION CHECKLIST

NERVES
☐ Trigeminal
   ☐ Mandibular (V3)
☐ Nervus intermedius
☐ Greater petrosal
☐ Facial
☐ Chorda tympani
☐ Vestibulocochlear
☐ Vagus

GANGLIA
☐ Trigeminal
☐ Geniculate

ARTERY
☐ Internal carotid

MUSCLES
☐ Tensor tympani
☐ Stapedius
☐ Auricularis

BONES
☐ Petrous part of temporal bone
☐ Tegmen tympani (roof)
☐ Auditory ossicles
   ☐ Malleus
   ☐ Incus
   ☐ Stapes

OTHER STRUCTURES
☐ External acoustic meatus
☐ Tympanic membrane
☐ Oval window

CARTILAGE
☐ Helix
☐ Antihelix
☐ Tragus
☐ Antitragus
☐ Auricular tubercle (of Darwin)

ATLAS REFERENCES

Netter: 45–52, 61, 142
McMinn: 58, 59, 73
Gray's Atlas: 566–571

DISSECTION STEPS

○ Exposure of the contents of the nasal cavity requires a midsagittal transection through the head (Fig. 26.1).

> **DISSECTION TIP**
>
> Electric saws are usually too small for transection of the head. Make sure that one of your classmates holds the cadaver head firmly as you cut with the saw.

○ Place the saw as close as possible to the midline. Begin the cut externally from the face toward the midportion of the head (Fig. 26.2).
○ Split the head in half, and choose one of the two halves to decapitate (Figs. 26.3 and 26.4).
○ Clean away soft tissues or any bony fragments after the hemisection (compare Fig. 26.4 with Fig. 26.5).

○ Identify several landmarks as indicated on the dissection photographs of the hemisected head.
○ The nasal cavities extend from the nares anteriorly to the choanae posteriorly, constituting the *nasal cavity proper.* Identify the superior, middle, and inferior nasal

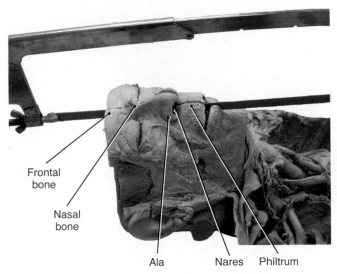

Fig. 26.2 Anterolateral view of face with previous craniotomy, demonstrating sagittal cut of nasal cavity.

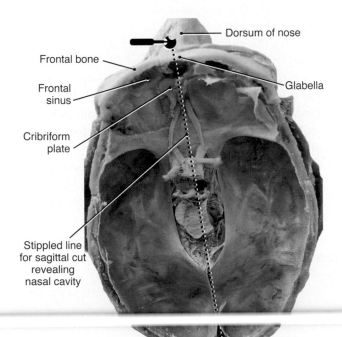

Fig. 26.1 Craniotomy view with *dashed line* for sagittal section.

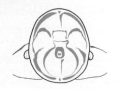

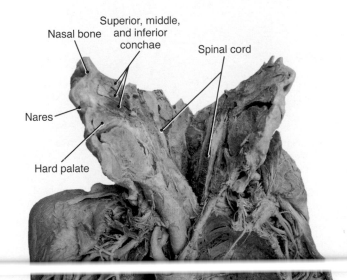

Fig. 26.3 Anterior view of sagittal cut of nasal and oral cavities revealing nasal septum with left and concha on right.

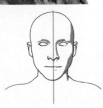

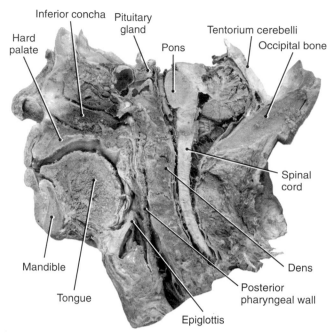

Fig. 26.4 Sagittal view of nasal and oral cavities revealing nasal bone, cartilage, concha, and openings. Structures of mouth and pharynx include hard palate, soft palate, tongue, mandible, epiglottis, and posterior pharyngeal wall.

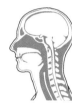

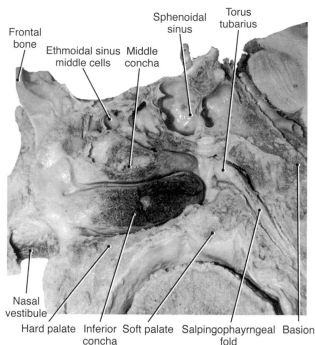

Fig. 26.6 Sagittal view of nasal cavity revealing sphenoidal, ethmoidal, and frontal sinuses; concha; nasal bone; torus tubarius; and salpingopharyngeal fold.

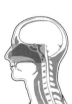

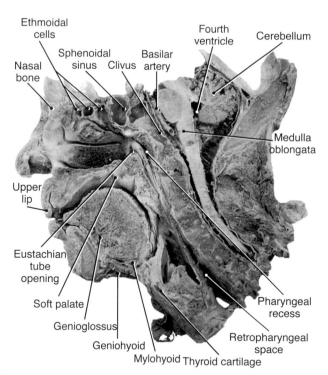

Fig. 26.5 Sagittal view of nasal and oral regions. Nasal region structures include sphenoidal sinus, ethmoidal sinus (anterior, middle, and posterior cells), nasal concha, and eustachian tube opening. Oral structures include lips, hard and soft palate, tongue, oral floor muscles (genioglossus, geniohyoid, mylohyoid), epiglottis, pharyngeal recess, and retropharyngeal space.

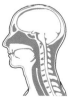

conchae, which are located within the nasal cavity proper (Figs. 26.6 and 26.7).

○ Identify the *superior meatus,* the space between the superior and middle conchae.

○ Continue inferiorly and identify the space between the middle and inferior conchae, the *middle meatus.*

○ Finally, identify the space between the inferior concha and the hard palate, the *inferior meatus* (see Figs. 26.6 and 26.7).

○ Posterior to the superior concha is a space referred to as the *sphenoethmoidal recess.* Identify the opening for the sphenoidal sinus into this recess (see Figs. 26.6 and 26.7).

DISSECTION **TIP**

Some specimens have an increased thickness of the nasal mucosa (see Figs. 26.6 and 26.7).

DISSECTION **TIP**

In most cadavers it is necessary to break away part of the thin, medial wall of the sphenoidal sinus to gain access to its interior. Some specimens may also have a "supreme" concha.

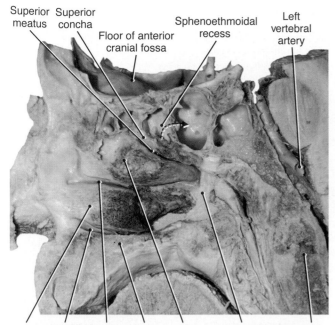

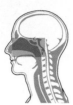

Fig. 26.7 Sagittal view of nasal cavity revealing sphenoidal and ethmoid sinuses and nasal concha highlighting drainage pathways that include sphenoethmoidal recess and meatus associated with superior, middle, and inferior conchae.

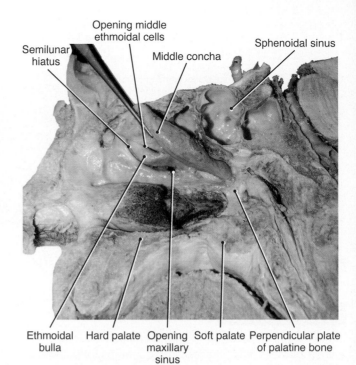

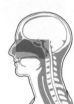

Fig. 26.8 Sagittal view of nasal cavity with middle concha reflected, revealing opening of ethmoidal cells, ethmoidal bulla, semilunar hiatus, and maxillary sinus opening.

○ With forceps, lift the middle meatus upward and identify the ethmoidal bulla.

ANATOMY **NOTE**

The ethmoidal bulla can be oversized from hypertrophy of the ethmoidal cells.

○ Locate the opening of the ethmoidal infundibulum into the semilunar hiatus (Fig. 26.8).
○ With scissors or a scalpel, cut the middle concha away from its junction with the lateral wall of the nasal cavity, and completely expose the middle meatus (Fig. 26.9).
○ Identify the anterior, middle, and posterior *ethmoidal cells.* In the superior meatus, find the ostia of the posterior ethmoidal cells (see Fig. 26.9 and Plate 26.1).

The *hiatus semilunaris* is the long, semicircular groove into which the frontonasal duct drains (drainage of frontal sinus through infundibulum), as well as the anterior ethmoidal cells.

○ Identify the opening of the maxillary sinus. Pass a probe into this opening.

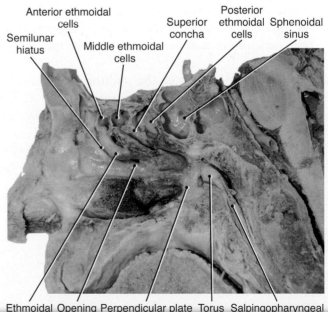

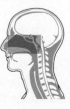

Fig. 26.9 Sagittal view of nasal cavity with superior concha cut and middle concha removed revealing sphenoidal sinus and posterior, middle, and anterior ethmoidal cells. Middle concha removed, highlighting ethmoidal bulla, semilunar hiatus, and maxillary sinus opening.

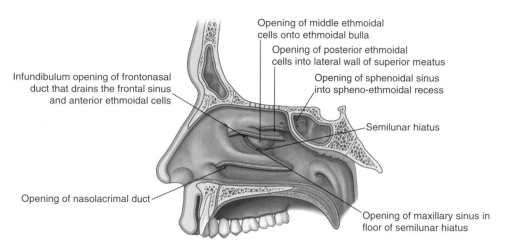

Opening of middle ethmoidal cells onto ethmoidal bulla

Opening of posterior ethmoidal cells into lateral wall of superior meatus

Opening of sphenoidal sinus into spheno-ethmoidal recess

Infundibulum opening of frontonasal duct that drains the frontal sinus and anterior ethmoidal cells

Semilunar hiatus

Opening of nasolacrimal duct

Opening of maxillary sinus in floor of semilunar hiatus

Plate 26.1 A lateral view of the structures of the nasal cavity, with conchae cut away.

DISSECTION **TIP**

Inspect the area of the middle meatus to determine whether there may be accessory openings for the maxillary sinus.

○ The *ethmoidal bulla* is formed by the bulging of ethmoidal cells into the middle meatus (see Fig. 26.9).

○ Remove the anterior half of the inferior nasal concha and identify the opening of the nasolacrimal duct (Fig. 26.10).

○ Place a probe in the nasolacrimal duct.

○ Before dissection of the pterygopalatine fossa, identify the opening to the auditory or pharyngotympanic tube *(eustachian tube)* and place a probe into it (see Fig. 26.10).

○ Identify the elevation of the auditory tube and its muscular ridge, the *salpingopharyngeal fold.* At the opening of the eustachian tube, dissect away the mucous membrane (Fig. 26.11).

○ Identify the *levator* veli palatini muscle (Fig. 26.12).

○ Anterior to the levator veli palatini, dissect out fat and other connective tissues (Fig. 26.13).

○ Identify the *tensor* veli palatini muscle (see Fig. 26.13).

DISSECTION **TIP**

The tensor veli palatini and levator veli palatini muscles are easy to distinguish because of the white, *tendinous* fibers of the *tensor* veli palatini (see Fig. 26.13).

○ Lift the soft tissues and mucous membranes at the space posterior to the nasal conchae and the tensor veli palatini (in essence, the posterior plate of the pterygoid process of the sphenoid bone) (Fig. 26.14).

○ Cut the posterior one third of the middle and superior conchae, and remove the mucosa and soft tissues to expose the palatine bone (Fig. 26.15).

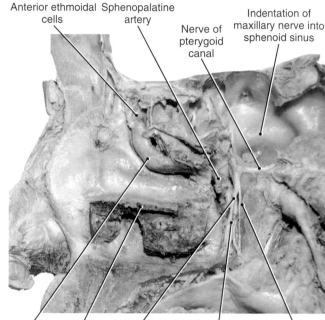

Anterior ethmoidal cells — Sphenopalatine artery — Nerve of pterygoid canal — Indentation of maxillary nerve into sphenoid sinus

Ethmoidal bulla — Inferior concha cut — Greater palatine nerve — Descending palatine artery — Lesser palatine nerve

Fig. 26.10 Sagittal view of nasal cavity with middle concha removed and inferior concha cut and partially removed, revealing drainage pathways of superior, middle, and inferior conchae (nasolacrimal duct) and osteotomy to pterygopalatine fossa. Pterygopalatine fossa includes ganglion, nerve of pterygoid canal, greater and lesser palatine nerves, and sphenopalatine and descending palatine arteries.

DISSECTION **TIP**

The palatine bone is thin, and you can identify the course of the greater and lesser palatine nerves and vessels before removing it.

○ With a small electric drill, cut away the palatine bone, making a vertical cut from the sphenoidal sinus to

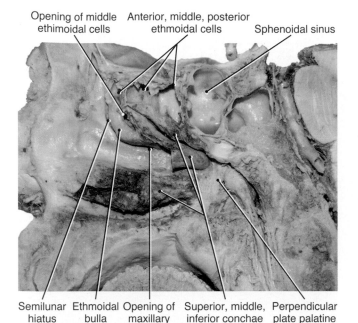

Opening of middle ethimoidal cells | Anterior, middle, posterior ethmoidal cells | Sphenoidal sinus

Semilunar hiatus | Ethmoidal bulla | Opening of maxillary sinus | Superior, middle, inferior conchae | Perpendicular plate palatine bone

Fig. 26.11 Sagittal view of nasal cavity revealing sphenoidal, posterior middle, and anterior ethmoidal cells. Middle concha removed, revealing semilunar hiatus, ethmoid bulla, maxillary sinus opening, and superior, middle, and inferior conchae, as well as the perpendicular plate of palatine bone.

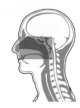

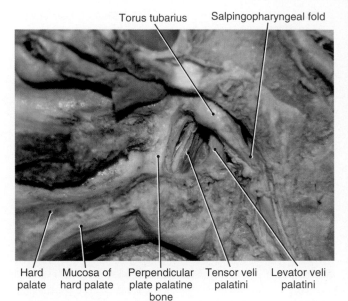

Torus tubarius | Salpingopharyngeal fold

Hard palate | Mucosa of hard palate | Perpendicular plate palatine bone | Tensor veli palatini | Levator veli palatini

Fig. 26.13 Sagittal view of nasal cavity highlighting hard palate and revealing tensor and levator veli palatini muscles, torus tubarius, and salpingopharyngeal fold.

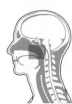

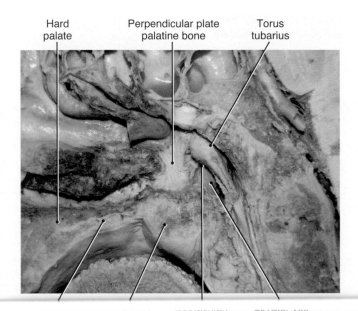

Hard palate | Perpendicular plate palatine bone | Torus tubarius

hard palate | tube opening | palatini

Fig. 26.12 Sagittal view of nasal cavity revealing hard and soft palate, torus tubarius, salpingopharyngeal fold, opening of eustachian tube, and levator veli palatini muscle.

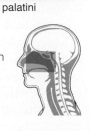

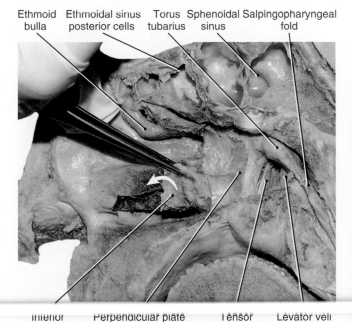

Ethmoid bulla | Ethmoidal sinus posterior cells | Torus tubarius | Sphenoidal sinus | Salpingopharyngeal fold

Inferior concha | Perpendicular plate palatine bone | Tensor veli palatini | Levator veli palatini

Fig. 26.14 Sagittal view of nasal cavity with superior, middle, and inferior concha cut, revealing perpendicular plate of palatine bone, tensor and levator veli palatini, torus tubarius, and salpingopharyngeal fold.

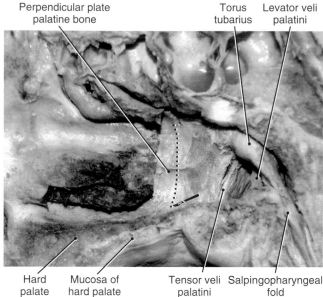

Perpendicular plate palatine bone — Torus tubarius — Levator veli palatini

Hard palate — Mucosa of hard palate — Tensor veli palatini — Salpingopharyngeal fold

Fig. 26.15 Sagittal view of nasal cavity highlighting perpendicular plate of palatine bone, tensor and levator veli palatini muscles, torus tubarius, and mucosa of hard palate.

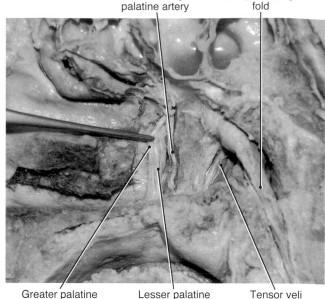

Descending palatine artery — Salpingopharyngeal fold

Greater palatine nerve retracted — Lesser palatine nerve retracted — Tensor veli palatini

Fig. 26.17 Sagittal view of nasal cavity with greater and lesser palatine nerves retracted, revealing descending palatine artery.

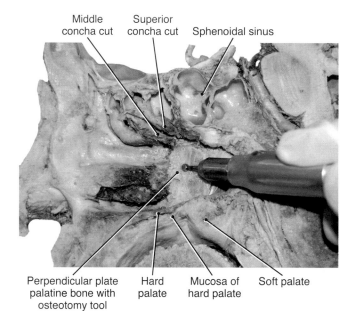

Middle concha cut — Superior concha cut — Sphenoidal sinus

Perpendicular plate palatine bone with osteotomy tool — Hard palate — Mucosa of hard palate — Soft palate

Fig. 26.16 Sagittal view of nasal cavity highlighting middle and superior conchae cut and perpendicular plate of palatine bone with small osteotomy to reveal pterygopalatine fossa structures.

the hard palate and posteriorly to the middle concha (see Figs. 26.15 and 26.16).

○ First, expose the greater and lesser palatine nerves, as well as the descending palatine artery and the greater and lesser palatine arteries (Figs. 26.17 and 26.18).

○ Continue drilling upward to the sphenoidal sinus. Identify the sphenopalatine artery and the pterygopalatine ganglion (Fig. 26.19 and Plate 26.2).

DISSECTION **TIP**

In this part of dissection, use fine forceps and scissors to separate the delicate nerves and arteries.

○ Continue drilling posteriorly to the pterygopalatine ganglion and inferior to the sphenoidal sinus. Expose the *vidian nerve* (nerve to pterygoid canal) (Fig. 26.20).

ANATOMY **NOTE**

The greater and deep petrosal nerves unite and form the nerve of the pterygoid canal. This nerve passes through the pterygoid canal of the sphenoid bone and then into the pterygopalatine fossa.

○ If time permits, drill away the sphenoidal sinus, and expose the connection of the pterygopalatine ganglion with the maxillary nerve (Fig. 26.21).

○ With scissors, reflect the oral mucosa from the hard palate, and identify the distribution of the greater and lesser palatine nerves (Fig. 26.22).

○ The lateral wall of the nasal cavity is dissected on one side of the head, as well as the pterygopalatine fossa. Dissect the nasal septum on the opposite side, i.e., the other hemisected part of the head (Fig. 26.23).

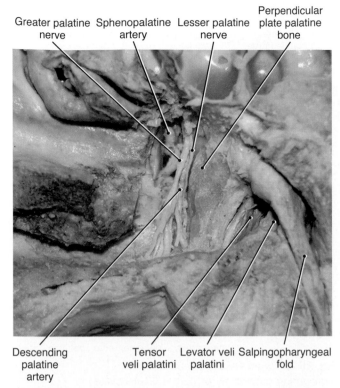

Greater palatine nerve   Sphenopalatine artery   Lesser palatine nerve   Perpendicular plate palatine bone

Descending palatine artery   Tensor veli palatini   Levator veli palatini   Salpingopharyngeal fold

Fig. 26.18 Sagittal view of nasal cavity highlighting osteotomy of perpendicular plate of palatine bone to reveal sphenopalatine artery, greater and lesser palatine nerves, and descending palatine artery.

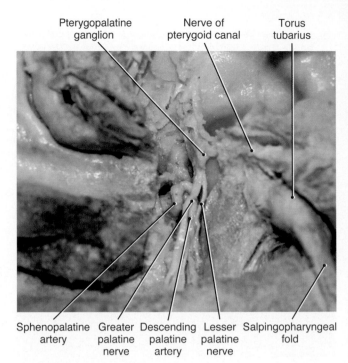

Pterygopalatine ganglion   Nerve of pterygoid canal   Torus tubarius

Sphenopalatine artery   Greater palatine nerve   Descending palatine artery   Lesser palatine nerve   Salpingopharyngeal fold

Fig. 26.19 Sagittal view of nasal cavity with osteotomy of perpendicular plate of palatine bone, revealing sphenopalatine artery, pterygopalatine ganglion, nerve of pterygoid canal, greater and lesser palatine nerves, and descending palatine artery.

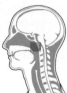

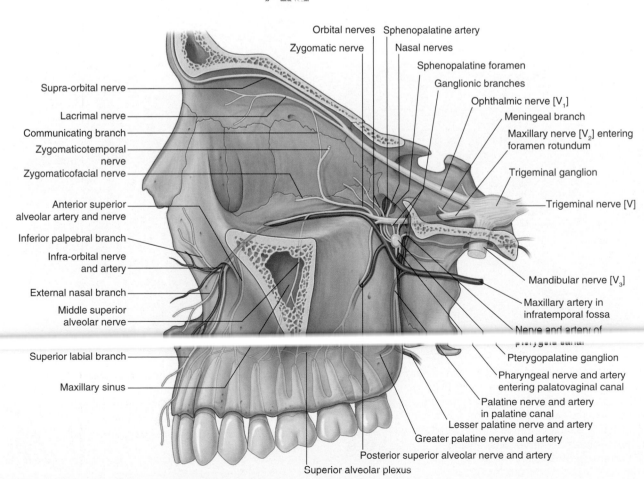

Orbital nerves   Sphenopalatine artery
Zygomatic nerve   Nasal nerves
Sphenopalatine foramen
Ganglionic branches
Ophthalmic nerve [V₁]
Meningeal branch
Maxillary nerve [V₂] entering foramen rotundum
Trigeminal ganglion
Trigeminal nerve [V]
Mandibular nerve [V₃]
Maxillary artery in infratemporal fossa
Nerve and artery of pterygoid canal
Pterygopalatine ganglion
Pharyngeal nerve and artery entering palatovaginal canal
Palatine nerve and artery in palatine canal
Lesser palatine nerve and artery
Greater palatine nerve and artery
Posterior superior alveolar nerve and artery
Superior alveolar plexus

Supra-orbital nerve
Lacrimal nerve
Communicating branch
Zygomaticotemporal nerve
Zygomaticofacial nerve
Anterior superior alveolar artery and nerve
Inferior palpebral branch
Infra-orbital nerve and artery
External nasal branch
Middle superior alveolar nerve
Superior labial branch
Maxillary sinus

Plate 26.2 Nerves and arteries of the pterygopalatine fossa.

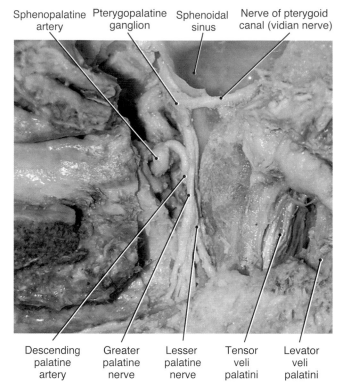

Sphenopalatine artery — Pterygopalatine ganglion — Sphenoidal sinus — Nerve of pterygoid canal (vidian nerve)

Descending palatine artery — Greater palatine nerve — Lesser palatine nerve — Tensor veli palatini — Levator veli palatini

Fig. 26.20 Sagittal view of nasal cavity with osteotomy of perpendicular plate of palatine bone, revealing pterygopalatine ganglion, nerve of pterygoid canal, greater and lesser palatine nerves, and descending palatine artery.

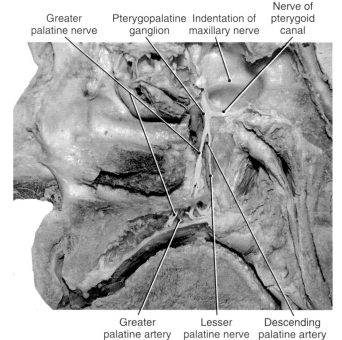

Greater palatine nerve — Pterygopalatine ganglion — Indentation of maxillary nerve — Nerve of pterygoid canal

Greater palatine artery — Lesser palatine nerve — Descending palatine artery

Fig. 26.21 Sagittal view of nasal cavity highlighting osteotomy of perpendicular plate of palatine bone and the sphenoidal sinus and revealing pterygopalatine fossa with pterygopalatine ganglion, nerve of pterygoid canal, greater palatine nerve, descending palatine artery, and maxillary nerve.

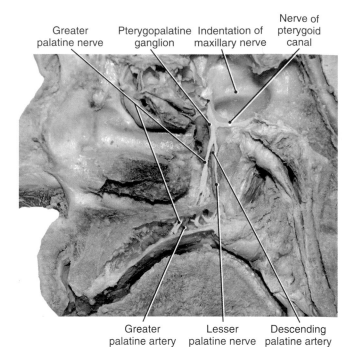

Greater palatine nerve — Pterygopalatine ganglion — Indentation of maxillary nerve — Nerve of pterygoid canal

Greater palatine artery — Lesser palatine nerve — Descending palatine artery

Fig. 26.22 Sagittal view of nasal cavity highlighting osteotomy of perpendicular plate of palatine bone, to show pterygopalatine fossa with pterygopalatine ganglion, nerve of pterygoid canal, greater and lesser palatine nerves and arteries, and descending palatine artery.

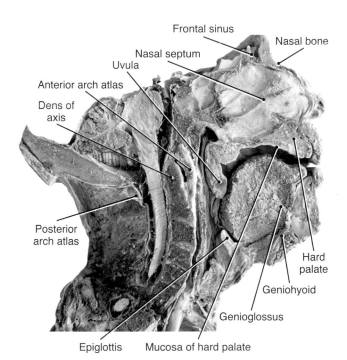

Frontal sinus — Nasal bone

Nasal septum — Uvula — Anterior arch atlas — Dens of axis

Posterior arch atlas

Epiglottis — Mucosa of hard palate — Geniohyoid — Genioglossus — Hard palate

Fig. 26.23 Sagittal view of nasal and oral cavities revealing nasal septum and sphenoidal/frontal sinuses. Oral cavity reveals hard palate, soft palate, uvula, pharynx, floor of tongue muscles (genioglossus, geniohyoid), and epiglottis.

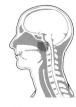
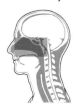
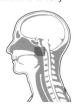

○ Remove the mucous membranes from the exposed surface of the nasal septum (Fig. 26.24).

○ Identify the septal cartilage, perpendicular plate of the ethmoid bone, and the vomer bone (Fig. 26.25).

DISSECTION **TIP**

Usually, it is difficult and time-consuming to find any of the nerves or vessels on the nasal mucosa, because of drying and shrinkage from fixation.

Identify the following:

○ 1. *Sphenoethmoidal recess,* posterior to the superior concha, the location of the opening for the sphenoidal sinus

○ 2. *Superior nasal meatus,* beneath the superior concha, the opening for the posterior ethmoidal cells

○ 3. *Middle nasal meatus,* the ethmoidal bulla, with openings for middle ethmoid cells and the maxillary sinus

○ 4. *Inferior nasal meatus,* the opening of the nasolacrimal duct

○ 5. *Ethmoidal infundibulum,* for the opening of the frontonasal duct from the frontal sinus

○ 6. *Hiatus semilunaris,* the semilunar hiatus, the long, crescent-shaped opening for the anterior ethmoidal cells

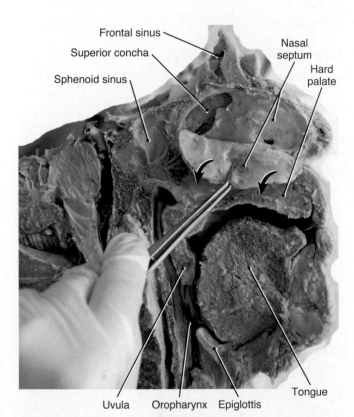

Frontal sinus
Superior concha
Sphenoid sinus
Nasal septum
Hard palate
Uvula   Oropharynx   Epiglottis
Tongue

Fig. 26.24 Sagittal view of nasal and oral cavities with nasal septum reflected, revealing superior concha, vomer bone, sphenoidal sinus, and frontal sinus. Oral cavity reveals tongue, floor of tongue muscles, uvula, epiglottis, and pharynx.

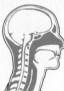

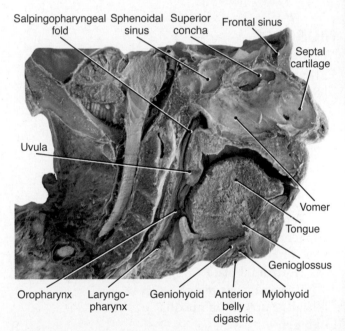

Salpingopharyngeal fold   Sphenoidal sinus   Superior concha   Frontal sinus
Septal cartilage
Uvula
Vomer
Tongue
Genioglossus
Oropharynx   Laryngo-pharynx   Geniohyoid   Anterior belly digastric   Mylohyoid

Fig. 26.25 Sagittal view of nasal and oral cavities revealing sphenoidal and frontal sinuses, septal cartilage, vomer bone, superior concha, and nasal pharynx. Oral cavity reveals uvula, tongue, and genioglossus, geniohyoid, mylohyoid, and anterior belly of digastric muscles.

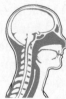

LABORATORY IDENTIFICATION CHECKLIST

NERVES
- ☐ Nerve of pterygoid canal
- ☐ Greater palatine
- ☐ Lesser palatine
- ☐ Maxillary

ARTERIES
- ☐ Sphenopalatine
  - ☐ Descending palatine
    - ☐ Greater palatine
    - ☐ Lesser palatine

MUSCLES
- ☐ Tensor veli palatini
- ☐ Levator veli palatini
- ☐ Salpingopharyngeus

BONES
- ☐ Nasal
- ☐ Frontal
- ☐ Ethmoid
  - ☐ Cribriform plate
  - ☐ Perpendicular plate
- ☐ Sphenoid
- ☐ Palatine
  - ☐ Horizontal plate
  - ☐ Perpendicular plate
- ☐ Palatine process of maxilla
- ☐ Vomer
- ☐ Conchae
  - ☐ Superior
  - ☐ Middle
  - ☐ Inferior

SINUSES
- ☐ Sphenoidal
- ☐ Ethmoidal
  - ☐ Posterior cells
  - ☐ Middle cells
  - ☐ Anterior cells
- ☐ Frontal
- ☐ Maxillary

DRAINAGE PATHWAYS
- ☐ Sphenoethmoidal recess
- ☐ Superior meatus
- ☐ Middle meatus
- ☐ Inferior meatus
- ☐ Ethmoidal bulla
- ☐ Semilunar hiatus
- ☐ Nasolacrimal duct
- ☐ Sphenopalatine foramen
- ☐ Maxillary sinus ostium
- ☐ Nares (nostrils)
  - ☐ Choanae
  - ☐ Vestibule

GANGLION
- ☐ Pterygopalatine

OTHER STRUCTURES
- ☐ Basion
- ☐ Clivus
- ☐ Dens
- ☐ Epiglottis
- ☐ Torus tubarius
- ☐ Uvula
- ☐ Septal cartilage

ATLAS REFERENCES

Netter: 65–72, 77, 81–86
McMinn: 46, 52
Gray's Atlas: 552–557, 572–582

DISSECTION STEPS

○ Identify the borders of the nasopharynx, oropharynx, and laryngopharynx on the cadaver (Fig. 27.1).

○ The tensor veli palatini and the levator veli palatini muscles have been identified during the dissection of the pterygopalatine fossa (see Fig. 27.1 and Chapter 26).

○ Identify the *torus tubarius,* a cartilaginous elevation of the auditory tube (see Figs. 27.4 and 27.1), and locate the pharyngeal tonsil superior to it.

○ Extending inferiorly from the torus tubarius is the *salpingopharyngeal fold,* formed by the underlying salpingopharyngeus muscle (see Fig. 27.3 and Plate 27.1).

○ Locate the borders of the tonsillar fossa in the oropharynx and identify the palatine tonsil bounded by two arches. Anteriorly, observe the *palatoglossal arch,* a mucosal fold formed by the palatoglossus muscle (see Fig. 27.1).

○ Posteriorly, a second arch, the *palatopharyngeal arch,* is formed by a mucosal fold from the underlying palatopharyngeus muscle (see Fig. 27.1).

○ In the tonsillar fossa, use your forceps to lift the mucous membrane and pull it off of the underlying musculature (Fig. 27.2).

○ Similarly, remove the mucous membrane and expose the palatopharyngeus muscle (see Fig. 27.2).

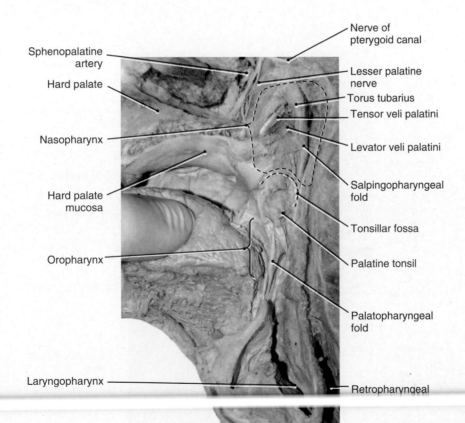

Sphenopalatine artery
Hard palate
Nasopharynx
Hard palate mucosa
Oropharynx
Laryngopharynx

Nerve of pterygoid canal
Lesser palatine nerve
Torus tubarius
Tensor veli palatini
Levator veli palatini
Salpingopharyngeal fold
Tonsillar fossa
Palatine tonsil
Palatopharyngeal fold
Retropharyngeal

Fig. 27.1 Sagittal view of oral cavity, including nasal and pharyngeal regions, revealing hard palate, nasopharynx region, hard palate mucosa, oral pharynx region, laryngopharynx region, retropharyngeal space, and salpingopharyngeal fold.

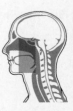

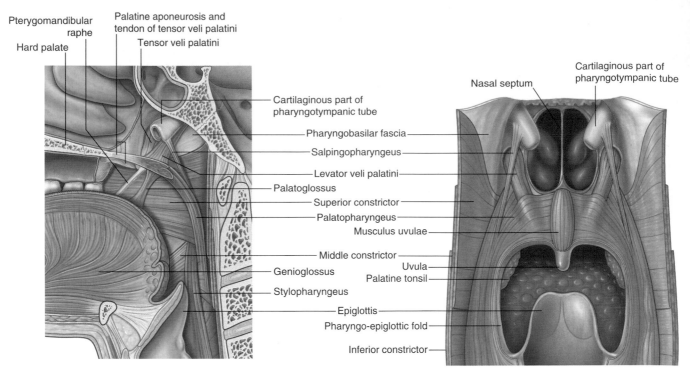

Plate 27.1 Muscles of soft palate, sagittal and posterior views.

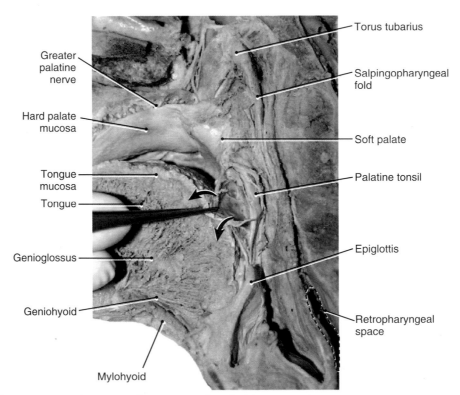

Fig. 27.2 Removal of mucous membranes and exposure of underlying musculature.

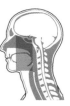

DISSECTION TIP

In the laryngopharynx, at the level of the epiglottis, the palatopharyngeus, salpingopharyngeus, and stylopharyngeus muscles give the impression that they blend and fuse with the posterior pharyngeal constrictor muscles (see Fig. 27.2). However, the posterior pharyngeal constrictors are separated from these muscles by a thin fascia, the *buccopharyngeal fascia.* In some specimens, this fascia may appear as a white vertical line.

○ Pull the palatine tonsil forward, and expose the palatopharyngeus muscle (Fig. 27.3).

○ Continue the dissection by removing the mucous membranes from the palatoglossal arch, and expose the palatoglossus muscle (Fig. 27.4).

○ Because this muscle is located deep and lateral to the tongue, pull the tongue forward and the palatine tonsil backward to expose it fully.

○ Divide the palatoglossus muscle, and identify the glossopharyngeal nerve (Fig. 27.5).

○ At the base of the tongue, identify the *lingual tonsil.*

DISSECTION TIP

To find the glossopharyngeal nerve, place your thumb at the lateral border of the epiglottis, between the palatine tonsil and the epiglottis. Split the palatoglossus muscle lateral to your thumb (see Fig. 27.5).

○ Identify the space between the epiglottis and the tongue. Look for a membranous ridge, the *median glossoepiglottic fold,* connecting the posterior surface of the tongue to the epiglottis (Fig. 27.6).

ANATOMY NOTE

This fold divides the area between the epiglottis and the tongue into two spaces, the *valleculae* (see Fig. 27.6).

INSPECTION

ANATOMY NOTE

The oral cavity occupies the space between the lips anteriorly and the palatoglossal folds posteriorly. For descriptive purposes, the oral cavity is also divided into the vestibule and the oral cavity proper. The *vestibule* includes the area between the external surfaces of the teeth and the internal surface of cheeks. The *oral cavity proper* is the space filled by the tongue.

○ Pull the tongue toward the midline and note the *vestibule.*

○ Identify the mucous membrane, the *frenulum,* between the inferior aspect of the tongue and the floor of the mouth (Fig. 27.7).

○ Lateral to the frenulum, identify multiple tributaries of the lingual veins and orifices of the submandibular glands, the *sublingual* papilla (sublingual *caruncle*).

○ Continue the inspection of the anterior surface of the tongue, and identify the *filiform* papillae.

○ Appreciate the much larger and sometimes reddish *fungiform* papillae.

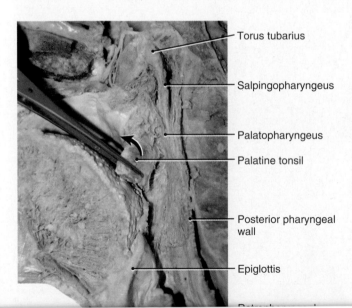

Fig. 27.3 Musculature of palatine tonsil reflected anteriorly, exposing the salpingopharyngeus, palatopharyngeus, and posterior pharyngeal wall.

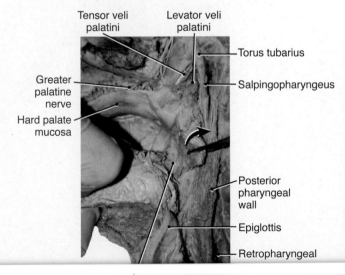

Fig. 27.4 Musculature of palatine tonsil reflected posteriorly, exposing the palatoglossal fold and palatoglossus muscle.

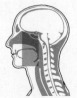

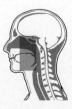

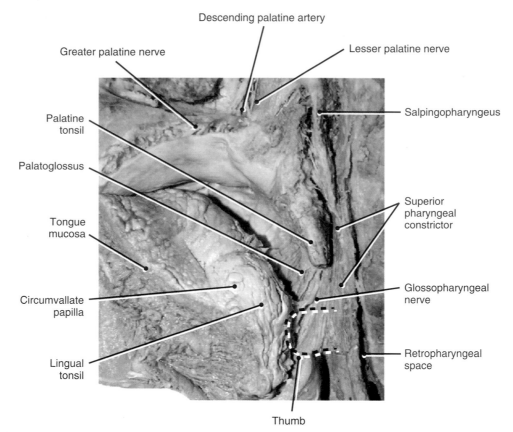

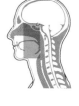

Fig. 27.5 To find the glossopharyngeal nerve, the thumb is placed *(dashed area)* lateral to the epiglottis between it and the palatine tonsil.

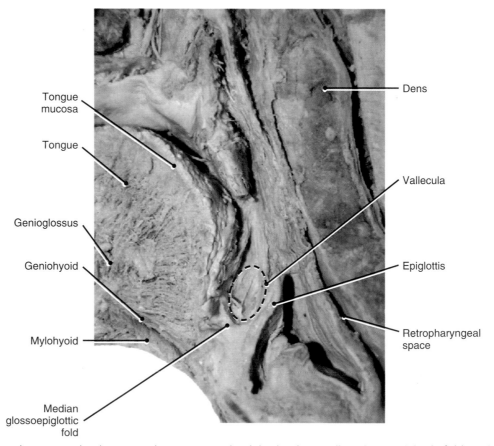

Fig. 27.6 Appreciate the connection between the tongue and epiglottis, the median glossoepiglottic fold, and spaces lateral to it (valleculae).

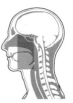

- At the posterior surface of the tongue, identify the sulcus terminalis and *vallate* papillae.
- At the midpoint of the sulcus terminalis, attempt to visualize the *foramen cecum* (Fig. 27.8 and Plate 27.2).
- Pull the tongue medially and make a shallow incision through the mucous membranes lateral to the tongue alongside the mandible (Fig. 27.9).

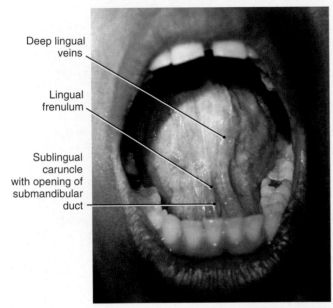

Fig. 27.7 Appreciate the lingual frenulum, deep lingual vein, and submandibular duct.

Deep lingual veins

Lingual frenulum

Sublingual caruncle with opening of submandibular duct

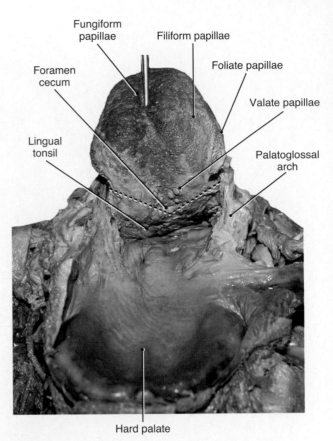

Fungiform papillae

Filiform papillae

Foliate papillae

Foramen cecum

Valate papillae

Lingual tonsil

Palatoglossal arch

Hard palate

Fig. 27.8 Hard palate reflected posteriorly with view from above revealing filiform, fungiform, and foliate papillae, and at the posterior third of the tongue, the sulcus terminalis (dashed line) and 10 to 12 vallate papillae.

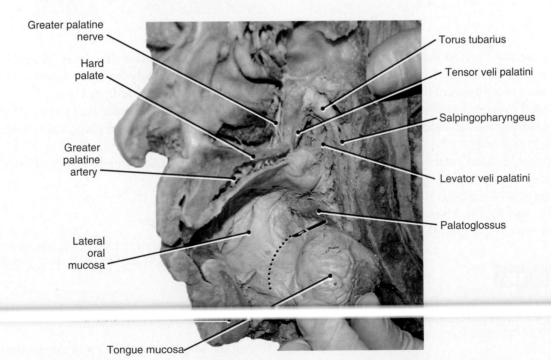

Greater palatine nerve

Hard palate

Greater palatine artery

Lateral oral mucosa

Torus tubarius

Tensor veli palatini

Salpingopharyngeus

Levator veli palatini

Palatoglossus

Tongue mucosa

Fig. 27.9 Tongue pulled medially with shallow incision *(dotted line)* through mucous membranes lateral to tongue alongside mandible.

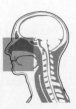

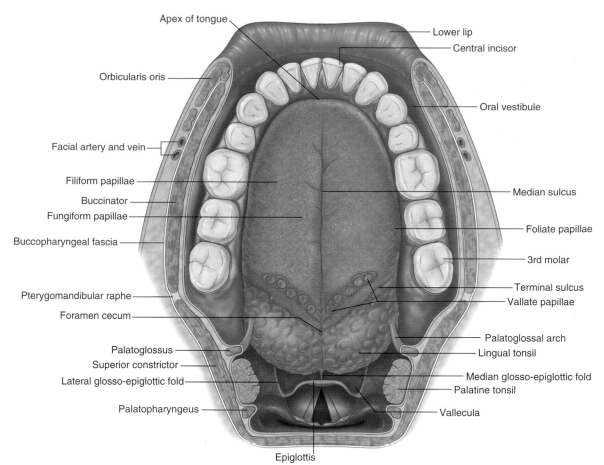

Apex of tongue
Orbicularis oris
Facial artery and vein
Filiform papillae
Buccinator
Fungiform papillae
Buccopharyngeal fascia
Pterygomandibular raphe
Foramen cecum
Palatoglossus
Superior constrictor
Lateral glosso-epiglottic fold
Palatopharyngeus
Epiglottis

Lower lip
Central incisor
Oral vestibule
Median sulcus
Foliate papillae
3rd molar
Terminal sulcus
Vallate papillae
Palatoglossal arch
Lingual tonsil
Median glosso-epiglottic fold
Palatine tonsil
Vallecula

Plate 27.2 Horizontal section showing superior view of tongue.

○ Extend the incision toward the palatoglossus but do not sever this muscle (Fig. 27.10).

○ Lift the mucous membranes of the vestibule and expose the mylohyoid muscle (Fig. 27.11).

○ Appreciate neuromuscular structures with the mylohyoid muscle exposed.

○ In the space between the palatoglossus and mylohyoid muscles, identify the *lingual nerve* descending from the infratemporal fossa into the floor of the mouth (Figs. 27.12 and 27.13). Clean the soft tissues and mucous membranes around the lingual nerve.

DISSECTION **TIP**

The dissection of the lingual nerve also continues from the floor of the mouth. Therefore do not attempt to dissect the nerve too deeply.

○ Make an incision through the mucous membrane of the floor of the mouth between the geniohyoid and mylohyoid muscles (Figs. 27.14 and 27.15), and identify the *lingual artery* (Fig. 27.16).

○ As the mucous membranes are reflected laterally from the midline, identify the *submandibular duct* (Wharton's duct) and the *sublingual gland.*

○ Expose the submandibular duct posteriorly to its origin from the submandibular gland, around the posterior edge of the mylohyoid muscle (Fig. 27.17).

○ Distal to the tortuous lingual artery, identify the lingual nerve.

ANATOMY **NOTE**

The lingual nerve passes medially toward the tongue as it crosses over the submandibular duct (Fig. 27.18).

○ Posterior to the tongue, expose the hypoglossal nerve.

○ Pull the tongue posteriorly and expose the mylohyoid muscle (Fig. 27.19).

○ Trace the lingual nerve as it descends from the infratemporal fossa between the palatoglossus and mylohyoid muscles. Note the submandibular duct crossing the lingual nerve (Fig. 27.20).

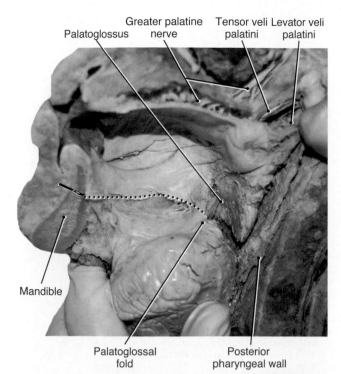

Palatoglossus — Greater palatine nerve — Tensor veli palatini — Levator veli palatini

Mandible

Palatoglossal fold — Posterior pharyngeal wall

Fig. 27.10 Incision extended toward palatoglossus muscle.

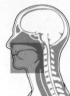

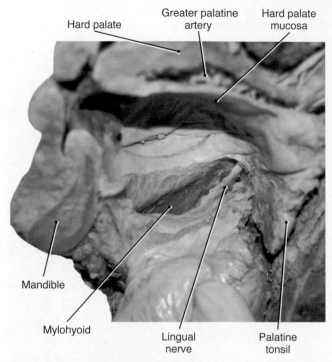

Hard palate — Greater palatine artery — Hard palate mucosa

Mandible

Mylohyoid — Lingual nerve — Palatine tonsil

Fig. 27.12 Appreciate the lingual nerve descending from the infratemporal fossa into the floor of the mouth, between palatoglossus and mylohyoid muscles.

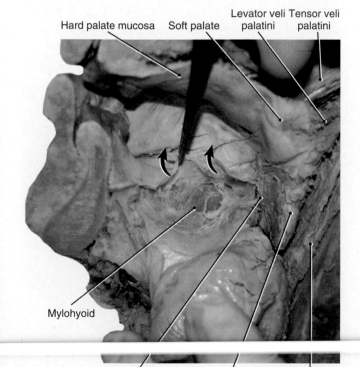

Hard palate mucosa — Soft palate — Levator veli palatini — Tensor veli palatini

Mylohyoid

Palatoglossus — Palatine tonsil — Posterior pharyngeal wall

Fig. 27.11 Mucous membranes of vestibule lifted, exposing the mylohyoid muscle.

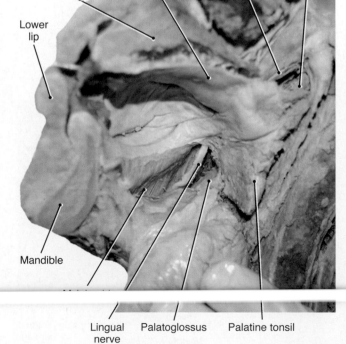

Hard palate — Hard palate mucosa — Tensor veli palatini — Levator veli palatini

Lower lip

Mandible

Lingual nerve — Palatoglossus — Palatine tonsil

Fig. 27.13 Soft tissues and mucous membranes cleaned around lingual nerve.

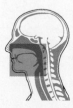

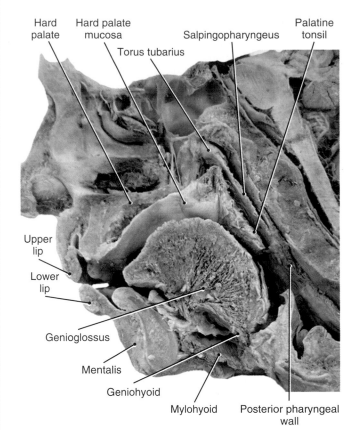

Hard palate | Hard palate mucosa | Salpingopharyngeus | Palatine tonsil
Torus tubarius

Upper lip

Lower lip

Genioglossus

Mentalis

Geniohyoid

Mylohyoid

Posterior pharyngeal wall

Fig. 27.14 Sagittal view of oral cavity, including nasal and pharyngeal regions, revealing hard palate mucosa, upper/lower lips, uvula, and mentalis, genioglossus, geniohyoid, mylohyoid, and salpingopharyngeus muscles.

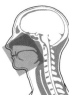

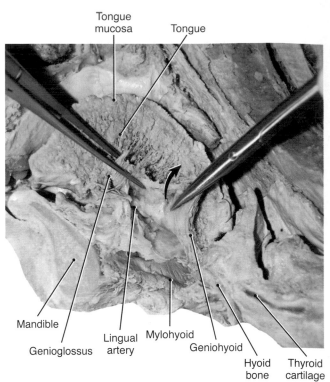

Tongue mucosa | Tongue

Mandible | Genioglossus | Lingual artery | Mylohyoid | Geniohyoid | Hyoid bone | Thyroid cartilage

Fig. 27.15 Geniohyoid muscle lifted upward to clean soft tissues underneath.

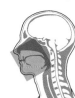

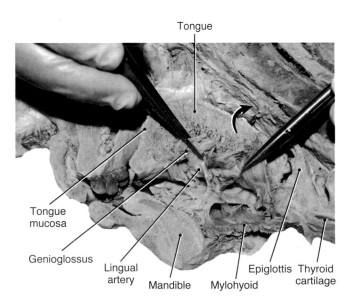

Tongue

Tongue mucosa

Genioglossus | Lingual artery | Mandible | Mylohyoid | Epiglottis | Thyroid cartilage

Fig. 27.16 Sagittal view of oral cavity revealing mucosa of tongue, tongue, genioglossus muscle, lingual artery, mandible, mylohyoid muscle, hyoid bone, and epiglottis.

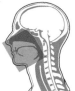

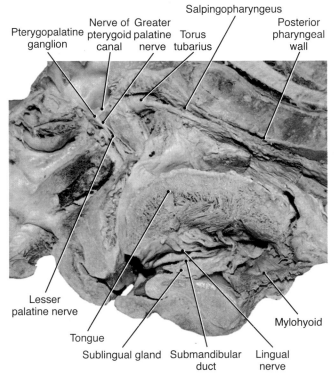

Pterygopalatine ganglion | Nerve of pterygoid canal | Greater palatine nerve | Torus tubarius | Salpingopharyngeus | Posterior pharyngeal wall

Lesser palatine nerve

Tongue | Sublingual gland | Submandibular duct | Lingual nerve | Mylohyoid

Fig. 27.17 Submandibular duct exposed posteriorly from origin at submandibular gland around posterior edge of the mylohyoid muscle

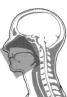

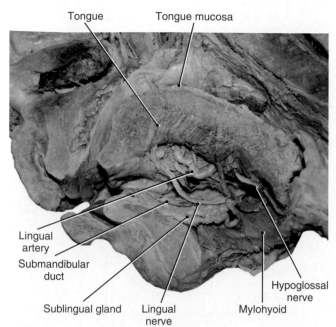

Fig. 27.18 Appreciate lingual nerve distal to tortuous lingual artery, passing medially toward tongue and crossing over submandibular duct, and hypoglossal nerve posteriorly.

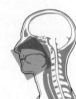

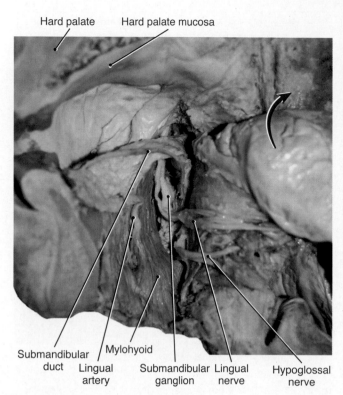

Fig. 27.20 Appreciate lingual nerve descending from infratemporal fossa and submandibular duct crossing over it.

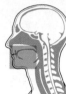

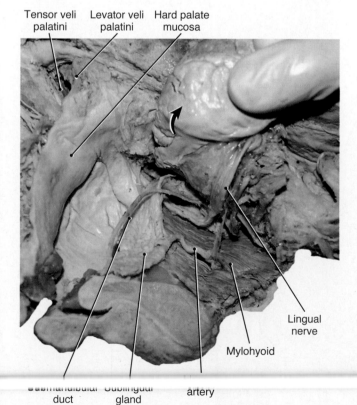

Fig. 27.19 Tongue pulled posteriorly, exposing mylohyoid muscle.

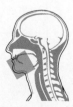

○ With the tongue pulled posteriorly, dissect between the lingual nerve and submandibular gland, and expose the *submandibular ganglion* (see Fig. 27.20).

DISSECTION TIP

The following landmarks help to identify the different structures in the floor of the mouth (Figs. 27.21 and 27.22):

- The *lingual artery* passes deep to the hyoglossus muscle and is often tortuous.
- The *hypoglossal nerve* passes superficial to the hyoglossus muscle and is seen at the posterior part of the tongue.
- Seen from the midline with the tongue in situ, the *lingual nerve* passes medially toward the tongue as it crosses over the submandibular duct (see Fig. 27.18).
- With the tongue reflected posteriorly, note the *submandibular duct* crossing over the lingual nerve (see Figs. 27.19 and 27.20 and Plate 27.3).

○ If time permits, separate and expose the hyoglossus, genioglossus, geniohyoid, styloglossus, and mylohyoid muscles.

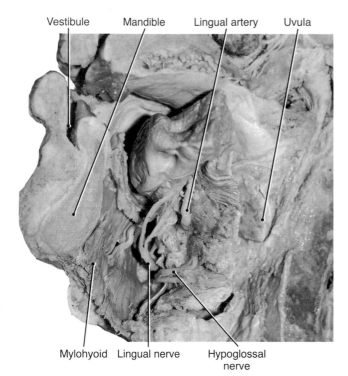

Vestibule Mandible Lingual artery Uvula

Mylohyoid Lingual nerve Hypoglossal nerve

Fig. 27.21 Sagittal view of oral cavity, including nasal and pharyngeal regions, revealing vestibule, lingual artery, hypoglossal nerve, lingual nerve, mylohyoid muscle, uvula, and hyoid bone.

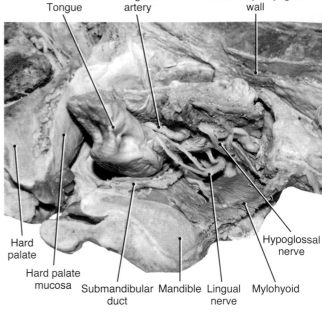

Tongue Lingual artery Posterior pharyngeal wall

Hard palate

Hard palate mucosa Submandibular duct Mandible Lingual nerve Mylohyoid Hypoglossal nerve

Fig. 27.22 Sagittal view of the oral cavity, highlighting hard palate and mucosa, tongue, hypoglossal nerve, lingual artery and nerve, mylohyoid muscle, and posterior pharyngeal wall.

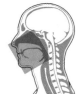

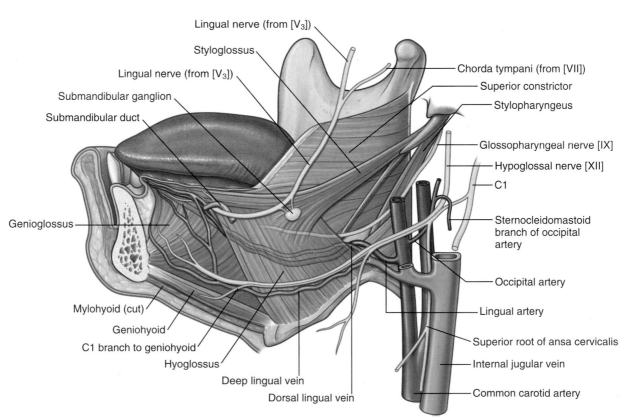

Lingual nerve (from [V₃])

Styloglossus

Lingual nerve (from [V₃])

Submandibular ganglion

Submandibular duct

Genioglossus

Mylohyoid (cut)

Geniohyoid

C1 branch to geniohyoid

Hyoglossus

Deep lingual vein

Dorsal lingual vein

Chorda tympani (from [VII])

Superior constrictor

Stylopharyngeus

Glossopharyngeal nerve [IX]

Hypoglossal nerve [XII]

C1

Sternocleidomastoid branch of occipital artery

Occipital artery

Lingual artery

Superior root of ansa cervicalis

Internal jugular vein

Common carotid artery

Plate 27.3 Arteries, veins, and nerves of the tongue.

DISSECTION **TIP**

To identify the following muscles, note their course:

- The *genioglossus* muscle runs from the mandible to the tongue.
- The *geniohyoid* runs from the mandible to the hyoid bone.
- The *hyoglossus* runs from the tongue to the hyoid bone.
- The *styloglossus* arises from the styloid process and enters the tongue posteriorly and passes under the palatoglossus to fuse with the hyoglossus muscle.

○ After you identify these muscles, make a small vertical cut near the tip of the tongue, and expose the vertical muscle fibers and intrinsic transverse muscle fibers.

○ Make another incision in the superficial tissue from the dorsum of the tongue, and expose the intrinsic longitudinal fibers (Fig. 27.23).

ANATOMY **NOTE**

In some cadavers, you may find some bony outgrowths in the oral cavity the torus palatinus and torus mandibularis. The *torus palatinus* and *torus mandibularis* are variant benign excrescences of the hard palate and mandible, respectively (Fig. 27.24).

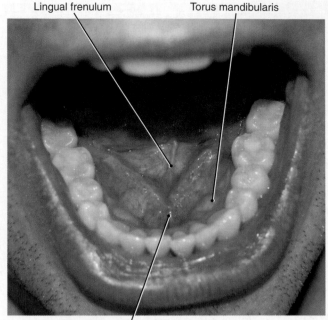

Fig. 27.24 Torus mandibularis is a benign, bony outgrowth of the mandible.

Lingual frenulum   Torus mandibularis

Sublingual caruncle with opening of submandibular duct

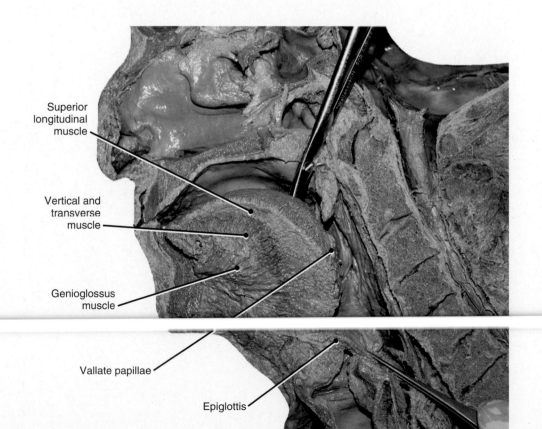

Superior longitudinal muscle

Vertical and transverse muscle

Genioglossus muscle

Vallate papillae

Epiglottis

Fig. 27.23 Midsagittal section of cadaveric head reveals intrinsic muscle of tongue.

LABORATORY IDENTIFICATION CHECKLIST

NERVES

- ☐ Lingual
- ☐ Hypoglossal
- ☐ Nerve to mylohyoid
- ☐ Glossopharyngeal

GANGLION

- ☐ Submandibular

ARTERY

- ☐ Lingual

VEIN

- ☐ Lingual

MUSCLES

- ☐ Digastric
  - ☐ Anterior belly
  - ☐ Posterior belly
- ☐ Mylohyoid
- ☐ Geniohyoid

- ☐ Genioglossus
- ☐ Tongue
  - ☐ Superior longitudinal fibers
  - ☐ Inferior longitudinal fibers
  - ☐ Horizontal fibers
  - ☐ Vertical fibers
  - ☐ Hyoglossus
  - ☐ Styloglossus

BONES

- ☐ Mandible
- ☐ Hyoid
- ☐ Temporal
  - ☐ Styloid process
  - ☐ Mastoid process

SALIVARY GLANDS

- ☐ Submandibular
  - ☐ Superficial and deep lobes
  - ☐ Submandibular duct (Wharton's duct)
- ☐ Sublingual

ATLAS REFERENCES
Netter: 89–93
McMinn: 48–50
Gray's Atlas: 558–562

BEFORE YOU BEGIN
The larynx occupies the space between the epiglottis superiorly and the inferior border of the cricoid cartilage.

INSPECTION
Technique 1

○ The inspection begins by examining the larynx in a hemisected head.
○ In a hemisected specimen, identify the epiglottis, laryngopharynx, thyroid cartilage, vallecula, uvula, posterior pharyngeal wall, cervical vertebrae, and trachea (Fig. 28.1 and Plate 28.1).
○ If the thyroid and cricoid cartilages are not hemisected, complete the hemisection and expose the contents of the larynx using scissors.

> ### DISSECTION TIP
> Do not cut directly in the midline of the cricoid and thyroid cartilages. Try to perform the cut as laterally as possible.

○ With your fingertips, keep the larynx open, and identify the supraglottic space, or *vestibule*, extending from the epiglottis to the vestibular folds (Fig. 28.2).
○ The *ventricle* is the space between the vestibular (false vocal) folds and the vocal (true vocal) folds (Plate 28.2).
○ Note the space between the vocal folds, the *rima glottidis* (Fig. 28.3).
○ Identify the infraglottic space between the vocal fold and the first tracheal ring.
○ Identify the *aryepiglottic fold,* the mucous membrane stretched between the epiglottis to the apex of the arytenoid cartilages.
○ With scissors, cut the remaining part of the larynx in the midsagittal plane (see Fig. 28.3).

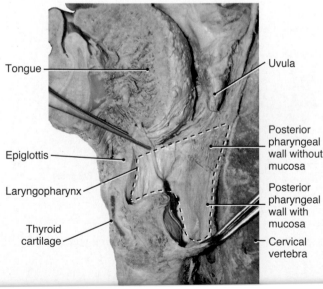

Tongue — Uvula
Epiglottis — Posterior pharyngeal wall without mucosa
Laryngopharynx — Posterior pharyngeal wall with mucosa
Thyroid cartilage — Cervical vertebra
Trachea

Fig. 28.1 Sagittal view of mouth and larynx, revealing tongue, epiglottis, laryngopharynx, thyroid cartilage, vallecula, uvula, posterior pharyngeal wall, cervical vertebrae, and trachea.

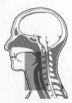

Epiglottis — Vestibule
Vestibular fold — Piriform recess
Vocal fold — Ventricle
Infraglottic space — Posterior cricoarytenoid muscle

Fig. 28.2 Sagittal view of mouth with open posterior view of larynx, highlighting epiglottis, vestibule/laryngeal inlet, vocal fold, vestibular fold, ventricle, posterior cricoarytenoid muscle, and piriform recess.

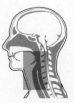

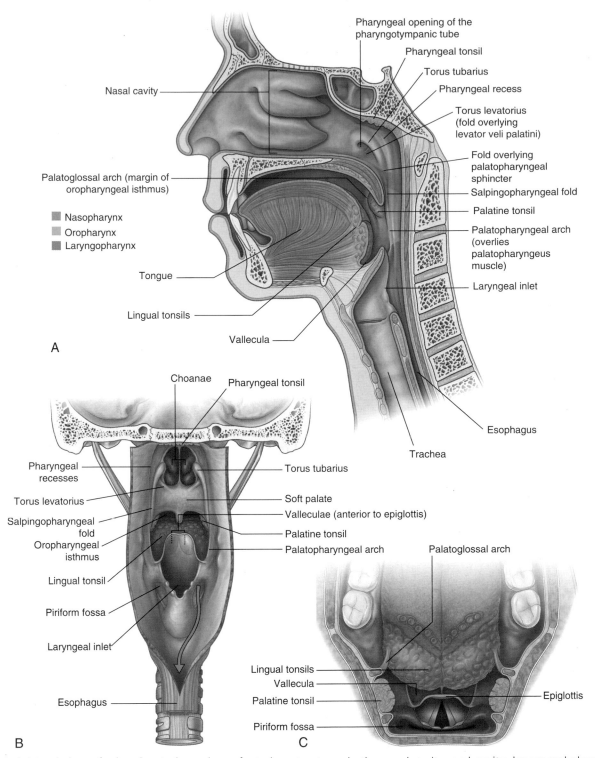

A

- Pharyngeal opening of the pharyngotympanic tube
- Pharyngeal tonsil
- Torus tubarius
- Pharyngeal recess
- Torus levatorius (fold overlying levator veli palatini)
- Fold overlying palatopharyngeal sphincter
- Salpingopharyngeal fold
- Palatine tonsil
- Palatopharyngeal arch (overlies palatopharyngeus muscle)
- Laryngeal inlet
- Esophagus
- Trachea

- Nasal cavity
- Palatoglossal arch (margin of oropharyngeal isthmus)

- Nasopharynx
- Oropharynx
- Laryngopharynx

- Tongue
- Lingual tonsils
- Vallecula

B

- Choanae
- Pharyngeal tonsil
- Pharyngeal recesses
- Torus levatorius
- Salpingopharyngeal fold
- Oropharyngeal isthmus
- Lingual tonsil
- Piriform fossa
- Laryngeal inlet
- Esophagus
- Torus tubarius
- Soft palate
- Valleculae (anterior to epiglottis)
- Palatine tonsil
- Palatopharyngeal arch

C

- Palatoglossal arch
- Lingual tonsils
- Vallecula
- Palatine tonsil
- Piriform fossa
- Epiglottis

Plate 28.1 A lateral view of a hemisected specimen featuring structures in the nasal cavity, oral cavity, larynx and pharynx.

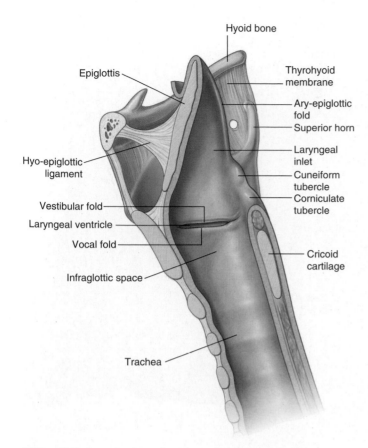

Plate 28.2 A sagittal section through laryngeal cavity showing vocal and vestibular folds.

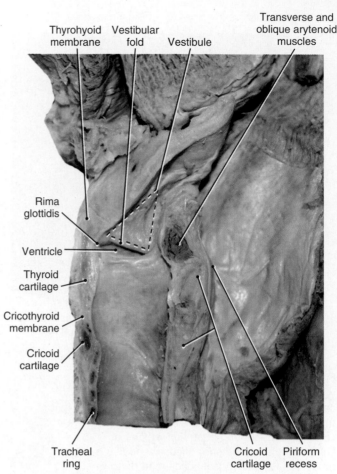

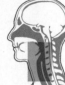

Fig. 28.4 Sagittal view with vestibule/ laryngeal inlet, vestibular fold, vocal fold, ventricle, thyroid and cricoid cartilages, tracheal ring, transverse arytenoid muscle, and piriform recess.

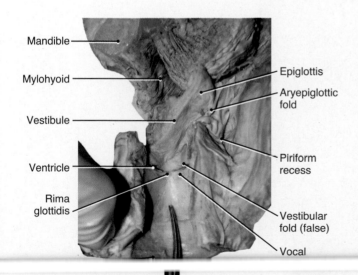

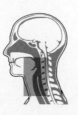

Fig. 28.3 Sagittal oral view with open posterior laryngeal view, revealing mandible, mylohyoid muscle, epiglottis, vestibule/ laryngeal inlet, piriform recess, vestibular fold, vocal fold, ventricle, and trachea.

○ Identify the epiglottis and the thyroid and cricoid cartilages (Fig. 28.4).

○ Note the thyroid cartilage and its attachment to the hyoid bone through the thyrohyoid membrane.

○ Identify the attachment of the thyroid cartilage to the cricoid cartilage by the cricothyroid membrane.

○ Palpate the arytenoid cartilages (Fig. 28.5) and at their free edge in the aryepiglottic fold, feel the corniculate and cuneiform cartilages.

○ Palpate the cricoid cartilage and make a midline incision along its posterior surface through the mucous muscle (see Fig. 28.5).

○ Superior to the posterior cricoarytenoid muscle, identify the transverse and oblique arytenoid muscles (Figs. 28.6 and 28.7).

○ Reflect the mucous membrane over the aryepiglottic fold, and expose the corniculate and cuneiform cartilages (see Fig. 28.7).

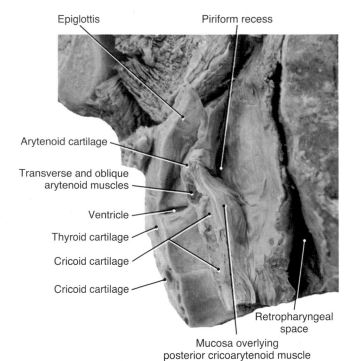

Epiglottis   Piriform recess

Arytenoid cartilage

Transverse and oblique
arytenoid muscles

Ventricle

Thyroid cartilage

Cricoid cartilage

Cricoid cartilage

Retropharyngeal
space

Mucosa overlying
posterior cricoarytenoid muscle

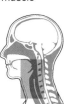

Fig. 28.5 Sagittal view of mouth and larynx
with posterior wall of pharynx reflected from
cervical vertebrae, revealing epiglottis,
transverse arytenoid muscle, ventricle, thyroid
cartilage, anterior and posterior regions of
cricoid cartilage, posterior cricoarytenoid
mucosa, retropharyngeal space, and piriform
recess.

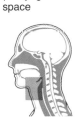

Vestibular   Transverse and
fold   oblique arytenoid
Ventricle   Vestibule muscles   Mucosa of
                                     pharynx

Vocal
fold

Thyroid
cartilage

Cricoid
cartilage

Retropharyngeal
space

Fig. 28.6 Sagittal view of laryngeal region,
revealing vestibule/laryngeal inlet, arytenoid
muscle, vestibular fold, vocal fold, ventricle,
cricoid cartilage, thyroid cartilage, mucosa of
the pharynx, and retropharyngeal space.

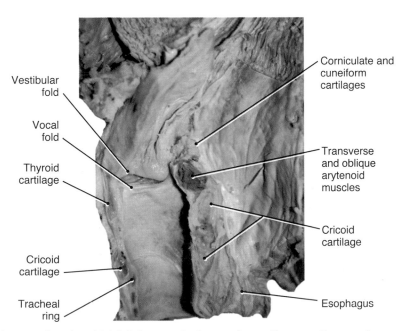

Vestibular
fold

Vocal
fold

Thyroid
cartilage

Cricoid
cartilage

Tracheal
ring

Corniculate and
cuneiform
cartilages

Transverse
and oblique
arytenoid
muscles

Cricoid
cartilage

Esophagus

Fig. 28.7 Sagittal view of laryngeal region, highlighting corniculate and cuneiform cartilages, pharyngeal
mucosa, and esophagus.

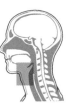

INSPECTION
Technique 2

○ Another technique for exposing the structures of the larynx is to remove the laryngopharynx and larynx en bloc from the cadaver and examine it.

○ Remove the laryngopharynx en bloc from the cadaver, and identify the aryepiglottic fold, piriform recess, and epiglottis (Fig. 28.8).

○ Palpate the greater horns (cornu) of the hyoid bone and thyroid cartilage, and remove the soft tissues around the larynx (Fig. 28.9).

○ Just inferior to the greater cornu of the hyoid bone, notice the internal branch of superior laryngeal nerve penetrating the thyrohyoid membrane (Fig. 28.10).

○ Reflect the mucosa over the posterior portion of the cricoid cartilage, and expose the posterior cricoarytenoid muscle (Fig. 28.11).

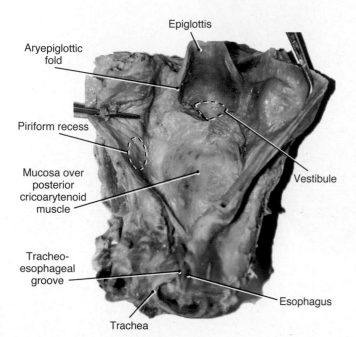

Fig. 28.8 Posterior view of larynx with posterior pharyngeal wall reflected from midline, revealing epiglottis, aryepiglottic fold, vestibule/laryngeal inlet, piriform recess, and tracheoesophageal groove.

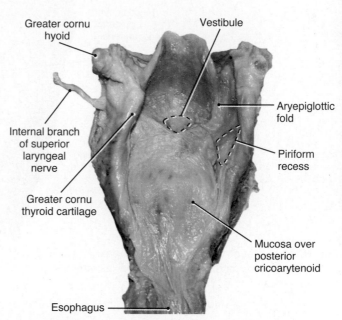

Fig. 28.10 Posterior view of larynx with posterior pharyngeal wall reflected, revealing vestibule/laryngeal inlet, greater cornu of hyoid and thyroid cartilage, and internal branch of superior laryngeal nerve.

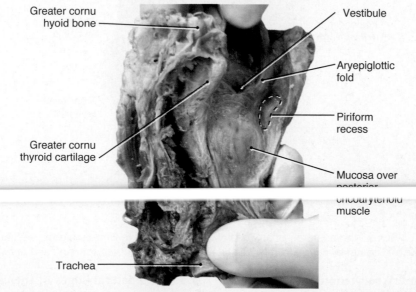

Fig. 28.9 Posterior view of larynx with posterior pharyngeal wall reflected from midline, highlighting horns (cornua) of hyoid and thyroid cartilage, mucosa over posterior cricoarytenoid muscle, aryepiglottic fold, and piriform recess.

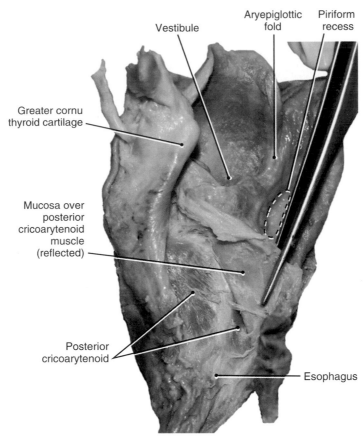

Fig. 28.11 Posterior view of larynx with pharyngeal wall cut from midline, revealing vestibule/laryngeal inlet, greater cornu of thyroid cartilage, posterior cricoarytenoid, esophagus, mucosa over posterior cricoarytenoid muscle, aryepiglottic fold, and piriform recess.

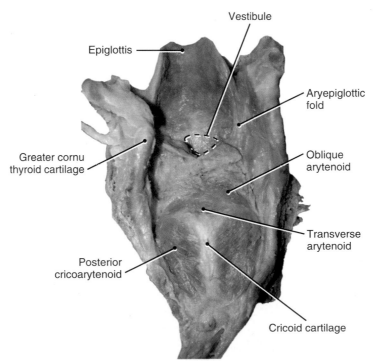

Fig. 28.12 Posterior view of larynx with posterior pharyngeal wall reflected, revealing epiglottis, vestibule/laryngeal inlet, posterior cricoarytenoid muscle, posterior cricoid cartilage, transverse and oblique arytenoids, and aryepiglottic fold.

○ Identify the posterior cricoarytenoid and transverse and oblique arytenoid muscles (Fig. 28.12).

○ Make a midline incision through the cricoid cartilage, and identify the vocal and vestibular folds (Fig. 28.13).

○ Pull the lateral edges of the cartilages open to fully expose the space between the vocal folds (Fig. 28.14).

○ Turn the specimen anteriorly and identify the *cricothyroid muscle*.

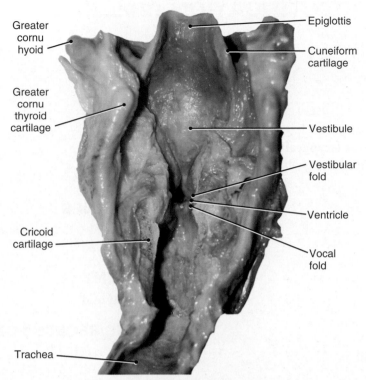

Fig. 28.13 Posterior midline view of larynx with cricoid cartilage reflected from midline, highlighting epiglottis, greater cornu (hyoid, thyroid cartilage), vocal and vestibular folds, cuneiform cartilage, ventricle, posterior region of cricoid cartilage, and trachea.

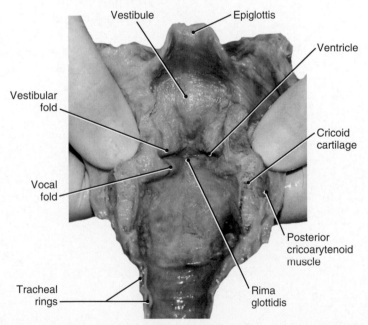

Fig. 28.14 Posterior view of larynx with cricoid cartilage reflected from midline, revealing epiglottis, vestibule/laryngeal inlet, vestibular fold, vocal fold, ventricle, posterior region of cricoid cartilage, posterior cricoarytenoid muscle, and tracheal rings.

○ Reflect the cricothyroid muscle anteriorly from the cricoid cartilage, and identify the median cricothyroid ligament in the midline between the thyroid and cricoid cartilages.

○ Identify the *thyroarytenoid muscle* lateral to the transverse and oblique arytenoids, ascending posteriorly from the midline to the arytenoid cartilage.

○ Inferior to the thyroarytenoid muscle, a small muscle, the *lateral cricoarytenoid muscle*, runs obliquely superior to the arytenoid cartilage.

DISSECTION **TIP**

If time permits, reflect the thyrohyoid membrane, and trace the course of the internal branch of superior laryngeal nerve to the piriform recess.

LABORATORY IDENTIFICATION CHECKLIST

NERVES
- ☐ Superior laryngeal
- ☐ External branch of superior laryngeal
- ☐ Internal branch of superior laryngeal
- ☐ Recurrent laryngeal
- ☐ Inferior laryngeal

ARTERIES
- ☐ Superior laryngeal

MUSCLES
- ☐ Uvula
- ☐ Cricothyroid
- ☐ Posterior cricoarytenoid
- ☐ Transverse cricoarytenoid
- ☐ Oblique cricoarytenoid
- ☐ Vocalis
- ☐ Lateral cricoarytenoid
- ☐ Thyroarytenoid

BONES
- ☐ Hyoid
  - ☐ Greater cornu

CARTILAGES
- ☐ Epiglottis
- ☐ Thyroid
  - ☐ Greater cornu
- ☐ Cricoid
- ☐ Arytenoid
- ☐ Corniculate
- ☐ Cuneiform
- ☐ Tracheal rings

MEMBRANES
- ☐ Thyrohyoid
- ☐ Cricothyroid

LIGAMENT
- ☐ Cricothyroid

SPACES/RECESS/FOLDS
- ☐ Piriform recess
- ☐ Vestibule
- ☐ Vocal folds
- ☐ Ventricle
- ☐ Vestibular folds
- ☐ Aryepiglottic folds
- ☐ Laryngopharynx

ATLAS REFERENCES

Netter: 75, 76, 79, 80, 86–88, 147, 148
McMinn: 45, 47
Gray's Atlas: 553–555, 565

BEFORE YOU BEGIN

Place the cadaver in the supine position, and identify the following landmarks in the postcraniotomy skull (Fig. 29.1):

- Anterior, middle, and posterior cranial fossae
- Transverse and sigmoid sinuses
- Confluence of sinuses

DISSECTION STEPS

○ With toothed forceps and a scalpel, remove the **dura mater** from the **posterior cranial fossa.**
○ With a mallet and chisel, make an inverted **V**–shaped cut (*dashed line* in Fig. 29.2) in the posterior cranial fossa (Plate 29.1).

○ Place the chisel 1 to 2 cm in the front of the **foramen magnum** at the midportion of the **clivus**, and make a deep cut.
○ Continue this cut laterally and posteriorly between the **jugular foramen** and the **hypoglossal canal** toward the edge of the **occipital bone** (Fig. 29.3).
○ Once the incisions are complete, pull the occipital bone backward to separate it from the skull base.
○ Use a scalpel to cut the soft tissues between the bone fragments.
○ Have a laboratory partner keep the head stable by holding it as shown in Fig. 29.4.

DISSECTION **TIP**

Be careful in making the separation in the region posterior to the jugular foramen. This is where the carotid sheath emerges, and aggressive dissection can damage its contents. As you pull the posterior cranial fossa backward (Fig. 29.5), place your finger in the opening you created at the clivus and pull backward (Fig. 29.6).

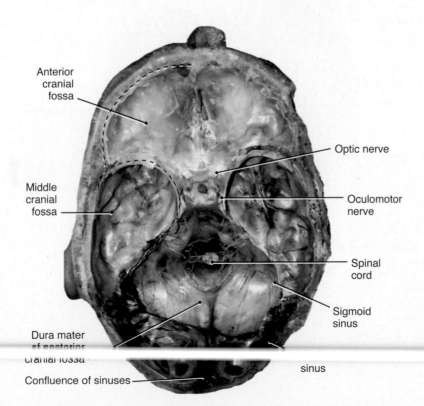

Anterior cranial fossa

Optic nerve

Middle cranial fossa

Oculomotor nerve

Spinal cord

Sigmoid sinus

Dura mater of posterior cranial fossa

sinus

Confluence of sinuses

Fig. 29.1 Horizontal section after craniotomy shows anterior, middle, and posterior cranial fossae, highlighting dura mater, dural venous sinuses (transverse, sigmoid, confluence), spinal cord, and cranial nerves (optic, oculomotor).

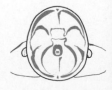

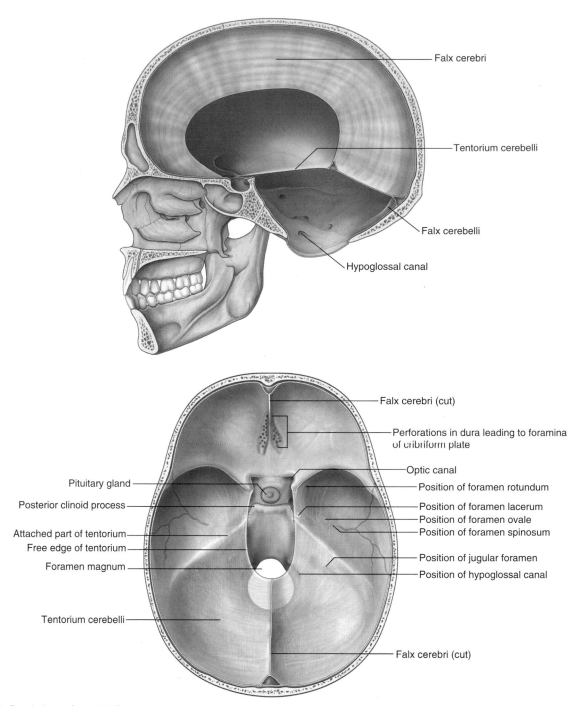

Plate 29.1 Depiction of cranial fossae, dura matter, and venous sinuses.

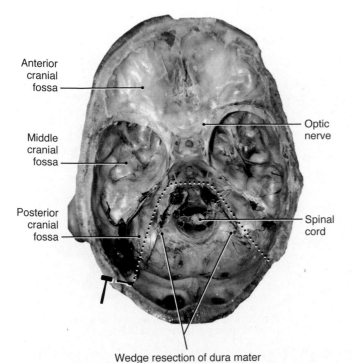

Anterior cranial fossa

Middle cranial fossa

Posterior cranial fossa

Optic nerve

Spinal cord

Wedge resection of dura mater

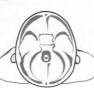

Fig. 29.2 Postcraniotomy horizontal section reveals anterior, middle, and posterior cranial fossae, with inverted-V–shaped section of dura mater removed from posterior cranial fossa, highlighting dural venous sinuses, spinal cord, and cranial nerves.

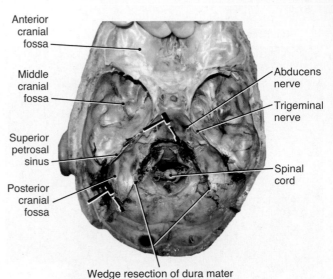

Anterior cranial fossa

Middle cranial fossa

Superior petrosal sinus

Posterior cranial fossa

Abducens nerve

Trigeminal nerve

Spinal cord

Wedge resection of dura mater

Fig. 29.3 Horizontal section after craniotomy reveals anterior, middle, and posterior cranial fossae, with section of dura mater removed from posterior cranial fossae, and a cut from clivus to occipital bone, highlighting dura mater, dural venous sinuses (superior petrosal), spinal cord, and cranial nerves (abducens, trigeminal).

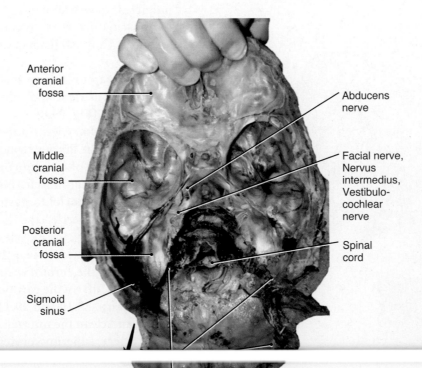

Anterior cranial fossa

Middle cranial fossa

Posterior cranial fossa

Sigmoid sinus

Abducens nerve

Facial nerve, Nervus intermedius, Vestibulo-cochlear nerve

Spinal cord

Wedge resection of posterior cranial fossa and dura mater

Fig. 29.4 Postcraniotomy horizontal section reveals anterior, middle, and posterior cranial fossae, with wedge resection from posterior cranial fossa reflected, highlighting dural venous sinuses (sigmoid sinus), spinal cord, and cranial nerves (abducens, facial, nervus intermedius, vestibulocochlear).

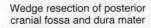

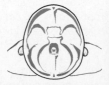

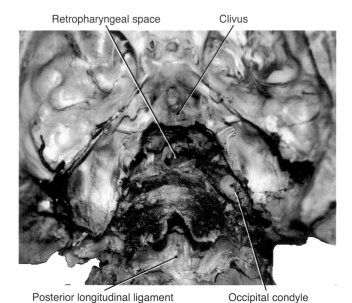

Fig. 29.5 Horizontal section after craniotomy, magnifying clival region of posterior cranial fossa and revealing small opening at retropharyngeal space.

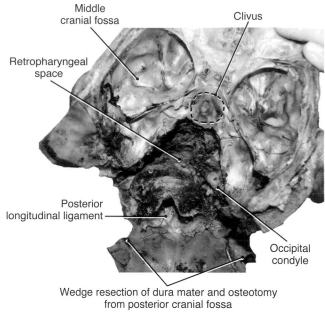

Fig. 29.7 Horizontal section after craniotomy of middle and posterior cranial fossae, with wedge osteotomy resection of posterior cranial fossa, revealing a large opening, the *retropharyngeal space.*

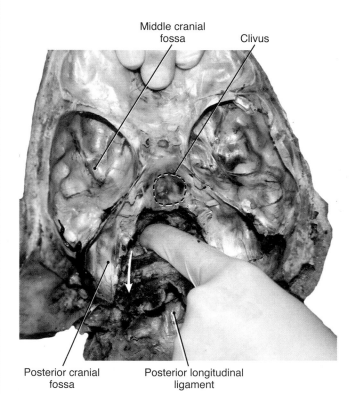

Fig. 29.6 Postcraniotomy horizontal section highlighting anterior, middle, and posterior cranial fossae, with wedge osteotomy resection of the posterior cranial fossa and finger in retropharyngeal space, pulling cranial fossa posteriorly.

○ Complete the separation of the posterior cranial fossa and musculature from the retropharyngeal space. Carefully cut any soft tissues obstructing the separation (Fig. 29.7).

○ Once the separation is complete, stabilize the head in the upright position, and fully expose the retropharyngeal space (Fig. 29.8).

○ Palpate the *pharyngeal tubercle,* which provides attachment to the fibrous raphe (seam) of the pharynx and is the point of attachment for the superior pharyngeal constrictor muscle (Fig. 29.9 and Plate 29.2).

○ Identify the **sternocleidomastoid muscle** laterally.

○ Beneath the tubercle, the *buccopharyngeal fascia* invests the constrictor muscles of the pharynx.

○ Lateral to this fascia, note a thickened, whitish condensed fascia, the *carotid sheath.*

○ With forceps, lift up the carotid sheath and expose its contents (Figs. 29.10 and 29.11).

○ Identify and clean the internal jugular vein, common carotid artery, superior cervical ganglion, and vagus nerve (Fig. 29.12).

○ Dissect the internal jugular vein, and identify the accessory nerve at its entrance into the sternocleidomastoid muscle (Fig. 29.13).

○ Trace the vagus nerve toward the base of the skull, and identify its inferior (nodose) ganglion and the jugular ganglion. The jugular ganglion of the vagus nerve is located superior to the nodose ganglion.

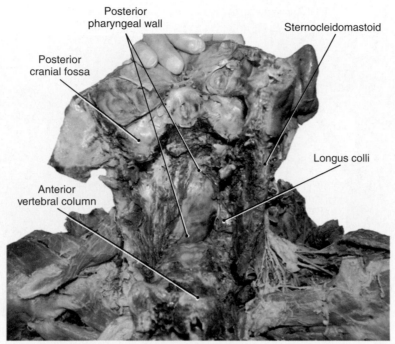

Fig. 29.8 Posterior view of pharynx after retropharyngeal dissection. Anterior view of vertebral column reveals fascia, sternocleidomastoid and longus colli muscles, and posterior cranial fossa.

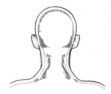

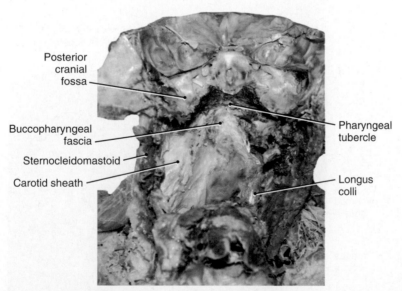

Fig. 29.9 Posterior view of pharynx with wedge osteotomy resection of posterior cranial fossa, highlighting buccopharyngeal fascia and pharyngeal tubercle.

○ Continue cleaning the carotid sheath and the buccopharyngeal fascia inferiorly (Fig. 29.14), and fully expose its contents (Fig. 29.15).

○ Identify the superior laryngeal nerve from its origin from the vagus nerve.

○ Trace the hypoglossal nerve from its emergence from the hypoglossal canal (Fig. 29.16). The *hypoglossal nerve* passes lateral to the internal carotid artery.

○ Medial to the internal carotid artery, identify the superior laryngeal nerve. Its internal branch travels

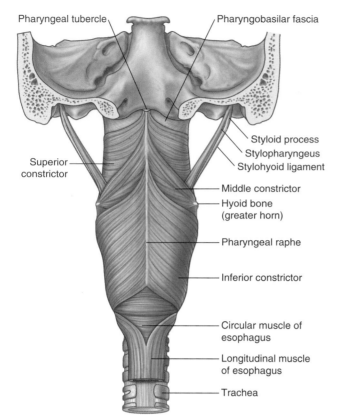

Plate 29.2 Depiction of the pharyngeal tubercle and superior, middle, and inferior constrictors (posterior view).

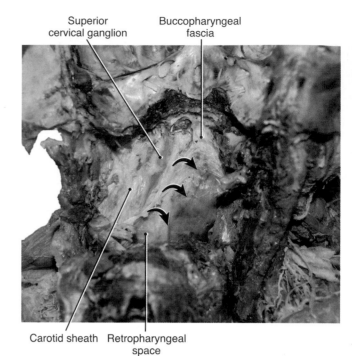

Fig. 29.10 Posterior view of pharynx with wedge osteotomy resection of posterior cranial fossa, revealing buccopharyngeal fascia, sternocleidomastoid muscle, and base of skull.

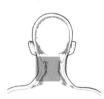

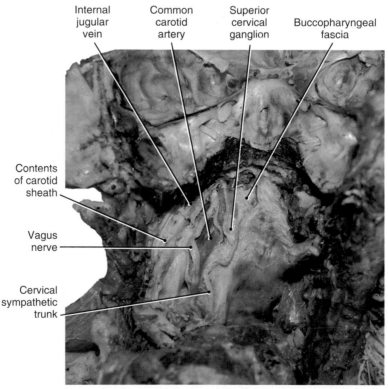

Fig. 29.11 Posterior view of pharynx with wedge osteotomy resection of posterior cranial fossa, revealing buccopharyngeal fascia, cervical sympathetic trunk, superior cervical ganglion, common carotid artery, internal jugular vein, and vagus nerve.

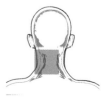

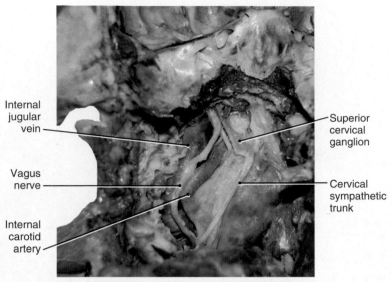

Fig. 29.12 Posterior view of pharynx with wedge osteotomy resection of posterior cranial fossa, highlighting contents of carotid sheath (internal jugular vein, common carotid artery, and vagus nerve), as well as superior cervical ganglion and cervical sympathetic trunk.

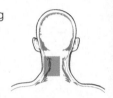

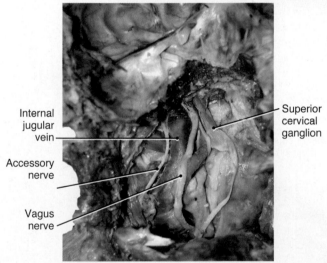

Fig. 29.13 Posterior view of pharynx with wedge osteotomy resection of posterior cranial fossa, revealing internal jugular vein, common carotid artery, inferior vagal ganglion (nodose ganglion), vagus nerve, superior cervical ganglion, and cervical sympathetic trunk.

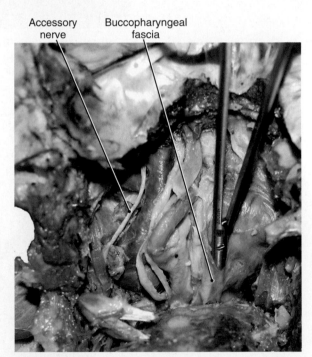

Fig. 29.14 Scissors removing remnants of carotid sheath and buccopharyngeal fascia, further exposing neurovascular structures and superior, middle, and inferior pharyngeal muscles.

tor muscles of the pharynx or the space between the external carotid artery and cornua of the hyoid bone.

DISSECTION TIP

You may encounter multiple lymph nodes around the internal jugular vein. After you identify these, remove them from the field of dissection (Fig. 29.17).

○ Lift the internal carotid artery to trace the pathway of the internal laryngeal artery and its division into internal and external branches (see Fig. 29.17).

○ Identify the superior, middle, and inferior pharyngeal constrictor muscles, and carefully clean the buccopharyngeal fascia and adipose tissue (see Fig. 29.17).

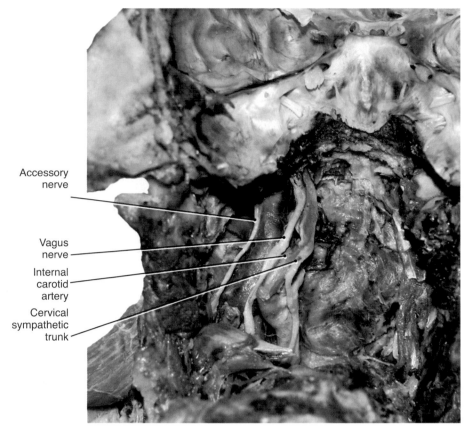

Accessory
nerve

Vagus
nerve

Internal
carotid
artery

Cervical
sympathetic
trunk

Fig. 29.15 Posterior view of pharynx with wedge osteotomy resection of posterior cranial fossa, highlighting accessory and vagus nerves and cervical sympathetic trunk, as well as internal jugular vein, common carotid artery, inferior (nodose) ganglion, vagus nerve, and superior cervical ganglion.

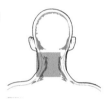

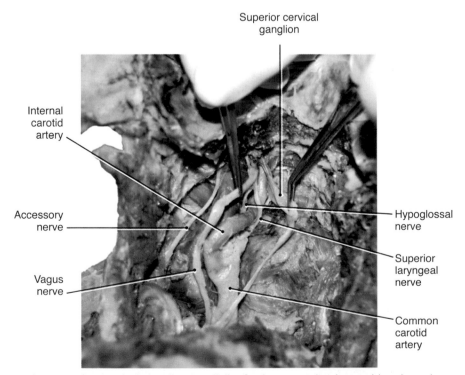

Superior cervical
ganglion

Internal
carotid
artery

Accessory
nerve

Vagus
nerve

Hypoglossal
nerve

Superior
laryngeal
nerve

Common
carotid
artery

Fig. 29.16 Forceps retracting superior cervical ganglion medially, further exposing internal jugular vein, common carotid artery, inferior (nodose) ganglion, vagus nerve, superior laryngeal nerve, and hypoglossal nerve.

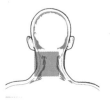

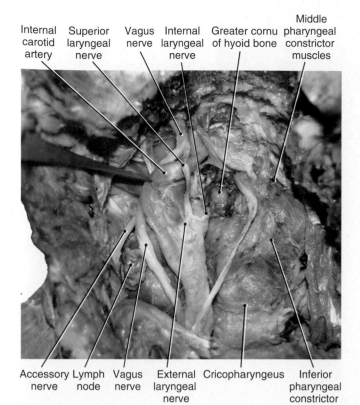

Internal carotid artery | Superior laryngeal nerve | Vagus nerve | Internal laryngeal nerve | Greater cornu of hyoid bone | Middle pharyngeal constrictor muscles

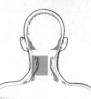

Accessory nerve | Lymph node | Vagus nerve | External laryngeal nerve | Cricopharyngeus | Inferior pharyngeal constrictor

Fig. 29.17 Posterior view of pharynx with wedge osteotomy resection of posterior cranial fossa revealing inferior pharyngeal constrictor (cricopharyngeus). Forceps retracting internal carotid artery laterally, further exposing division of superior laryngeal nerve into internal and external branches.

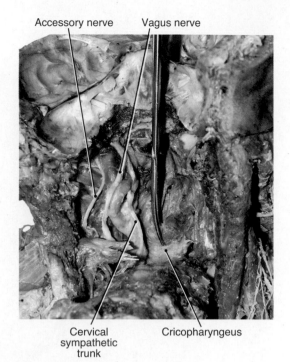

Accessory nerve | Vagus nerve

Cervical sympathetic trunk | Cricopharyngeus

Fig. 29.18 Midsagittal incision at midline of superior middle and inferior pharyngeal constrictors, exposing internal aspect of pharynx.

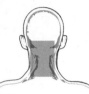

○ Make a midsagittal incision at the midline of the pharyngeal constrictor muscles to expose the internal aspect of the pharynx and to visualize such structures as the cervical sympathetic trunk and the epiglottis (Figs. 29.18 and 29.19).

DISSECTION OF UNDIVIDED SPECIMEN

○ A different method of dissection of the retropharyngeal space is through the suboccipital region. In this approach, all the musculature of the back, as well as the cervical vertebrae and spinal cord are removed, exposing the retropharyngeal space (Fig. 29.20 and Plates 29.3 and 29.4).

○ The pharyngeal constrictor muscles are especially useful landmarks that aid in dissecting methods as follows:

○ *Superior pharyngeal constrictor:* Identify the gap between the upper border of the superior pharyngeal constrictor muscle and the base of the skull. Clean the pharyngobasilar fascia that occupies this space, and expose the levator veli palatini muscle, auditory tube, and ascending palatine artery (Fig. 29.21).

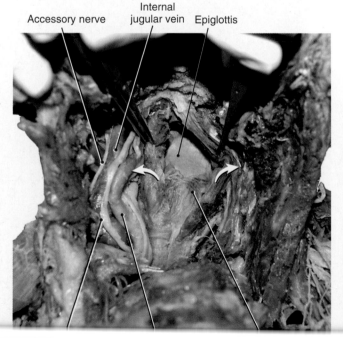

Accessory nerve | Internal jugular vein | Epiglottis

Vagus nerve | Internal carotid artery | Posterior cricoarytenoid muscle

Fig. 29.19 Vertical incision of pharynx with pharyngeal wall reflected, revealing epiglottis and posterior cricoarytenoid muscle.

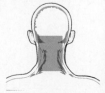

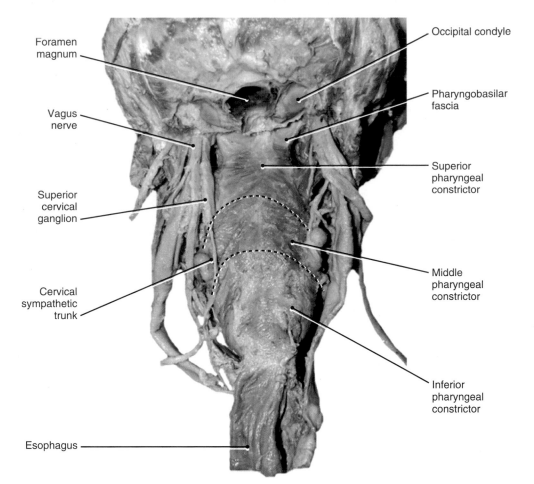

Fig. 29.20 Posterior view of pharynx and base of skull, revealing foramen magnum, occipital condyle, pharyngobasilar fascia, and superior, middle, and inferior pharyngeal constrictors, as well as superior cervical ganglion and cervical sympathetic trunk.

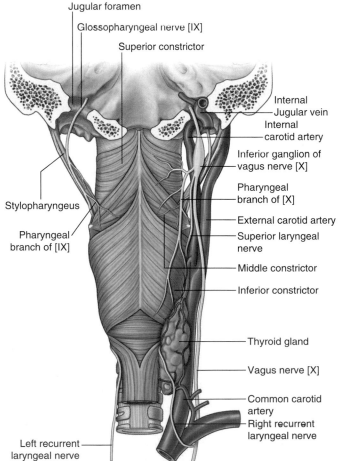

Plate 29.3 Posterior view of retropharyngeal space, with vast majority of neurovascular structures and muscles exposed.

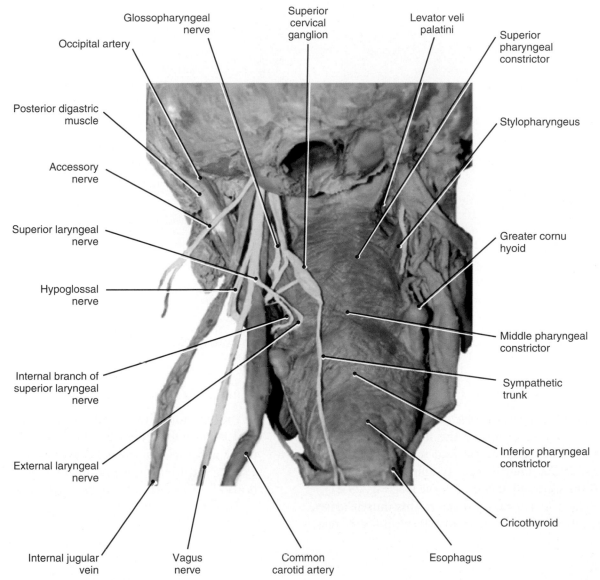

Occipital artery

Posterior digastric muscle

Accessory nerve

Superior laryngeal nerve

Hypoglossal nerve

Internal branch of superior laryngeal nerve

External laryngeal nerve

Internal jugular vein

Glossopharyngeal nerve

Superior cervical ganglion

Levator veli palatini

Superior pharyngeal constrictor

Stylopharyngeus

Greater cornu hyoid

Middle pharyngeal constrictor

Sympathetic trunk

Inferior pharyngeal constrictor

Cricothyroid

Vagus nerve

Common carotid artery

Esophagus

Fig. 29.21 View of retropharyngeal space, with vast majority of neurovascular structures and muscles exposed.

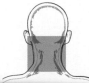

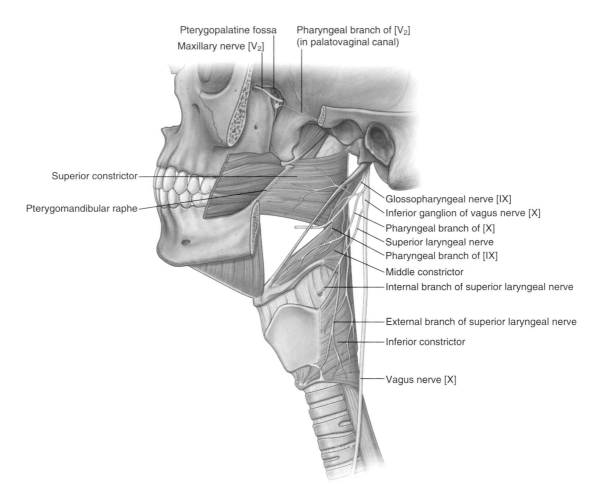

Pterygopalatine fossa
Maxillary nerve [V₂]

Pharyngeal branch of [V₂]
(in palatovaginal canal)

Superior constrictor

Pterygomandibular raphe

Glossopharyngeal nerve [IX]
Inferior ganglion of vagus nerve [X]
Pharyngeal branch of [X]
Superior laryngeal nerve
Pharyngeal branch of [IX]
Middle constrictor
Internal branch of superior laryngeal nerve

External branch of superior laryngeal nerve
Inferior constrictor

Vagus nerve [X]

Plate 29.4 Lateral view of retropharyngeal space, with majority of neurovascular structures and muscles exposed.

○ *Middle pharyngeal constrictor:* This muscle attaches to the greater cornu of the hyoid bone. At the junction of the superior and middle pharyngeal constrictors, identify the stylopharyngeus muscle and the glossopharyngeal nerve (see Fig. 29.21).

○ *Inferior pharyngeal constrictor:* This muscle arises from the sides of the thyroid and cricoid cartilages.

At the junction of the middle and inferior pharyngeal constrictors, identify the internal laryngeal nerve and the superior laryngeal artery (see Fig. 29.21). The inferior part of the inferior constrictor is also known as the *cricopharyngeus* muscle.

LABORATORY IDENTIFICATION CHECKLIST

NERVES
- [ ] Sympathetic trunk
- [ ] Vagus
  - [ ] Recurrent laryngeal
  - [ ] Inferior laryngeal
- [ ] Accessory
- [ ] Hypoglossal
- [ ] Glossopharyngeal

GANGLIA
- [ ] Superior cervical
- [ ] Middle cervical

ARTERIES
- [ ] Common carotid
- [ ] Internal carotid
- [ ] External carotid
- [ ] Vertebral

VEIN
- [ ] Internal jugular

MUSCLES
- [ ] Sternocleidomastoid
- [ ] Stylopharyngeus
- [ ] Superior constrictor
- [ ] Middle constrictor
- [ ] Inferior constrictor
- [ ] Longus colli

BONES
- [ ] Occipital
- [ ] Temporal
  - [ ] Mastoid process
  - [ ] Styloid process
- [ ] Hyoid
- [ ] Atlas (C1)
- [ ] Axis (C2)
- [ ] C3 to C7

CARTILAGES
- [ ] Thyroid
- [ ] Cricoid

LIGAMENTS
- [ ] Transverse, of atlas
- [ ] Alar

GLANDS
- [ ] Thyroid
- [ ] Parathyroid

FASCIAE
- [ ] Buccopharyngeal
- [ ] Retropharyngeal
- [ ] Prevertebral

CLINICAL APPLICATIONS

CRICOTHYROTOMY

Gray's Anatomy for Students: 536, 541, 543
Netter: 78, 83

Clinical Application

Procedure creates an emergent airway through the cricothyroid membrane.

Anatomic Landmarks (Figs. VIII.1 and VIII.2)

Palpation of midline structures
- Hyoid cartilage
- Thyroid cartilage
- Cricoid cartilage

Skin/subcutaneous tissue
- Cricothyroid arteries and small veins (may traverse the cricothyroid membrane)
- Cricothyroid membrane

TRACHEAL INTUBATION

Gray's Anatomy for Students: 552, 553, 560
Netter: 68, 75, 77–79

Clinical Application

Procedure maintains and controls definitive airway by introducing a tube orally that passes through the larynx between the vocal cords, stopping before the tracheal bifurcation.

Anatomic Landmarks (Fig. VIII.3)

- Mouth
  Incisor teeth
  Anterior arch: palatoglossus muscle
  Palatine tonsil
  Posterior arch: palatopharyngeus muscle
- Oral pharynx
- Epiglottis
- Vallecula

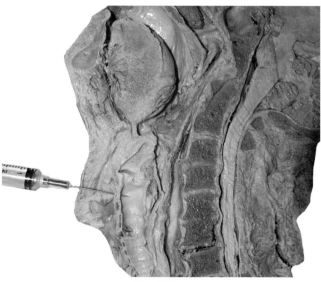

Fig. VIII.1

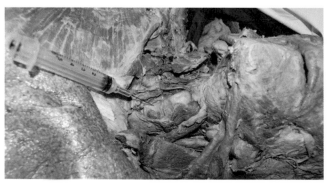

Fig. VIII.2

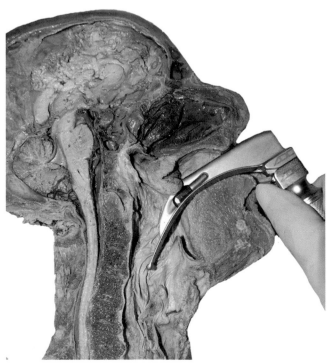

Fig. VIII.3

- Piriform recess
- Vocal cords
- Trachea

NASOTRACHEAL INTUBATION

Gray's Anatomy for Students: 552
Netter: 68, 75, 77–79

Clinical Application

Procedure maintains and controls an airway by introducing a tube nasally that passes through the oral pharynx and larynx between the vocal cords, stopping short of the tracheal bifurcation.

Anatomic Landmarks

- Right or left nostril
- Concha or turbinates
- Nasopharynx
- Oropharynx
- Laryngopharynx
- Trachea

BURR HOLES FOR CRANIOTOMY

Gray's Anatomy for Students: 490
Netter: 16

Clinical Application

Procedure creates a hole in the skull to evacuate blood from an epidural or subdural hemorrhage.

Anatomic Landmarks

- Scalp
- Skin
- Connective tissue
- Aponeurosis
- Loose areolar tissue
- Periosteum
- Bones of the calvaria
- Dura mater

AKINOSI TECHNIQUE: TRIGEMINAL-MANDIBULAR NERVE BLOCK

Gray's Anatomy for Students: 576
Netter: 133

Clinical Application

Procedure allows a local anesthetic to be deposited near the mandibular division of the trigeminal nerve, when opening the mouth is prohibited.

Anatomic Landmarks

- Oral vestibule
- Mucosa medial to ramus
- Maxillary bone and mucosa
- Trigeminal nerve–mandibular nerve branches

INDEX